Fruits, Vegetables, and Herbs

Fruits, Vegetables, and Herbs

Bioactive Foods in Health Promotion

Edited by

Ronald Ross Watson

University of Arizona, Tucson, AZ, United States

Victor R. Preedy

King's College London, London, United Kingdom

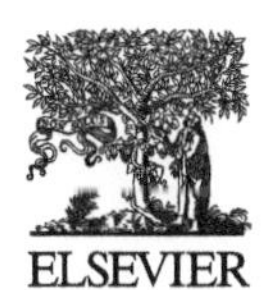

AMSTERDAM • BOSTON • HEIDELBERG • LONDON
NEW YORK • OXFORD • PARIS • SAN DIEGO
SAN FRANCISCO • SINGAPORE • SYDNEY • TOKYO
Academic Press is an imprint of Elsevier

Academic Press is an imprint of Elsevier
125 London Wall, London EC2Y 5AS, UK
525 B Street, Suite 1800, San Diego, CA 92101-4495, USA
50 Hampshire Street, 5th Floor, Cambridge, MA 02139, USA
The Boulevard, Langford Lane, Kidlington, Oxford OX5 1GB, UK

Notices
Knowledge and best practice in this field are constantly changing. As new research and experience broaden our understanding, changes in research methods, professional practices, or medical treatment may become necessary.

Practitioners and researchers must always rely on their own experience and knowledge in evaluating and using any information, methods, compounds, or experiments described herein. In using such information or methods they should be mindful of their own safety and the safety of others, including parties for whom they have a professional responsibility.

To the fullest extent of the law, neither the Publisher nor the authors, contributors, or editors, assume any liability for any injury and/or damage to persons or property as a matter of products liability, negligence or otherwise, or from any use or operation of any methods, products, instructions, or ideas contained in the material herein.

ISBN: 978-0-12-802972-5

British Library Cataloguing-in-Publication Data
A catalogue record for this book is available from the British Library

Library of Congress Cataloging-in-Publication Data
A catalog record for this book is available from the Library of Congress

For information on all Academic Press publications
visit our website at https://www.elsevier.com/

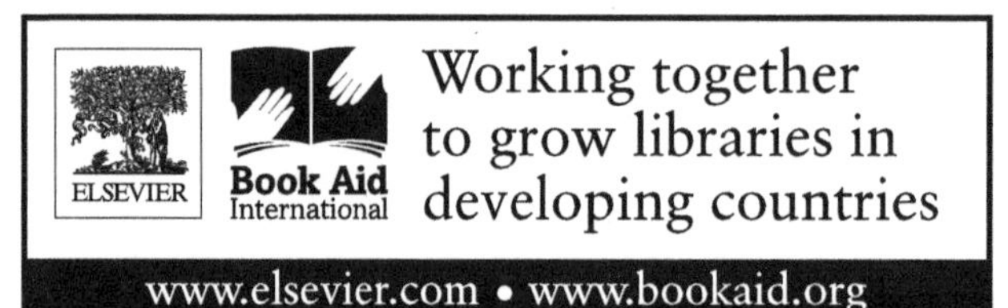

Publisher: Nikki Levy
Acquisition Editor: Megan Ball
Editorial Project Manager: Karen R. Miller
Production Project Manager: Julie-Ann Stansfield
Designer: Maria Inês Cruz

Typeset by MPS Limited, Chennai, India

Contents

SECTION 3 VEGETABLES IN HEALTH AND DISEASES

SECTION 4 HERBS IN HEALTH AND DISEASES

List of Contributors

Sulaiman O. Aljaloud
North Carolina Agricultural and Technical State University, Greensboro, NC, United States; King Saud University, Riyadh, Saudi Arabia

Elena Antonini
University of Urbino "Carlo Bo", Urbino, Italy

Greg Arnold
Complete Chiropractic Healthcare, Hauppauge, NY, United States

Bahlouli Aziz
Ibn Tofail University, Kenitra, Morocco

Neela Badrie
The University of the West Indies, St. Augustine, Trinidad and Tobago, West Indies

Kylie Ball
Deakin University, Burwood, VIC, Australia

Kalyani H. Barve
Shobhaben Pratapbhai Patel School of Pharmacy & Technology Management, SVKM's NMIMS, Mumbai, Maharashtra, India

Sa'eed Halilu Bawa
The University of the West Indies, St. Augustine, Trinidad and Tobago, West Indies; Warsaw University of Life Sciences, Warsaw, Poland

Tarik Bor
North Carolina Agricultural and Technical State University, Greensboro, NC, United States

Amy C. Brown
University of Hawaii at Manoa, Honolulu, HI, United States

Gene Bruno
Huntington College of Health Sciences, Knoxville, TN, United States

Mohd Hanafi Ahmad Damanhuri
Universiti Kebangsaan Malaysia, Kuala Lumpur, Malaysia

Lina Wati Durani
Shiga University of Medical Science, Otsu, Japan; Universiti Kebangsaan Malaysia, Kuala Lumpur, Malaysia

Akram Elembaby
University of Arizona, Tucson, AZ, United States

Ibrahim Elmadfa
University of Vienna, Vienna, Austria

A. Ross Ferguson
The New Zealand Institute for Plant & Food Research Limited, New Zealand

Alessandra Frati
University of Urbino "Carlo Bo", Urbino, Italy

Anil B. Gaikwad
Birla Institute of Technology and Science, Pilani, Rajasthan, India

Mayuresh S. Garud
Shobhaben Pratapbhai Patel School of Pharmacy & Technology Management, SVKM's NMIMS, Mumbai, Maharashtra, India

R.S. Gaud
Shobhaben Pratapbhai Patel School of Pharmacy & Technology Management, SVKM's NMIMS, Mumbai, Maharashtra, India

S.D. Ghate
Mangalore University, Mangalagangotri, Mangalore, Karnataka, India

Hajjaj Ghizlane
Mohammed V University, Rabat, Morocco

Marian Glick-Bauer
City University of New York, New York, NY, United States

Ajai P Gupta
CSIR-Indian Institute of Integrative Medicine, Jammu, India

Suphla Gupta
CSIR-Indian Institute of Integrative Medicine, Jammu, India

Rabin Gyawali
North Carolina Agricultural and Technical State University, Greensboro, NC, United States

Hamizah Shahirah Hamezah
Shiga University of Medical Science, Otsu, Japan; Universiti Kebangsaan Malaysia, Kuala Lumpur, Malaysia

Denise C. Hunter
The New Zealand Institute for Plant & Food Research Limited, New Zealand

Nor Faeizah Ibrahim
Shiga University of Medical Science, Otsu, Japan; Universiti Kebangsaan Malaysia, Kuala Lumpur, Malaysia

Salam A. Ibrahim
North Carolina Agricultural and Technical State University, Greensboro, NC, United States

Marcello Iriti
Milan State University, Milan, Italy

Dan Ju
University of Hawaii Cancer Center, Honolulu, HI, United States

N.C. Karun
Mangalore University, Mangalagangotri, Mangalore, Karnataka, India

Saima Khan
CSIR-Indian Institute of Integrative Medicine, Jammu, India

Yogesh A. Kulkarni
Shobhaben Pratapbhai Patel School of Pharmacy & Technology Management, SVKM's NMIMS, Mumbai, Maharashtra, India

Karen Lamb
Deakin University, Burwood, VIC, Australia

Sajad A Lone
CSIR-Indian Institute of Integrative Medicine, Jammu, India

Gertraud Maskarinec
University of Hawaii Cancer Center, Honolulu, HI, United States

Alexa L. Meyer
University of Vienna, Vienna, Austria

Malik Muzafar
CSIR-Indian Institute of Integrative Medicine, Jammu, India

Wan Zurinah Wan Ngah
Universiti Kebangsaan Malaysia, Kuala Lumpur, Malaysia

Paolino Ninfali
University of Urbino "Carlo Bo", Urbino, Italy

V.R. Niveditha
Mangalore University, Mangalagangotri, Mangalore, Karnataka, India

Dana Lee Olstad
Deakin University, Burwood, VIC, Australia

Manisha J. Oza
Shobhaben Pratapbhai Patel School of Pharmacy & Technology Management, SVKM's NMIMS, Mumbai, Maharashtra, India; SVKM's Dr. Bhanuben Nanavati College of Pharmacy, Mumbai, Maharashtra, India

Anuradha Pandey
Birla Institute of Technology and Science, Pilani, Rajasthan, India

Pankaj Pandotra
CSIR-Indian Institute of Integrative Medicine, Jammu, India

Yikyung Park
Washington University School of Medicine, St. Louis, MO, United States

Asif Khurshid Qazi
CSIR-Indian Institute of Integrative Medicine, Jammu, India

Lawrence W. Sanchez
University of Arizona, Tucson, AZ, United States

Alexander G. Schauss
AIBMR Life Sciences, Puyallup, WA, United States; University of Arizona, Tucson, AZ, United States

Margot A. Skinner
The University of Auckland, Auckland, New Zealand

Danfeng Song
AUI Fine Foods, Gaithersburg, MD, United States

K.R. Sridhar
Mangalore University, Mangalagangotri, Mangalore, Karnataka, India

Hiroyasu Taguchi
Shiga University of Medical Science, Otsu, Japan

Youcai Tang
Zhengzhou University, Zhengzhou, Henan, China; Saint Louis University School of Medicine, St. Louis, MO, United States

Lukar Thornton
Deakin University, Burwood, VIC, Australia

Ikuo Tooyama
Shiga University of Medical Science, Otsu, Japan

Elena Maria Varoni
Milan State University, Milan, Italy

Ronald Ross Watson
University of Arizona, Tucson, AZ, United States

Seren Wechsler
City University of New York, New York, NY, United States

Daijiro Yanagisawa
Shiga University of Medical Science, Otsu, Japan

Ming-Chin Yeh
City University of New York, New York, NY, United States

Preface

SECTION 1: OVERVIEW OF FRUITS, VEGETABLES, AND HERBS IN HEALTH

The U.S. National Cancer Institute estimates that cancer prevention is promoted by eating five servings of fruits and/or vegetables per day, but most eat an insufficient two or three servings. There is a major unmet need for more fruit and vegetable consumption, yet it is within the reach and control of most adults. In this book, multiple experts define the data supporting benefits of various fruits, vegetables, and herbs in health and disease prevention. This information will encourage further research as well as providing the basis for changes in diets of families and groups, like school children, to promote greater use and research on benefits of specific foods. This book begins with research on inequalities in consumption of plant materials. This is followed by discussion of the effects of industrial freezing, cooking and storage on antioxidant nutrients which are then described as indicators of consumption in aged humans. Hajjaj and Aziz describe pharmacological properties of nonfood agents from medicinal plants. Kulkarni and colleagues discuss some of these flavonoid agents in diabetics. A specific example, curcumin, is reviewed for its epigenetic actions as a therapeutic constituent.

SECTION 2: FRUITS IN HEALTH AND DISEASES

The expert reviews in this section provide readers with valuable evidence-based conclusions and recommendations that provide a helpful basis for beneficial dietary modifications for implementation by government and the public. Schauss describes recent advances in acai research for mechanisms of action. Iriti and Celoria discuss other bioactive agents from grapes as do Hunter and colleagues on kiwifruit in health. Maskarinec describes, in detail, an increasingly popular medicinal food, cocoa, and evidence on health benefits. Pomegranate extracts are reviewed by Bruno, and berries and their impact on blood pressure are assessed by Arnold. Functional fruit development and delivery is important in health promotion and disease prevention. These reviews define and support the actions of some foods' bioactive constituents like bioflavonoids and other vegetable compounds.

SECTION 3: VEGETABLES IN HEALTH AND DISEASES

This section reviews and presents new hypotheses and conclusions on the effects of different bioactive components of vegetables to prevent disease and improve the health of various populations. Researchers in Hawaii review a traditional food, poi, for its uses and implications on disease prevention. Karun concludes with description of mushrooms found in India. Research on such common and novel foods provides information while promoting further study.

SECTION 4: HERBS AND THEIR CONSTITUENTS IN HEALTH AND DISEASES

Extensive research focuses on the growing body of knowledge on the role of various foods as well as their constituents *in reducing disease*. Yeh and colleagues discuss consumption patterns of such materials in US assistance programs. Bawa and Badrie describe and define the components and actions of okra. The multitude of biomolecules in such vegetables plays crucial roles in health maintenance. They may, therefore, be more effective and certainly have different actions beyond their nutrient content. As described by Park, the bioavailability of plants' nonnutritive constituents play a key role in their effectiveness. For example, fiber consumption can impact the prevention of cardiovascular disease. In vitro studies are early ways to investigate new uses of constituents. Thus curcumin is studied in liver cells and reviewed. This is followed by human studies relative to brain composition and health including amyloid pathology. Next, a group of authors review new data on natural herbal products in treatment of cancer via tubulin inhibition. Finally, reviews describe antimicrobial actions of spices and foods.

Diet and nutrition are vital keys to controlling or promoting morbidity and mortality from chronic diseases. A frequent goal of foods is to reduce oxidative damage and cancer promotion. Fruits, vegetables, herbs and their constituents as dietary supplements are now a multibillion-dollar business which is built upon moderate but increasing research data. For example, the U.S. Food and Drug Administration are pushing this industry, with the support of Congress, to base its claims and products on scientific research. It takes very substantial research data to allow labeling of food packages with health claims. However, many people are interested in early research to alter government food programs as well as their own lifestyle. This book will be useful to laymen who apply it to modify their lifestyles, as well as to the growing nutrition, food science, and natural product community. Each vegetable contains thousands of different biomolecules, some with the potential to promote health or retard disease and cancer. Specific foods, individual fruits or vegetables and their byproducts are biomedicines with expanded understanding and use. However, which biomolecules in vegetables or fruits are best to prevent with disease or promote health? This book will focus on the role of natural products to produce active agents from dietary fruits and vegetables.

Ronald Ross Watson and Victor R. Preedy

Acknowledgments

The work of Dr. Watson's editorial assistant, Bethany L. Stevens, in communicating with authors and working on the manuscripts was critical to the successful completion of this book. The support of Karen R. Miller and Jaclyn Truesdell is very much appreciated. Support for Ms. Stevens' and Dr. Watson's work was graciously provided by Natural Health Research Institute (www.naturalhealthresearch.org), which is an independent, nonprofit organization that supports science-based research on natural health and wellness. It is committed to informing about scientific evidence on the usefulness and cost-effectiveness of diet, supplements, and a healthy lifestyle to improve health and wellness and reduce disease. Finally, the work of librarian of the Arizona Health Science Library, Mari Stoddard, was vital and very helpful in identifying key researchers who participated in this book.

Section 1

Overview of Fruits, Vegetables, and Herbs in Health

Chapter 1

Socioeconomic inequalities in fruit and vegetable intakes

Lukar Thornton, Dana Lee Olstad, Karen Lamb and Kylie Ball
Deakin University, Burwood, VIC, Australia

CHAPTER OUTLINE

Fruits, Vegetables, and Herbs.
DOI: http://dx.doi.org/10.1016/B978-0-12-802972-5.00001-9

INTRODUCTION

Socioeconomic position (SEP) refers to an individual's social and economic ranking within society based on access to resources (such as material and social assets, including income, wealth, and educational credentials) and prestige (ie, an individual's status in a social hierarchy, linked for instance to their occupation, income, or education level) (Krieger et al., 1997). Individual SEP can be measured using a variety of indicators which commonly include education, occupation, and income (Galobardes et al., 2006). Composite measures are frequently used when examining neighborhood level measures of SEP and are commonly created by combining census data on a range of indicators.

Although SEP has been measured in different ways, studies have demonstrated with reasonable consistency an increased risk of low or inadequate fruit and vegetable consumption among those of lower SEP compared with those of higher SEP. This chapter provides an overview of evidence pertaining to socioeconomic inequalities in fruit and vegetable consumption in children, adolescents, adults, and older adults (see "Overview of Evidence on Socioeconomic Inequalities in Fruit and Vegetable Consumption" section). Guided by a socioecological framework, in the "Mechanisms Underlying Socioeconomic Inequalities in Fruit and Vegetable Consumption" section, we explore the underlying mechanisms that may be driving these differences. Findings from these sections are used to inform recommendations for future research (see "Future Research Directions" section) and policy (see "Implications for Practice" section).

OVERVIEW OF EVIDENCE ON SOCIOECONOMIC INEQUALITIES IN FRUIT AND VEGETABLE CONSUMPTION

While SEP can be measured and defined in multiple ways, it is common for studies to consider a single indicator when examining associations between SEP and fruit and vegetable intake (Turrell et al., 2003). Although indicators of SEP can be correlated, each measures a different aspect of social stratification so it may be appropriate to examine more than one SEP indicator within a single study. Furthermore, these indicators can be measured in different ways which can influence study findings, relevance, and interpretability. For example, education can be quantified in a variety of ways, including years of education completed or categories detailing the highest level of education attained (eg, trade certificate/college qualification/bachelor degree); indicators of work status can be measured using employment status (eg, employed/unemployed/retired) or job classification (eg, white collar/blue collar); income can be measured using either individual or household income (Shavers, 2007). Measures also differ between age groups. For example, when considering the SEP of a child, parental education and occupation have been the most frequently used indicators, although other measures have included indicators of SEP at the school (eg, percentage receiving free school meals) or neighborhood level (eg, median household income of the neighborhood of residence) (Zarnowiecki et al., 2014b). It is important to be mindful of these measurement differences when interpreting the literature on links between SEP and fruit and vegetable intake.

The following overview of existing evidence on socioeconomic inequalities in fruit and vegetable consumption is largely restricted to evidence from developed countries, primarily because these countries typically have more established systems of nutrition monitoring and reporting of inequalities in diet. Furthermore, factors affecting food supply, diets, and socioeconomic variations in diet are likely to be substantially different between developed and developing countries.

Children

Children's SEP is primarily determined on the basis of indicators of parental SEP. A comprehensive review of studies that have examined fruit and vegetable consumption among children and adolescents in relation to SEP concluded that, although SEP was operationalized differently across studies, low SEP was consistently associated with less frequent intake of fruits and vegetables, especially when family income was the indicator of interest (Rasmussen et al., 2006). These early findings have been largely verified by more recent analyses. An Australian study showed that in general, lower SEP was associated with lower intake of fruits and vegetables among children aged 9–13 years using a variety of SEP indicators (Zarnowiecki et al., 2014a). A similar conclusion was reached in a national, cross-sectional study of 2–16 year olds in Australia, which identified socioeconomic gradients in fruit and vegetable intakes using several indicators (Cameron et al., 2012). While a limited number of studies have shown null findings (eg, indices of SEP (parental income, education, child-reported family affluence) were unrelated to children' fruit and vegetable intake in one Canadian province (Attorp et al., 2014)); on the whole, there is generally strong evidence of socioeconomic gradients in children's fruit and vegetable intakes.

In other studies using a more limited range of single SEP indicators, children (10–15 years) with more highly educated parents were more likely to consume vegetables daily than those with less educated parents (Ahmadi et al., 2015). The frequency of fruit intake was higher among children whose parents were employed in higher status occupations compared to those whose parents were employed in mid or low status occupations in another study (Sandvik et al., 2010).

Some evidence also suggests that SEP variations in children's fruit and vegetable intakes may be increasing over time. An analysis of two cross-sectional groups of 10–12 year olds (n = 1488 in 2001; n = 1339 in 2008) in Norway found that fruit and vegetable intake among 10–12 year olds of less educated parents was lower in 2008 than in 2001, whereas the reverse was found among children whose parents were more highly educated (Hilsen et al., 2011). Thus the difference in the frequency of fruit and vegetable intake between children with lower and more highly educated parents was 0.9 times/week in 2001, but had widened to 2.4 times/week by 2008.

Adolescents

Like children, adolescent SEP is most often measured on the basis of parental SEP. As previously described, two studies that included both children and adolescents found evidence of socioeconomic gradients in fruit and vegetable consumption among adolescents (Rasmussen et al., 2006; Cameron et al., 2012). Studies conducted exclusively among adolescents support these findings.

In Australia, adolescents (12–15 years) with more highly educated mothers consumed fruit more frequently than those with less educated mothers (Ball et al., 2009). In Norway, adolescents (mean age 12.5 years in 2002; mean age 15.5 years in 2005) with more highly educated parents and higher household incomes consumed fruits and vegetables more often than those with less educated parents and from lower income households (Bere et al., 2008). In Canada, the proportion of adolescents (12–19 years) consuming the recommended amounts of fruits and vegetables increased from 34.2% in the lowest category of household income to 42.1% in the highest category (Riediger et al., 2007). Data from 33 countries in Europe, North America, and Israel collected as part of the 2001–02 Health Behavior in School-Aged Children study showed that daily fruit and vegetable consumption was less common among 13 and 15 year olds from low affluent families compared to more affluent families (the family affluence scale includes four different factors) (Richter et al., 2009).

A representative national survey from Australia showed that adolescents (12–17 years) residing in high SEP neighborhoods were more likely to report eating the recommended number of daily servings of fruits and vegetables compared to those living in lower SEP neighborhoods (Morley et al., 2012).

Adults

Many studies of adult populations show differences by SEP in the quantity and/or variety of fruits and vegetables consumed. For example, systematic reviews of socioeconomic variations in diet across Europe showed that higher SEP was consistently associated with greater consumption of both fruits and vegetables (De Irala-Estevez and Groth, 2000; Giskes et al., 2010). Similarly, socioeconomic gradients in fruit and vegetable consumption among adults have been reported in studies in the United States (Dubowitz et al., 2008; Wang et al., 2014), Canada (Riediger and Moghadasian, 2008; Dehghan et al., 2011), multiple European countries (Boylan et al., 2011), the United Kingdom (Billson et al., 1999), and Australia (Ball et al., 2004; Giskes et al., 2002a,b; Mishra et al., 2010). Even within a disadvantaged population (low-income women living in socioeconomically disadvantaged areas), inequalities exist in fruit and vegetable consumption based on other socioeconomic factors such as education (Thornton et al., 2014). Findings are also consistent with evidence from low- to middle-income countries as reported through both a systematic review (Mayen et al., 2014) and a separate analysis of World Health Organization Survey data (Hosseinpoor et al., 2012).

An important point to note is that inequalities exist in both men and women, with low SEP men often showing the poorest diets of any population group (Giskes et al., 2004; Worsley et al., 2004). Relative to women, however, studies on men's fruit and vegetable consumption are less common. Of further concern are findings from prospective studies showing that socioeconomic inequalities in adults' fruit and vegetable consumption may actually be widening over time (Wang et al., 2014; Wrieden et al., 2004).

Older adults

Fruit and vegetable intake among the elderly is an important indicator of nutritional risk (de Morais et al., 2013). Greater adherence to dietary guidelines can result in a higher quality of life among older adults (Gopinath et al., 2014). While fewer studies exist which examine older population groups compared to other age groups, there has been increased research interest in examining socioeconomic inequalities in fruit and vegetable intake among the elderly in recent times (Nicklett and Kadell, 2013), likely due to the aging population in many high-income countries. A multination European study restricted to adults aged 60 years and older found educational attainment to be positively related to consumption of a vegetable-based diet (Bamia et al., 2005). However, in the Netherlands, studies have shown conflicting findings in the strength of associations between SEP indicators and fruit and vegetable intake in older populations (van Rossum et al., 2000; Dijkstra et al., 2014, 2015). In a UK cohort, the variety of fruit and vegetables consumed was found to be positively related to a number of SEP indicators; however, the quantity consumed across SEP groups was similar (Conklin et al., 2014). The authors noted that such results emphasize the need to promote the importance and benefits of consuming a wider range of fruits and vegetables. In North America the proportion of Canadian adults aged $\geq$ 65 years consuming fruits and vegetables five or more times a day was higher among those with higher income and education levels (Riediger and Moghadasian, 2008), while in the United States, higher fruit and vegetable consumption has been linked to higher income among those aged 60 years and older (Bowman, 2007). Inadequate fruit and vegetable intake was also associated with lower education among older adults in South Africa (Peltzer and Phaswana-Mafuya, 2012).

Summary

The evidence summarized above demonstrates the existence of socioeconomic inequalities in fruit and vegetable consumption, such that persons of low SEP are at increased risk of consuming relatively lower quantities and fewer varieties of fruits and vegetables than their higher SEP peers. These socioeconomic inequalities have been observed relatively consistently among children, adolescents, adults, and older adults across multiple nations. It is important to consider the possibility of overreporting of fruit and vegetable intakes by those of high SEP as a potential explanatory factor for socioeconomic gradients in intakes. However, it is unlikely that such a reporting bias would completely account for the relatively consistent findings across multiple studies. Socioeconomic inequalities in fruit and vegetable consumption parallel inequalities in health outcomes, and represent one potential pathway by which low SEP might lead to poorer health. In order to address this situation, an understanding of the mechanisms underlying socioeconomic inequalities in fruit and vegetable consumption is required.

MECHANISMS UNDERLYING SOCIOECONOMIC INEQUALITIES IN FRUIT AND VEGETABLE CONSUMPTION

While there is an increasing body of evidence on factors associated with fruit and vegetable intake, findings on the determinants of socioeconomic inequalities in these intakes have been slower to emerge. As such, we do not yet have a good understanding of why people of lower SEP tend to eat less fruits and vegetables. Qualitative studies and quantitative descriptive studies have shed some light on possible explanations, but until recently very few quantitative studies had empirically tested the contribution of different factors to explaining or mediating socioeconomic inequalities. In recent years, several quantitative studies have capitalized on advances in the understanding and application of statistical methods related to mediation pathways and have begun to provide insights into the mechanisms by which lower SEP might lead to lower consumption of fruits and vegetables.

An overview of the literature on potential determinants of socioeconomic inequalities in fruit and vegetable consumption in different age groups is provided below. Some of this literature reports on determinants of particular relevance to low SEP groups; other research explicitly examines the mediating role of particular determinants in explaining socioeconomic variations in consumption. These determinants are categorized in accordance with social–ecological conceptual models of health behavior (Stokols, 1996), which posit the importance of influences within intrapersonal, social, and environmental domains.

Children

Intrapersonal determinants

A small number of intrapersonal determinants have been associated with fruit and vegetable consumption among low SEP children. Among Norwegian children whose parents were employed in low status occupations, children's attitudes toward, and self-efficacy for, eating fruit were related to their intentions to consume fruit and subsequently their fruit consumption (Sandvik et al., 2010). Also in Norway an increasing disparity in children's preferences for fruits and vegetables partly mediated an increase in socioeconomic disparities in fruit and vegetable intake from 2001 to 2008, as children with more highly educated parents had a steeper increase in preference for fruits and vegetables over time compared to those with less educated parents (Hilsen et al., 2011).

Social determinants

Parental influences have been associated with children's consumption of fruits and vegetables in several studies. Parental modeling of fruit and vegetable consumption appears potentially important, with one study, for example, showing parental consumption norms partially mediated associations between parental education and children's vegetable intake (Ahmadi et al., 2015). In another study, parental fruit consumption explained up to

45% of the association between parental education and child fruit consumption (Rodenburg et al., 2012). Familial support for eating fruits and vegetables is another important factor that has been positively associated with fruit and vegetable consumption among children from low-income families (Donnelly and Springer, 2015). These findings are supported by results from a qualitative study among disadvantaged mothers and children, where both parental modeling and support for fruit and vegetable consumption were described as key factors that influenced children's consumption of fruits and vegetables (Williams et al., 2011). Other important determinants of children's fruit and vegetable intakes in that study included parental control and rules related to the amount and type of food consumed.

Environmental determinants

The availability and accessibility of fruits and vegetables may influence their consumption among children of low SEP. In studies among mother–child pairs living in socioeconomically disadvantaged neighborhoods in Australia, the availability of fruits and vegetables in the home was described as an important determinant of children's consumption of fruits and vegetables (Williams et al., 2011), and also mediated associations between mothers' nutrition knowledge and children's fruit and vegetable intakes (Campbell et al., 2013). Interestingly in Norway, larger increases in the accessibility of fruits and vegetables within the homes of children with more highly educated, compared to those with less educated parents, partially mediated an increase in socioeconomic disparities in fruit and vegetable intakes over 7 years (Hilsen et al., 2011).

Adolescents

Intrapersonal determinants

Several intrapersonal determinants of fruit and vegetable consumption among low SEP adolescents were identified in three separate analyses based on a survey of 12- to 15-year-old Australian adolescents. First, greater perceived importance of health was associated with more frequent fruit and vegetable intake among low SEP adolescents (Stephens et al., 2011). In longitudinal analyses, disadvantaged adolescents who consumed fruits and vegetables frequently at baseline were more likely to remain frequent consumers at follow-up 2 years later. Girls had 72% higher odds of frequent fruit consumption at follow-up than did boys (Stephens et al., 2014). When compared to adolescents who reported having ≥$20 of spending money per week at baseline, adolescents who had $5–$9 of weekly spending money were 66% less likely to consume vegetables frequently 2 years later (Stephens et al., 2014). In mediation analyses among a sample of adolescents from varied socioeconomic backgrounds, cognitive factors, including self-efficacy for increasing fruit and reducing "junk food" consumption, and the perceived importance of health behaviors partly mediated socioeconomic variations in fruit intakes (Ball et al., 2009).

Social determinants

Familial influences are important in explaining socioeconomic variations in adolescents' fruit and vegetable intakes. Similar to findings among children, parental modeling has been shown to mediate associations between SEP and fruit and vegetable intake among adolescents in both cross-sectional (Ball et al., 2009) and longitudinal studies (Bere et al., 2008). Also as has been found in children, familial support for fruit and vegetable consumption was associated with low-income adolescents' fruit and vegetable consumption (Di Noia and Byrd-Bredbenner, 2013), and partially mediated socioeconomic variations in adolescent fruit intakes (Ball et al., 2009).

Environmental determinants

The availability of healthy and unhealthy foods has been shown to influence adolescents' fruit and vegetable intakes, just as it has in children. Within the home, availability of fruits and vegetables and energy-dense snack foods partially mediated socioeconomic variations in fruit and vegetable intakes among adolescents (Ball et al., 2009; Bere et al., 2008). In schools, availability of vending machines was important, as those who reported hardly ever purchasing items from school vending machines at baseline were nearly three times as likely to frequently consume fruit at follow-up compared to those who more often purchased items from vending machines (Stephens et al., 2011).

Adults

Intrapersonal mediators

Lower levels of nutrition knowledge, and lower prioritization of health during food selection have been implicated as potential explanatory factors in the association of SEP with diet quality among adults (Ball et al., 2006; Turrell, 1997). For example, Ball et al. showed that women with lower levels of education had less knowledge about the nutrient sources and health effects of different foods, and reported giving less consideration to health when making food purchasing choices, and these factors partly explained their lower intakes of fruits and vegetables (Ball et al., 2006). In trying to explain socioeconomic disparities in fruit and vegetable consumption among a Finnish sample, findings from one study suggested that price and familiarity of foods were driving food choices among less educated consumers, while those with higher income were motivated by health considerations (Konttinen et al., 2013).

Some have suggested that the poorer diets of adults of low SEP are attributable to a lack of cooking skills or interest in cooking among these groups, but evidence of socioeconomic differentials in these constructs is equivocal (Caraher and Lang, 1999; McLaughlin et al., 2003). Other potential explanations for the lower intakes of fruits and vegetables among adults of low SEP include lower perceived palatability of fruits and vegetables (Darmon and Drewnowski, 2008), apathy toward nutrition messages (Patterson et al., 2001), or lack of motivation or misperceptions about the adequacy of one's diet (Dibsdall et al., 2003). These factors may also be important in promoting resilience to unhealthy eating behaviors among low SEP groups (Thornton et al., 2015; Williams et al., 2010). A recent study highlighted that little is known regarding factors that mediate fruit consumption among men (Pechey et al., 2015).

Social mediators

Some data suggest that people of low SEP receive less social support from their families to eat healthily (Inglis et al., 2005), which may impede their efforts to eat more fruits and vegetables. This is supported by analyses conducted by Ball et al. who found that family and friends' support partially mediated educational differences in women's fruit and vegetable intake (Ball et al., 2006). Time pressures associated with long or inflexible working hours have also been implicated as barriers to shopping for and preparing healthy foods in low SEP groups (Inglis et al., 2005).

Environmental mediators

With regards to home environments, a study from the Netherlands found that availability of vegetables at home partially mediated the relationship between education level and vegetable consumption (Springvloet et al., 2014). Others, however, have found home environment factors to be unrelated to inequalities in fruit and vegetable consumption (Giskes et al., 2009).

At the neighborhood level, there is limited evidence supporting the hypothesis that availability and accessibility of fruits and vegetables explain socioeconomic inequalities in fruit and vegetable consumption (Giskes et al., 2011). Some studies that have explicitly tested the role of food availability and access in mediating associations of individual SEP with diet have found limited evidence of a mediating effect (Ball et al., 2006; Giskes et al., 2008). Although lower consumption of vegetables was reported among women living in disadvantaged neighborhoods in Melbourne, differences were not attributable to the food environment in these neighborhoods (Thornton et al., 2010). While there is limited available evidence on the role of objective environmental measures in dietary inequalities, quantitative research suggests that lower SEP women may perceive the environment as less supportive and this may contribute to the observed inequalities (Williams et al., 2012). This is not supported, however, by findings from several qualitative studies which have demonstrated that availability of and access to good quality healthy foods are not perceived as significant barriers to healthy eating among low SEP groups (Inglis et al., 2005; Dibsdall et al., 2002).

Another environmental factor considered has been food cost. Several authors have argued that the poorer diet quality among individuals of low SEP is attributable to the relatively higher costs of a healthy diet (Darmon and Drewnowski, 2008). While some experimental studies support this hypothesis (An, 2013), it is not reinforced by all available evidence. For example, recent work suggests broader pricing policies may have more limited benefits for low-income groups, potentially leading to increased inequalities, and that pricing policies should therefore be designed and targeted to low-income groups (Darmon et al., 2014). In a quasi-experimental study, Inglis et al. showed that socioeconomic inequalities in the healthfulness of food choices (including fruits and vegetables) were not reduced through (theoretically) manipulating the food budgets available to low- and high-income women (Inglis et al., 2009). Others who have examined objectively-assessed food prices found that these did not impact on food purchasing decisions or explain inequalities in purchasing of healthy and less healthy foods (although this study did not specifically assess fruit and vegetable purchasing) (Giskes et al., 2007).

Older adults

Intrapersonal, social, and environmental mediators

While a wide range of factors associated with fruit and vegetable intake among older adults has recently been reviewed (Nicklett and Kadell, 2013), work focusing on potential mediators of socioeconomic difference in this age group is more limited. Two Dutch studies investigated factors linked to socioeconomic differences in food choice; however, neither investigated if these mediated differences in dietary inequalities. Firstly, Kamphius et al. found that the healthiness of food was rated more important among higher educated and higher income participants than among those of lower education and lower income (Kamphuis et al., 2015). In the second study, compared to those of higher SEP, prevention of disease was less likely to be reported as a motivating factor to eat healthfully by low SEP participants; however, feeling fit was more of a motivating factor among low-income participants, and current health was reportedly more motivating among lower educated participants (Dijkstra et al., 2014). Whether and how such factors mediate inequalities in diet among older adults remains largely unknown. In another Dutch sample, cost concerns were identified as one of the key mediators of differences in fruit intake but no mediating factors were found for vegetable intake (Dijkstra et al., 2015).

While access to transport, social support, and other indicators of social isolation may influence diets among the elderly (Locher et al., 2005), little is known about their associations with fruit and vegetable intake (Donkin et al., 1998) or whether these factors help explain socioeconomic differences.

Summary

This review describes a growing body of evidence that has identified selected intrapersonal, social, and (less consistently) environmental factors that may be important in explaining the lower intakes of fruit and vegetables among socioeconomically disadvantaged groups. However, it also highlights that evidence remains patchy, particularly in certain areas such as understanding mediators of inequalities among older adults, or the importance of environmental mediators. Additional priorities for future research in this field are described in the "Future Research Directions" section.

FUTURE RESEARCH DIRECTIONS

Measures of socioeconomic position

Although SEP indicators may be selected on the basis of data availability, education is often preferred due to the ease with which this indicator can be measured. However, limitations on the reliance on single measures of SEP have been raised (Galobardes et al., 2006). For example, existing occupational indicators may have limited relevance due to changes in work practices over time, and that income, as well as being a potentially sensitive measure which can suffer from nonresponse, can also be highly variable over time (Galobardes et al., 2006). Future studies should more carefully consider and justify the choice of appropriate SEP indicators and their measurement. Ideally, these choices should be based on theories around plausible causal relationships linking socioeconomic characteristics to fruit and vegetable consumption, bearing in mind that the most suitable indicator may depend on the relevant population under consideration

(Shavers, 2007). Furthermore, using neighborhood level measures of SEP as proxies for individual SEP can misestimate associations between individual SEP and fruit and vegetable intake, as all individuals within the same neighborhood are assigned the same level of SEP. When considered alongside individual level SEP, neighborhood SEP measures can provide estimates of contextual effects on fruit and vegetable intake.

Measures of fruit and vegetable intake

The variety of methods used to classify fruit and vegetable intake can present challenges in comparing findings. Outcomes considered have included, for example, the number of times fruit or vegetables were consumed per day, the mean number of daily servings, consumption of at least one serve per day, grams consumed per day, quartiles of intake, and high versus low consumers (Giskes et al., 2011). Recently, Roark and Niederhauser (2013) raised some of the challenges associated with measuring fruit and vegetable intake, namely capturing accurate intake data and deciding which types of produce should be considered within each food group.

Rasmussen et al. (2006) discussed challenges in comparing studies that vary in how fruit and vegetable intake is defined, suggesting that different factors may be associated with different aspects of dietary intake; that is, some indicators of SEP may be important for determining frequency of intake, while others may be important for determining the variety or amount. Similarly, different associations could be observed between SEP indicators and fruit and vegetable indicators if considered separately. The choice of intake measure should be determined by the aims of the research. For example, if it is the magnitude of differences between SEP groups that is of interest, then continuous measures such as the number of servings of fruit and vegetables should be considered. Where arbitrary categorization of continuous measures has been used, this may lead to a loss of power to detect associations and can cause difficulties in comparing studies across different contexts (Lamb and White, 2015).

UNDERSTUDIED POPULATIONS

More work is required to examine factors that lead to socioeconomic disparities in the eating behaviors of men. Adult men display some of the lowest rates of fruit and vegetable consumption and are therefore an important population group to target for interventions. Unfortunately, with few studies specifically investigating men, data to inform such interventions are currently lacking. Likewise a focus on the eating behaviors of older adults has been quite recent and further work is needed in this population group to assist the elderly to maintain a high quality of life as they age. As mentioned earlier, this overview was largely limited to high-income countries and there is a need for additional research in low/middle-income countries to improve dietary behaviors in these nations.

Improvements to study design and statistical analysis

Longitudinal studies are required to help elucidate pathways through which SEP influences fruit and vegetable intakes and to appropriately account for the fact that mediating processes take time to unfold (Preacher, 2015; Richiardi et al., 2013). Directed acyclic graphs (also known as causal diagrams), rarely used in social epidemiology, could also be used when examining associations between SEP and fruit and vegetable intake to determine potential sources of bias (Glymour, 2006; Greenland et al., 1999). Intervention studies which attempt to influence hypothesized mediators of inequalities in fruit and vegetable intakes may also help to establish more conclusively those determinants that might best be targeted in efforts to reduce socioeconomic inequalities in fruit and vegetable intakes at different life stages.

IMPLICATIONS FOR PRACTICE

The available literature on the existence of socioeconomic differentials in fruit and vegetable consumption across the life course points to several clear practice implications. Persons of low SEP are likely to require additional assistance to enable them to better meet health recommendations regarding consumption of fruits and vegetables. However, the factors that mediate socioeconomic inequalities in fruit and vegetable intakes and that might therefore be targeted in nutrition promotion interventions remain poorly understood. In the absence of strong evidence of mediating factors, it is difficult to recommend public health strategies or policies that might be implemented in order to reduce socioeconomic discrepancies in fruit and vegetable consumption. Using the limited existing evidence, several strategies could be considered, at least for adolescents and adults. Among adolescents, strategies aimed at increasing self-efficacy, at promoting the importance of healthy eating, and at promoting increased availability of fruits and vegetables in the home may help in supporting those of low SEP to consume more fruits and vegetables. Among adults, such strategies might include nutrition education and messages aimed at promoting the importance of health when making food purchasing choices; advice on engaging family and garnering support for making healthy food choices; and tips on time-efficient preparation of fruits and vegetables.

While broader policies ensuring the equitable provision of healthy foods in all neighborhoods across the socioeconomic spectrum are clearly important, further research is necessary before advocating for this as a specific strategy for reducing socioeconomic inequalities in fruit and vegetable consumption. In any case, available evidence suggests that such environmental strategies should be supplemented with education and support to enable individuals to make healthy dietary choices, regardless of their SEP.

CONCLUSION

This overview of the scientific literature shows that there are consistent socioeconomic differentials in intakes of fruits and vegetables, by which individuals of low SEP are at increased risk of inadequate consumption of these foods. These findings are relatively robust across age groups and SEP indicators. However, this field would benefit from a greater understanding of the mechanisms underlying associations of SEP with fruit and vegetable consumption. In particular, there is a dearth of information on mediating factors among older adults and adult men.

REFERENCES

Ahmadi, N., Black, J.L., Velazquez, C.E., Chapman, G.E., Veenstra, G., 2015. Associations between socio-economic status and school-day dietary intake in a sample of grade 5–8 students in Vancouver, Canada. Public Health Nutr. 18, 764–773.

An, R., 2013. Effectiveness of subsidies in promoting healthy food purchases and consumption: a review of field experiments. Public Health Nutr. 16, 1215–1228.

Attorp, A., Scott, J.E., Yew, A.C., Rhodes, R.E., Barr, S.I., Naylor, P.J., 2014. Associations between socioeconomic, parental and home environment factors and fruit and vegetable consumption of children in grades five and six in British Columbia, Canada. BMC Public Health 14, 150.

Ball, K., Mishra, G.D., Thane, C.W., Hodge, A., 2004. How well do Australian women comply with dietary guidelines? Public Health Nutr. 7, 443–452.

Ball, K., Crawford, D., Mishra, G., 2006. Socio-economic inequalities in women's fruit and vegetable intakes: a multilevel study of individual, social and environmental mediators. Public Health Nutr. 9, 623–630.

Ball, K., MacFarlane, A., Crawford, D., Savige, G., Andrianopoulos, N., Worsley, A., 2009. Can social cognitive theory constructs explain socio-economic variations in adolescent eating behaviours? A mediation analysis. Health Educ. Res. 24, 496–506.

Bamia, C., Orfanos, P., Ferrari, P., Overvad, K., Hundborg, H.H., Tjonneland, A., et al., 2005. Dietary patterns among older Europeans: the EPIC-Elderly study. Br. J. Nutr. 94, 100–113.

Bere, E., van Lenthe, F., Klepp, K.I., Brug, J., 2008. Why do parents' education level and income affect the amount of fruits and vegetables adolescents eat? Eur. J. Public Health 18 (6), 611–615.

Billson, H., Pryer, J.A., Nichols, R., 1999. Variation in fruit and vegetable consumption among adults in Britain. An analysis from the dietary and nutritional survey of British adults. Eur. J. Clin. Nutr. 53, 946–952.

Bowman, S., 2007. Low economic status is associated with suboptimal intakes of nutritious foods by adults in the National Health and Nutrition Examination Survey 1999-2002. Nutr. Res. 27, 515–523.

Boylan, S., Lallukka, T., Lahelma, E., Pikhart, H., Malyutina, S., Pajak, A., et al., 2011. Socio-economic circumstances and food habits in Eastern, Central and Western European populations. Public Health Nutr. 14, 678–687.

Cameron, A.J., Ball, K., Pearson, N., Lioret, S., Crawford, D.A., Campbell, K., et al., 2012. Socioeconomic variation in diet and activity-related behaviours of Australian children and adolescents aged 2-16 years. Pediatr. Obes. 7, 329–342.

Campbell, K.J., Abbott, G., Spence, A.C., Crawford, D.A., McNaughton, S.A., Ball, K., 2013. Home food availability mediates associations between mothers' nutrition knowledge and child diet. Appetite 71, 1–6.

Caraher, M., Lang, T., 1999. Can't cook, won't cook: a review of cooking skills and their relevance to health promotion. Int. J. Health Promotion Educ. 37, 89–100.

Conklin, A.I., Forouhi, N.G., Suhrcke, M., Surtees, P., Wareham, N.J., Monsivais, P., 2014. Variety more than quantity of fruit and vegetable intake varies by socioeconomic status and financial hardship. Findings from older adults in the EPIC cohort. Appetite 83, 248–255.

Darmon, N., Drewnowski, A., 2008. Does social class predict diet quality? Am. J. Clin. Nutr. 87, 1107–1117.

Darmon, N., Lacroix, A., Muller, L., Ruffieux, B., 2014. Food price policies improve diet quality while increasing socioeconomic inequalities in nutrition. Int. J. Behav. Nutr. Phys. Act. 11, 66.

Dehghan, M., Akhtar-Danesh, N., Merchant, A.T., 2011. Factors associated with fruit and vegetable consumption among adults. J. Hum. Nutr. Diet. 24, 128–134.

De Irala-Estevez, J., Groth, M., 2000. A systematic review of socio-economic differences in food habits in Europe: consumption of fruit and vegetables. Eur. J. Clin. Nutr. 54 (9), 706–714.

Dibsdall, L.A., Lambert, N., Frewer, L.J., 2002. Using interpretative phenomenology to understand the food-related experiences and beliefs of a select group of low-income UK women. J. Nutr. Educ. Behav. 34, 298–309.

Dibsdall, L.A., Lambert, N., Bobbin, R.F., Frewer, L.J., 2003. Low-income consumers' attitudes and behaviour towards access, availability and motivation to eat fruit and vegetables. Public Health Nutr. 6, 159–168.

Dijkstra, S., Neter, J.E., Brouwer, I.A., Huisman, M., Visser, M., 2014. Motivations to eat healthily in older Dutch adults—a cross sectional study. Int. J. Behav. Nutr. Phys. Act. 11, 141.

Dijkstra, S.C., Neter, J.E., van Stralen, M.M., Knol, D.L., Brouwer, I.A., Huisman, M., et al., 2015. The role of perceived barriers in explaining socio-economic status differences in adherence to the fruit, vegetable and fish guidelines in older adults: a mediation study. Public Health Nutr. 18, 797–808.

de Morais, C., Oliveira, B., Afonso, C., Lumbers, M., Raats, M., de Almeida, M.D.V., 2013. Nutritional risk of European elderly. Eur. J. Clin. Nutr. 67, 1215–1219.

Di Noia, J., Byrd-Bredbenner, C., 2013. Adolescent fruit and vegetable intake: influence of family support and moderation by home availability of relationships with afrocentric values and taste preferences. J. Acad. Nutr. Diet. 113, 803–808.

Donkin, A.J., Johnson, A.E., Morgan, K., Neale, R.J., Page, R.M., Silburn, R.L., 1998. Gender and living alone as determinants of fruit and vegetable consumption among the elderly living at home in urban Nottingham. Appetite 30, 39–51.

Donnelly, R., Springer, A., 2015. Parental social support, ethnicity, and energy balance-related behaviors in ethnically diverse, low-income, urban elementary schoolchildren. J. Nutr. Educ. Behav. 47, 10–18.

Dubowitz, T., Heron, M., Bird, C.E., Lurie, N., Finch, B.K., Basurto-Davila, R., et al., 2008. Neighborhood socioeconomic status and fruit and vegetable intake among whites, blacks, and Mexican Americans in the United States. Am. J. Clin. Nutr. 87, 1883–1891.

Galobardes, B., Shaw, M., Lawlor, D.A., Lynch, J.W., Davey Smith, G., 2006. Indicators of socioeconomic position (part 1). J. Epidemiol. Community Health 60, 7–12.

Giskes, K., Turrell, G., Patterson, C., Newman, B., 2002a. Socioeconomic differences among Australian adults in consumption of fruit and vegetabls and intakes of vitamins A, C and folate. J. Hum. Nutr. Diet. 15, 375–385.

Giskes, K., Turrell, G., Patterson, C., Newman, B., 2002b. Socio-economic differences in fruit and vegetable consumption among Australian adolescents and adults. Public Health Nutr. 5, 663–669.

Giskes, K., Lenthe, Fv. F., Brug, H.J., Mackenbach, J., 2004. Dietary intakes of adults in the Netherlands by childhood and adulthood socioeconomic position. Eur. J. Clin. Nutr. 58, 871–880.

Giskes, K., Van Lenthe, F.J., Brug, J., Mackenbach, J.P., Turrell, G., 2007. Socioeconomic inequalities in food purchasing: the contribution of respondent-perceived and actual (objectively measured) price and availability of foods. Prev. Med. 41 (1), 41–48.

Giskes, K., van Lenthe, F., Kamphuis, C., Huisman, M., Brug, J., Mackenbach, J.P., 2009. Household and food shopping environments: do they play a role in socioeconomic inequalities in fruit and vegetable consumption? A multilevel study among Dutch adults. J. Epidemiol. Community Health 63 (2), 113–120.

Giskes, K., Avendano, M., Brug, J., Kunst, A.E., 2010. A systematic review of studies on socioeconomic inequalities in dietary intakes associated with weight gain and overweight/obesity conducted among European adults. Obes. Rev. 11, 413–429.

Giskes, K., van Lenthe, F., Avendano-Pabon, M., Brug, J., 2011. A systematic review of environmental factors and obesogenic dietary intakes among adults: are we getting closer to understanding obesogenic environments? Obes. Rev. 12, e95–e106.

Glymour, M.M., 2006. Using causal diagrams to understand common problems in social epidemiology. In: Oakes, J.M., Kaufman, J.S. (Eds.), Methods in Social Epidemiology Jossey-Bass, San Francisco, CA.

Gopinath, B., Russell, J., Flood, V.M., Burlutsky, G., Mitchell, P., 2014. Adherence to dietary guidelines positively affects quality of life and functional status of older adults. J. Acad. Nutr. Diet. 114, 220–229.

Greenland, S., Pearl, J., Robins, J.M., 1999. Causal diagrams for epidemiologic research. Epidemiology 10, 37–48.

Hilsen, M., van Stralen, M.M., Klepp, K.I., Bere, E., 2011. Changes in 10-12 year old's fruit and vegetable intake in Norway from 2001 to 2008 in relation to gender and socioeconomic status—a comparison of two cross-sectional groups. Int. J. Behav. Nutr. Phys. Act. 8, 108.

Hosseinpoor, A.R., Bergen, N., Kunst, A., Harper, S., Guthold, R., Rekve, D., et al., 2012. Socioeconomic inequalities in risk factors for non communicable diseases in low-income and middle-income countries: results from the World Health Survey. BMC Public Health 12, 912.

Inglis, V., Ball, K., Crawford, D., 2005. Why do women of low socioeconomic status have poorer dietary behaviours than women of higher socioeconomic status? A qualitative exploration. Appetite 45, 334–343.

Inglis, V., Ball, K., Crawford, D., 2009. Does modifying the household food budget predict changes in the healthfulness of purchasing choices among low- and high-income women? Appetite 52, 273–279.

Kamphuis, C.B.M., de Bekker-Grob, E.W., van Lenthe, F.J., 2015. Factors affecting food choices of older adults from high and low socioeconomic groups: a discrete choice experiment. Am. J. Clin. Nutr. 101 (4), 768–774.

Konttinen, H., Sarlio-Lahteenkorva, S., Silventoinen, K., Mannisto, S., Haukkala, A., 2013. Socio-economic disparities in the consumption of vegetables, fruit and energy-dense foods: the role of motive priorities. Public Health Nutr. 16, 873–882.

Krieger, N., Williams, D.R., Moss, N.E., 1997. Measuring social class in US public health research: concepts, methodologies, and guidelines. Annu. Rev. Public Health 18, 341–378.

Lamb, K.E., White, S.R., 2015. Categorisation of built environment characteristics: the trouble with tertiles. Int. J. Behav. Nutr. Phys. Act. 12, 19.

Locher, J.L., Ritchie, C.S., Roth, D.L., Baker, P.S., Bodner, E.V., Allman, R.M., 2005. Social isolation, support, and capital and nutritional risk in an older sample: ethnic and gender differences. Soc. Sci. Med. 60, 747–761.

Mayen, A.L., Marques-Vidal, P., Paccaud, F., Bovet, P., Stringhini, S., 2014. Socioeconomic determinants of dietary patterns in low- and middle-income countries: a systematic review. Am. J. Clin. Nutr. 100, 1520–1531.

McLaughlin, C., Tarasuk, V., Kreiger, N., 2003. An examination of at-home food preparation activity among low-income, food-insecure women. J. Am. Diet. Assoc. 103, 1506–1512.

Mishra, G.D., McNaughton, S.A., Ball, K., Brown, W.J., Giles, G.G., Dobson, A.J., 2010. Major dietary patterns of young and middle aged women: results from a prospective Australian cohort study. Eur. J. Clin. Nutr. 64, 1125–1133.

Morley, B., Scully, M., Niven, P., Baur, L.A., Crawford, D., Flood, V., et al., 2012. Prevalence and socio-demographic distribution of eating, physical activity and sedentary behaviours among Australian adolescents. Health Promot. J. Austr. 23, 213–218.

Nicklett, E.J., Kadell, A.R., 2013. Fruit and vegetable intake among older adults: a scoping review. Maturitas 75, 305–312.

Patterson, R.E., Satia, J.A., Kristal, A.R., Neuhouser, M.L., Drewnowski, A., 2001. Is there a consumer backlash against the diet and health message? J. Am. Diet. Assoc. 101, 37–41.

Pechey, R., Monsivais, P., Ng, Y.-L., Marteau, T.M., 2015. Why don't poor men eat fruit? Socioeconomic differences in motivations for fruit consumption. Appetite 84, 271–279.

Peltzer, K., Phaswana-Mafuya, N., 2012. Fruit and vegetable intake and associated factors in older adults in South Africa. Glob. Health Action 5. http://dx.doi.org/10.3402/gha.v5i0.18668.

Preacher, K.J., 2015. Advances in mediation analysis: a survey and synthesis of new developments. Annu. Rev. Psychol. 66, 825–852.

Rasmussen, M., Krolner, R., Klepp, K.I., Lytle, L., Brug, J., Bere, E., et al., 2006. Determinants of fruit and vegetable consumption among children and adolescents: a review of the literature. Part I: quantitative studies. Int. J. Behav. Nutr. Phys. Act. 3, 22.

Richiardi, L., Bellocco, R., Zugna, D., 2013. Mediation analysis in epidemiology: methods, interpretation and bias. Int. J. Epidemiol. 42, 1511–1519.

Richter, M., Erhart, M., Vereecken, C.A., Zambon, A., Boyce, W., Nic Gabhainn, S., 2009. The role of behavioural factors in explaining socio-economic differences in adolescent health: a multilevel study in 33 countries. Soc. Sci. Med. 69, 396–403.

Riediger, N.D., Moghadasian, M.H., 2008. Patterns of fruit and vegetable consumption and the influence of sex, age and socio-demographic factors among Canadian elderly. J. Am. Coll. Nutr. 27, 306–313.

Riediger, N.D., Shooshtari, S., Moghadasian, M.H., 2007. The influence of sociodemographic factors on patterns of fruit and vegetable consumption in Canadian adolescents. J. Am. Diet. Assoc. 107, 1511–1518.

Roark, R.A., Niederhauser, V.P., 2013. Fruit and vegetable intake: issues with definition and measurement. Public Health Nutr. 16, 2–7.

Rodenburg, G., Oenema, A., Kremers, S.P., van de Mheen, D., 2012. Parental and child fruit consumption in the context of general parenting, parental education and ethnic background. Appetite 58, 364–372.

Sandvik, C., Gjestad, R., Samdal, O., Brug, J., Klepp, K.I., 2010. Does socio-economic status moderate the associations between psychosocial predictors and fruit intake in schoolchildren? The Pro Children study. Health Educ. Res. 25, 121–134.

Shavers, V.L., 2007. Measurement of socioeconomic status in health disparities research. J. Natl. Med. Assoc. 99, 1013–1023.

Springvloet, L., Lechner, L., Oenema, A., 2014. Can individual cognitions, self-regulation and environmental variables explain educational differences in vegetable consumption? A cross-sectional study among Dutch adults. Int. J. Behav. Nutr. Phys. Act. 11, 149.

Stephens, L.D., McNaughton, S.A., Crawford, D., MacFarlane, A., Ball, K., 2011. Correlates of dietary resilience among socioeconomically disadvantaged adolescents. Eur. J. Clin. Nutr. 65, 1219–1232.

Stephens, L.D., McNaughton, S.A., Crawford, D., Ball, K., 2014. Longitudinal predictors of frequent vegetable and fruit consumption among socio-economically disadvantaged Australian adolescents. Appetite 78, 165–171.

Stokols, D., 1996. Translating social ecological theory into guidelines for community health promotion. Am. J. Health Promotion 10, 282–298.

Thornton, L.E., Crawford, D.A., Ball, K., 2010. Neighbourhood-socioeconomic variation in women's diet: the role of nutrition environments. Eur. J. Clin. Nutr. 64, 1423–1432.

Thornton, L.E., Pearce, J.R., Ball, K., 2014. Sociodemographic factors associated with healthy eating and food security in socio-economically disadvantaged groups in the UK and Victoria, Australia. Public Health Nutr. 17, 20–30.

Thornton, L.E., Lamb, K.E., Tseng, M., Crawford, D.A., Ball, K., 2015. Does food store access modify associations between intrapersonal factors and fruit and vegetable consumption? Eur. J. Clin. Nutr. 69 (8), 902–906.

Turrell, G., 1997. Educational differences in dietary guideline food practices: are they associated with educational differences in food and nutrition knowledge? Aust. J. Nutr. Diet. 54, 25–33.

Turrell, G., Hewitt, B., Patterson, C., Oldenburg, B., 2003. Measuring socio-economic position in dietary research: is choice of socio-economic indicator important? Public Health Nutr. 6, 191–201.

van Rossum, C.T., van de Mheen, H., Witteman, J.C., Grobbee, E., Mackenbach, J.P., 2000. Education and nutrient intake in Dutch elderly people. The Rotterdam Study. Eur. J. Clin. Nutr. 54, 159–165.

Wang, D.D., Leung, C.W., Li, Y., Ding, E.L., Chiuve, S.E., Hu, F.B., et al., 2014. Trends in dietary quality among adults in the United States, 1999 through 2010. JAMA Intern. Med. 174, 1587–1595.

Williams, L., Ball, K., Crawford, D., 2010. Why do some socioeconomically disadvantaged women eat better than others? An investigation of the personal, social and environmental correlates of fruit and vegetable consumption. Appetite 55, 441–446.

Williams, L.K., Veitch, J., Ball, K., 2011. What helps children eat well? A qualitative exploration of resilience among disadvantaged families. Health Educ. Res. 26, 296–307.

Williams, L.K., Thornton, L., Crawford, D., Ball, K., 2012. Perceived quality and availability of fruit and vegetables are associated with perceptions of fruit and vegetable affordability among socio-economically disadvantaged women. Public Health Nutr. 15, 1262–1267.

Worsley, A., Blasche, R., Ball, K., Crawford, D., 2004. The relationship between education and food consumption in the 1995 Australian National Nutrition Survey. Public Health Nutr. 7, 649–663.

Wrieden, W.L., Connaghan, J., Morrison, C., Tunstall-Pedoe, H., 2004. Secular and socio-economic trends in compliance with dietary targets in the north Glasgow MONICA population surveys 1986-1995: did social gradients widen? Public Health Nutr. 7, 835–842.

Zarnowiecki, D., Ball, K., Parletta, N., Dollman, J., 2014a. Describing socioeconomic gradients in children's diets—does the socioeconomic indicator used matter? Int. J. Behav. Nutr. Phys. Act. 11, 44.

Zarnowiecki, D.M., Dollman, J., Parletta, N., 2014b. Associations between predictors of children's dietary intake and socioeconomic position: a systematic review of the literature. Obesity Rev. 15, 375–391.

Chapter 2

Industrial freezing, cooking, and storage differently affect antioxidant nutrients in vegetables

Alessandra Frati, Elena Antonini and Paolino Ninfali
University of Urbino "Carlo Bo", Urbino, Italy

CHAPTER OUTLINE

INTRODUCTION

In fresh vegetables, the phenolic compounds are important phytonutrients, able to defend the body from aging (Finkel and Holbrook, 2000) and chronic diseases (Block, 1992; Boeing et al., 2012; Gil et al., 1999; Lampe, 1999). Every day, our body is subjected to the attach from many radical species (reactive oxygen species (ROS)), formed not only during the physiological metabolism of energetic nutrients but also under infection, smoking, and pollution threaten (Dean et al., 1997; Finkel and Holbrook, 2000). When the normal antioxidant defenses are overwhelmed, the ROS give rise to a condition of oxidative stress (Halliwell and Cross, 1994), which means that ROS attack and oxidize portions of lipids, nucleic

Fruits, Vegetables, and Herbs.
DOI: http://dx.doi.org/10.1016/B978-0-12-802972-5.00002-0

acids, and proteins, with consequent impairment of physiological functions and arising of pathologies (Dean et al., 1997; Halliwell and Gutteridge, 1990). For rescuing the body from oxidative stress conditions, it becomes of vital importance the contribute of antioxidant nutrients (Sun et al., 2002). Fresh vegetables are relevant reservoirs of vitamins C, A, and E, as well as of phenol compounds (Rickman et al., 2007a). If introduced in the body at every meal (Ninfali et al., 2005), those nutrients provide consistent protection to physiological macromolecules by increasing the antioxidant capacity of the plasma (Prior et al., 2007).

Many people are not able to consume fresh vegetables every day, due to job conditions, distance from the markets of fresh products, or very less time for shopping and cooking (Bertuccioli and Ninfali, 2014). Therefore they buy frozen vegetables and consume them every day.

The question that arises is: "How much antioxidants are present in the frozen vegetables in respect to the correspondent fresh products?" This question has attracted the interest of the food technologists and nutritionists, and many efforts have been made to provide an answer (Rickman et al., 2007a,b).

The antioxidant nutrients and their antioxidant capacity have been often analyzed in most of the frozen vegetables, and guideline tables have been published for consumer's aid (www.istitutosurgelati.it). Guidelines were also provided by international organizations for the control of the industrial preparation of vegetables, including freezing (FAO, 1995).

Early work performed in our laboratory (Ninfali and Bacchiocca, 2003), regarded the phenolic content and antioxidant capacity of fresh and frozen vegetables, such as beet green, spinach, broccoli, and carrots. The study showed that frozen vegetables provided 30–50% less of antioxidants with respect to fresh vegetables. Moreover, we and others provided evidence that the vegetable cultivar is an important genetic determinant of antioxidants content and vegetable capacity to undergo processing (Kurilich et al., 2002; Ninfali and Bacchiocca, 2003). The decay of antioxidants was interpreted as mainly due to the blanching process, which precedes the freezing step (Ng et al., 1998). Blanching is a mild heat treatment, accomplished with hot water, steam, hot air, or microwave, which may result in nutrient losses. For instance, 72% of the phenol concentration is lost in the florets and 43% in the stems by boiling broccoli for 5 min (Zhang and Hamauzu, 2004). The retained antioxidant activity measured by 2,2-diphenyl-1-picrylhydrazyl (DPPH) method was about 35%, both in the florets and in the stems; by microwaving, the retained phenols were the same as by boiling (Zhang and Hamauzu, 2004).

Ismail et al. (2004) found that thermal treatment decreased the total phenols by 14% in spinach, 20% in cabbage, and 12% in kale.

On the contrary, other authors showed that total phenols significantly increased to various extent in green beans, spinach, and broccoli, depending on the type of cooking (Turkmen et al., 2005). In general, Turkmen et al. (2005) found that cooking did not cause any deleterious effect on the phenol pool.

Ewald et al. (1999) analyzed the content of some major flavonoids in onion, green beans, and peas, before and after heat treatments. The authors found that the loss of quercetin ranged between 25% and 41% and kaempferol from 0.35% to 0.96% after steaming (Ewald et al., 1999). Further processing by cooking, frying, or warming had only small effects on the flavonoid content (Ewald et al., 1999).

An important review on antioxidant losses with domestic cooking methods was published by Ruiz-Rodriguez et al. (2008), considering several nutrient, including antioxidants.

From all cited papers, it appears evident that most of the authors found a phenol loss and a consequent antioxidant activity decay with cooking. Only sporadic reports showed that the phenols were stable to thermal treatments.

Nowadays, most industries are actively involved in the characterization of the nutritional value of their frozen products. In the meantime, industries are searching for mild technologies of transformation in order to save the most delicate nutrients, including vitamin C and polyphenols (Rickman et al., 2007b).

In this work, we compared total phenols and antioxidant activity in three types of fresh and frozen vegetables, chosen on the basis of their different texture: spinach, green beans, and broccoli. The antioxidant nutrients were also evaluated after boiling or heating the vegetables. In addition, total phenols and antioxidant activity were studied during storage in domestic refrigerators.

THE INDUSTRIAL PROCESSING OF FROZEN VEGETABLES

The industry controls all aspects of the productive chain of the frozen vegetables. Fig. 2.1 shows the flowchart of the industrial processing subdivided in preharvest, harvest, and handling for freezing. Opportune vegetable cultivars are selected on the basis of a compromise among nutrient

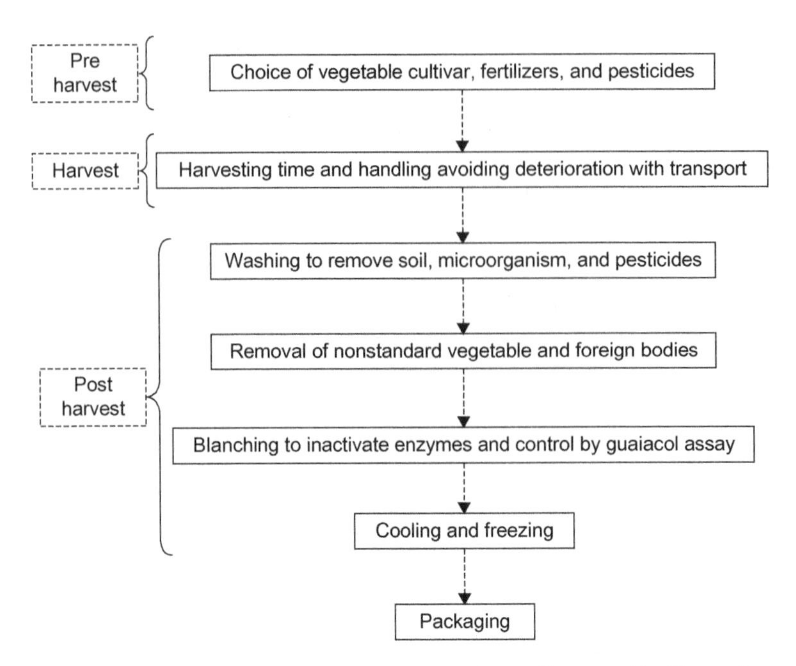

■ **FIGURE 2.1** Flowchart of the control steps in the industrial production of frozen vegetables. Efficiency of blanching is controlled by testing the residual peroxidase activity with guaiacol and hydrogen peroxide substrates.

content, low need of chemical fertilizers, and pesticides, as well as resistance to the mechanical stress (Kader, 2009).

At harvest, the maturity of the vegetables and the mechanical methods for harvesting are accurately identified. Time of postharvest storage and transport to the industry plant are as short as possible to avoid spoilage and fermentation of the vegetable. Once arrived to the industry, the vegetable is treated immediately. To avoid the effect of the browning, the endogenous enzymes are inactivated during processing by blanching, which is strictly necessary for almost all vegetables to be frozen (Williams et al., 1986). If vegetables are not blanched enough, the enzymes continue to be active during frozen storage, causing off-colors, off-flavors, and toughening (De Corcuera et al., 2007; Rickman et al., 2007a,b). Blanching time is crucial, as it varies with the type of vegetable and the size of the pieces to be frozen, which should be homogenous as much as possible. For this reason, the blanching step requires frequent controls of the inactivation of the peroxidases, as well as the search for defects in organoleptic properties and microorganism's concentration (Rickman et al., 2007a; Williams et al., 1986).

PHENOL OXIDIZING ENZYMES AND BLANCHING

The enzymatic oxidation of polyphenols, and particularly of flavonoids, occurs when the integrity of the vegetable cells is altered. Three major enzyme groups participate to the oxidation of the flavonoids: the laccases (EC 1.10.3.2), the catechol oxidases (EC 1.12.3.1), and the peroxidases (POD) (EC 1.11.1.7).

The laccases are multicopper glycoproteins, which catalyze the oxidation of diphenolic substrates in the presence of oxygen. They react with both *o*- and *p*-diphenols, and therefore they are endowed of little specificity (Pourcel et al., 2007).

The catechol oxidases catalyze the oxidation of the sole *o*-diphenols, to the correspondent quinones (Siegbahn, 2004). They are moderately glycosylated proteins, binding copper in two different domains and utilizing oxygen as molecular cofactor (Pourcel et al., 2007).

The peroxidases are a group of proteins, which contain, in the catalytic center, a metal, commonly iron or copper. The cofactor indispensable for the activity is the heme group (Thongsook et al., 2007). They catalyze the oxidation of phenols associated to reduction of hydrogen peroxide.

The plants have three classes of POD, which differ for the localization within the cell: class I groups soluble intracellular enzymes, which protect the cell from toxic peroxides; class II, are monomeric glycoproteins deputed to the lignin degradation (lignin peroxidase); class III groups the secreted peroxidases, which have many tissue specific functions, such as, removal of peroxides from the cytosol and chloroplasts, biosynthesis of the cell wall, and biosynthesis of the ethylene (Pourcel et al., 2007).

The pH interval for peroxidase reaction ranges from 3.5 to 9 (Koksal, 2011). Methanol and acetone inhibit the enzyme activity, when used at percentages higher than 60% (Pourcel et al., 2007).

Some authors (Bahceci et al., 2005) proposed to optimize blanching operation for green beans by targeting the inactivation of the lipoxygenase (LOX, EC.1.13.11.45). LOX activity is related to off-flavor development and color change, due to radical formation by oxidation of lipids. The formed radicals can destroy chlorophyll and carotenes during frozen storage (Morales-Blancas et al., 2002).

Ramirez and Whitaker (1998) proposed to use the cystine lyase as a blanching indicator in broccoli, but other researchers found that it is more heat labile than POD and LOX (Barrett et al., 2000).

From this short description, it appears evident that there are many phenol oxidizing enzymes in vegetables and their inactivation must be carefully controlled during the processing, to avoid undesired browning and nutrient losses.

The controls for the proper blanching are carried out quickly, along the productive plant. An assay of the residual activity in the blanched vegetable is routinely performed with the guaiacol, as substrate, for its high reactivity for the peroxidases (Lepedus et al., 2004). In the reduced form, the guaiacol has a peak of absorbance at 275 nm, but when it is oxidized, it provides a double peak, growing with the reaction time, with a maximum at 417 and 470 nm (Pourcel et al., 2007).

The activity of guaiacol peroxidases may be determined by measuring spectrophotometrically the absorbance increase at 470 nm of the vegetable juice. Alternatively, staining of vegetable cross sections can be orientatively used by adding the substrates on the sections (Lepedus et al., 2004).

OPTIMIZATION OF THE TOTAL PHENOLS EXTRACTION AND ANALYSIS

Several methods are available in the literature for phenol extraction from vegetables (Johnson, 2013; Naczk and Shahidi, 2006). In some cases, only organic solvents are used; in other cases, acid or basic treatments are preferred in combination with an organic solvent. For comparative studies between fresh and frozen vegetables, it is necessary to utilize an efficient extraction method. In fact, due to the different texture of raw and processed vegetables, the use of the organic solvent alone, could be unable to completely extract the phenols in the raw vegetable, though it could be enough in processed vegetables.

It is worth to note that, in the vegetable cell, part of the phenolic compounds is bound to cellulose, pectin, and proteins. These bound phenols could be hardly extractable from the raw produce. Occasionally, it has been observed in the literature that the phenol concentration of blanched vegetables is the same or even higher than the row vegetables. These results could be partially due to the softer texture of the heat-treated vegetables, which allows higher extraction of phenols from blanched vegetables, in respect to the raw.

In our laboratory, the extraction of the phenols was performed by grating the vegetable and treating the whole vegetable pulp with perchloric acid (PCA) and acetone, as reported (Ninfali and Bacchiocca, 2003). Two repeated extractions of the phenols with 5% PCA and two with 70%

acetone were consecutively applied; then, the four supernatants were combined and neutralized by potassium carbonate and phosphate buffer, pH 7.2. After centrifugation the neutralized extract was used for phenol and antioxidant capacity analysis.

In our extraction method, the PCA caused softening of the vegetable texture, thus facilitating the access of the acetone, inside to the vegetable matrices, allowing the extraction of most of the bound phenols. Furthermore, PCA inactivated the POD and LOX enzymes, thus avoiding the enzymatic oxidation of the phenols and increasing the yield.

A second important methodological aspect, for the comparison between fresh and frozen vegetables, regards the need to express the data on dry weight basis as it should be taken into account the changes of internal water. The dry weight was determined by us, drying samples at 110°C for 20h, and the percent of water was drawn to be utilized in the result calculation.

Concerning the domestic conservation of fresh vegetables, we utilized the cold room of our laboratory, with the temperature fixed at +6°C and humidity at 50%.

For simulation of the domestic cooking, we boiled 7min the spinach and 20min both green beans and broccoli (about 100g each) in 1L of hot water.

The phenolic compounds were assayed with the Folin–Ciocalteu method, as reported (Singleton et al., 1999), and the antioxidant capacity was determined by the oxygen radical absorbance capacity (ORAC) method (Ninfali et al., 2005).

COMPARISON AMONG VEGETABLES: SPINACH, BROCCOLI, AND GREEN BEANS

The spinach (*Spinacia oleracea*) is one of the most consumed green leafy vegetables. The family name of spinach is the *Amaranthaceae* and the *Chenopodiaceae* is the subfamily. Spinach is rich in vitamin C, β-carotene equivalents, vitamin K, folates as well as of phenolic compounds (http://phenol-explorer.eu). The spinach leaves are ovate to triangular-based, very variable in size, and surface type (smooth or bullous) depending on the cultivar.

The companies involved in frozen vegetable production, generally utilize cultivars with smooth leaves, which are preferred for their minor retention of water.

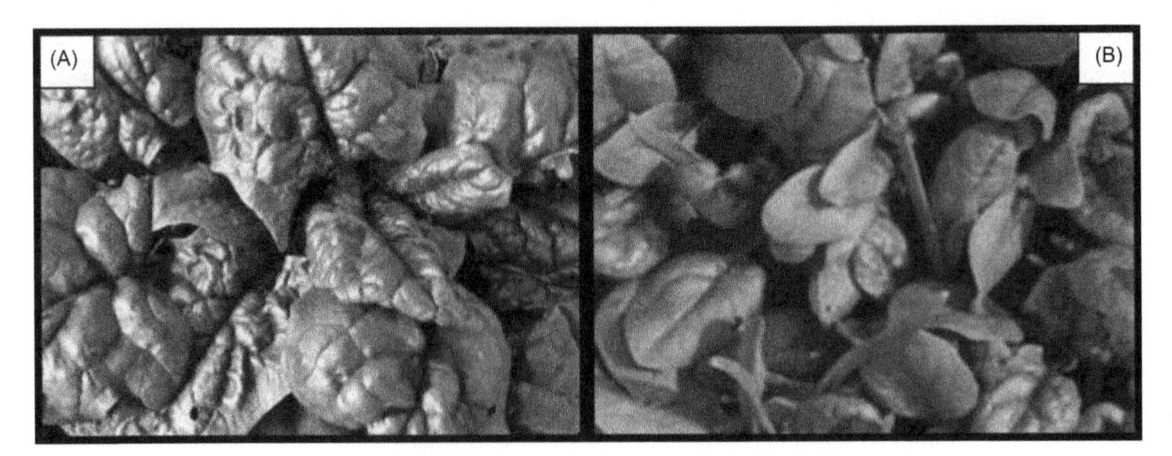

■ **FIGURE 2.2** Spinach cultivars with different leaves: the ***Matador*** cv. (Fig. 2.2A) and the ***Mississipi*** cv. (Fig. 2.2B).

Fig. 2.2 shows two spinach cultivars with different types of leaves. Fig. 2.2A shows the *Matador* cv. with bullous leaves and Fig. 2.2B the *Mississipi* cv. with smooth leaves.

Following the flowchart (Fig. 2.1), the spinach are collected by machine, early in the morning, and transferred immediately to the industry. The processing includes washing and cleaning, then blanching for 3–5 min by boiling. The control of the peroxidase activity is performed during processing, to avoid changes in quality. After precooling, followed by draining of the water, the spinach is chilled, transformed into small cubes, and packaged. The frozen spinach is distributed with a shelf life of 24 months at −20°C. The instructions for the consumers suggest to heat the vegetable in an oven or with a spoon of oil in a pan.

Broccoli (*Brassica oleracea*) belongs to the family of the *Brassicaceae*. It has large flower heads, usually green in color, arranged in a tree-like structure on branches.

Broccoli is high in vitamin C (Singh et al., 2007) and carotenoids as well as in lutein (Galgano et al., 2007; Park et al., 2012). Broccoli contains multiple nutrients with potent antiviral, antibacterial, and anticancer activity (Chang et al., 2006; Marques et al., 2014; Vallejo et al., 2003). Ingestion of raw broccoli produces indole-3-carbinol, which boosts DNA repair and blocks the growth of cancer cells (Brandi et al., 2003). Broccoli also contains glucoraphanin, which can be processed into sulforaphane, an anticancer compound (Davis and Ross, 2007; Jeffery and Araya, 2009). Unfortunately, boiling broccoli reduces the levels of sulforaphane, with losses of 20–30% after 5 min and 40–50% after 10 min (Dosz and Jeffery, 2013).

Concerning the industrial freezing, broccoli is collected by hand, the leaves are removed, and the heads carefully disposed into aerated cassettes, then transported to the industry. Here, broccoli is separated into florets, partially by automatic cutters and partially by hand. The florets are selected to obtain homogeneous sizes. After the washing, the blanching into boiling water is then performed. The blanching time is protracted proportionally to the size and hardness of the florets, which generally are no more than 2–4 cm across. It becomes important to inactivate most of the peroxidase and lipoxygenase activity in the internal side of the florets, as the former enzyme can have a degree of reactivation (Thongsook et al., 2007) and the latter is very resistant to thermal treatments (Morales-Blancas et al., 2002). The cooled florets are then drained, promptly frozen, and packaged.

Green beans (*Leguminosae*) are the unripe fruit of various cultivars of the common bean (*Phaseolus vulgaris*), selected especially for the flavor or sweetness of their pods. Although green beans are not always high in their concentration of phenolic compounds or vitamin C, they have impressive antioxidant capacity (Turkmen et al., 2005), likely due to some flavonoids found in green beans, which include: quercetin, kaempferol, catechins, epicatechins, and procyanidins. Several antioxidant carotenoids are also present in green beans, including: lutein, β-carotene, violaxanthin, and neoxanthin (Bahceci et al., 2005).

Regarding to the industrial freezing, the green beans are collected early in the morning, by an harvest machine. The developmental stage is carefully chosen, as it is the most important determinant of the texture. The right stage for harvesting is when the pods cease the elongation and the seeds, inside the pods, begin the maturation (Stolle-Smits et al., 1999).

Once harvested, green beans are immediately transferred to the industry. Here, they are washed and selected, and then blanched by steaming, with an accurate control for the peroxidase inactivation (Bahceci et al., 2005). After precooling, the freezing is applied, followed by the packaging in plastic bags.

EXPERIMENTAL DATA OBTAINED IN OUR LABORATORY

Studies were earlier performed in our lab on different vegetables, before and after the industrial freezing. The analyzed samples were drawn along the productive plant, in such a way to obtain a correspondence between the fresh and frozen products.

Fig. 2.3 shows the total phenols and the antioxidant capacity of spinach, green beans, and broccoli, before and after the freezing process. Fig. 2.3

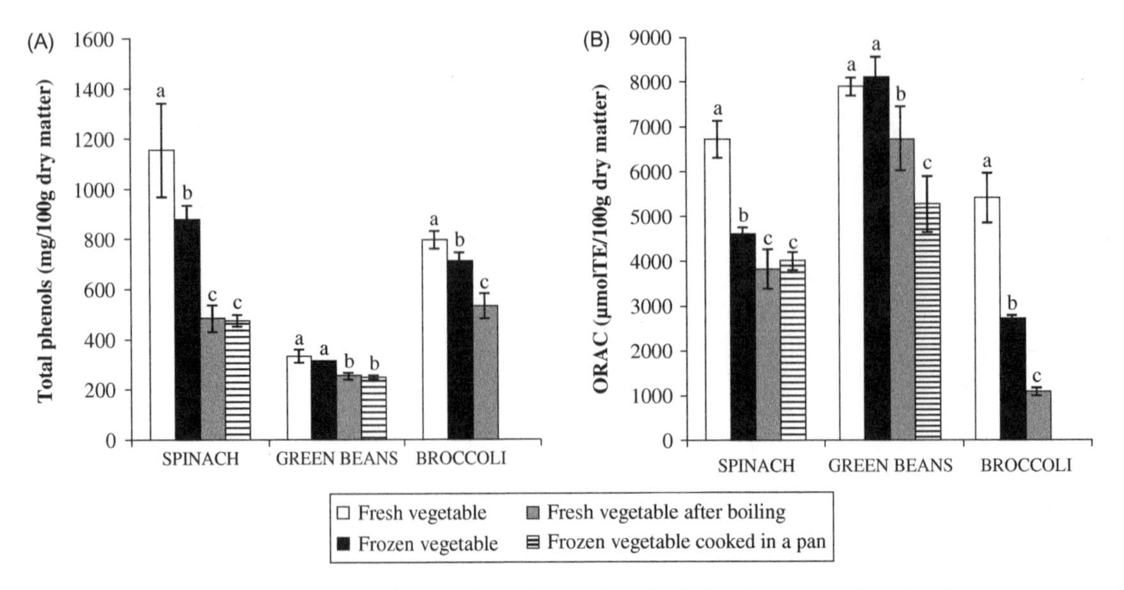

■ **FIGURE 2.3** Total phenols (A) and antioxidant capacity (B) in spinach, green beans, and broccoli under fresh, frozen, boiled, and cooked conditions. Values were referred on dry weight basis and were the means ±SD of six different assays. Different letters indicate statistically significant differences by the student's T-test with the significance level set at $P \leq 0.05$.

also shows results obtained from fresh vegetables after boiling and, in two cases, the same parameters regard the vegetables heated in a pan.

Fig. 2.3A shows the total phenol concentration of the three vegetables. Frozen spinach showed a marked reduction of the phenols, as compared to the fresh product. The value is further reduced in spinach, when the fresh vegetable is boiled. The frozen spinach cooked in a pan, showed a phenol concentration lower than the frozen spinach.

The spinach ORAC values (Fig. 2.3B) approximately reflect the pattern of the phenols, although the discrepancy between the ORAC of the frozen versus the ORAC of the fresh products is a little higher than that observed in total phenols.

The total phenols of green beans (Fig. 2.3A) showed a moderate decay in the transformation from fresh to frozen products. The fresh green beans boiled in water were quite stable in antioxidant parameters, as well as the frozen green beans heated in a pan.

The ORAC values of the green beans, during processing, showed more relevant differences than the phenol values (Fig. 2.3B). However, the most striking aspect is the very high value of the green beans ORAC, in respect to the other vegetables. The green beans ORAC reaches 8000 units in both fresh and frozen vegetables, despite the low concentration of phenols. The high ORAC value means that green beans have phenols endowed with a very high antiperoxyl radical activity (Prior et al., 2007).

We must underlie the stability of the ORAC value of green beans after the freezing processing. This may be due to particular structure of the vegetable, which contains phenols both in the pods and in the internal seeds. It may be sought that the pods exert a protection on the internal seeds during blanching.

In the broccoli, we observed a moderate decay of total phenols from fresh to frozen or boiled product (Fig. 2.3A). Indeed, this decay is more pronounced by considering the ORAC parameter (Fig. 2.3B), thus indicating that processing oxidizes the compounds with the most relevant antioxidant activity, making them ineffective. It has been previously demonstrated by others (Kurilich et al., 2002), that about 95% of the antioxidant capacity, measured with the ORAC assay, lies in the hydrophilic extract and only 5% or less in the lipophilic extract.

Overall, the results show the particular behavior of each vegetable for the antioxidant loss during the freezing processing. The evaluation of the total phenols, combined with the ORAC assay, provides a more complete picture of the antioxidant nutrient losses.

Fig. 2.4 shows total phenols (Fig. 2.4A) and ORAC values (Fig. 2.4B) of the three vegetables along 1 week of storage at +6°C. The spinach shows

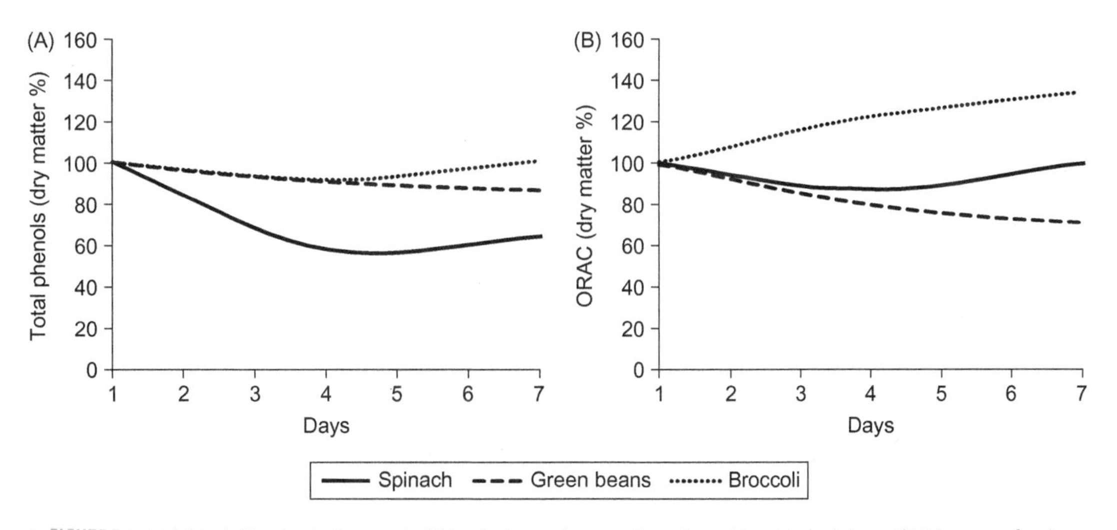

■ **FIGURE 2.4** Total phenols (A) and antioxidant capacity (B) in spinach, green beans, and broccoli stored 1 week in the dark at +6°C. Values were referred on dry weight basis and were the means ±SD of six different assays.

a 40% decay of total phenols from 1 to 4 days, then the values remained constant from 4 to 7 days (Fig. 2.4A). Total phenols of green beans and broccoli were stable till to 4 days, then broccoli, but not green beans phenols, showed a tendency to increase from 4 to 7 days. In the ORAC values, the green beans showed a slow progressive decay, the spinach a very small decay, followed by a recovery, whereas the broccoli showed a progressive increase during the storage (Fig. 2.4B).

These results can be interpreted by considering that the vegetables, stored in the dark at +6°C, change their secondary metabolism, with production of new metabolites with different antioxidant capacity. These metabolic modifications are vegetable specific and very likely also tissue specific (Santos et al., 2014). In a first instance, it looks better to store fresh vegetables 1 week in the fridge instead of buying frozen vegetables. However, the results of Fig. 2.4, though showing a relative stability of the antioxidant parameters, highlight the modification of secondary metabolites. The consequences of this modification lie into organoleptic changes, dehydration, loss of firmness, fermentation, and mold formation, with losses in the sanitary quality.

CONCLUSIONS

In the industrial freezing, the losses of phenols were found markedly different from one vegetable to the other and sometime lower than those due to differences between cultivars (Bacchiocca et al., 2006; Ninfali et al., 2005).

The spinach was more vulnerable to the freezing process than broccoli and green beans. However, the losses of antioxidants of all vegetables were found moderate (Fig. 2.5).

The reason of this moderate decay of antioxidants is certainly due to the improvement of the processing plants, in respect to the past (Ninfali and Bacchiocca, 2003). Nowadays, the industries operate in a continuous manner, with a strict control of all steps. The fresh vegetables enter the plant from one side and get out frozen from the other side, transported by conveyor belts, with a minimum intervention of the workers. The microbiological quality is also very good as contamination is tested by drawing samples at every step.

The blanching is the most delicate aspect to be controlled for reducing vitamins and polyphenols losses, which are due to a double process: the leaching into the water of the more polar compounds (Makris and Rossiter, 2001); breakdown of native phenolic compounds with formation

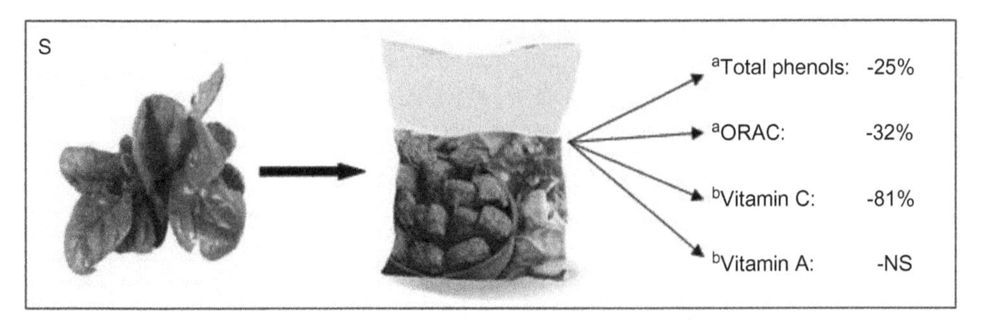

B
aTotal phenols: -11%
aORAC: -50%
bVitamin C: -35%
cSulforaphane: -40%

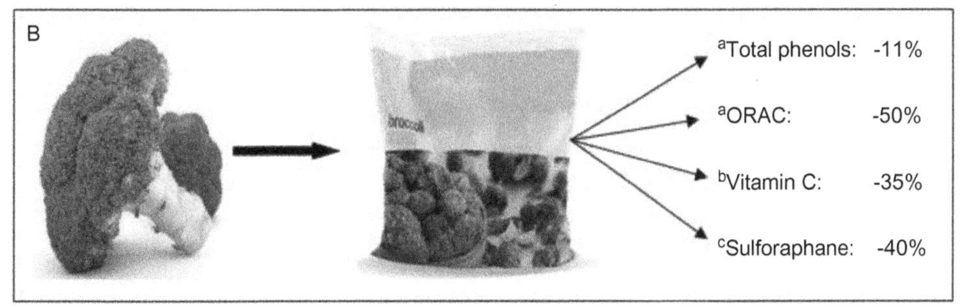

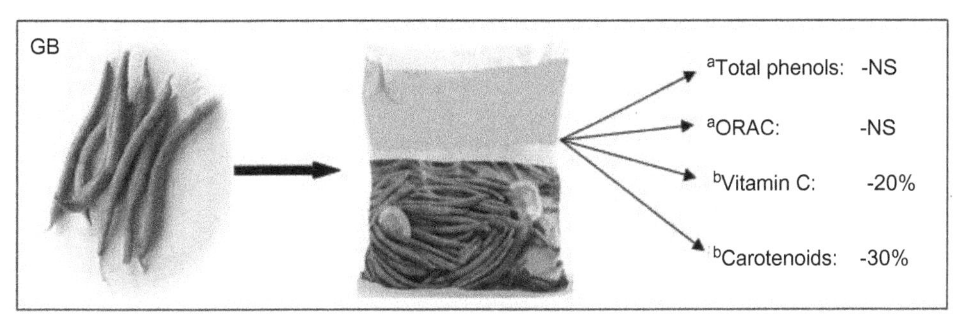

■ **FIGURE 2.5** Summary of the nutrient decay in frozen vegetables: *S*, spinach; *B*, broccoli; *GB*, green beans. (a) Our data presented in this paper, (b) data from Rickman et al. (2007a,b), (c) data from Dosz and Jeffery (2013).

of degradation products, from the heat labile secondary metabolites (Ruiz-Rodriguez et al., 2008). Efforts made to improve this step, were not able to completely eliminate the losses of nutrients.

In the broccoli, the blanching inactivates both the POD and the LOX, but also the myrosinase enzyme (EC 3.2.1.147), which generates bioactive molecules, during the chewing of raw brassica vegetables (Leoni et al., 1997).

Some authors have highlighted these problems and found a solution. For example, to recovery the health potential of the frozen broccoli, Dosz and Jeffery (2013) suggested to sprinkle 0.25% of daikon radish powder on the frozen broccoli, in order to add the myrosinase of the radish to the broccoli. This interesting example of food integration is functional to restore the lost myrosinase and provide bioactive molecules in the frozen vegetable.

To save nutrients, when boiling fresh and frozen vegetables in the domestic preparations, it is important to reduce the time of cooking and the volume of water. The highest retention of nutrients was observed with little water (Leskova et al., 2006). Interestingly, addition of vegetable extracts, or powders, as well as spices or citric acid to the boiling water, significantly reduced the losses of phenolic compounds in the boiling water (Ruiz-Rodriguez et al., 2008).

Steaming provokes a minor loss of nutrients than boiling (Ninfali et al., 2005), whereas microwaving strictly depends on the time of permanence in the oven (Ruiz-Rodriguez et al., 2008). In the case of microwaved broccoli, a remarkable loss of phenolic compounds and antioxidant activity was described by Vallejo et al. (2003).

The domestic storage of the vegetables for a week in the fridge exposes the product to metabolic modifications and fermentations, which lead to a slight decrease in total phenols, with varying losses depending on the vegetable. Major modifications in the secondary metabolites occur after 4 days of storage, with changes in the composition of the antioxidant pool and increases in the microbiological contamination. To describe these changes, the high-performance liquid chromatography pattern of secondary metabolites, repeated every day, could show the modifications of the endogenous phenolic compounds (Ruiz-Rodriguez et al., 2008).

In conclusion, improvements in the processing of frozen vegetables are still possible, but they can be obtained through the concerted action of food technologists and nutrition experts. Improvements in the final product can be reached by restoring nutrients lost in the processing, with the aid of dressings or additions of the lost enzymes able to provide bioactive compounds. The responsible attention of the consumers, in choosing the produce, cooking and dressing it at home, is strictly necessary to ameliorate the nutritional quality of the processed vegetables.

REFERENCES

Bacchiocca, M., Biagiotti, E., Ninfali, P., 2006. Nutritional and technological reasons for evaluating the antioxidant capacity of vegetable products. Ital. J. Food Sci. 18, 209–217.

Bahceci, K.S., Serpen, A., Gokmen, V., Acar, J., 2005. Study of lipoxygenase and peroxidase as indicator enzymes in green beans: change of enzyme activity, ascorbic acid and chlorophylls during frozen storage. J. Food Eng. 66, 187–192.

Barrett, D.M., Garcia, E.L., Russell, G.F., Ramirez, E., Shirazi, A., 2000. Blanch time and cultivar effects on quality of frozen and stored corn and broccoli. J. Food Sci. 65, 534–540.

Bertuccioli, A., Ninfali, P., 2014. The Mediterranean Diet in the era of globalization: the need to support knowledge of healthy dietary factors in the new socio-economical framework. Mediterr. J. Nutr. Metab. 7, 75–86.

Block, G., 1992. The data support a role for antioxidants in reducing cancer risk. Nutr. Rev. 50, 207–213.

Boeing, H., Bechthold, A., Bub, A., Ellinger, S., Haller, D., Kroke, A., et al., 2012. Critical review: vegetables and fruit in the prevention of chronic diseases. Eur. J. Nutr. 51, 637–663.

Brandi, G., Paiardini, M., Cervasi, B., Fiorucci, C., Filippone, P., De Marco, C., et al., 2003. A new indole-3-carbinol tetrameric derivative inhibits cyclin-dependent kinase 6 expression, and induces G(1) cell cycle arrest in both estrogen-dependent and estrogen-independent breast cancer cell lines. Cancer Res. 63, 4028–4036.

Chang, X.F., Firestone, G.L., Bjeldanes, L.F., 2006. Inhibition of growth factor-induced ras signaling in vascular endothelial cells and angiogenesis by 3,3′-diindolylmethane. Carcinogenesis 27, 541–550.

Davis, C.D., Ross, S.A., 2007. Dietary components impact histone modifications and cancer risk. Nutr. Rev. 65, 88–94.

De Corcuera, J.I.R., Cavalieri, R.P., Powers, J.R., 2007. Blanching of foods. In: Heldman, D. (Ed.), Encyclopedia of Agricultural, Food, and Biological Engineering Mercel Dekker Inc., Washington, DC. http://dx.doi.org/10.1081/E-EAFE-120030417.

Dean, R.T., Fu, S.L., Stocker, R., Davies, M.J., 1997. Biochemistry and pathology of radical-mediated protein oxidation. Biochem. J. 324, 1–18.

Dosz, E.B., Jeffery, E.H., 2013. Commercially produced frozen broccoli lacks the ability to form sulforaphane. J. Funct. Foods 5, 987–990.

Ewald, C., Fjelkner-Modig, S., Johansson, K., Sjoholm, I., Akesson, B., 1999. Effect of processing on major flavonoids in processed onions, green beans, and peas. Food Chem. 64, 231–235.

FAO, 1995. Fruit and vegetable processing. FAO Agricultural Services Bulletin, 119. Rome.

Finkel, T., Holbrook, N.J., 2000. Oxidants, oxidative stress and the biology of ageing. Nature 408, 239–247.

Galgano, F., Favati, F., Caruso, M., Pietrafesa, A., Natella, S., 2007. The influence of processing and preservation on the retention of health-promoting compounds in broccoli. J. Food Sci. 72, S130–S135.

Gil, M.I., Ferreres, F., Tomas-Barberan, F.A., 1999. Effect of postharvest storage and processing on the antioxidant constituents (flavonoids and vitamin C) of fresh-cut spinach. J. Agric. Food Chem. 47, 2213–2217.

Halliwell, B., Gutteridge, J.M.C., 1990. Role of free-radicals and catalytic metal-ions in human-disease—an overview. Methods Enzymol. 186, 1–85.

Halliwell, B., Cross, C.E., 1994. Oxygen-derived species—their relation to human-disease and environmental-stress. Environ. Health Perspect. 102, 5–12.

Ismail, A., Marjan, Z.M., Foong, C.W., 2004. Total antioxidant activity and phenolic content in selected vegetables. Food Chem. 87, 581–586.

Jeffery, E.H., Araya, M., 2009. Physiological effects of broccoli consumption. Phytochem. Rev. 8, 283–298.

Johnson, I.T., 2013. Phytochemicals and health. In: Tiwari, B.K., Brunton, N.P., Brennan, C.S. (Eds.), Handbook of Plant Food Phytochemicals: Sources, Stability and Extraction John Wiley & Sons Ltd, Oxford. http://dx.doi.org/10.1002/9781118464717.ch3.

Kader, A.A., 2009. Effects on nutritional quality. In: Yahia, E.M. (Ed.), Modified and Controlled Atmospheres for the Storage, Transportation, and Pakaging of Horticulural Commodities Taylor and Francis Group, Boca Raton, FL. http://dx.doi.org/10.1201/9781420069587.ch6.

Koksal, E., 2011. Peroxidase from leaves of spinach (*Spinacia oleracea*): partial purification and some biochemical properties. Int. J. Pharmacol. 7, 135–139.

Kurilich, A.C., Jeffery, E.H., Juvik, J.A., Wallig, M.A., Klein, B.P., 2002. Antioxidant capacity of different broccoli (*Brassica oleracea*) genotypes using the oxygen radical absorbance capacity (ORAC) assay. J. Agric. Food Chem. 50, 5053–5057.

Lampe, J.W., 1999. Health effects of vegetables and fruit: assessing mechanisms of action in human experimental studies. Am. J. Clin. Nutr. 70, 475S–490S.

Leoni, O., Iori, R., Palmieri, S., Esposito, E., Menegatti, E., Cortesi, R., et al., 1997. Myrosinase-generated isothiocyanate from glucosinolates: isolation, characterization and in vitro antiproliferative studies. Bioorg. Med. Chem. 5, 1799–1806.

Lepedus, H., Cesar, V., Krsnik-Rasol, M., 2004. Guaiacol Peroxidases in carrot (*Daucus carota* L.) root. Food Technol. Biotechnol. 42, 33–36.

Leskova, E., Kubikova, J., Kovacikova, E., Kosicka, M., Porubska, J., Holcikova, K., 2006. Vitamin losses: retention during heat treatment and continual changes expressed by mathematical models. J. Food Compost. Anal. 19, 252–276.

Makris, D.P., Rossiter, J.T., 2001. Domestic processing of onion bulbs (*Allium cepa*) and asparagus spears (*Asparagus officinalis*): effect on flavonol content and antioxidant status. J. Agric. Food Chem. 49, 3216–3222.

Marques, M., Laflamme, L., Benassou, I., Cissokho, C., Guillemette, B., Gaudreau, L., 2014. Low levels of 3,3′-diindolylmethane activate estrogen receptor a and induce proliferation of breast cancer cells in the absence of estradiol. BMC Cancer 14, 524.

Morales-Blancas, E.F., Chandia, V.E., Cisneros-Zevallos, L., 2002. Thermal inactivation kinetics of peroxidase and lipoxygenase from broccoli, green asparagus and carrots. J. Food Sci. 67, 146–154.

Naczk, M., Shahidi, F., 2006. Phenolics in cereals, fruits and vegetables: occurrence, extraction and analysis. J. Pharm. Biomed. Anal. 41, 1523–1542.

Ng, A., Smith, A.C., Waldron, K.W., 1998. Effect of tissue type and variety on cell wall chemistry of onion (*Allium cepa* L.). Food Chem. 63, 17–24.

Ninfali, P., Bacchiocca, M., 2003. Polyphenols and antioxidant capacity of vegetables under fresh and frozen conditions. J. Agric. Food Chem. 51, 2222–2226.

Ninfali, P., Mea, G., Giorgini, S., Rocchi, M., Bacchiocca, M., 2005. Antioxidant capacity of vegetables, spices and dressings relevant to nutrition. Br. J. Nutr. 93, 257–266.

Park, W.T., Kim, J.K., Park, S., Lee, S.W., Li, X., Kim, Y.B., et al., 2012. Metabolic profiling of glucosinolates, anthocyanins, carotenoids, and other secondary metabolites in kohlrabi (*Brassica oleracea* var. gongylodes). J. Agric. Food Chem. 60, 8111–8116.

Pourcel, L., Routaboul, J.M., Cheynier, V., Lepiniec, L., Debeaujon, I., 2007. Flavonoid oxidation in plants: from biochemical properties to physiological functions. Trends Plant Sci. 12, 29–36.

Prior, R.L., Go, L.W., Wu, X.L., Jacob, R.A., Sotoudeh, G., Kader, A.A., et al., 2007. Plasma antioxidant capacity changes following a meal as a measure of the ability of a food to alter in vivo antioxidant status. J. Am. Coll. Nutr. 26, 170–181.

Ramirez, E.C., Whitaker, J.R., 1998. Cystine lyases in plants: a comprehensive review. J. Food Biochem. 22, 427–440.

Rickman, J.C., Barrett, D.M., Bruhn, C.M., 2007a. Nutritional comparison of fresh, frozen and canned fruits and vegetables. Part 1. Vitamins C and B and phenolic compounds. J. Sci. Food Agric. 87, 930–944.

Rickman, J.C., Bruhn, C.M., Barrett, D.M., 2007b. Nutritional comparison of fresh, frozen, and canned fruits and vegetables-II. Vitamin A and carotenoids, vitamin E, minerals and fiber. J. Sci. Food Agric. 87, 1185–1196.

Ruiz-Rodriguez, A., Marín, F.R., Ocaña, A., Soler-Rivas, C., 2008. Effect of domestic processing on bioactive compounds. Phytochem. Rev. 7, 345–384.

Santos, J., Herrero, M., Mendiola, J.A., Oliva-Teles, M.T., Ibanez, E., Delerue-Matos, C., et al., 2014. Fresh-cut aromatic herbs: nutritional quality stability during shelf-life. LWT-Food Sci. Technol. 59, 101–107.

Siegbahn, P.E.M., 2004. The catalytic cycle of catechol oxidase. J. Biol. Inorg. Chem. 9, 577–590.

Singh, J., Upadhyay, A.K., Prasad, K., Bahadur, A., Rai, M., 2007. Variability of carotenes, vitamin C, E and phenolics in Brassica vegetables. J. Food Compost. Anal. 20, 106–112.

Singleton, V.L., Orthofer, R., Lamuela-Raventos, R.M., 1999. Analysis of total phenols and other oxidation substrates and antioxidants by means of Folin-Ciocalteu reagent. Oxid. Antioxid. Pt A 299, 152–178.

Stolle-Smits, T., Beekhuizen, J.G., Kok, M.T.C., Pijnenburg, M., Recourt, K., Derksen, J., et al., 1999. Changes in cell wall polysaccharides of green bean pods during development. Plant Physiol. 121, 363–372.

Sun, J., Chu, Y.F., Wu, X.Z., Liu, R.H., 2002. Antioxidant and anti proliferative activities of common fruits. J. Agric. Food Chem. 50, 7449–7454.

Thongsook, T., Whitaker, J.R., Smith, G.M., Barrett, D.M., 2007. Reactivation of broccoli peroxidases: structural changes of partially denatured isoenzymes. J. Agric. Food Chem. 55, 1009–1018.

Turkmen, N., Sari, F., Velioglu, Y.S., 2005. The effect of cooking methods on total phenolics and antioxidant activity of selected green vegetables. Food Chem. 93, 713–718.

Vallejo, F., Garcia-Viguera, C., Tomas-Barberan, F.A., 2003. Changes in broccoli (*Brassica oleracea* L. var. italica) health-promoting compounds with inflorescence development. J. Agric. Food Chem. 51, 3776–3782.

Williams, D.C., Lim, M.H., Chen, A.O., Pangborn, R.M., Whitaker, J.R., 1986. Blanching of vegetables for freezing—which indicator enzyme to choose. Food Technol. 40, 130–140.

Zhang, D.L., Hamauzu, Y., 2004. Phenolics, ascorbic acid, carotenoids and antioxidant activity of broccoli and their changes during conventional and microwave cooking. Food Chem. 88, 503–509.

Chapter 3

Pharmacological properties of some medicinal plants, its components and using fields

Hajjaj Ghizlane[1] and Bahlouli Aziz[2]
[1]*Mohammed V University, Rabat, Morocco*
[2]*Ibn Tofail University, Kenitra, Morocco*

CHAPTER OUTLINE

INTRODUCTION

Herbal remedies have been used for thousands of years. Early in human history, people practiced herbal medicine as a magical or religious healing art (Backer, 1965). Today, a lot of people use herbal medicine or rely on them. Of the 252 drugs considered as basic and essential by the World Health Organization (WHO), 11% are exclusively of plant origin and a significant number are synthetic drugs obtained from natural precursors. Natural compounds can be lead compounds, allowing the design and rational planning of new drugs, biomimetic synthesis development and the discovery of new therapeutic properties not yet attributed to known

Fruits, Vegetables, and Herbs.
DOI: http://dx.doi.org/10.1016/B978-0-12-802972-5.00003-2

compounds (Hamburger and Hostettmann, 1991). In recent years, there has been growing interest in alternative therapies and the therapeutic use of natural products, especially those derived from plants (Goldfrank et al., 1982; Vulto and Smet, 1988; Mentz and Schenkel, 1989). There is now considerable scientific evidence that a large number of herbal medicines exert their effect on different body systems, and this supports and confirms the extensive empirical testimony gained over the years. This increasing body of evidence reinforces the case for including herbal medicines in the mainstream therapy of a number of chronic disorders, either alone, or as part of a programme of integrative medicine.

In this chapter we present a number of studies which have been conducted on the phytochemical, pharmacological, and toxicological aspects of *Matricaria chamomilla* L., *Ormenis mixta* L., *Pistacia atlantica* Desf., *Papaver rhoeas* L. and their uses in traditional medicine.

SOME OF THE PLANTS THAT HAVE CONTRIBUTED TO THE DISCOVERY OF DRUGS FOR USE IN MODERN MEDICINE

Matricaria chamomilla *L.*

Chamomile is a solar herb, meaning that its energetic associations are with the sun; The Egyptians valued the herb as a cure for malaria and dedicated chamomile to their sun god, Ra. Chamomile was one of the nine sacred herbs that the Anglo-Saxons believed had special powers. The chamomiles have long been used in European herbal medicine for their relaxing and soothing properties and for stomach complaints and women's problems. In the middle ages, chamomile was a popular strewing herb and in folk culture it has been called the "plant doctor" because it seems to help other plants growing near it. This plant is a widely recognized herb in Western culture and it is known as Baboon in Morocco belongs to the Asteraceae family. Its medicinal usage dates back to antiquity where such notables as Hippocrates, Galen, and Asclepius made written reference to it (Thorne research, 2008).

Description

Chamomile is an annual plant with thin spindle shaped roots only penetrating flatly into the soil. The branched stem is erect, heavily ramified, and grows to a height of 10–80 cm. The long and narrow leaves are bi- to tripinnate. The flower heads are placed separately, they have a diameter of 10–30 mm, and they are pedunculate and heterogamous. The golden yellow tubular florets with 5 teeth are 1.5–2.5 mm long, ending always in a glandulous tube. The 11–27 white plant flowers are 6–11 mm long, 3.5 mm wide, and arranged concentrically. The receptacle is 6–8 mm wide, flat in the beginning and conical, cone-shaped later, hollow the latter being a very important distinctive characteristic of *M. chamomilla* L. and without paleae. The fruit is a yellowish brown achene (Franke, 2005) (Fig. 3.1).

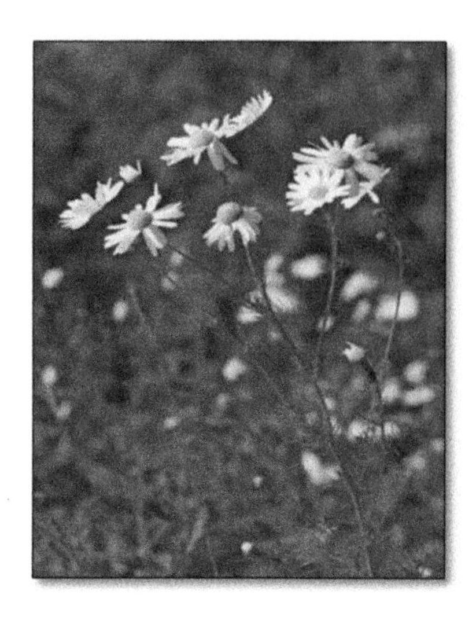

■ **FIGURE 3.1** ***Matricaria chamomilla*** **L.**
http://en.wikipedia.org/wiki/Chamomile

Traditional use

Today, chamomile is one of the most widely used herbs in the world. It is generally considered as safe and gentle herbal remedy that may be used daily as a calming tea. It has been extensively used in traditional medicine for hay fever, inflammation, muscle spasms, menstrual disorders, ulcers, wounds, gastrointestinal disorders, rheumatic pain, and hemorrhoids. In the form of an aqueous extract *M. chamomilla* L. has been frequently used as a mild sedative to calm nerves and reduce anxiety, to treat hysteria, nightmares, insomnia, and other sleep problems (Forster et al., 1980).

Chemical constituents

Matricaria chamomilla L. contains a large number of therapeutically interesting and active compound classes. The most important are the components of the essential oil and the flavonoid fraction. Apart from them, the following compound classes were detected and characterized: mucins, coumarins, phenol carboxylic acids (phenyl substituted carboxylic acids), amino acids, phytosterols, choline, and mineral substances (Frank and Schilcher, 2005). The chamomile constituents are best categorized according to their lipophilicity (Schilcher, 1987). The lipophilic fraction includes individual components of the essential oil, coumarins, methoxylated flavone aglyca, phytosterols, and "lipidic and waxy substances." The hydrophilic fraction consists of flavonoids, mucilage, phenyl carboxylic acids, amino acids, and choline.

In a study, the essential oil of *M. chamomilla* L. from Morocco was analyzed by capillary gas chromatography with mass spectrometric detector (GC-MS). Twenty-five compounds were identified in the essential oils and the main constituents of the essential oils were chamazulene (25.21%), *cis*-β-farnesene (12.51%), eucalyptol (9.19%), coumarin (7.72%), galaxolide (6.28%), and camphor (4.3%) (Hajjaj et al., 2013a,b).

Pharmacological properties

In several studies *M. chamomilla* L. has been reported to exhibit antiinflammatory, antispasmodic, antioxidative, antibacterial, antifungal, anticancer, antiallergic, hypoglycemic, analgesic, immunomodulatory, antistress, antiulcerogenic, antihypertensive, CNS depressant, hepatoprotective, chemopreventive, radioprotective, antitumor, and antipyretic (Ompal et al., 2011).

Toxicological study

In a study the acute and Subchronic toxicity (90 days) of *M. chamomilla* L. water extract (MCWE) via oral route rodent models were investigated. For the acute toxicity study, water extract of *M. chamomilla* L. administrated to mice at doses ranging from 300 to 2000 mg/kg. General behavior, adverse effects, mortality were recorded for up to 14 days posttreatment for this study, the median lethal dose (LD50) of MCWE was found to be higher than 2 g/kg. In the Subchronic toxicity study, *M. chamomilla* L. water extract was administrated orally to rats at doses of 300 and 600 mg/kg for 90 days. MCWE at different doses used, did not induce any statistically significant changes in body weight gain or organs weight compared to control group. It also showed no significant alteration in hematological parameters in treatment groups. However, biochemical parameters showed a significant ($P < 0.05$) decrease in blood sugar and rise in serum urea suggesting degenerative changes in the kidney. Histopathological analyses revealed adverse changes in the architecture of kidney, lung, and spleen for the treated groups. In this study no-observed adverse effect level (NOAEL) for repeated dose administration of MCWE was considered to be under 300 mg/kg body weight however MCWE may have long-term toxic effects on the kidney, lung, and spleen (Hajjaj et al., 2015).

Analgesic activity

The effects of *M. chamomilla* L. aqueous extract (200, 400, and 600 mg/kg p.o.) and essential oil (100, 200, and 300 mg/kg p.o.) on the antinociceptive activity in rodent models were evaluated in a study. The analgesic effect was evaluated using acetic acid induced writhing and Tail immersion test. In the acetic acid-induced writhing model, both extracts had a good analgesic effect characterized by a reduction in the number of writhes when compared to the control and reference drug (aspirin). For the Tail immersion test, essential oil of chamomile exhibited significant analgesic activity at low dose of 200 mg/kg comparable to the aqueous extract at higher a dose of 600 mg/kg. The results of this study indicated that the aqueous extract and essential oil of *M. chamomilla* L. possesses potential antinociceptive activity at both the peripheral and central levels which are mediated through central inhibitory mechanism (Hajjaj et al., 2014).

Antiinflammatory activity

In a study, the effect of *M. chamomilla* L. aqueous extract on antiinflammatory activity in vivo properties was investigated by using carrageenan and experimental trauma-induced hind paw edema in rodents at doses of 300 and 500 mg/kg body weight. Indomethacin was used as standard.

The results showed that *M. chamomilla* L. aqueous extract possesses a significant activity comparable to the control and reference drug used in both models. This study demonstrated that aqueous extract of *M. chamomilla* L. exhibited significant antiinflammatory activity (Hajjaj et al., 2013a,b).

Central nervous system activity

In a study, the essential oil of *M. chamomilla* L. (EOMC) was investigated on central nervous system (CNS) using different models based on mice and rats behavior. The results of the psychopharmacological screening revealed that EOMC produced significant sedative effect at the doses of 300, 400, and 500 mg/kg (p.o.). It affected curiosity (Hole-Board Test, chimney Test), and caused a remarkable decrease in muscle relaxant activity (Rota-Rod and Traction Tests), also potentiate the hypnotic effects of sodium thiopental in rats but did not present any hypnotic action or catalepsy effect (Hajjaj et al., 2013a,b).

Ormenis mixta *L.*

Moroccan Chamomile (*O. mixta* L.) was originally known as Anthemis mixta and is correctly called (*Chamaemelum mixtum*), this plant belong to the family Asteraceae. The plant is an annual and is probably a native of northwest Africa and evolved from a very common ormenis species which grows all over the Mediterranean countries.

Moroccan chamomile cannot be used as a replacement for either German or Roman chamomile. In the world of essential oils, there are three chamomiles: one is German, another is Roman, and the last one though these siblings have much in common, they do have differences that go beyond their point of origin (Coste, 1980; Gamisans and Jeanmonod, 1998).

This plant used almost exclusively in the fragrance trade as a topnote in colognes. Moroccan chamomile oil is pale to brownish yellow in color with a sweet, tenacious balsamic undertone reminiscent of ambra. It blends well with a range of oils, including artemisia oils, cypress, vetiver, lavender, and olibanum. The essential oil is an excellent skin care remedy of this plant; it has many of the same qualities as Roman chamomile, except that its antiinflammatory properties are greater because of a higher percentage of azulene (Lawrence, 1993).

Description

Flowers comprise yellow capitula and white bracts and the branched stem is erect and smooth and grows to a high of 15–60 cm. The long and the narrow leaves are bipinnate or tripinnate (Coste, 1980) (Fig. 3.2).

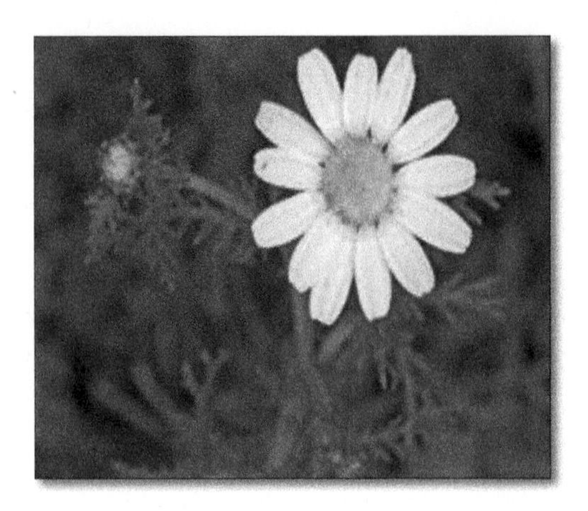

■ FIGURE 3.2 *Ormenis mixta* L. *http://www.jardinsauvage.fr/FLORE/GROUPEMENTS/TOLPION.html*

Traditional use

Ormenis mixta L. used by naturopaths and herbalists as an analgesic, antiallergenic, antiinflammatory, antispasmodic, carminative, hepatic, digestive, febrifuge, fungicidal, nerve sedative, sudorific, vermifuge, a stimulant of leucocyte production and as a vulnerary agent. The plant is well known and cultivated for the extraction of essential oil from its aerial parts, which is sold and used in aromatherapy as an aphrodisiac, antibacterial, and anxiolytic (Lahsissene et al., 2009).

Chemical constituents

Three studies have investigated the chemical composition of *O. mixta* L. essential oils from Morocco, in which santolina alcohol (27.9–32%), α-pinene (3.6–15%), germacrene D (3.3–10.2%), yomogi alcohol (2.8–4.5%), and (E)-β-farnesene (2.5–4.5%) have been identified as the main components (Toulemonde and Beauverd, 1984).

In another study the air-dried aerial parts of *O. mixta* (L.) Dumort. ssp. multicaulis collected from two different regions of Morocco (Kénitra and Salé) were hydrodistilled yielding averagely 0.4% essential oil. The oils were qualitatively similar and characterized by an important percentage of irregular monoterpenic alcohols (Zrira et al., 2007).

Pharmacological properties

Moroccan chamomile has antispasmodic properties and is a great oil for relieving period pains. It has excellent relaxing properties and can be used to help treat the symptoms of depression, irritability, and anxiety (Lahsissene et al., 2009).

Antiproliferative effect

In the course to contribute to development of new anticancer drugs against cervical cancer, the human cervical carcinoma SiHa and HeLa cell lines, has been used as a model system in a study for screening promising plant materials from folk Moroccan medicine possessing anticancer effect. The methanol extract of *O. mixta* L. was tested for its potential cytotoxic effects, SiHa and HeLa cells were treated with different concentrations ranging of methanolic extract from 15 to 500 μg/mL for 48 h. The cells viability were determined by MTT assay.

The methanolic extract of *O. mixta* L. has lower cytotoxic effect on the cancer cell lines tested. Their IC50 values were 383 $\pm$ 26 μg/mL in SiHa cells and 311 $\pm$ 14 μg/mL in HeLa cells, respectively (Nawal et al., 2009).

Pistacia atlantica *Desf.*

The resiniferous pistachio tree belongs to *Pistacia*, a genus of 11 species in the Anacardiaceae family distributed in the Mediterranean and Middle Eastern areas (Yari et al., 2007). Greece is one of the most important pistachio producing countries, along with Iran, Turkey, and India. Pistachios are commercially used as in-shell snacks, in confectionery, in ice creams, candies, bakery goods, and as a flavoring. *Pistacia* oil is nutritive and of excellent quality and has a fluid consistency and nice odor and savor (Koutsoudaki et al., 2005). Recent taxonomic verifications showed the existence in north Africa of a subspecies, called *P. atlantica* Desf. subsp. Atlantica. Its leaves are used as a stomachic, while its fruits and oleoresin are used in medicine.

Description

The leaves of pistachio tree are alternate, pinnately compound, and can be either evergreen or deciduous depending on species. Baneh tree or wild pistachio with scientific name of *P. atlantica* (Betoum) is a tree which can reach 25 m in height. It is the most characteristic plant species of the pre-Saharian regions of the country. This plant has also been used for the treatment of peptic ulcer and as mouth freshener (de Vartavan, 2007).

Traditional use

The aerial part has traditionally been used as a stimulant, for its diuretic properties, and to treat hypertension, coughs, sore throats, eczema, stomach aches, kidney stones, and jaundice (Palevitch and Yaniv, 2000). "Gum" mastic, oleoresin exudates from the stem of this plant (Dogan et al., 2003) is a source of traditional medicinal agent for the relief of upper abdominal discomfort, stomach aches, dyspepsia, and peptic ulcer (Benhammou et al., 2008).

Chemical constituents

Chemical studies on *Pistacia* genus have led to discovering diverse secondary metabolites in addition to high level of vitamins and minerals. Exudate gums of the tree contain resins and volatile oil and pinenes, sabinene, and limonene are the main ingredients of its oil (Sharifi and Hazell, 2011; Sharifi and Hazell, 2012).

In a study the chemical composition of the essential oil of this plant reveals the presence of several main compounds: myrcene (19–25%), α-pinene (16%), terpinen-4-ol (22%) (Picci et al., 1987), d-3-carene (65%) (De Poote et al., 1991), myrcene, limonene, terpinen-4-ol, α-pinene, β-pinene, α-phellandrene, sabinene, para-cymene, and γ-terpinene (Castola et al., 2000).

The chemical composition of the fruits of the north Algerian ecotype *P. atlantica* subsp. atlantica was determined and compared to other fruits of different species in the genus growing in south Algeria and other Mediterranean regions. These fruits were analyzed for their dry matter, protein, crude oil, ash, fatty acids, and phytosterol content. The main fatty acids identified by gas chromatography were oleic (54.15%), linoleic (28.84%), and palmitic (12.21%) acids. The fruits of the north ecotype were found to be rich in protein, oil, fiber, and unsaturated fatty acids, suggesting that they may be valuable for food uses. The sterols isolated were campesterol, stigmasterol, β-sitosterol, and Δ5-avenasterol with β-sitosterol as the major constituent (85 ± 0.85%). The biochemical data indicated an elevated MUFA rate (~56%) in *Pistacia* oil which may be important against certain pathologies for its nutritional and preventive virtues (Benhassaini et al., 2007).

Pharmacological properties

Different parts of *Pistacia* species have been investigated for various pharmacological activities. Amongst its therapeutic properties, it has been implicated in the relief of upper abdominal discomfort, stomachaches, dyspepsia, and peptic ulcer (Al-Said et al., 1986; Huwez and Al-Habbal, 1986). *Pistacia* species have also been reported to possess stimulant and diuretic properties (Bentleyand and Trimon, 1980).

Toxicological study

In a toxicological study by Hossein M. and coworkers revealed that the LD50 of the intraperitoneal injection of the *P. atlantica* methanolic extract was 2.43 g/kg and the maximum nonfatal dose was 1.66 g/kg. Obtained results showed potential of *P. atlantica* extract as a natural source with no significant toxicity for producing a new scolicidal agent for use in hydatid cyst surgery (Hossein et al., 2015).

Antiinflammatory activity

In a study the antiinflammatory effect of *P. atlantica* Desf. volatile oil and gum on acetic acid-induced acute colitis in rat. Three doses of gum (100, 200, and 400 mg/kg) were administered both orally (p.o.) and intrarectally (i.r.) while volatile oil was administered p.o. with doses 100, 200, and 400 μL/kg for four constitutive days. Antiinflammatory effects of the test compounds were compared with oral prednisolone and hydrocortisone enema. Wet colon weight/length ratio and tissue damage scores and area as well as indices of colitis and tissue myeloperoxidase activity were evaluated for each specimen. The therapeutic effects of *Pistacia* in applied doses of oral gum as well as volatile oil reduce all indices of colitis and myeloperoxidase activity (Minaiyan et al., 2015).

Antimicrobial activity

In a study the essential oil from the gum of *P. atlantica* Desf. grown in Algeria was obtained by the hydrodistillation method, and its antimicrobial activities against the growth of clinical isolates of *Staphylococcus aureus*, *Escherichia coli*, and *Streptococcus pyogenes* were evaluated using three different methods: agar disc diffusion; dilution broth methods; and minimum inhibitory concentration (MIC), which was subsequently determined. The results of this study revealed that essential oil resin of *P. atlantica* Desf. has antimicrobial activity against Gram-positive and -negative bacteria which are resistant to commonly used antimicrobial agents and they were considerably dependent on concentration (Ghalem and Mohamed, 2009).

Antioxidant activity

In a study the antioxidant activity of *P. atlantica* Desf. leaf oils from diverse origins of Algeria showed higher antioxidant capacity relative to the antioxidant of reference ascorbic acid when measured using the FRAP assay (Gourine et al., 2010). The best activity was found in the oil obtained from Laghouat, mainly constituted by α-pinene+ α-thujene, camphene, and spathulenol.

Radical scavenging and antiacetylcholinesterase activities

In a work the radical scavenging activity, acetylcholinesterase inhibition, and proline content of an aqueous extract from wild pistachio

(*P. atlantica* Desf.) leaves were investigated. The effect of aqueous extract on superoxide radical scavenging, hydroxyl radical scavenging, N,N-dimethyl-1,4-phenylendiammoniumdichloride (DMPD) radical scavenging, ABTS radical scavenging, nitric oxide scavenging, and β-carotene bleaching activities were examined. This study found that the aqueous extract possesses considerable amounts of flavonoids (33.52 ± 2.04 μg catechin equivalents/mg of extract). The effect of this extract in scavenging activity of hydroxyl radical and DMPD was significantly better than that of ascorbic acid and butylated hydroxyanisole (BHA). The effect of the extract in superoxide and ABTS was significantly similar than that of tested standard antioxidants. The proline content of the extract was found to be 0.54± 0.01 μg proline/mg of extract. Aqueous extract of *P. atlantica* Desf. inhibited acetylcholinesterase activity effectively with IC50 value of 58.05± 0.12 μg/mL (Aysegul et al., 2013).

Effect in acetic acid induced colitis in rats

In a study the effect of the *P. atlantica* Desf. fruit oil extract in treating experimentally induced colitis in a rat model was investigated. The finding of this investigation demonstrated that *P. atlantica* Desf. fruit oil extract reduces colonic injury by suppressing oxidative damage. The pathogenesis of the disease was assessed by evaluating different parameters such as macroscopic score, microscopic score, and oxidative stress markers like malondialdehyde (MDA) level.

An improvement and lower MDA levels in the groups treated with the high dose of fruit extract compared with the untreated group was observed. Histological and macroscopic data confirmed that both oral and rectal administration of *P. atlantica* Desf. fruit oil extract could alleviate bowel inflammation. Asacole was used as the standard drug, which produced no significant difference in the above parameters in comparison with *Pistacia* at doses 600 mg/kg (orally) and 20% gel form (rectally) (Nader et al., 2014).

Papaver rhoeas *L.*

Papaver rhoeas L. belongs to the Papaveraceae family, and is commonly known as "corn poppy." The plant is found wild in various parts of Europe, northern Africa, and western Asia (GRIN database, 2009).

Description

Papaver rhoeas L. is a grassy plant with red flower and with height 25–90 cm growing in different parts of world (Zargari, 1994a,b).

Chemical constituents

A phytochemical study showed that *P. rhoeas* L. leaves contain several flavonols, like quercetin, kaempferol, myricetin, and isorhamnetin, as well as minerals, like potassium, sodium, and calcium (Trichopoulou et al., 2000). *Papaver* have different alkaloids for example rhoeadine, rhoeadic acid, papaveric acid, mekoid acid, mucilage, and sugar (El-Masry et al., 1981). In another study phytochemical analysis has revealed that the plant extract contains several alkaloids including rhoeadine, rhoeadic acid, papaveric acid, rhoeagenine, and anthocyanins (Zargari, 1995; Balabanli et al., 2006; Kalav and Sariyar, 1989). Modern pharmacology revealed that its extract contains several alkaloids such as rhoeadine, rhoeadic acid, papaveric acid, rhoeagenine, and anthocyanins.

Traditional use

The plant has been used for medicinal proposes a long time ago for treatment of a wide range of diseases including inflammation, diarrhea, sleep disorders, treatment of cough, analgesia, and also to reduce the withdrawal signs of opioid addiction (Zargari, 1994a,b). It is also claimed that *P. rhoeas* exhibits sedative, narcotic, and emollient effects (Zargari, 1994). Furthermore, it is known to claim intestinal and urinary irritation and to be useful in various conditions such as bronchitis, pneumonia, and rash fever (Valnet, 1992).

Pharmacological properties

Pharmacological studies have shown that the plant extract may have some radical scavenging properties (Williams et al., 2001). Investigations also indicated that the *P. rhoeas* L. extract also possess antiulcergenic property (El and Karakaya, 2004).

Studies in animal models have shown that *P. rhoeas* L. extract can reduce morphine-induced place preference, sensitization, locomotor activity, and locomotor and pain tolerance. Furthermore, it has been shown that the extract also reduces stress-induced alterations in plasma corticosterone levels and induces analgesic and antiinflammatory effects in mice (Gürbüz et al., 2003).

Toxicological study

It must be mentioned that toxicological study by Soulimani R. and coworkers revealed that the plant extract has no toxic effects in mice and perhaps in human as well (Gürbüz et al., 2003).

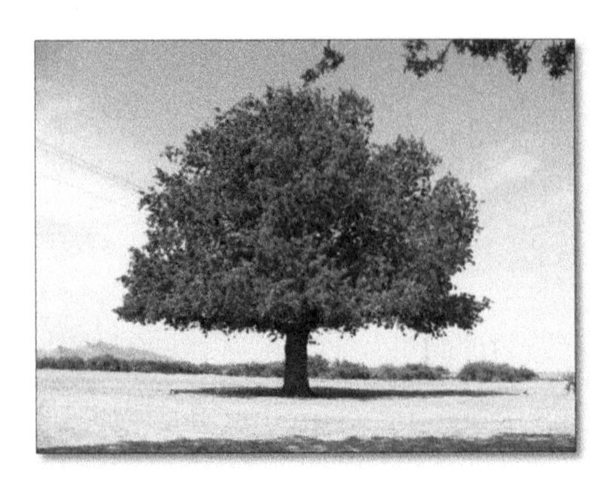

■ FIGURE 3.3 *Pistacia atlantica* Desf. *https://www.flickr.com/photos*

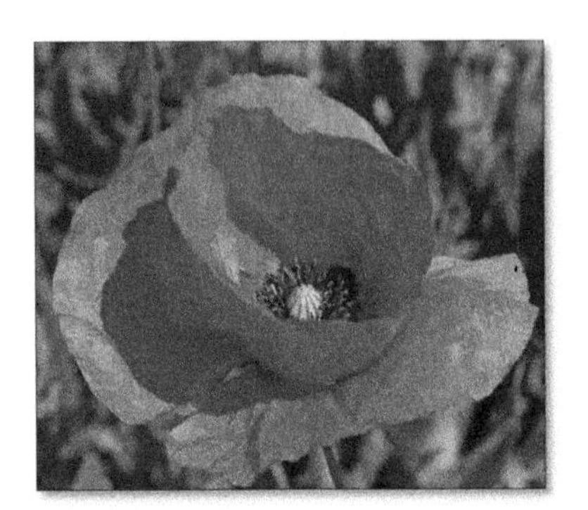

■ FIGURE 3.4 *Papaver rhoeas* L. *https://upload.wikimedia.org/wikipedia/commons/0/02/Coquelicot%281%29.JPG*

Antiinflammatory and antinociceptive effects

Experiments have shown that the extract not only inhibits both pain phases of formalin test, but can also inhibit inflammation induced by formalin (Gürbüz et al., 2003). These effects may be due to the activity of *P. rhoeas* L. extract on opioid, glutamate, and nitric oxide systems (Gürbüz et al., 2003). In addition, *P. rhoeas* L extract has been shown to elevate plasma corticosterone concentration indicating that the antiinflammatory effects of the extract can also be indirect (Gürbüz et al., 2003). Considering the fact that the *P. rhoeas* L extract did not induce dependence and addition in animal models (Gürbüz et al., 2003), its antinociceptive properties is in the high value and some clinical trials in this regard may be useful. Even though, it may open a new line of investigation in pain management and relief (Figs. 3.3 and 3.4).

Antigenotoxic capacity

In a study anticytotoxic and antigenotoxic potential of *P. rhoeas* L. water leaf extract against the radiomimetic zeocin in two types of test-systems—*Hordeum vulgare* and human lymphocytes in vitro was provided. Mitotic index (MI) was used as an endpoint for cytotoxicity, the frequency of chromosome aberrations (MwA) and the number of induced micronuclei (MN)—as endpoints for genotoxicity/clastogenicity. Formation of aberration "hot spots" was also used as an indicator for genotoxicity in *Hordeum vulgare*.

The results showed that *P. rhoeas* L. leaf extract has weak cytotoxic and genotoxic effects depending on the concentrations. Human lymphocytes are more sensitive than *Hordeum vulgare*. By applying two types of experimental designs with split treatment we found that *P. rhoeas* L. leaf extract possesses anticytotoxic and antigenotoxic potential against the oxidative stress induced by the radiomimetic zeocin in both test-systems. The effect is more pronounced with 4 h inter-treatment time between treatments which may indicate induction of adaptive response (AR) (Hassan and Hedayat, 2014).

Antimicrobial activity

The in vitro antimicrobial activity of ethanol extract of *P. rhoeas* L. was tested against a panel of laboratory control strains belonging to the American Type Culture Collection Maryland, USA. Antibacterial activity was evaluated against two Gram-positive (*Bacillus subtilis* ATCC 6633 and *Staphylococcus aureus* ATCC 6538) and three Gram-negative bacteria (*Escherichia coli* ATCC 8739, *Pseudomonas aeruginosa* ATCC 9027, and *Salmonella* abony NCTC 6017). The antifungal activity was tested against two organisms *Aspergillus niger* ATCC 16404 and *Candida albicans* ATCC 10231.

Papaver rhoeas L. ethanolic extract showed antimicrobial activity against all tested microorganisms, with the exception both of bacteria *B. subtilis* and mould *A. niger*. This study suggests that the investigated extracts of plant *P. rhoes* L. could be potentially applied as antimicrobial agents (Svetla et al., 2014).

In conclusion *M. chamomilla* L., *O. mixta* L., *P. atlantica* Desf., *P. rhoeas* L. are a potential medicinal and aromatic plants, until now they have been utilized in the world by people in medicine and pharmacology (antitumor, antibacterial, antimicrobial, antispasmodic and antioxidant, painful menstruation, colds, headaches, insomnia, mild sedative, and antidepressant), in food industry and in cosmetic industry. It might be concluded that these plants have emerged up as novel therapeutic agents and treats variety of aliments very efficiently. However, to guarantee their safety, further toxicity studies need to be performed as well as assays to clarify the mechanism of action and possible interactions with other compounds. The optimization of formulations, the establishment of optimal concentrations for clinical applications, and the search for possible side-effects are together research lines that need to be highlighted.

REFERENCES

Al-Said, M.S., Ageel, A.M., Parmar, N.S., Tariq, M., 1986. Evaluation of mastic, a crude drug obtained from *Pistacia lentiscus* for gastric and duodenal anti-ulcer activity. J. Ethnopharmacol. 15, 271–278.

Aysegul, P., Inci, A., Refiye, Y., 2013. Radical scavenging and anti-acetylcholinesterase activities of aqueous extract of wild pistachio (*Pistacia atlantica* Desf.) leaves. Food Sci. Biotechnol. 22 (2), 515–522.

Backer, H.G., 1965. Plant and Civilization. Wadsworth Publishing Company, Inc., Belmont, CA.145–157.

Balabanli, C., Albayrak, S., Türk, M., Yüksel, O., 2006. Some weeds are found in Turkey's pasture and its impact on animals. J. Fac. Forestry 2, 89–96.

Benhammou, N., Bekkara, F.A., Panovska, T.K., 2008. Antioxidant and antimicrobial activities of the *Pistacia lentiscus* and *Pistacia atlantica* extracts. Afr. J. Pharm. Pharmacol. 2 (2), 022–028.

Benhassaini, H., Bendahmane, M., Benchalgo, N., 2007. The chemical composition of fruits of *Pistacia atlantica* desf. subsp. atlantica from Algeria. Chem. Nat. Comp. 43 (2).

Bentleyand, R.Y., Trimon, H., 1980. Medicinal Plants. J. & A. Churchill, London. 68.

Castola, V., Bighelli, A., Casanova, J., 2000. Intraspecific chemical variability of the essential oil of *Pistacia lentiscus* L. from Corsica. Biochem. Syst. Ecol. 28, 79–88.

Coste, H., 1980. Flore Descriptive et Illustrée de la France, de la Corse et des Contrées Limitrophes II. Librairie Scientifique et Technique Albert Blanchart, Paris, France. 627.

De Poote, H.L., Schamp, N.M., Aboutabl, E.A., El Tohamy, S.F., Doss, S.L., 1991. Essential oils from the leaves of three *Pistacia* species grown in Egypt. Flav. Fragr. J. 6, 229–232.

de Vartavan, C.T., 2007. Pistacia species in relation to their use as varnish and incense in pharaonic Egypt. C.BP and MOS 2, 63–92.

Dogan, O., Baslar, S., Aydin, H., Mert, H.H., 2003. A study of the soil-plant interactions of *Pistacia lentiscus* L. distributed in the western Anatolian part of Turkey. Acta Bot. Croat. 62 (2), 73–88.

El, S.N., Karakaya, S., 2004. Radical scavenging and iron-chelating activities of some greens used as traditional dishes in Mediterranean diet. Int. J. Food Sci. Nutr. 55 (1), 67–74.

El-Masry, S., El-Ghazooly, M.G., Omar, A.A., Khafagy, S.M., Phillipson, J.D., 1981. Alkaloids from Egyptian *Papaver rhoeas*. Planta Medica. 41, 61–64.

Forster, H.B., Niklas, H., Lutz, S., 1980. Antispasmodic effects of some medicinal plants. Planta Med. 40, 309–319.

Frank, R., Schilcher, H., 2005. Chamomile, Industrial Profile. Taylor and Francis, New York. 278.

Franke, R., 2005. Chamomile: industrial profiles Plant Sources, first ed. CRC Press, Boca Raton. 39–42.

Gamisans, J., Jeanmonod, D., 1998. Complements au Prodrome de la Flore Corse: Asteraceae – II. Editions des Conservatoires et Jardins botaniques de la Ville de Geneve, Geneve, Switzerland. 340.

Ghalem, B.R., Mohamed, B., 2009. Essential oil from gum of *Pistacia atlantica* Desf.: screening of antimicrobial activity. Afr. J. Pharm. Pharmacol. 3 (3), 087–091.

Goldfrank, L., et al., 1982. The pernicious panacea: herbal medicine. Hosp. Physician 10, 64–86.

Gourine, N., Yousfi, M., Bombarda, I., Nadjemi, B., Stocker, P., Gaydon, E.M., 2010. Antioxidant activities and chemical composition of essential oil of *Pistacia atlantica* from Algeria. Ind. Crop. Prod. 31, 203–208.

GRIN database, 2009. Germplasm Resources Information Network-(GRIN). National Germplasm Resources Laboratory, Beltsville, Maryland, Retrieved from <http:/www.ars-grin.gov/cgibin/html/tax> (accessed 25.11.09.).

Gürbüz, I., Ustün, O., Yesilada, E., Sezik, E., Kutsal, O., 2003. Anti-ulcerogenic activity of some plants used as folk remedy in Turkey. J. Ethnopharmacol. 88 (1), 93–97.

Hajjaj, G., Bounihi, A., Tajani, M., Cherrah, Y., Zellou, A., 2013a. Anti-inflammatory evaluation of aqueous extract of *Matricaria chamomilla* L. (asteraceae) in experimental animal models from Morocco. World J. Pharm. Res. 2 (5), 1218–1228.

Hajjaj, G., Bounihi, A., Tajani, M., Cherrah, Y., Zellou, A., 2013b. Evaluation of CNS activities of *Matricaria chamomilla* L. essential oil in experimental animals from Morocco. Int. J. Pharm. Pharm. Sci. 5 (2), 530–534.

Hajjaj, G., Bounihi, A., Tajani, M., Cherrah, Y., Zellou, A., 2014. In vivo analgesic activity of essential oil and aqueous extract of *Matricaria chamomilla* L. (asteraceae). World J. Pharm. Pharm. Sci. 3 (5), 01–13.

Hajjaj, G., Bounihi, A., Tajani, M., Chebraoui, L., Bouabdellah, M., Cherradi, N., et al., 2015. Acute and sub-chronic oral toxicity of standardized water extract of *Matricaria chamomilla* L. in Morocco. Int. J. Universal Pharm. Bio Sci. 4 (1), 1–14.

Hamburger, M., Hostettmann, K., 1991. Bioactivity in plants: the link between phytochemistry and medicine. Phytochemistry 30, 3864–3874.

Hassan, G., Hedayat, S., 2014. Pharmacological Properties of *Papaver rhoeas* L., (16-31 December). Annu. Res. Rev. Biol. 4 (24).

Hossein, M., Farnaz, K., Mehdi, G., Amir Tavakoli, K.A., Yarahmadi, M., 2015. Chemical composition, protoscolicidal effects and acute toxicity of Pistacia atlantica Desf. fruit extract. Nat. Prod. Res 7, 1–4.

Huwez, F.U., Al-Habbal, M.J., 1986. Mastic in treatment of benign gastric ulcers. Gastroenterol. Jpn. 21, 273–274.

Kalav, Y.N., Sariyar, G., 1989. Alkaloids from Turkish *Papaver rhoeas* L. Planta Medica. 55, 488.

Koutsoudaki, C., Kresk, M., Rodger, A., 2005. Chemical composition and antibacterial activity of the essential oil and the gum of *Pistacia lentiscus* Var. chia. J. Agric. Food Chem. 53, 7681–7685.

Lahsissene, H., Kahouadji, A., Tijane, M., Hseini, S., 2009. Catalogue des plantes médicinales utilisées dans la région de Zaer (Maroc Occidental), 186. Rev. Bot., Lejeunia.

Lawrence, B.M., 1993. A planning scheme to evaluate new aromatic plants for the flavour and fragrance industries. In: Janick, J., Simon, J.E. (Eds.), New Crops Wiley, New York, pp. 620–627.

Mentz, L.A., Schenkel, E.P., 1989. A coerenciae a confiabilidade das indicacoes terapeuticas. Caderno de Farmacia 5 (1/2), 93–119.

Minaiyan, M., Karimi, F., Ghannadi, A., 2015. Anti-inflammatory effect of *Pistacia atlantica* subsp. kurdica volatile oil and gum on acetic acid-induced acute colitis in rat. Res. J. Pharmacognosy (RJP) 2 (2), 1–12.

Nader, T., Masoumi, S., Massood, H., Ali Reza, S., Hoda, E., Omid, K.H., et al., 2014. Healing effect of *Pistacia atlantica* fruit oil extract in acetic acid-induced colitis in rats. Iran J. Med. Sci. 39 (6), 522–528.

Nawal, M., Laïla, B., Saaid, A., Hamid, M., El mzibri, M., 2009. Cytotoxic effect of some Moroccan medicinal plant extracts on human cervical cell lines. J. Med Plants Res. 3 (12), 1045–1050.

Ompal, S., Zakia, K., Neelam, M., Manoj, K., 2011. Chamomile (*Matricaria chamomilla* L.): an overview. Pharmacogn Rev. 5 (9), 82–95.

Palevitch, D., Yaniv, Z., 2000. The effects of aqueous extracts prepared from the leaves of *Pistacia lentiscus* in experimental liver disease, Medicinal Plants of the Holy Land., Modan Publishing House, Tel Aviv, Israel. In: Ljubuncic et al. (Eds.). J. Ethnopharmacol. pp. 198–204.

Picci, V., Scotti, A., Mariani, M., Colombo, E., 1987. Composition of the volatile oil of *Pistacia lentiscus* L. of sardinian origin. In: Martens, Flavour Science and Technology Wiley, New York, pp. 107–110.

Schilcher, H. (Hrsg), 1987. die kamille. Handbuch fur arzte, apotheker und andere naturwissen-schaftler wissenschaftliche verlagsgesellschaft mbH struttgart.

Sharifi, M.S., Hazell, S.L., 2011. GC-MS analysis and antimicrobial activity of the essential oil of the trunk exudates from *Pistacia atlantica* kurdica. J. Pharm. Sci. Res. 3, 1364–1367.

Sharifi, M.S., Hazell, S.L., 2012. Isolation, analysis and antimicrobial activity of the acidic fractions of mastic, kurdica, mutica and cabolica gums from genus *Pistacia*. Glob. J. Health Sci. 4, 217–228.

Svetla, G., Gabriele, J., Alexander, S., Fridrich, G., 2014. Antigenotoxic capacity of *Papaver rhoeas* L. extract. Int. J. Pharm. Pharm. Sci. 6 (1), 717–723.

Thorne research, 2008. alternative medicine review. volume 13, Number 1.

Toulemonde, B., Beauverd, D., 1984. Contribution a l'étude d'une camomille sauvage du Maroc: L'huile essentielle d'*Ormenis mixta* L. 1er Colloque International sur les Plantes Aromatiques et Médicinales du Maroc. Centre National de Coordination et de Planification de la Recherche Scientifique et Technique, Rabat, Morocco.169–173.

Trichopoulou, A., Vasilopoulou, E., Hollman, P., Chamalides, C.H., Foufa, E., Kaloudis, T.R., et al., 2000. Nutritional composition and flavonoid content of edible wild greens and green pies: a potential rich source of antioxidant nutritients in the Mediterranean diet. Food Chem. 70, 319–323.

Valnet, J., 1992. Phytotherapie, sixth ed. Maloine, Paris, France.

Vulto, A.G., Smet, P.A.G.M., 1988. Drugs used in non-orthodox medicine. In: Dukes, M.M.G. (Ed.), Meyler's Side Effects of Drugs, eleventh ed. Elsevier, Amsterdam, pp. 999–1005.

Williams, J.T., Christie, M.J., Manzoni, O., 2001. Cellular and synaptic adaptations mediating opioid dependence. Physiol. Rev. 81, 299–343.

Yari, K.Y., Amanlou, M., Esmaeelian, B., Moradi, B.S., Saheb, J.M., 2007. Inhibitory effects of a flavonoid-rich extract of *Pistacia vera* hull on growth and acid production of bacteria involved in dental plaque. Inter. J. harmacol. 3 (3), 219–226.

Zargari, A., 1994a. Medical Plants, vol. 1. Tehran University, Tehran. 91–102.

Zargari, A., 1994b. Medicinal Plants, fourth ed. Tehran University Press, Tehran, Iran.231–234

Zargari, A., 1995. Medical Plants, vol. 1. Tehran University, Tehran, Iran.

Zrira, S., Menut, C., Bessiere, J.M., Benjilalii, B., 2007. Chemical composition of the essential oils of Moroccan *Ormenis mixta* (L.) Dumort. ssp. Multicaulis. Essent. Oil Bearing Plants 10, 378–385.

Chapter 4

Nutritional indicators and health aspects of fruit and vegetable consumption in aged adults

Ibrahim Elmadfa and Alexa L. Meyer
University of Vienna, Vienna, Austria

CHAPTER OUTLINE

INTRODUCTION

Medical progress, improved living conditions and higher food security and food safety have greatly extended the life expectancy especially in high-income countries. Moreover, elderly today are on average healthier and fitter than earlier generations (Freedman et al., 2002). This along with declining birth rates leads to an increased aging of populations in many countries and particularly in the European region. Indeed, by 2040, the percentage of individuals aged 65 years or more is projected to reach about 20% in Northern America (Kinsella et al., 2009) and 27% in the European

Fruits, Vegetables, and Herbs.
DOI: http://dx.doi.org/10.1016/B978-0-12-802972-5.00004-4

Union (EU-28) (Eurostat, 2013). Although overall, a good health status can be maintained longer, the increasing number of elderly will be associated with higher morbidity and will present a heavy burden on the health care system. Moreover, the rising number of obese persons is likely to contribute to an increase in noncommunicable diseases that are already the leading death cause worldwide and are associated with both, an excessive body weight and higher age (Manton, 2008; National Institute on Aging et al., 2011). Maintaining health and well-being in the elderly population for as long as possible is therefore of great importance and nutrition plays a crucial role in this endeavor.

Fruits and vegetables are central components of a healthy balanced diet being rich sources of essential nutrients and bioactive health-promoting components.

While an adequate intake of fruits and vegetables is important for the entire population, they play a paramount role in the nutrition of groups that have a particular risk for nutritional deficiencies such as the elderly for instance. Indeed, they offer a number of components that can play essential parts in the fight against age-related health problems. This chapter is intended to provide an overview of some of these positive impacts.

THE AGING BODY

Aging is associated with a number of physiological changes that may affect the nutritional status of an individual. While the basal requirements of most nutrients do not appear to change markedly with age, age-related degenerative and/or pathological processes can influence the body's capacity to absorb and metabolize nutrients, their storage and distribution, as well as other factors like redox balance for instance. The latter is particularly related to changes in the immunological response. Indeed, it is known that with increasing age, low-grade inflammatory events occur more frequently or become even chronic, a phenomenon that has been termed inflamm-aging (Franceschi et al., 2007).

This increased inflammation is associated with higher oxidative stress and the resulting tissue damage is repaired less efficiently in the old organism (Burton and Krizhanovsky, 2014). Indeed, most of the diseases commonly related to aging are also associated with excessive generation of reactive molecules and low-grade chronic inflammation even though there is still a lack of knowledge about causal relationships (Cannizzo et al., 2011). However, an alternative theory has recently been proposed that the increase in reactive molecules like reactive oxygen and nitrogen species (RONS) could be a stress reaction of the body to damage to proteins and DNA accumulating over the life span. In accord with their role in signal transduction, reactive oxygen species (ROS) in this model would induce protective and repair mechanisms to counteract this damage, but eventually, their increased production might result in oxidative damage and disease itself (Hekimi et al., 2011).

Another crucial change is the loss of lean body mass, mainly in the form of muscle, and the increase of fat tissue, leading to a decline in metabolic activity and hence of energy expenditure. Additionally, changes occur in the composition of the lean body mass with a reduction of metabolically active tissues to the benefit of extracellular mass and water. In turn, the metabolic activity of the organ tissue seems not reduced (Bosy-Westphal et al., 2003). A tendency toward lower physical activity contributes further to the decrease of energy requirements (Elia et al., 2000).

Together with the reduction in organ mass, aging entails functional losses in many organs such as the kidneys for instance. Starting at about the fourth decade of age, a steady decrease in the glomerular filtration rate and renal blood flow occurs despite a high individual variability. The ability to concentrate or dilute the urine to maintain the electrolyte balance and pH value of the body is impaired resulting in a higher obligatory urine volume and higher electrolyte losses. At the same time, the increasing permeability of the glomerular basal membrane can lead to proteinuria especially in the presence of hypertension (Silva, 2005; Weinstein and Anderson, 2010).

Among the many other body parts and function affected by aging, the decline in bone mineral mass is noteworthy that can lead to osteoporosis and a higher risk for bone fractures (Eastell and Lambert, 2002).

All these functions are affected by the nutritional status and can be positively influenced by a healthy food choice and a diet rich in fruits and vegetables (see Table 4.1, p. 60).

FRUITS AND VEGETABLES AND THEIR SPECIAL ROLE IN THE NUTRITION OF THE ELDERLY

Generally, nutrition of the elderly is characterized by a coexistence of overweight and obesity on the one hand and a high risk of under- and malnutrition on the other hand, the latter gaining in importance with increasing age. The aforementioned decline in energy expenditure promotes body weight gain particularly when food intake and appetite are yet uncompromised. The prevalence of overweight and obesity culminates in the 60- to

Table 4.1 Overview of the Role of Components in Fruits and Vegetables in Health Promotion and Disease Prevention and (Putative) Underlying Mechanisms (for Details See Text)

Component	Effect/Mechanism	Outcome
Micronutrients	High nutrient density	Improved nutritional status while preventing obesity
	Source of K, Mg, vitamin C	Preservation of bone mass
	Source of folate	Prevention of hyperhomocysteinemia and low hemoglobin concentration
Antioxidants	Scavenging of free radicals	Protection from oxidative stress and damage
Phytochemicals	Regulation of xenometabolic enzymes (phase 1 and phase 2)	Detoxification of cancerogens, inhibition of procancerogen activation
	Hormetic stimulation of antioxidant enzymes and antistress genes	Activation of antistress defense mechanisms
	Stimulation of bone anabolism	Preservation of bone mass
Dietary fiber	Increasing bowel function	Prevention of constipation
	Improvement of gut flora	Prevention of inflammatory bowel disease
	Fermentation to short-chain fatty acids	Promotion of endothelial function
		Better nutrient absorption
		Antiinflammatory effects
	Binding of cholesterol and bile acids	Prevention of hypercholesterolemia
	Delayed carbohydrate absorption	Improved glucose tolerance
Water	Contribution to fluid/water intake	Prevention of dehydration

70-year-olds to decline thereafter. As in younger persons, obesity in the elderly is associated with a number of health impairments, but at the same time, a moderately higher body mass index (up to $30\,kg/m^2$) is generally associated with a lower mortality in this age group, a phenomenon that has been ascribed to the lower risk of malnutrition and sarcopenia associated with a higher bodyweight (Heiat et al., 2001; Gulsvik et al., 2009). In turn, underweight presents a serious health issue in geriatric patients and is mostly due to an overall insufficient food intake (Mathus-Vliegen and Obesity Management Task Force of the European Association for the Study of Obesity, 2012; Jahangir et al., 2014).

However, the requirements of most micronutrients do not markedly change with aging, making an adequate supply even more difficult when energy intake is reduced and appetite declining. Both groups, underweight as well overweight elderly are therefore threatened by deficiencies of certain macro- and micronutrients, notably iron, zinc, calcium, vitamins of the B group and vitamin D, and protein in frail elderly (Montgomery et al., 2014; Bernstein et al., 2012).

Fruits and vegetables as nutrient-rich, low-energy foods

With their abundance in many vitamins, minerals, and trace elements together with their low-energy content, fruits and vegetables can improve the supply of these essential micronutrients while preventing excessive weight gain. Moreover, even though low-energy content is less beneficial in undernourished elderly, these latter still benefit from an abundant consumption of fruits and vegetables and their richness in micronutrients and bioactive plant compounds. As such, vegetables and fruits are particularly good sources of magnesium, potassium, folate, vitamin C, vitamin K, as well as carotenoids.

Some vegetables like broccoli and other Brassicaceae varieties also contain notable amounts of calcium (Mangels, 2014). All of these nutrients have been reported as marginal at least in certain groups of elderly across Europe (Elmadfa et al., 2009). Thus, magnesium intake of 65- to 80-year-old men and women was on average below the respective recommended amount in the Austrian Nutrition Report 2012 (Elmadfa et al., 2012). In the UK National Diet and Nutrition Survey 2008/2009–2011/2012, mean intake of magnesium and potassium of persons aged 65 years and over was also below the reference nutrient intake (87% and 81% of RNI, respectively) (NatCen Social Research et al., 2015).

All these micronutrients also play a major role for bone health. Indeed, their intake was positively related to bone mineral density and negatively to the excretion of biomarkers of bone resorption in a number of studies. In these surveys, fruits and vegetables were major sources of these nutrients (Tucker et al., 1999; New et al., 2000). Furthermore, a higher consumption of fruits and vegetables was itself associated with higher bone mineral density (Tucker et al., 2002).

However, other constituents of fruits and vegetables, namely bioactive secondary phytochemicals, have also been suggested as active agents in the positive effects on bone health. Isoflavones from soy for instance, stimulate osteoblasts and inhibit osteoclasts by binding to estrogen receptors and bone anabolic effects have also been observed for other flavonoids found in fruits and vegetables (Horcajada and Offord, 2012). Other health-promoting effects of phytochemicals will be discussed in the following paragraph.

The high vitamin C content of many vegetables and fruits can improve the bioavailability of iron from the diet (Lane and Richardson, 2014). Iron-deficiency anemia is common in elderly people and even though chronic diseases and inflammatory processes are strong causative factors, improvement of the body's iron status contributes to its therapy (Andrès et al., 2008; Bross et al., 2010; Elmadfa et al., 2014).

Folate deficiency is another potential cause of anemia in the elderly albeit to a lesser degree than iron deficiency (Andrès et al., 2008; Bross et al., 2010). However, it is also associated with cognitive impairment, Alzheimer's disease, dementia, and depression in elderly. A possible relationship exists with hyperhomocysteinemia that has also been described as a cardiovascular risk factor (Araújo et al., 2015). Although the evidence for effects of supplementation with folate and other B vitamins associated with cognitive function on mental health in the elderly is so far equivocal, fruits and vegetables being major sources of folate may be protective by contributing to adequate intake of folate (Malouf and Grimley Evans, 2008; Bermejo et al., 2007).

With their high water content (80–90% of fresh weight in most varieties) vegetables and fruits can also contribute to fluid intake. As mentioned before, the age-related decline in kidney function entails a higher obligatory urine excretion. While this is compensated through lower losses from sweating under normal climatic conditions, high temperatures can lead to dehydration (Manz et al., 2012; Maughan, 2012). Additionally, fluid intake in elderly people is often inadequate for various reasons such as reduced thirst sensation, incontinence, and cognitive impairment (Schols et al., 2009). While to the authors' knowledge no studies focused on the contribution of vegetables and fruits to hydration status, a positive relationship has been shown in children (Montenegro-Bethancourt et al., 2013).

Antioxidants and bioactive plant components

Besides micronutrients, a large variety of other bioactive components in vegetables and fruits have been shown to exert health-promoting effects. Many of these phytochemicals act as antioxidants, and as mentioned earlier, oxidative stress increases with aging even though it may not be its initial cause but rather the consequence of the body's reaction to accumulating oxidative degenerative damage to lysosomal and mitochondrial membranes, DNA, and proteins that gets out of control in the aged individual. Indeed, ROS like hydrogen peroxide (H_2O_2), for instance, serve as signaling molecules in the regulation of enzymes and transcription factors that are central to the maintenance of redox balance (Hekimi et al., 2011). This might explain why supplementation with large doses of antioxidants has often failed to counteract aging and extend life span and even shown detrimental effects (Bjelakovic et al., 2012; Sadowska-Bartosz and Bartosz, 2014). Certain long living mutants of *Caenorhabditis elegans* were shown to produce higher H_2O_2 levels than the wild type and treatment with the antioxidants N-acetyl-cysteine and vitamin C abolished or at least diminished the differences in life span between the mutants and the wild type (Yang and Hekimi, 2010). These results do not refute the important role of an adequate antioxidant status though. Rather, they show the complexity of the physiological redox system, the lack of a gold standard to assess the oxidative status and the need to differentiate between individuals and population groups as well as particular bioactive molecules. They also call for caution with antioxidant supplementation. In this context, it has to be considered that antioxidants in the body form a network of substances interacting with each other (Serafini, 2006; Ndhlala et al., 2010; Halliwell, 2012). A diet rich in fruits and vegetables provides a wide selection of antioxidative molecules (Chu et al., 2002; Sun et al., 2002).

However, the effects of phytochemicals are not solely attributable to direct RONS scavenging. In fact, it has become increasingly evident that their impact on the oxidative balance is part of a stress resistance program initiated by the body to protect itself from potentially harmful phytochemicals produced by the plants to repel predators and pests. Generally, the small amounts of these substances that occur in a natural diverse diet are well tolerated by the organism equipped with an efficient machinery for their detoxification. On the contrary, their regular consumption appears to stimulate the metabolism and degradation of xenobiotics including certain cancerogens. This adaptive process also known as hormesis enables individuals exposed to low levels of stress to become more resistant against heavier burdens and this is supposed to be a major mechanism of health-promotion through phytochemicals (Calabrese et al., 2012; Murugaiyah and Mattson, 2015).

Thus, polyphenols like flavonoids, isoflavonoids, and anthocyanidins, as well as isothiocyanates of which a wide variety is found in fruits and vegetables, can influence the transcription of genes for phase-1 and phase-2 metabolic enzymes of the cytochrome P450 (CYP450) family that are involved in detoxification by binding to transcription factors and nuclear receptors. Agonistic as well as antagonistic effects of polyphenols have been reported depending on the chemical structure but also on the experimental conditions, and thus, anticancerogenic effects reported for some polyphenols could arise either from the stimulation of the degradation of cancerogens or the inhibition of their formation from inactive precursors. The latter could also be mediated through a direct interaction of phytochemicals with metabolic enzymes (Mandlekar et al., 2006).

Furthermore, phytochemicals have been shown to stimulate the production of enzymes and molecules acting as antioxidants and regulators and sensors of oxygen homeostasis like glutathione reductase, heme oxygenases, catalase, thioredoxin, NAD(P)H quinone oxidoreductase through activation of nuclear factor erythroid 2-related factor 2 (Nfr2) and its subsequent binding to antioxidant response elements (ARE) of the genes for these enzymes (Calabrese et al., 2012). Antiinflammatory and anticancerogenic properties of phytochemicals are also mediated through modulation of the transcription factors NF-κB and AP-1 with effects differing between healthy and cancerous cells (Gopalakrishnan and Tony Kong, 2008). Another mechanism is via the activation of the AMP-activated protein kinase (AMPK)/sirtuin (SIRT) pathway regulating the cells' energy homeostasis and nutrient metabolism. SIRT proteins have also been associated with cellular stress resistance and longevity (Murugaiyah and Mattson, 2015). Antiinflammatory effects have been found for anthocyanins that are present in high amounts in berries. These effects are ascribed to the modulation of cell signaling pathways by for example, interacting with redox-sensitive kinases or directly with transcription factors (Joseph et al., 2014).

Maintenance of these pathways of cellular homeostasis is crucial for longevity and healthy aging. Aging is associated with impairments in the function of metabolic and redox-regulating enzymes resulting in an increase in inflammatory processes and cancerogenesis (Suh et al., 2004; Li and Fukagawa, 2010). Through their effects on these metabolic pathways, phytochemicals from a healthy varied diet rich in fruits and vegetables can mitigate these developments.

Dietary fiber

Aging is frequently associated with constipation partly due to lower intake of dietary fiber and altered gut microflora (Britton and McLaughlin, 2013; Woodmansey, 2007).

Both factors are related as especially soluble fermentable fiber serves as energy source for lactobacilli and bifidobacteria and its intake can thus contribute to the maintenance of a healthy gut flora. Age-related changes in the gut microbiome have been observed although no clear pattern could be identified. Contrary results reported from different countries may arise from environmental factors that play an important role in the composition of the gut microflora (Biagi et al., 2013). Moreover, differences are also seen within the group of elderly with very old persons showing greater changes than younger ones whose flora often does not differ from that in young adults (Biagi et al., 2010). The same was also observed in frail elderly or those living in long-term care institutions compared to community-living persons (Claesson et al., 2012). However, a shift toward a bacterial population dominated by facultative anaerobic species that are more pathogenic has been repeatedly described (Biagi et al., 2013). It could also be shown that the diet has a marked effect on the composition of the microflora with a pattern based on a higher and more variable consumption of fruits and vegetables promoting a healthier gut flora (Claesson et al., 2012). This is of particular relevance in relationship to aging as the intestinal bacteria have been associated with the local immune system and its function as well as dysfunction that can lead to inflammatory bowel diseases. Occurrence of the latter increases with aging and the prevalence of elevated inflammatory markers like C-reactive protein (CRP), cytokines interleukin (IL)-6 and IL-8, was found to be higher in older individuals especially the very old and frail and to correlate with changes in the gut microflora (Biagi et al., 2010; Claesson et al., 2012). Intestinal microorganisms might contribute to an increase of inflammation in the gut when the senescent immune system fails to adequately control the commensal bacteria resulting in overgrowth and loss of tolerance to harmless species. A predominance of more harmful species furthers this development and the local processes can even contribute to the systemic inflammation observed with aging (Schiffrin et al., 2010).

Some gut microbe strains are producers of short-chain fatty acids (SCFA) that have shown antiinflammatory and anticarcinogenic effects (Roy et al., 2006). Aging has been associated with a decline in SCFA production (Claesson et al., 2012; Hippe et al., 2011). In turn, intake of dietary fiber was correlated with production of SCFA in elderly individuals. Apples and oranges contributed notably to SCFA production including butyrate (Cuervo et al., 2013). Both fruit varieties are rich in pectin that is a major substrate for bacterial fermentation and SCFA release (Titgemeyer et al., 1991). SCFAs serve as energy substrate to enterocytes, thereby contributing to the maintenance of a healthy endothelium (Cook and Sellin, 1998) and thus aiding intestinal micronutrient absorption that can be impaired by aging, for example in the case of vitamin B_{12} and often related to inflammatory diseases of the gut (Holt, 2007). Indeed, in frail institutionalized elderly receiving a fiber-enriched diet over 12 weeks the status of vitamin B_6, B_{12}, and folate improved and the use of laxatives could be reduced (Sturtzel et al., 2010). It has also been suggested that SCFA are, at least partly, responsible for the improvement of mineral absorption by prebiotics (Roy et al., 2006).

Finally, dietary fiber in the diet has other health-promoting effects. Epidemiological data support that consuming a fiber-rich diet can lower the risk for cardiovascular disease although this is most evident for cereal fiber. Especially soluble fiber has been repeatedly shown to lower total and LDL cholesterol in the blood of human subjects. Furthermore, there is also some evidence for beneficial effects on glucose tolerance and prevention of diabetes mellitus type 2 (Slavin, 2008; Theuwissen and Mensink, 2008).

INTAKE OF FRUITS AND VEGETABLES IN ELDERLY ACROSS EUROPE

To date, most countries more or less regularly conduct nutritional surveys at the population level providing important data about dietary intake and consumption patterns. A compilation of data from recent nutrition surveys from several countries of the European Union is presented by the European Food Safety Authority (EFSA) in its Comprehensive European Food Consumption Database (EFSA, 2015). It contains intake amounts of various foods and food groups for different age groups including elderly persons giving an overview of fruit and vegetable consumption in the European Union. Generally, intake amounts did not meet the recommendations of nutrition societies or the World Health Organization. The latter advises a consumption of at least 400 g/day of fruits and vegetables while other entities suggest even higher quantities (eg, 650 g/day from the German Nutrition Society) (World Health Organization, 2003; Boeing et al., 2012). Notable exceptions were elderly in Romania and Italy (see Fig. 4.1). However, when compared to the intakes of younger adults, elderly above 65 years did consume comparable or even higher amounts of fruits and vegetables. Especially the younger elderly aged 65–74 years had a relatively better intake pattern while consumption declined again with increasing age (see Fig. 4.2). It must however be noted that the threshold for older elderly was set rather low at 75 years.

With the exception of Romania, higher amounts of fruits than vegetables were consumed or about equal amounts of both in Ireland, Italy, the Netherlands, and the United Kingdom.

The percentage of consumers was generally high, ranging from about 88% to 100% with the exception of vegetable consumption in Austria that was only reported by 70% of the respondents (EFSA, 2015).

A higher vegetable and fruit consumption in the elderly compared to younger individuals was also observed in the German Health Interview and Examination Survey for Adults (DEGS1) in which the oldest participants (60–79 years) had the highest average intake. Moreover, women and men aged 60–69 years and men aged 70–79 years were more likely to meet

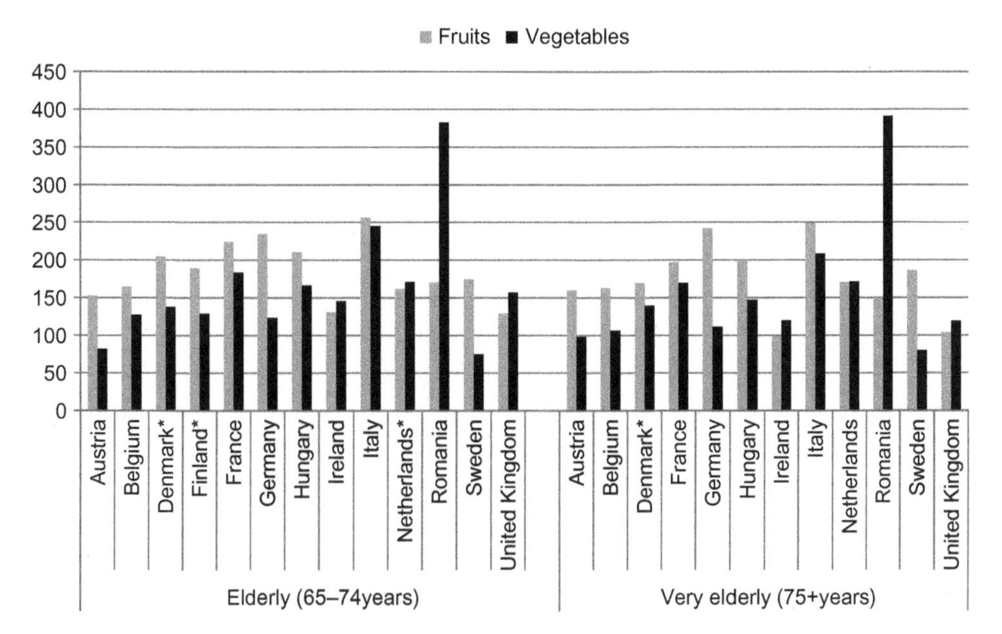

■ **FIGURE 4.1 Intake of fruits and vegetables in elderly adults from countries of the European Union.** Data are taken from the European Food Safety Authority's Comprehensive European Food Consumption Database (EFSA, 2015), a compilation of food consumption data from 32 different dietary surveys using 24 h or 48 h recalls or food records carried out in 22 different Member States of the European Union. Data for elderly and very elderly were available from 13 and 12 countries, respectively. **Mean of two surveys.*

the recommended intake of five or more portions of vegetables and fruits per day. In turn, consumption of raw vegetables was higher in the younger age groups. Nevertheless, more than half of the men and the women aged 60–79 years consumed less than three portions of vegetables and fruits per day and less than 20% of the women and less than 12% of the men ate five or more portions per day, the average amount corresponding to 3.7 and 3.2 daily portions in 60- to 69-year-old and 70- to 79-year-old women, respectively, and to 2.8 and 2.6 in men of the respective age groups. Fruit consumption was higher than that of vegetables (Mensink et al., 2013).

In the Austrian Study on Nutrition Status (ASNS) 2012 (Elmadfa et al., 2012), consumption of fruits and vegetables was also too low in the elderly participants (65–80 years) amounting on average to 128 g/day and 152 g/day, respectively, in men and to 113 g/day and 143 g/day, respectively, in women. These amounts were somewhat lower than in the younger adults especially for fruits. Mean intake covered about 30% and 40–50% of the respective national recommendations for vegetable and fruit intake. The unsatisfactory consumption was mirrored in low plasma concentrations of

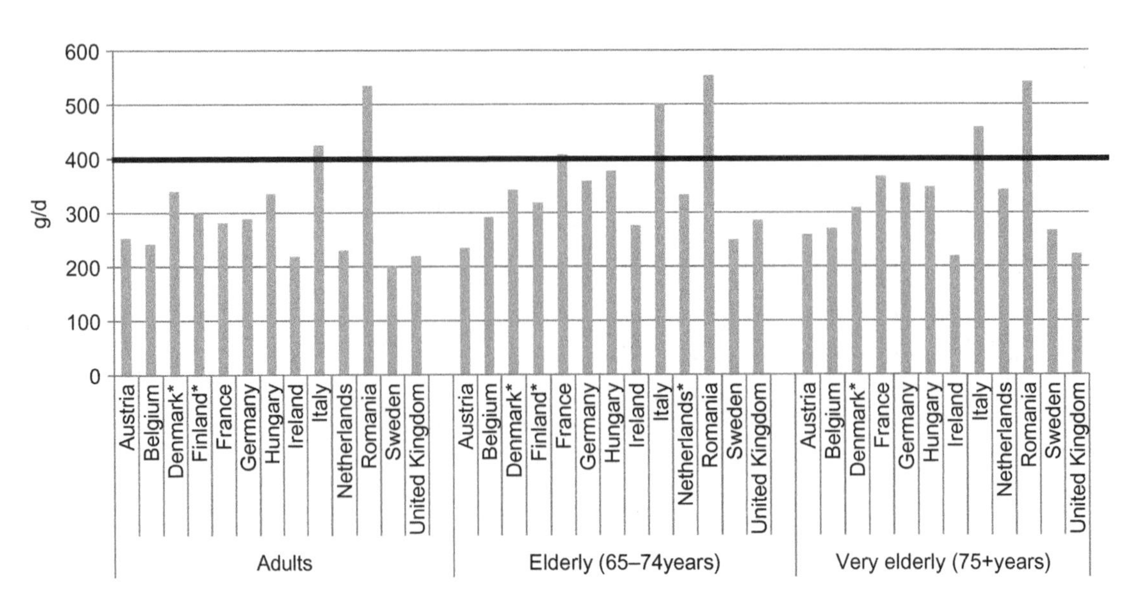

■ **FIGURE 4.2 Combined intake of fruits and vegetables in elderly adults compared to younger adults (18–64 years) from countries of the European Union.** Data are taken from the European Food Safety Authority's Comprehensive European Food Consumption Database (EFSA, 2015), a compilation of food consumption data from 32 different dietary surveys using 24 h or 48 h recalls or food records carried out in 22 different Member States of the European Union. Data for elderly and very elderly were available from 13 and 12 countries, respectively, and are here compared to data from adults from the same countries. The black line marks the lower value of the range of daily fruit and vegetable consumption recommended by the World Health Organization (400–500 g/day) (World Health Organization, 2003). **Mean of two surveys.*

carotenoids that have been described as possible biomarkers of fruit and vegetable intake. Thus, more than half (56%) of the 65- to 80-year-old women and two-thirds (67%) of the men had plasma levels of β-carotene below the cut-off value of 0.373 μmol/L, suggested by Sauberlich et al. as the threshold for satisfactory status (Sauberlich et al., 1974). Accordingly, only about 41% of the women and 33% of the men met the target level of 0.4 μmol/L or more considered as desirable for health optimization and primary prevention of cardiovascular disease and cancer (Gey, 1998). It has to be kept in mind, though, that carotenoid levels show a high variability. Nevertheless, only about 11% of the elderly women and about 8% of the men in the ASNS 2012 had plasma levels of β-carotene exceeding 0.745 μmol/L as recommended by Elmadfa et al. (Elmadfa et al., 2012). In turn, concentrations of this order are found in populations with higher fruit and vegetable consumption such as vegetarians and have been associated with lower risk for cardiovascular diseases and certain cancer types (Sesso et al., 2005; Eliassen et al., 2012).

Low intakes of fruits and vegetables in elderly have also been reported from outside Europe. Thus, in the US Federal Government's National Health and Nutrition Examination Study (NHANES) 1999–2002, average daily intake of fruits and vegetables was 1.4 cups and 1.8 cups, respectively, in male and 1.3 cups and 1.5 cups, respectively, in female elderly aged 65 years and older, these amounts being below those recommended by the USDA. While intake amounts of vegetables were slightly higher in younger adults, elderly were more likely to consume fruits and showed a preference for whole fruits over juice. The pattern of vegetable intake was less satisfactory with a predominance of starchy varieties (U.S. Department of Agriculture and Center for Nutrition Policy and Promotion, 2007).

A survey in Canadian elderly aged 65 years and older showed that less than 50% of the participants met the guideline to consume at least five portions of fruits and vegetables per day (Riediger and Moghadasian, 2008).

Overall, fruit and vegetable intake is too low in elderly individuals even though it is comparable to the situation in younger adults. Indeed, there is even a trend toward healthier nutrition in older persons.

FACTORS INFLUENCING FRUIT AND VEGETABLE CONSUMPTION IN ELDERLY

Considering the particular health benefits of fruits and vegetables for aged persons, their consumption should be promoted. While many of the factors influencing their intake are the same as in younger individuals, they might gain more weight with aging as for example, financial hardship after retirement or difficulties in purchasing, transporting, and preparing fruits and vegetables (Dijkstra et al., 2014).

Additionally, some age-related physiological changes specifically affect the dietary pattern of elder persons. A most notable alteration is the impairment of the capacity to chew and swallow. Both are particular barriers to the consumption of fibrous or hard foods such as varied vegetables and fruits. Indeed, impaired chewing ability has been associated with lower intake of fruits and vegetables (Tada and Miura, 2014). Nevertheless, a study comparing the classification of fruits and vegetables as difficult or easy to eat based on textural properties by young and elderly persons from the United Kingdom and Finland revealed only small differences between both age groups (Roininen et al., 2004).

Food intake of aged individuals is also modified by anorexia of aging that can be due to various causes such as impaired gastrointestinal function, constipation, reduced salivation, neurological alterations, chronic inflammatory processes, and medications. Anorexia of aging has been associated with a lower consumption of fruits and vegetables in particular (Donini et al., 2013; Tracey, 2010).

An influence of the way people perceive aging in general and their health behavior has been described in a German study. Participants who had a more positive view of aging, accorded more importance to physical activity for healthy aging and were more active had a healthier dietary pattern than people with a more pessimistic perception of aging and a more passive comportment. Even though the participants in this study were aged between 50 and 70 years and thus rather young, it shows the importance of motivational factors and of the overall picture of aging suggesting that current antiaging trends can have a positive effect on nutritional behavior (Huy et al., 2010).

Introducing new varieties of fruits and vegetables was described as a possible approach to increase overall intake of these food groups in an Australian collective. Other successful means were informing the participants about adequate intake amounts and at-home delivery of fruits and vegetables (Dixon et al., 2004).

Most available surveys on fruit and vegetable intake and on how to increase their consumption were conducted in predominantly independently living elderly populations and this may explain the lack of marked differences to younger adults. Frailty and loss of independence increase the risk of malnutrition (Volkert et al., 2010) and are also likely to have a negative impact on fruit and vegetable intake.

CONCLUSION

With their high contents of various health-promoting nutrients and bioactive compounds, fruits and vegetables are a central ingredient in the diet of elderly persons that are threatened by a number of diseases and degenerative processes. Notably, while antioxidative micronutrients as well as bioactive phytochemicals have shown many health-promoting effects, supplementation of single isolated compounds has sometimes resulted in negative outcomes, especially at high doses. In turn, vegetables and fruits contain a large diversity of different substances in rather low amounts so that the regular consumption of a variety of these foods covers a wide range of benefits while at the same time limiting negative effects.

To be successful, approaches to promote the consumption of fruits and vegetables must take into account the specific needs and physiological characteristics of the elderly.

REFERENCES

Andrès, E., Federici, L., Serraj, K., Kaltenbach, G., 2008. Update on nutrient-deficient anemia in elderly patients. Eur. J. Intern. Med. 19, 488–493.

Araújo, J.R., Martel, F., Borges, N., Araújo, J.M., Keating, E., 2015. Folates and aging: role in mild cognitive impairment, dementia and depression. Ageing Res. Rev. 22, 9–19.

Bermejo, L.M., Aparicio, A., Andrés, P., López-Sobaler, A.M., Ortega, R.M., 2007. The influence of fruit and vegetable intake on the nutritional status and plasma homocysteine levels of institutionalised elderly people. Public Health Nutr. 10, 266–272.

Bernstein, M., Munoz, N., Academy of Nutrition and Dietetics, 2012. Position of the Academy of Nutrition and Dietetics: food and nutrition for older adults: promoting health and wellness. J. Acad. Nutr. Diet. 112, 1255–1277.

Biagi, E., Candela, M., Turroni, S., Garagnani, P., Franceschi, C., Brigidi, P., 2013. Ageing and gut microbes: perspectives for health maintenance and longevity. Pharmacol. Res. 69, 11–20.

Biagi, E., Nylund, L., Candela, M., Ostan, R., Bucci, L., Pini, E., et al., 2010. Through ageing, and beyond: gut microbiota and inflammatory status in seniors and centenarians. PLoS One 5, e10667.

Bjelakovic, G., Nikolova, D., Gluud, L.L., Simonetti, R.G., Gluud, C., 2012. Antioxidant supplements for prevention of mortality in healthy participants and patients with various diseases. Cochrane Database Syst. Rev. 3, CD007176.

Boeing, H., Bechthold, A., Bub, A., Ellinger, S., Haller, D., Kroke, A., et al., 2012. Critical review: vegetables and fruit in the prevention of chronic diseases. Eur. J. Nutr. 51, 637–663.

Bosy-Westphal, A., Eichhorn, C., Kutzner, D., Illner, K., Heller, M., Müller, M.J., 2003. The age-related decline in resting energy expenditure in humans is due to the loss of fat-free mass and to alterations in its metabolically active components. J. Nutr. 133, 2356–2362.

Britton, E., McLaughlin, J.T., 2013. Ageing and the gut. Proc. Nutr. Soc. 72, 173–177.

Bross, M.H., Soch, K., Smith-Knuppel, T., 2010. Anemia in older persons. Am. Fam. Physician 82, 480–487.

Burton, D.G.A., Krizhanovsky, V., 2014. Physiological and pathological consequences of cellular senescence. Cell Mol. Life Sci. 71, 4373–4386.

Calabrese, V., Cornelius, C., Dinkova-Kostova, A.T., Iavicoli, I., Di Paola, R., Koverech, A., et al., 2012. Cellular stress responses, hormetic phytochemicals and vitagenes in aging and longevity. Biochim. Biophys. Acta. 1822, 753–783.

Cannizzo, E.S., Clement, C.C., Sahu, R., Follo, C., Santambrogio, L., 2011. Oxidative stress, inflamm-aging and immunosenescence. J. Proteomics 74, 2313–2323.

Chu, Y.F., Sun, J., Wu, X., Liu, R.H., 2002. Antioxidant and antiproliferative activities of common vegetables. J. Agric. Food Chem. 50, 6910–6916.

Claesson, M.J., Jeffery, I.B., Conde, S., Power, S.E., O'Connor, E.M., Cusack, S., et al., 2012. Gut microbiota composition correlates with diet and health in the elderly. Nature 488, 178–185.

Cook, S.I., Sellin, J.H., 1998. Short chain fatty acids in health and disease. Aliment. Pharmacol. Ther. 12, 499–507.

Cuervo, A., Salazar, N., Ruas-Madiedo, P., Gueimonde, M., González, S., 2013. Fiber from a regular diet is directly associated with fecal short-chain fatty acid concentrations in the elderly. Nutr. Res. 33, 811–816.

Dijkstra, S.C., Neter, J.E., van Stralen, M.M., Knol, D.L., Brouwer, I.A., Huisman, M., et al., 2014. The role of perceived barriers in explaining socio-economic status differences in adherence to the fruit, vegetable and fish guidelines in older adults: a mediation study. Public Health Nutr. 18, 797–808.

Dixon, H., Mullins, R., Wakefield, M., Hill, D., 2004. Encouraging the consumption of fruit and vegetables by older Australians: an experimental study. J. Nutr. Educ. Behav. 36, 245–249.

Donini, L.M., Poggiogalle, E., Piredda, M., Pinto, A., Barbagallom, M., Cucinotta, D., et al., 2013. Anorexia and eating patterns in the elderly. PLoS ONE 8, e63539.

Eastell, R., Lambert, H., 2002. Strategies for skeletal health in the elderly. Proc. Nutr. Soc. 61, 173–180.

Elia, M., Ritz, P., Stubbs, R.J., 2000. Total energy expenditure in the elderly. Eur. J. Clin. Nutr. 54, S92–S103.

Eliassen, A.H., Hendrickson, S.J., Brinton, L.A., Buring, J.E., Campos, H., Dai, Q., et al., 2012. Circulating carotenoids and risk of breast cancer: pooled analysis of eight prospective studies. J. Natl. Cancer Inst. 104, 1905–1916.

Elmadfa, I., Meyer, A., Nowak, V., Hasenegger, V., Putz, P., Verstraeten, R., et al., 2009. European Nutrition and Health Report 2009. Forum Nutr. 62, 1–405. (cited on p. 60).

Elmadfa, I., Hasenegger, V., Wagner, K., Putz, P., Weidl, N.M., Wottawa, D., et al., 2012. Österreichischer Ernährungsbericht 2012 [Austrian Nutrition Report 2012], first ed. Commissioned by the Federal Ministry of Health, Vienna.

Elmadfa, I., Sturtzel, B., Ohrenberger, G., 2014. Intervention mit eisenreichen Lebensmitteln – Einfluss auf den Status ausgewählter Mikronährstoffe und die Anämie-Prävalenz geriatrischer Patienten [Intervention with iron-rich foods – Effect on the status of selected micronutrients and anemia prevalence in geriatric patients, in German]. Abstract from the Proceedings of the Annual Meeting of the Austrian Nutrition Society 2014. Ernährung/Nutrition 38, 16.

European Food Safety Authority, 2015. European Food Safety Authority: EFSA comprehensive food consumption database. <http://www.efsa.europa.eu/en/datexfoodcdb/datexfooddb.htm> (accessed 12.06.15.).

Eurostat, 2013. Europe in figures - Eurostat yearbook. Available from <http://ec.europa.eu/eurostat/statistics-explained/index.php/Europe_in_figures_-_Eurostat_yearbook> (accessed 12.06.15.).

Franceschi, C., Capri, M., Monti, D., Giunta, S., Olivieri, F., Sevini, F., et al., 2007. Inflammaging and anti-inflammaging: a systemic perspective on aging and longevity emerged from studies in humans. Mech. Ageing Dev. 128, 92–105.

Freedman, V.A., Martin, L.G., Schoeni, R.F., 2002. Recent trends in disability and functioning among older adults in the United States: a systematic review. JAMA 288, 3137–3146.

Gey, K.F., 1998. Vitamins E plus C and interacting co-nutrients required for optimal health. BioFactors 7, 113–174.

Gopalakrishnan, A., Tony Kong, A.N., 2008. Anticarcinogenesis by dietary phytochemicals: cytoprotection by Nrf2 in normal cells and cytotoxicity by modulation of transcription factors NF-κB and AP-1 in abnormal cancer cells. Food Chem. Toxicol. 46, 1257–1270.

Gulsvik, A.K., Thelle, D.S., Mowé, M., Wyller, T.B., 2009. Increased mortality in the slim elderly: a 42 years follow-up study in a general population. Eur. J. Epidemiol. 24, 683–690.

Halliwell, B., 2012. The antioxidant paradox: less paradoxical now? Br. J. Clin. Pharmacol. 75, 637–644.

Heiat, A., Vaccarino, V., Krumholz, H.M., 2001. An evidence-based assessment of federal guidelines for overweight and obesity as they apply to elderly persons. Arch. Intern. Med. 161, 1194–1203.

Hekimi, S., Lapointe, J., Wen, Y., 2011. Taking a “good” look at free radicals in the aging process. Trends Cell Biol. 21, 569–576.

Hippe, B., Zwielehner, J., Liszt, K., Lassl, C., Unger, F., Haslberger, A.G., 2011. Quantification of butyrylCoA:acetateCoA-transferase genes reveals different butyrate production capacity in individuals according to diet and age. FEMS Microbiol. Lett. 316, 130–135.

Holt, P.R., 2007. Intestinal malabsorption in the elderly. Dig. Dis. 25, 144–150.

Horcajada, M.N., Offord, E., 2012. Naturally plant-derived compounds: role in bone anabolism. Curr. Mol. Pharmacol. 5, 205–218.

Huy, C., Schneider, S., Thiel, A., 2010. Perception of aging and health behavior: determinants of a healthy diet in an older German population. J. Nutr. Health Aging 14, 381–385.

Jahangir, E., De Schutter, A., Lavie, C.J., 2014. Low weight and overweightness in older adults: risk and clinical management. Prog. Cardiovasc. Dis. 57, 127–133.

Joseph, S.V., Edirisinghe, I., Burton-Freeman, B.M., 2014. Berries: anti-inflammatory effects in humans. J. Agric. Food Chem. 62, 3886–3903.

Kinsella, K., Wan, H., U.S. Census Bureau, 2009. An Aging World: 2008. International Population Reports, P95/09-1. U.S. Government Printing Office, Washington, DC.

Lane, D.J., Richardson, D.R., 2014. The active role of vitamin C in mammalian iron metabolism: much more than just enhanced iron absorption!. Free Radic. Biol. Med. 75, 69–83.

Li, M., Fukagawa, N.K., 2010. Age-related changes in redox signaling and VSMC function. Antioxid. Redox. Signal. 12, 641–655.

Malouf, R., Grimley Evans, J., 2008. Folic acid with or without vitamin B12 for the prevention and treatment of healthy elderly and demented people. Cochrane Database Syst. Rev. 4, CD004514.

Mandlekar, S., Hong, J.L., Kong, A.N.T., 2006. Modulation of metabolic enzymes by dietary phytochemicals: a review of mechanisms underlying beneficial versus unfavorable effects. Curr. Drug Metab. 7, 661–675.

Mangels, A.R., 2014. Bone nutrients for vegetarians. Am. J. Clin. Nutr. 100 (suppl), 469S–475S.

Manton, K.G., 2008. Recent declines in chronic disability in the elderly U.S. population: risk factors and future dynamics. Annu. Rev. Public Health. 29, 91–113.

Manz, F., Johner, S.A., Wentz, A., Boeing, H., Remer, T., 2012. Water balance throughout the adult lifespan in a German population. Br. J. Nutr. 107, 1673–1681.

Mathus-Vliegen, E.M., Obesity Management Task Force of the European Association for the Study of Obesity, 2012. Prevalence, pathophysiology, health consequences and treatment options of obesity in the elderly: a guideline. Obes. Facts. 5, 460–483.

Maughan, R.J., 2012. Hydration, morbidity, and mortality in vulnerable populations. Nutr. Rev. 70, S152–S155.

Mensink, G.B.M., Truthmann, J., Rabenberg, M., Heidemann, C., Haftenberger, M., Schienkiewitz, A., et al., 2013. Fruit and vegetable intake in Germany. Results of the German Health Interview and Examination Survey for Adults (DEGS1). Bundesgesundheitsbl 56, 779–785.

Montenegro-Bethancourt, G., Johner, S.A., Remer, T., 2013. Contribution of fruit and vegetable intake to hydration status in school children. Am. J. Clin. Nutr. 98, 1103–1112.

Montgomery, S.C., Streit, S.M., Beebe, M.L., Maxwell 4th, P.J., 2014. Micronutrient needs of the elderly. Nutr. Clin. Pract. 29, 435–444.

Murugaiyah, V., Mattson, M.P., 2015. Neurohormetic phytochemicals: An evolutionary—bioenergetic perspective. Neurochem. Int. 89, 271–280.

NatCen Social Research, MRC Human Nutrition Research, University College London Medical School, 2015. National Diet and Nutrition Survey Years 1-4, 2008/09-2011/12, seventh ed. UK Data Archive, Colchester, Essex, SN: 6533.

National Institute on Aging, National Institutes of Health, U.S. Department of Health and Human Services and World Health Organization, 2011. Global Health and Aging. NIH Publication, Bethesda, MD, 11–7737.

Ndhlala, A., Moyo, M., Van Staden, J., 2010. Natural antioxidants: fascinating or mythical biomolecules? Molecules 15, 6905–6930.

New, S.A., Robins, S.P., Campbell, M.K., Martin, J.C., Garton, M.J., Bolton-Smith, C., et al., 2000. Dietary influences on bone mass and bone metabolism: further evidence of a positive link between fruit and vegetable consumption and bone health? Am. J. Clin. Nutr. 71, 142–151.

Riediger, N.D., Moghadasian, M.H., 2008. Patterns of fruit and vegetable consumption and the influence of sex, age and socio-demographic factors among Canadian elderly. J. Am. Coll. Nutr. 27, 306–313.

Roininen, K., Fillion, L., Kilcast, D., Lähteenmäki, L., 2004. Exploring difficult textural properties in fruit and vegetables for the elderly in Finland and the United Kingdom. Food Qual. Prefer. 15, 517–530.

Roy, C.C., Kien, C.L., Bouthillier, L., Levy, E., 2006. Short-chain fatty acids: ready for prime time? Nutr. Clin. Pract. 21, 351–366.

Sadowska-Bartosz, I., Bartosz, G., 2014. Effect of antioxidants supplementation on aging and longevity. Biomed. Res. Int. 2014, 404680.

Sauberlich, H.E., Dowdy, R.P., Skala, J.H., 1974. Laboratory Tests for the Assessment of Nutritional Status. CRC Press, Boca Raton, FL.

Schiffrin, E.J., Morley, J.E., Donnet-Hughes, A., Guigoz, Y., 2010. The inflammation status of the elderly: the intestinal contribution. Mutat. Res. 690, 50–56.

Schols, J.M.G.A., De Groot, C.P.G.M., Van der Cammen, T.J.M., Olde Rikkert, M.G.M., 2009. Preventing and treating dehydration in the elderly during periods of illness and warm weather. J. Nutr. Health Aging 13, 150–157.

Serafini, M., 2006. Back to the origin of the "antioxidant hypothesis": the lost role of the antioxidant network in disease prevention. J. Sci. Food Agric. 86, 1989–1991.

Sesso, H.D., Buring, J.E., Norkus, E.P., Gaziano, J.M., 2005. Plasma lycopene, other carotenoids, and retinol and the risk of cardiovascular disease in men. Am. J. Clin. Nutr. 81, 990–997.

Silva, F.G., 2005. The aging kidney: a review – Part I. Int. Urol. Nephrol. 37, 185–205.

Slavin, J.L., 2008. Position of the American Dietetic Association: health implications of dietary fiber. J. Am. Diet. Assoc. 108, 1716–1731.

Sturtzel, B., Dietrich, A., Wagner, K.H., Gisinger, C., Elmadfa, I., 2010. The status of vitamins B6, B12, folate, and of homocysteine in geriatric home residents receiving laxatives or dietary fiber. J. Nutr. Health Aging 14, 219–223.

Suh, J.H., Shenvi, S.V., Dixon, B.M., Liu, H., Jaiswal, A.K., Liu, R.M., et al., 2004. Decline in transcriptional activity of Nrf2 causes age-related loss of glutathione synthesis, which is reversible with lipoic acid. Proc. Natl. Acad. Sci. USA. 101, 3381–3386.

Sun, J., Chu, Y.F., Wu, X., Liu, R.H., 2002. Antioxidant and antiproliferative activities of common fruits. J. Agric. Food Chem. 50, 7449–7454.

Tada, A., Miura, H., 2014. Systematic review of the association of mastication with food and nutrient intake in the independent elderly. Arch. Gerontol. Geriatr. 59, 497–505.

Theuwissen, E., Mensink, R.P., 2008. Water-soluble dietary fibers and cardiovascular disease. Physiol. Behav. 94, 285–292.

Titgemeyer, E.C., Bourquin, L.D., Fahey Jr., G.C., Garleb, K.A., 1991. Fermentability of various fiber sources by human fecal bacteria in vitro. Am. J. Clin. Nutr. 53, 1418–1424.

Tracey, K.J., 2010. Understanding immunity requires more than immunology. Nat. Immunol. 11, 561–564.

Tucker, K.L., Chen, H., Hannan, M.T., Cupples, L.A., Wilson, P.W., Felson, D., et al., 2002. Bone mineral density and dietary patterns in older adults: the Framingham Osteoporosis Study. Am. J. Clin. Nutr. 76, 245–252.

Tucker, K.L., Hannan, M.T., Chen, H., Cupples, L.A., Wilson, P.W., Kiel, D.P., 1999. Potassium, magnesium, and fruit and vegetable intakes are associated with greater bone mineral density in elderly men and women. Am. J. Clin. Nutr. 69, 727–736.

U.S. Department of Agriculture and Center for Nutrition Policy and Promotion, 2007. Fruit and vegetable consumption by older Americans. Nutr. Insight 34 Available online at <http://www.cnpp.usda.gov/sites/default/files/nutrition_insights_uploads/Insight34.pdf> (accessed 18.06.15.).

Volkert, D., Saeglitz, C., Gueldenzoph, H., Sieber, C.C., Stehle, P., 2010. Undiagnosed malnutrition and nutrition-related problems in geriatric patients. J. Nutr. Health Aging 14, 387–392.

Weinstein, J.R., Anderson, S., 2010. The aging kidney: physiological changes. Adv. Chronic Kidney Dis. 17, 302–307.

Woodmansey, E.J., 2007. Intestinal bacteria and ageing. J. Appl. Microbiol. 102, 1178–1186.

World Health Organization, 2003. Diet, nutrition and the prevention of chronic diseases. Report of a Joint FAO/WHO Expert Consultation. WHO Technical Report Series, No. 916. World Health Organization, Geneva, <http://www.who.int/iris/bitstream/10665/42665/1/WHO_TRS_916.pdf?ua=1> (accessed 12.06.15.).

Yang, W., Hekimi, S., 2010. A mitochondrial superoxide signal triggers increased longevity in Caenorhabditis elegans. PLoS Biol. 8, e1000556.

Chapter 5

Diabetes, diabetic complications, and flavonoids

Yogesh A. Kulkarni[1], Mayuresh S. Garud[1], Manisha J. Oza[1,2], Kalyani H. Barve[1] and Anil B. Gaikwad[3]
[1]*Shobhaben Pratapbhai Patel School of Pharmacy & Technology Management, SVKM's NMIMS, Mumbai, Maharashtra, India*
[2]*SVKM's Dr. Bhanuben Nanavati College of Pharmacy, Mumbai, Maharashtra, India*
[3]*Birla Institute of Technology and Science, Pilani, Rajasthan, India*

CHAPTER OUTLINE

INTRODUCTION

Diabetes mellitus (DM) is among the most prevalent diseases with which a large population of world is suffering from. Incidence of diabetes is on rise all over the world. According to International Diabetes Federation (IDF), 387 million people were living with diabetes in year 2014, which is expected to increase by more 205 million till 2035 (IDF, 2013). World Health Organization (WHO) has reported that DM is becoming a lead cause of mortality and morbidity worldwide. Although there are numerous

Fruits, Vegetables, and Herbs.
DOI: http://dx.doi.org/10.1016/B978-0-12-802972-5.00005-6

options for diagnosis and treatment of diabetes, 50% of the population does not know that they are suffering from it and one person dies because of diabetes every 7 s (IDF, 2013).

DM is a group of metabolic disorders which is final result of hyperglycemia. Reduced insulin secretion, decreased glucose utilization, and increased glucose production are the etiological factors which contribute to hyperglycemia.

Poor-controlled chronic hyperglycemia is known to initiate diabetic vascular complications via many metabolic and structural dysregulation. The prevalence of complications increases with prolonged duration of diabetes. Dysregulations include increased generation of reactive oxygen species (ROS; Zhou et al., 2012); elevated production of advanced glycation end products (AGEs; Ojima et al., 2012); abnormal activation of signaling cascades such as activation of polyol pathway, protein kinase C pathway, hexosamine (Juan et al., 2012; Riedl et al., 2011); and abnormal stimulation of hemodynamic regulatory mechanisms like the renin–angiotensin system (Singh et al., 2003; Garud and Kulkarni, 2014). These derangements and abnormal functioning can cause many secondary pathophysiologic changes leading to various complications. Diabetic complications have great share in the morbidity and mortality of patients related with diabetes.

Complications of diabetes are majorly classified under two classes, that is, microvascular complications which involve small vessels and capillaries and macrovascular complications which involve large vessels, such as arteries and veins. Retinopathy, nephropathy, neuropathy, etc., are microvascular complications while macrovascular complications include coronary artery disease, atherosclerosis, peripheral vascular disease, etc.

Nephropathy is one of the progressive complications of diabetes. Most earlier and typical manifestation of diabetic nephropathy is microalbuminuria, which further progresses to albuminuria and ultimately to renal failure (Drummond and Mauer, 2002). Diabetic nephropathy is one of the leading cause of end-stage renal disease and chronic kidney disease (Brenner et al., 2001). Characteristic physiological changes in kidney include thickening of glomerular basement membranes and glomerular hyperfiltration, causing mesangial extracellular matrix expansion. These changes further increase urinary albumin excretion and accelerate progression of glomerular and tubular sclerosis and renal failure (Chen et al., 2001; Van Dijk and Berl, 2004).

Diabetic retinopathy causes visual disability and blindness in the person suffering from it (Harding, 2003). The severity of diabetic retinopathy ranges from nonproliferative and preproliferative to severe proliferative diabetic retinopathy (Harding, 2003). The severity can increase to such an extent that it can lead to total or partial vision loss via a vitric hemorrhage or retinal detachment, as well as central vision loss can happen via retinal vessel leakage and subsequent macular edema (Sheetz and King, 2002).

Nearly 50% of the people with diabetes suffer from some kind of peripheral neuropathy, which can be polydiabetic or monodiabetic neuropathy (Dyck et al., 1993). Among the characteristic manifestations of diabetic neuropathy, autonomic dysfunction is one of the sign which can be life-threatening. Autonomic neuropathy includes cardiovascular autonomic dysfunction which is expressed as abnormal heart rate and vascular control (Vinik et al., 2003). Diabetic neuropathy is manifested with pain, autonomic disturbances, and trophic changes in the feet. Some patients with diabetes show development of focal and multifocal neuropathies involving cranial nerve and also include limb and truncal neuropathies (Vinik et al., 2003).

Cardiovascular disorders are the foremost cause of death in people with type 2 diabetes. Diabetic patients have a fourfold more risk for having cardiovascular disorders even after controlling traditional risk factors, such as age, obesity, tobacco use, dyslipidemia, and hypertension (Bonora et al., 2002; Buyken et al., 2007). The risk is so high that, about 70% of the deaths caused by diabetes are accounted to its cardiovascular complications (Laakso, 1999). Hyperglycemia is also one of the causative factor for stroke. Diabetes-related factors like proteinuria, microalbuminuria, and hyperuricemia are also associated with increased risk for stroke (Sasaki et al., 1995; Guerrero-Romero and Rodriguez-Moran, 1999; Lehto et al., 1998). Elevated blood concentration of chronic inflammatory markers in diabetic patient makes them more prone to stroke (Cade, 2008).

Management and treatment of diabetes and related complications is of prime importance. Finding of new drugs and betterment of current therapeutic regimen is necessary to achieve the target of decreasing the mortalities and morbidities related with the diabetes and its complications.

Plants have served as a great source of medicines for variety of diseases and aliments including diabetes and its complications. Various groups of phytochemicals derived from plant are identified and reported to have antidiabetic activity along with having potential to treat complications of it. This chapter focuses on use of flavonoids, an important class of phytochemicals, in treatment and management of diabetes and its complications

FLAVONOIDS

In the year of 1930, rutin was isolated from oranges which at that time was believed to be a vitamin and was named as vitamin P. Further research showed that rutin is not a vitamin and is a type of flavonoid. More than 4000 several flavonoids have been identified. Structurally, flavonoids are made up of skeleton of 15-carbon which consists two benzene rings (ring A and B) linked via a heterocyclic pyrane ring (Fig. 5.1).

Flavonoids can be divided into various classes based on level of oxidation and pattern of substitution of the pyrane ring. Whereas, flavonoids in individual class differ in the substitution of the A and B rings (Middleton, 1998). Flavonoids can be divided into several classes depending on their chemical structures which include anthocyanins, flavones, flavonols, flavanones, dihydroflavonols, chalcones, aurones, flavonons, flavan and proanthocyanidins, isoflavonoids, isoflavones, isoflavonones, isoflavons, isoflavene, biflavonoids, neoflavonoids, flavonoid alkaloids, etc. (Tsukasa, 2000).

Flavonoids are reported to have wide range of pharmacological activities like antibacterial, antiviral, antiallergic, antiinflammatory activity, etc. (Cushnie and Lamb, 2005; Cook and Samman, 1996). They have shown antitumor activity, vasodilatory action and also found effective in treatment of neurodegenerative diseases (Tsuchiya, 2010; Chebil et al., 2006). Flavonoids are also found to inhibit cyclooxygenase and lipoxygenase enzyme activities, lipid peroxidation, platelet aggregation, and capillary permeability. Activities shown by flavonoids can be assigned to their antioxidants, free radical scavenging potential (Chebil et al., 2006; Kulkarni and Garud, 2015). Various enzyme inhibitory activities of flavonoids like inhibition of hydrolases, hyalouronidase, alkaline phosphatise, arylsulfatase, cyclic adenosine monophosphate (cAMP) phosphodiesterase, lipase, α-glucosidase, and kinase are reported (Narayana et al., 2001).

In following text we have discussed the various subclasses of flavonoids in context of their antidiabetic activity along with their potential in management and treatment of diabetic complications.

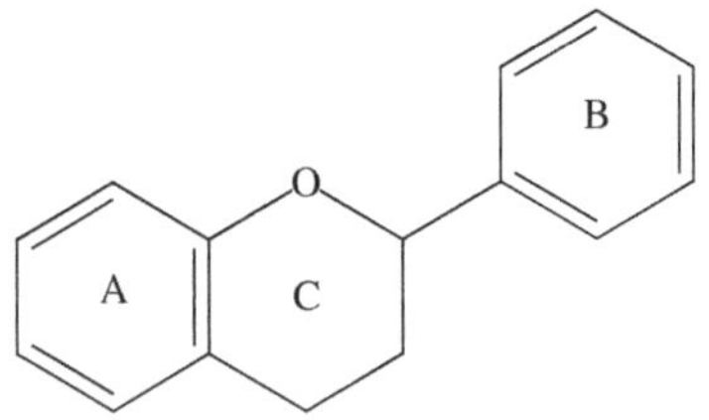

A C B O

■ FIGURE 5.1 Common structure of flavonoids.

Flavonol

Flavonols are biologically active subclass of flavonoid which mainly includes galangin, kaempferol, quercetin, and myricetin. All these flavonols possess identical chemical structures except number of hydroxyl group on the B ring (Neveu et al., 2010). It has been reported that a mixture of flavonols such as quercetin, kaempferol, myricetin, and galangin increased cellular glucose metabolism via increasing expression of GLUT1 in HepG2 cells (Kerimi et al., 2015). They are also reported to be a strong inhibitor of AGEs formation as specially formation of pentosidine in collagen (Urios et al., 2007; Ghaffari and Mojab, 2007). Galangin, a flavonol present in *Alpinia galangal*, has been reported to have antioxidant, hypolipidemic, and pancreatic lipase inhibitory activity, thus it may be considered to find its therapeutic potential in diabetes (Kumar and Alagawadi, 2013).

Kaempferol

It is a 3,5,7-trihydroxy-2-(4-hydroxy phenyl)-4H-1-benzopyran-4-one present in various fruits, vegetables, and medicinal plants such as grapes, strawberries, leek, beans, cabbage, tea, broccoli, Moringaspps, *Sophora japonica*, Propolis, *Ginkgo biloba*, Tiliaspps (Rajendran et al., 2014). It is reported that kaempferol prevents the glycosylation of hemoglobin at desirable concentration by its antioxidant mechanism (Asgary et al., 1999). Furthermore, kaempferol was found to increase insulin sensitivity and produced hypoglycemic effect in type 2 diabetic rats (Andrade et al., 2000). In addition, kaempferol derivative was found to reduce blood glucose by increasing glucose uptake in muscles (Jorge et al., 2004). Flavonol including kaemfperol was reported to inhibit formation of pentosidine (AGEs) in collagen (Urios et al., 2007). It also inhibited glycation of low-density lipoprotein in human-blood sample probably by antioxidant mechanism (Ghaffari and Mojab, 2007; Wu et al., 2009). Kaempferol also inhibited protein glycosylation with reducing sugar, 2-deoxy-D-ribose in MC3T3-E1 mouse osteoblastic cell line, and inhibited osteoblastic cell damage (Suh et al., 2009). Kaempferol increased glucose uptake and reduced hyperglycemia through partial agonistic action on PPAR-γ in 3T3-L1 cells (Fang et al., 2008; Zhang and Liu, 2011). Furthermore, it also reduces hyperlipidemia and insulin resistance in type 2 diabetic rats by downregulating SREBP-1C and PPAR-γ (Zang et al., 2015). In an in vitro study conducted by Saifudin et al. (2013) observed that kaempferol derivative isolated from *Zingiber aromaticum* inhibited protein tyrosine phosphatase 1β an enzyme associated with type 2 diabetes and obesity. A recent mechanistic study uncovered the role of kaempferol in protection of pancreatic beta cells from hyperlipidemia-induced damage. Kaempferol increased the expression of pancreatic and duodenal homeobox-1 and subsequently stimulated cAMP production and protein kinase A as well as cAMP response element-binding protein (CREB) activation in INS-1E cells (Zhang et al., 2013).

Rutin

It is a 5,7,3′,4′-hydroxy-3-rutinose, the glycoside of quercetin (Nakamura et al., 2000). It is present in many plants but buckwheat, black tea, and apples are considered to be a major source of it. It has wide range of pharmacological actions including anticancer, cytoprotective, antiplatelet, antithrobotic, and antioxidant (Sheu et al., 2004; Trumbeckaite et al., 2006). Recent reports also showed that rutin possesses anti-AGEs and antioxidant properties so can be used to treat diabetic and its complications (Cervantes-Laurean et al., 2006; Stanley Mainzen and Kamalakkannan, 2006). Rutin rich fraction of *Phyllanthus sellowianus* as well as rutin was studied in streptozotocin (STZ)-induced diabetic rats and showed hypoglycemic effect in diabetic rats (Hnatyszyn et al., 2002; Kamalakkannan and Prince, 2006). Moreover, rutin also regulated glucose homeostasis by regulating carbohydrate metabolism and antioxidant status in diabetic rats (Stanley Mainzen and Kamalakkannan, 2006; Kamalakkannan and Stanely Mainzen, 2006). In addition rutin also increased insulin-independent and insulin-dependent glucose uptake in skeletal muscles by CaMKII-mediated GLUT4 translocation and insulin receptor kinase-mediated GLUT4 translocation, respectively (Kappel et al., 2013; Hsu et al., 2014). Both IRS2 and AMPK signaling play a critical role in maintaining integrity of pancreatic β-cells and insulin resistance in type 2 diabetics. Rutin has been shown to activate both IRS2 and AMPK signaling and protects pancreatic β-cells damage from glucotoxicity and also reduced insulin resistance (Cai and Lin, 2009). It is also reported to regulate enzymes associated with lipoprotein and lipid metabolism by antioxidant mechanism (Stanely Mainzen and Kannan, 2006). Rutin inhibited AGE formation with goat eye lens proteins (Sumbul et al., 2011). G-rutin, a transglycosylated form of rutin, suppressed formation of AGE in muscles and kidney in diabetic rats (Nagasawa et al., 2003). Furthermore, rutin was found to be a strong inhibitor of pentosidine (AGEs) formation in collagen and protects from vascular complications in diabetes (Urios et al., 2007). Besides it also inhibits glycation of low-density lipoprotein in human-blood sample probably by antioxidant mechanism (Ghaffari and Mojab, 2007). It was found that rutin has been protected diabetic rats against lung damage and neuropathy by reducing oxidative stress (Je et al., 2002). It also provided neuroprotection in retina of diabetic rats by its antiapoptotic activity and increasing Bcl2 level as well as decreasing caspase-3 level in retina (Ola et al., 2015). In another study it was reported to protect type 1 and type 2 diabetic rat from cardiomyopathy by reducing oxidative stress, inflammation, cell death, and inhibiting aldose reductase (Krishna et al., 2005; Wang et al., 2015). Moreover, it has been also shown cardioprotective effect in experimental myocardial infarction in diabetic rats partly via its antioxidant mechanism and partly by increasing synthesis of NO via enhanced activation of nitric oxide synthase (Challa et al., 2011). It also attenuated myocardial dysfunction in STZ-induced diabetic rats (Guimaraes et al., 2015). Tissue growth factor (TGF)-β is considered to be a critical factor in the development of renal diseases. Hyperglycemia-induced TGF-β signaling abnormalities are the leading cause of functional disturbance of mesangial cells. A study by Tang et al. (2011a) andHao et al. (2012) reported that rutin has been delayed the development of glomerulosclerosis of diabetic nephropathy in rat mesangial cells and in STZ-induced diabetic rats by inhibiting cell hypertrophy and reducing TGF-β/Smads-mediated accumulation of ECM.

Myricetin

It is a natural flavone present in fruits, vegetables, tea, berries, and medicinal plants generally in the form of glycoside. It has been reported to have antioxidant, anticancer, antimutagenic, cardioprotective, and antidiabetic activity (Ong and Khoo, 1997). It has been found that myricetin-reduced insulin resistance in type 2 diabetic rats by reducing obesity and proinflammatory cytokines levels in rats (Choi et al., 2014). A study by Ozcan et al. (2012) demonstrated that myricetin has beneficial role in diabetic nephropathy by normalizing impaired renal functions, reduction in glomerulosclerosis and normalization of glutathione peroxidase and xanthine oxidase activity.

Quercetin

The first report on antidiabetic effect of quercetin was published in 1958. Quercetin was found to reduce blood sugar level in alloxan, STZ-induced and in type 2 diabetic db/db mice diabetic rats (Di Maggio and Ciaceri, 1958; Vessal et al., 2003; Jeong et al., 2012). Later it was reported as aldose reductase inhibitor as well as PPAR-γ agonist which plays an important role in reducing hyperglycemia (Fang et al., 2008). Quercetin has been reported to improve liver and pancreas function via inhibiting Cdkn1a expression which is generally involved in cell proliferation (Kobori et al., 2009). In diabetic neuropathy, normal size and density of neurons get altered which impair the functions of neurons. In one of the studies quercetin was found to maintain density and mass of myenteric neurons and glia cell in the cecum of rat (Ferreira et al., 2013). It was also reported to attenuate memory dysfunction in diabetic rats (Bhutada et al., 2010). It has also been demonstrated protective effect in osteopenia in diabetic rat by reducing bone loss via its antioxidant effect (Liang et al., 2011). Quercetin treatment also reduced testicular damage by reducing apoptosis and increasing proliferating cell nuclear antigen expression in tissue of testis (Kanter et al., 2012). Diabetic nephropathy is another major complication of diabetes. Quercetin also provided nephroprotection to diabetic rats by ameliorating oxidative stress and renal dysfunctions (Gomes et al., 2014; Elbe et al., 2015). In the mechanistic study carried out by Huang et al. (2005) it reduced expression of platelet-derived growth factor-B and vascular endothelial growth factor-1 in kidney of STZ-induced diabetic rats. Furthermore, quercetin has been reported to reduce Smad 2/3 expression, type-IV collagen, laminin, and TGF-β1 mRNA level in rat mesangial cells, as well as TGF-β1 and connective TGF in diabetic rats which are involved in the progression of diabetic nephropathy (Tang et al., 2011b; Lai et al., 2012). In addition it also regulated activation of renal NLRP3 inflammasome which has been responsible for upregulation of inflammatory cytokines IL-1β and IL-18 in diabetic rats (Wang et al., 2012a). Epithelial to mesenchymal transition plays a critical role in the pathogenesis of renal fibrosis in diabetic nephropathy. Lu et al. (2015) reported that quercetin inhibited epithelial to mesenchymal transition of HK-2 and NRK-52E cells via inhibiting transcription facts such as snail and twist and mTORC1/p70S6K signaling. Hyperglycemia-induced oxidative stress in diabetics activates various signaling pathways including NF-kβ, which increases lipid peroxidation, protein nitration, and LDL oxidation by increasing expression of inducible nitric oxide synthase. Quercetin was reported to reduce NF-kβ activation and overexpression of iNOs via eradicating IκB kinase (IKK)/NF-kβ signaling pathway (Dias et al., 2005). In addition it also reduced NF-kβ p65 expression in type 2 diabetic rats which are associated with diabetic nephropathy (Chen et al., 2012). oxidative stress in diabetes also plays a major role in the development of endothelial dysfunction. In one of the studies quercetin was found to improve vascular reactivity and endothelial function in blood vessels through increasing bioavailability of endothelial nitric oxide (Ajay et al., 2006; Machha et al., 2007). It has been also reported to show cardioprotection against myocardial infarction in diabetic rats via antioxidant mechanism (Annapurna et al., 2009). AMP-activated protein kinase is a well-known target for metabolic disorder including diabetes. Activation of AMPK leads to increased substrate uptake capacity of cells and restoration of energy homeostasis and this provides beneficial effect in metabolic stress. Quercetin has been found to activate AMPK

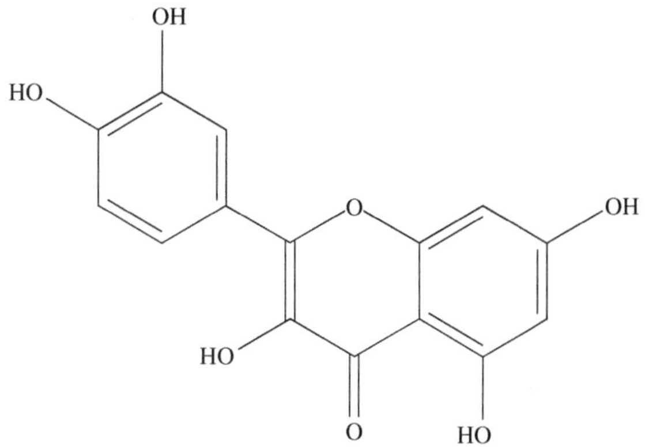

■ **FIGURE 5.2** Structure of quercetin.

pathway in C2C12 muscle cells, L6 skeletal muscle cells as well as in H4IIE hepatocytes and increased GLUT4 translocation which ultimately increased glucose uptake in cells (Eid et al., 2010, 2015). Monocyte chemoattractant protein-1 is involved in the initial stages of atherosclerosis processes in various cells including smooth muscle cells, macrophages cells, and endothelial cells. In diabetes due to hyperglycemic condition level of circulating MCP-1 gets increased and promotes atherosclerosis. A study by Panicker et al. (2010) revealed that quercetin-reduced expression of MCP-1 in aortic endothelial cells via regulating NF-kβ and AP-1 pathways which are responsible for the expression of MCP-1. Quercetin was found to protect endothelial progenitor cells from hyperglycemia-induced damage via Sirt-1-dependent upregulation of Endothelial NOS (eNOS) in endothelial progenitor cells (Zhao et al., 2014) (Fig. 5.2).

Flavonones

Hesperidin

Jung et al. (2004) and Akiyama et al. (2010) reported that hesperidin-reduced hyperglycemia through increasing hepatic glycolysis and reducing hepatic gluconeogenesis in type 2 diabetic rats and hypolipidemic effect in type 1 diabetic rats. It also reduced oxidative injury by improving antioxidant potential in osteoblasts MC3T3-E1 cells suggesting its beneficial role in diabetic bone diseases (Choi and Kim, 2008). Hyperglycemia-induced ROS plays a pivotal role in the production of proinflammatory mediators and development of atherosclerosis and associated risk of myocardial infarction. Hesperidin was found to protect against myocardial infarction as well as diabetic neuropathy in diabetic rats by improving lipid profile and blood sugar level, by regulating PPAR-γ function, and by reducing proinflammatory mediators (Kakadiya et al., 2010; Mahmoud et al., 2012; Agrawal et al., 2014). It has been also reported to have a protective role in diabetic retinopathy via antiapoptosis, antiangiogenic, and antioxidant effect (Kumar et al., 2013; Shi et al., 2012).

Flavones

They have a double bond between positions 2 and 3 and a ketone in position 4 of the C ring. Most flavones of vegetables and fruits have a hydroxyl group in position 5 of the A ring, while the hydroxylation in other positions for the most part in position 7 of the A ring or 3′ and 4′ of the B ring may vary according to the taxonomic classification of the particular vegetable or fruit. Glycosylation occurs primarily on positions 5 and 7, methylation and acylation on the hydroxyl groups of the B ring. Some flavones, such as nobiletin and tangeretin, are polymethoxylated.

Apigenin

Apigenin has been reported to reduce serum insulin and thyroid hormone along with reducing hyperglycemia and hepatic glucose 6-phaspatase activity in diabetic rats (Rauter et al., 2010). In addition it also showed improvement in antioxidant status in rats and reduced lipid peroxidation in alloxan-induced diabetic rats (Panda and Kar, 2007). Additionally it has been reported to protect pancreatic β-cells from oxidative damage (Suh et al., 2012). Furthermore a mechanistic study uncovered the role of apigenin in reducing blood sugar level in rats. It was found that apigenin stimulated insulin secretion in diabetic rats glucose uptake in soleus muscle of rat by regulating insulin transduction mechanism (Cazarolli et al., 2009). It is well known that increased cellular NAD + level has a beneficial role in the metabolic disorder including diabetes, due to activation of Sirtuin and inhibition of CD38 which is associated with regulation of protein acetylation/deacetylation processes. Apigenin was found to reduce global protein acetylation and increased NAD + level in obese mice (Escande et al., 2013). Moreover it is also reported to have DPP-IV inhibitory activity which is nowadays considered as a major therapeutic target for the type 2 diabetes treatment (Fan et al., 2013). Vicenin-2, a glycoside of apigenin, was also found to reduce formation of AGE which plays a major role in the development of diabetes and associated complications (Islam et al., 2014). It has also been found to induce FOXO1 which is an important mediator of insulin signal transduction (Bumke-Vogt et al., 2014). Hyperglycemia-induced endothelial dysfunction is an early stage of development of atheroscloric vascular diseases. In the initial stage various adhesion molecules such as vascular cell adhesion molecule-1, platelet/endothelial cell adhesion molecule-1, and intercellular adhesion molecule-1 expressed on the endothelial cell surface. In addition increased plasma level of TNF-α in diabetes activates leukocyte migration to endothelium which ultimately affects endothelial cells junctions and cytoskeleton. Apigenin was reported to suppressed adhesion of U937 cells by inhibiting expression of VCAM1, IKKα, and IKKε/IKKi as well as by regulating NF-kβ activation (Yamagata et al., 2010).

Luteolin

Luteolin 5-*O*-beta rutinoside was found to reduce glycemia level and increased insulin level in blood of STZ-induced diabetic rats (Zarzuelo et al., 1996). Alpha-glycosidase is involved in the carbohydrate metabolism and hence its inhibitors reduce postprandial glucose by delaying absorption of glucose. Luteolin was found to be a strong inhibitor of α-glucosidase, and also reduced insulin resistance by suppressing SREBP1 expression as well as protects pancreatic β-cell functions and reduce gluconeogenic capacity in diabetics (Kwon et al., 2015; Bumke-Vogt et al., 2014). Kim et al. (2014) reported that luteolin inhibited NF-kβ activation and subsequently reduced production of proinflammatory cytokines which plays a major role in diabetic complications. Chronic hyperglycemia leads to generation of ROS; this damages the function of various bioactive mediators in endothelium such as nitric oxide, endothelin, and prostacyclin which ultimately affects endothelial functions. Luteolin has been reported to protect against endothelial dysfunctions by reducing risk of impaired endothelial-dependent relaxation in diabetic rats via NOS-NO pathway (Qian et al., 2010; El-Bassossy et al., 2013) and improved cardiac function as well as lipid profile by reducing mitochondrial oxidative stress (Azevedo et al., 2010; Sun et al., 2012). In addition it was also found to reduce risk of cardiomyopathy in diabetes (Wang et al., 2012b). A study by Wang et al. (2011) reported that luteolin protects against oxidative stress-induced diabetic nephropathy via its antioxidant mechanism. Moreover it was also found to improve neuronal functions in diabetic encephalopathy and wound healing in diabetic rats (Liu et al., 2013; Lodhi and Singhai, 2013).

Baicalein

It was found to protect against diabetes via regulation of pancreatic β-cell function (Fu et al., 2014). it has been also found that baicalein reduced hypertension in diabetics by reducing formation of AGEs, as well as decreased NF-kβ activity and TNF α level in blood, and vascular inflammation by reducing oxidative stress, expression of cell adhesion molecules, monocyte adhesion, and vascular permeability in diabetic condition (Ku and Bae, 2015). It was found to reduce abnormality in vascular tissue and ganglion cells in diabetic retina (Yang et al., 2009). Furthermore, it was also reported to protect renal function via its antioxidant, antihyperglycemic, and antiinflammatory effect in diabetic animals (Ahad et al., 2014). It has been also studied in diabetic neuropathy and it was found to attenuated diabetic neuropathy via inhibiting activation of p38 MAPK and reducing oxidative stress (Yorek, 2011). Recently it has been reported to protect against cognitive deficit in diabetic rat through regulating PI3K/Akt/GSK3β signaling pathway (Qi et al., 2015).

Isoflavones

Isoflavones are phytoestrogens found mainly in the plants belonging to family Fabaceae (ie, Leguminosae). Different legumes belonging to this family such as soy beans, barley, fava beans, kudzu, lupine, broccoli, peanut, and cauliflower are the major sources of the natural isoflavones (Prasad et al., 2010). Genistin, daidzin, and glycetin are the main isoflavones which are present in glycosylated form (Coward et al., 1993; Axelson et al., 1984). The genistein, daidzein, and glycitein are the biologically active aglycones of these isoflavones, respectively (Heinonen et al., 2003). Other isoflavones present in legumes are biochanin A and formononetin which gets converted to the more potent genistein and daidzein after 4′-*O*-demethylation (Tolleson et al., 2002).

Various studies have reported the antidiabetic activity of isoflavones. It is also reported to have their effectiveness in management of various complications of diabetes. Following are the isoflavones showing effectiveness in diabetes and its complications.

Genistein

Genistein, an important isoflavone, is reported to possess antidiabetic activity. Numerous studies which have carried out the mechanistic have demonstrated that genistein has direct effects on β-cell proliferation and glucose-stimulated insulin secretion (Gilberta and Liu, 2013; Liu et al., 2006; Fu et al., 2010). Genistein is also found effective in treatment of diabetes-related renal dysfunctions (Ibrahim et al., 2010) (Fig. 5.3).

Chalcones

Chalcones (1,3-diaryl-2-propen-1-ones) are the first isolable open chained compounds formed in flavonoid biosynthesis, having two aromatic rings connected by three carbon α,β-unsaturated carbonyl systems. They are abundantly found in citrus fruits, vegetables, and various plant genera such

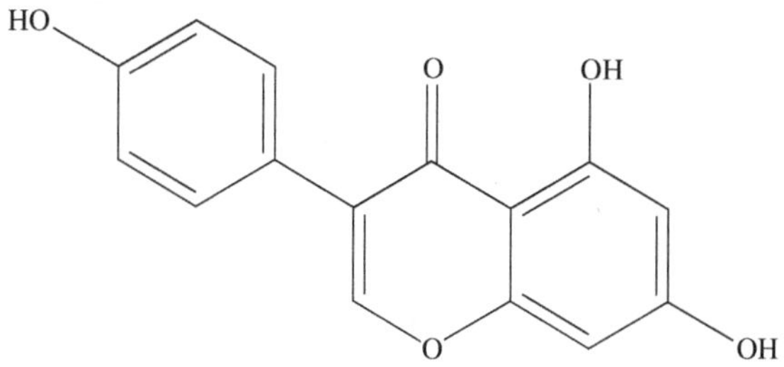

FIGURE 5.3 Structure of genistein.

as *Glycyrrhiza, Humulus, Sophora, Angelica, Scutellaria, Ficus, Morus, Dorstenia, Artocarpus*, and many more. This class of flavonoids attribute interesting spectrum of biological activity includes antioxidant, antifungal, antiviral, antibacterial, antiprotozoal, antitumor, cytotoxic, antidiabetic, cardioprotective, and neuroprotective (Di Carlo et al., 1999; Yadav et al., 2011).

Aspalathin

Aspalathin is a dihydrochalcone present in the South African plant species *Aspalathus linearis* (Rooibos). Several studies are stated to antidiabetic effect of aspalathin. Impaired carbohydrate metabolism is the leading cause of hyperglycemia in diabetes. It is observed that aspalathin improved glucose homeostasis in type 2 diabetic rats by stimulating insulin secretion from β-cells and increased glucose uptake in muscle tissues (Kawano et al., 2009; Muller et al., 2012). It also reduced glucose production and lipogenesis by reducing gene expression of related hepatic enzymes in vitro. Furthermore it also activated AMPK and stimulated GLUT4 translocation to plasma membrane (Son et al., 2013). Increased level of free fatty acids such as palmitate in skeletal muscle is responsible for insulin resistance and damage glucose disposal from peripheral circulation. Mazibuko et al. (2013) reported that aspalathin-rich fraction and aspalathin both down regulated PKC Θ activation which is responsible for palmitate-induced insulin resistance in C2C12 skeletal muscle cells. Diabetes is an independent risk factor for the diabetic cardiomyopathy. Uncontrolled hyperglycemia increases oxidative stress and damages myocardium which ultimately leads to cardiomyocytes apoptosis and myocardial dysfunctions. Recently it is reported that aqueous extract of fermented rooibos (rich in aspalathin) protects cardiomyocytes of diabetic rats by reducing oxidative stress and ischemia (Dludla et al., 2014). Uncontrolled hyperglycemia leads to vascular inflammation in diabetes and damage vascular tissues. NF-kβ is a transcription factor involved in inflammatory processes. It induces proinflammatory cytokines and chemokines and affects cell adhesion molecules. Aspalathin reduced vascular inflammation by inhibiting NF-kβ in human endothelial cells (Ku et al., 2015).

Butein

It is a 3,4,2,4′-tetrahydrochalcone derived from *Rhus verniciflua.* It is reported to have antiinflammatory, antioxidant, anticancer, antiparasitic, and analgesic activity. It is also shown to have antidiabetic activity and tested in diabetic complications (Kang et al., 2004; Yu et al., 1995; Lim et al., 2001). Inducible nitric oxide synthase is one of the factor responsible for pancreatic β-cell damage. Jeong et al. (2011) studied effect of butein on INS-1 cell and reported that it prevents inducible nitric oxide synthase expression, NF-kβ translocation, cytokine-induced nitric oxide production and also inhibited glucose-induced insulin secretion thus it can be used to prevent pancreatic β-cell damage in type 1 diabetes (Jeong et al., 2011). In similar study it inhibited adipocyte inflammation by inhibiting NF-kβ/MAPK-dependent transcriptional activity. It also enhances leptin signaling and also reduced glucose intolerance by inhibiting IKKβ/NF-κB signaling. Inflammation in adipose tissue is common in type 2 diabetes, and nowadays it is considered as therapeutic target for type 2 diabetes so butein may considered as therapeutic agent to treat adipocyte inflammation associated with type 2 diabetes (Wang et al., 2014).

Isoliquiritigenin

It is a 2′,4′4′-three hydroxyl chalcone isolated from liquorice and has been described to have antiallergic, antitumor, antiplatelet, and vasorelaxant activity (Chen et al., 2009). Isoliquiritigenin inhibited aldose reductase an enzyme which plays a crucial role in development of diabetic angiopathy by accumulating sorbitol via polyol pathway (Aida et al., 1990). A potent vasodilator, prostacyclin, has been reduced in diabetic condition, this leads to development of atherosclerotic vascular complications in diabetics (Kazama et al., 1987). Wakasugi et al. (1991) reported that isoliquiritigenin increased vascular synthesis of prostacyclin. cAMP levels get reduced peripheral nerves in diabetic neuropathy. It has been reported that isoliquiritigenin increased cAMP level in peripheral nerve via regulating polyol pathway (Shindo et al., 1992). Mesangial fibrosis and glomerulosclerosis in diabetic nephropathy results in end-stage renal failure. Li et al. (2010) reported that isoliqiritigenin retarded TGF-β1-SMAD signaling transduction and reduced mesangial matrix accumulation so it may provide protection against renal damage. Furthermore isoliquiritigenin isolated from heartwood of *Dalbergia odorifera* inhibited α-glucosidase, which is activated in type 2 diabetes (Zhao et al., 2013).

Phloretin/phloridzin

It is a dihydrochalcone with C6-C3-C6 skeleton structure with a β-D-glucopyranose moiety at secondary position. It was used as antipyretic agent and first time isolated from stem bark of apple tree. It has been reported to have antioxidant, antiobesity, and antidiabetic activity. It is extensively studied for effects on glucose uptake and diabetes (Gosch et al., 2010). Phlorizin is a competitive inhibitor of sodium-glucose linked transporter 1 (SGLT1) (in intestine) and SGLT2 (in kidney) (Panayotova-Heiermann et al., 1995).

BIFLAVONOIDS

Biflavonoids are dimer of various classes of flavonoids which are connected with either C-C or C-O-C bond. The most commonly observed biflavonoid in nature is of flavone–flavone, flavone–flavonol, and flavonone–flavone type. They are less widely distributed in nature. Only limited species of the plants have biflavonoid, and the most common plant species which contain biflavonoids are *Selaginella* species, *G. biloba* and *Garcinia kola.* This class of flavonoids has multiple types of biological and pharmacological properties emanating from different types of chemical substitution such as hydroxyl and methoxyl groups. They are reported to possess antimicrobial, antioxidant, antiinflammatory, antiviral, antifungal, antiacetylcholinesterase, hepatoprotective, antiallergic, immunosuppressive activity, and many other activities (Lakey-Beitia et al., 2014; Thapa and Chi, 2015). Biflovonoids are also reported to have antidiabetic activity (Adaramoye and Adeyemi, 2006). There are numerous biflavonoids such as ginkgetin, sequoiaflavone, bilobetin, sciadopitysin, taiwanhomoflavone-A, cryptomerin B, podoverinine B, morelloflavone, and many more isolated from various plant species. Majority of these biflavonoids having antioxidant activity but limited biflavonoids are investigated in diabetic and its complications, and this includes amentoflavone and kolaviron.

Amentoflavone

It is a biflavonoid of apigenin(3′,8″-bisapigenin) present in *Selaginella tamariscina*, *Biophytum sensitivum*, *Calophyllum flavoramulum*, *Cycas pectinata*, and many other plant species (Liao et al., 2015; Ferchichi et al., 2012). It is reported to possess various pharmacological activity which includes antiviral, antidepressant, antioxidant, antiinflammatory, nitric oxide synthase inhibitor, inhibit lipid peroxidation, and also inactivate NF-kβ (Woo et al., 2005; Banerjee et al., 2002; Lin et al., 1999; Cholbi et al., 1991; Baureithel et al., 1997). Recently it is reported that amentoflavone is a potent antidiabetic agent by inhibiting α-glucosidase and α-amylase enzymes in diabetic rats. α-glucosidase and α-amylase are the two major enzymes which are associated with carbohydrate metabolism. Inhibition of these two enzymes by amentoflavone leads to reduction in glucose absorption and ultimately normalizes blood glucose level (Laishram et al., 2015). AGE is always a major factor involved in pathogenesis of diabetes and its vascular complications. Amentoflavone also demonstrated anti-AGEs activity by its antioxidant mechanism which includes free radical scavenging and divalent metal ion chelation (Ferchichi et al., 2012).

Kolaviron

It is potent antioxidant biflavonoid complex (GB 1 + GB 2+ kolaflavanone) present in seeds of *G. kola.* It has been demonstrated to be an anti-inflammatory, antigenotoxic, and hepatoprotective agent (Farombi et al., 2013; Ijomone and Obi, 2013). It is also reported to have antidiabetic and antilipidemic activity. Kolaviron complex demonstrated significant antidiabetic effect when studied in STZ-induced diabetic rat and alloxan diabetic rabbit. It also improved cardiac, renal, and liver marker in diabetic rats and inhibited aldose reductase in alloxan diabetic rabbit (Adaramoye, 2012; Iwu et al., 1990).

ANTHOCYANINS

Anthocyanins are water-soluble glycosides or acylglycosides of polyhydroxyl. They are derivatives of 2-phenylbenzopyrylium or flavylium salts, which forms an important group of biosynthesized pigments via phenylpropanoid pathway. Nearly, 700 different anthocyanins have been identified so far (Andersen and Jordheim, 2010; Li et al., 2013) (Fig. 5.4).

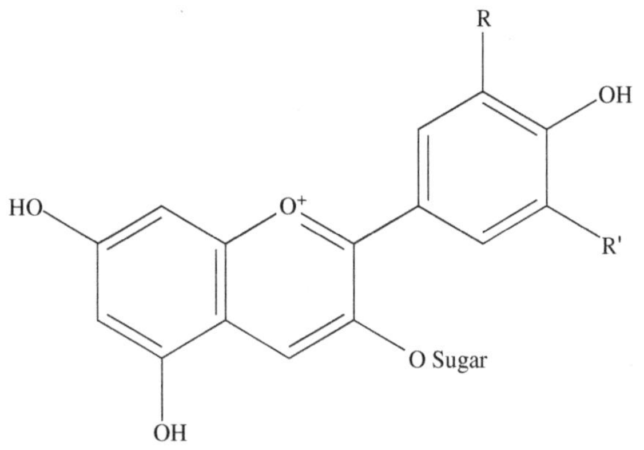

■ **FIGURE 5.4** Common structure of anthocyanins.

Recently Jayaprakasam et al. (2005) showed that anthocyanins and anthocyanidins can induce insulin release from pancreatic β-cells. Anthocyanins are reported to have potential for treatment of diabetic retinopathy (Nabavi et al., 2015). Anthocyanin protects against diabetes-related endothelial dysfunction as well as increases adiponectin secretion (Liu et al., 2014).

SUMMARY

Diabetes and hence the diabetic complications are highly prevalent, demanding special attention towards finding most effective drugs. From ages, nature has provided numerous drugs for treatment of a range of disorders which includes diabetes. Chemical compounds from natural source have also served as lead molecules for development of new chemical entities which are developed into medicine. Plants are rich source of variety of chemical compounds which are classified under various phytochemical classes. Flavonoid is one of the most important classes of phytochemicals reported to have several biological activities. Studies showed that different compounds from subclasses of flavonoids possess potential to treat the diabetes and to manage the complications of it. Exploring the use of different flavonoids and finding the molecular mechanisms for its antidiabetic activity and effect in diabetic complications will help to develop a better treatment regimen.

REFERENCES

Adaramoye, O.A., 2012. Antidiabetic effect of kolaviron, a biflavonoid complex isolatedfrom *Garcinia kola* seeds, in Wistar rats. Afr. Health Sci. 12 (4), 498–506.

Adaramoye, O.A., Adeyemi, E.O., 2006. Hypoglycaemic and hypolipidaemic effects offractions from kolaviron, a biflavonoid complex from *Garcinia kola* instreptozotocin-induced diabetes mellitus rats. J. Pharm. Pharmacol. 58 (1), 121–128.

Agrawal, Y.O., Sharma, P.K., Shrivastava, B., Arya, D.S., Goyal, S.N., 2014. Hesperidin blunts streptozotocin-isoproternol induced myocardial toxicity in rats by altering of PPAR-γ receptor. Chem. Biol. Interact. 219, 211–220.

Ahad, A., Mujeeb, M., Ahsan, H., Siddiqui, W.A., 2014. Prophylactic effect of baicaleinagainst renal dysfunction in type 2 diabetic rats. Biochimie 106, 101–110.

Aida, K., Tawata, M., Shindo, H., Onaya, T., Sasaki, H., Yamaguchi, T., et al., 1990. Isoliquiritigenin: a new aldose reductase inhibitor from glycyrrhizae radix. Planta Med. 56 (3), 254–258.

Ajay, M., Achike, F.I., Mustafa, A.M., Mustafa, M.R., 2006. Effect of quercetin on alteredvascular reactivity in aortas isolated from streptozotocin-induced diabetic rats. Diabetes Res. Clin. Pract. 73 (1), 1–7.

Akiyama, S., Katsumata, S., Suzuki, K., Ishimi, Y., Wu, J., Uehara, M., 2010. Dietary hesperidin exerts hypoglycemic and hypolipidemic effects in streptozotocin-induced marginal type 1 diabetic rats. J. Clin. Biochem. Nutr. 46 (1), 87–92.

Andersen, M., Jordheim, M., 2010. Chemistry of flavonoid-based colors in plants. In: Mander, L.N., Liu, H.W. (Eds.), Comprehensive Natural Products II: Chemistry and Biology Elsevier, Oxford, pp. 547–614.

Andrade, C.A., Wiedenfeld, H., Revilla, M.C., Sergio, I.A., 2000. Hypoglycemic effect of *Equisetum myriochaetum* aerial parts on streptozotocin diabetic rats. J. Ethnopharmacol. 72 (1–2), 129–133.

Annapurna, A., Reddy, C.S., Akondi, R.B., Rao, S.R., 2009. Cardioprotective actions of two bioflavonoids, quercetin and rutin, in experimental myocardial infarction in both normal and streptozotocin-induced type I diabetic rats. J. Pharm. Pharmacol. 61 (10), 1365–1374.

Asgary, S., Naderi, G., Sarrafzadegan, N., Ghassemi, N., Boshtam, M., Rafie, M., et al., 1999. Anti-oxidant effect of flavonoids on hemoglobin glycosylation. Pharm. Acta Helv. 73 (5), 223–226.

Axelson, M., Sjövall, J., Gustafsson, B.E., Setchell, K.D., 1984. Soya—a dietarysource of the non-steroidal oestrogenequol in man and animals. J. Endocrinol. 102, 49–56.

Azevedo, M.F., Camsari, C., Sá, C.M., Lima, C.F., Fernandes-Ferreira, M., Pereira-Wilson, C., 2010. Ursolic acid and luteolin-7-glucoside improve lipid profiles and increase liver glycogen content through glycogen synthase kinase-3. Phytother. Res. 2, S220–S224.

Banerjee, T., Valacchi, G., Ziboh, V.A., van der Vliet, A., 2002. Inhibition of TNFalpha-induced cyclooxygenase-2 expression by amentoflavone through suppression of NF-kappaB activation in A549 cells. Mol. Cell Biochem. 238, 105–110.

Baureithel, K.H., Buter, K.B., Engesser, A., Burkard, W., Schaffner, W., 1997. Inhibition of benzodiazepine binding in vitro by amentoflavone, a constituent of various species of Hypericum. Pharm. Acta Helv. 72 (3), 153–157.

Bhutada, P., Mundhada, Y., Bansod, K., Bhutada, C., Tawari, S., Dixit, P., et al., 2010. Ameliorative effect of quercetin on memory dysfunction in streptozotocin-induced diabetic rats. Neurobiol. Learn. Mem. 94 (3), 293–302.

Bonora, E., Formentini, G., Calcaterra, F., et al., 2002. HOMA-estimated insulin resistance is an independent predictor of cardiovascular disease in type 2 diabetic subjects: prospective data from the Verona Diabetes Complications Study. Diabetes Care 25, 1135–1141.

Brenner, B.M., Cooper, M.E., de Zeeuw, D., et al., 2001. Effects of losartan on renal and cardiovascular outcomes in patients with type 2 diabetes and nephropathy. N. Engl. J. Med. 345, 861–869.

Bumke-Vogt, C., Osterhoff, M.A., Borchert, A., Guzman-Perez, V., Sarem, Z., Birkenfeld, A.L., et al., 2014. The flavones apigenin and luteolin induce FOXO1 translocation but inhibit gluconeogenic and lipogenic gene expression in human cells. PLoS One 9 (8), e104321.

Buyken, A.E., Von, E.A., Schulte, H., et al., 2007. Type 2 diabetes mellitus and risk of coronary heart disease: results of the 10-year follow-up of the PROCAM Study. Eur. J. Cardiovasc. Prev. Rehabil. 14, 230–236.

Cade, W.T., 2008. Diabetes-related microvascular and macrovascular diseases in the physical therapy setting. Phys. Ther. 88 (11), 1322–1335.

Cai, E.P., Lin, J.K., 2009. Epigallocatechingallate (EGCG) and rutin suppress the glucotoxicity through activating IRS2 and AMPK signaling in rat pancreatic beta cells. J. Agric. Food Chem. 57 (20), 9817–9827.

Cazarolli, L.H., Folador, P., Moresco, H.H., Brighente, I.M., Pizzolatti, M.G., Silva, F.R., 2009. Mechanism of action of the stimulatory effect ofapigenin-6-C-(2″-O-alpha-l-rhamnopyranosyl)-beta-L-fucopyranoside on 14C-glucoseuptake. Chem. Biol. Interact. 179 (2–3), 407–412.

Cervantes-Laurean, D., Schramm, D.D., Jacobson, E.L., Halaweish, I., Bruckner, G.G., Boissonneault, G.A., 2006. Inhibition of advanced glycation end product formation on collagen by rutin and its metabolites. J. Nutr. Biochem. 17, 531–540.

Challa, S.R., Akula, A., Metla, S., Gopal, P.N., 2011. Partial role of nitric oxide in infarctsize limiting effect of quercetin and rutin against ischemia-reperfusion injuryin normal and diabetic rats. Indian J. Exp. Biol. 49 (3), 207–210.

Chebil, L., Humeau, C., Falcimaigne, A., Engasser, J., Ghoul, M., 2006. Enzymatic acylation of flavonoids. Process Biochem. 41, 2237–2251.

Chen, G., Zhu, L., Liu, Y., Zhou, Q., Chen, H., Yang, J., 2009. Isoliquiritigenin, a flavonoidfrom licorice, plays a dual role in regulating gastrointestinal motility in vitro and in vivo. Phytother. Res. 23 (4), 498–506.

Chen, P., Chen, J.B., Chen, W.Y., Zheng, Q.L., Wang, Y.Q., Xu, X.J., 2012. Effects of quercetin onnuclear factor-κB p65 expression in renal ubiquitin-proteasome system of diabeticrats. Zhonghua Nei Ke Za Zhi 51 (6), 460–465.

Chen, S., Hong, S.W., Iglesias-de la Cruz, M.C., et al., 2001. The key role of the transforming growth factor-beta system in the pathogenesis of diabetic nephropathy. Ren. Fail. 23, 471–481.

Choi, E.M., Kim, Y.H., 2008. Hesperetin attenuates the highly reducing sugar-triggered inhibition of osteoblast differentiation. Cell Biol. Toxicol. 24 (3), 225–231.

Choi, H.N., Kang, M.J., Lee, S.J., Kim, J.I., 2014. Ameliorative effect of myricetin on insulin resistance in mice fed a high-fat, high-sucrose diet. Nutr. Res. Pract. 8 (5), 544–549.

Cholbi, M.R., Paya, M., Alcaraz, M.J., 1991. Inhibitory effects of phenolic compounds on CCl4-induced microsomal lipid peroxidation. Experientia 47 (2), 195–199.

Cook, N.C., Samman, S., 1996. Flavonoids: chemistry, metabolism, cardioprotective effects and dietary sources. Nutr. Biochem. 7, 66–76.

Coward, L., Barnes, N.C., Setchell, K.D.R., Barnes, S., 1993. Genistein, daidzein, andtheir beta-glycoside conjugates: antitumor isoflavones in soybean foods from American and Asian diets. J. Agric. Food Chem. 41, 1961–1967.

Cushnie, T.P.T., Lamb, A.J., 2005. Antimicrobial activity of flavonoids. Int. J. Antimicrob. Agents 26, 343–356.

Dias, A.S., Porawski, M., Alonso, M., Marroni, N., Collado, P.S., González-Gallego, J., 2005. Quercetin decreases oxidative stress, NF-kappaB activation, and iNOS over expression in liver of streptozotocin-induced diabetic rats. J. Nutr. 135 (10), 2299–2304.

Di Carlo, G., Mascolo, N., Izzo, A.A., Capasso, F., 1999. Flavonoids: old and new aspects of a class of natural therapeutic drugs. Life Sci. 65, 337–353.

Di Maggio, G., Ciaceri, G., 1958. Effect of quercetin on blood sugar levels inalloxan diabetes. Rass. Clin. Ter. 57 (1), 14–16.

Dludla, P.V., Muller, C.J., Louw, J., Joubert, E., Salie, R., Opoku, A.R., et al., 2014. The cardioprotective effect of an aqueous extract of fermented rooibos (*Aspalathus linearis*) on cultured cardiomyocytes derived from diabetic rats. Phytomedicine 21 (5), 595–601.

Drummond, K., Mauer, M., 2002. The early natural history of nephropathy in type 1 diabetes, II: early renal structural changes in type 1 diabetes. Diabetes 51, 1580–1587.

Dyck, P.J., Kratz, K.M., Karnes, J.L., et al., 1993. The prevalence by staged severity of various types of diabetic neuropathy, retinopathy, and nephropathy in a population-based cohort: the Rochester Diabetic Neuropathy Study. Neurology 43, 817–824.

Eid, H.M., Martineau, L.C., Saleem, A., Muhammad, A., Vallerand, D., Benhaddou-Andaloussi, A., et al., 2010. Stimulation of AMP-activated protein kinase and enhancement of basal glucose uptake in musclecells by quercetin and quercetin glycosides, active principles of the antidiabetic medicinal plant *Vaccinium vitis-idaea*. Mol. Nutr. Food Res. 54 (7), 991–1003.

Eid, H.M., Nachar, A., Thong, F., Sweeney, G., Haddad, P.S., 2015. The molecular basis of theantidiabetic action of quercetin in cultured skeletal muscle cells and hepatocytes. Pharmacogn. Mag. 11 (41), 74–81.

El-Bassossy, H.M., Abo-Warda, S.M., Fahmy, A., 2013. Chrysin and luteolin attenuate diabetes-induced impairment in endothelial-dependent relaxation: effect on lipid profile, AGEs and NO generation. Phytother. Res. 27 (11), 1678–1684.

Elbe, H., Vardi, N., Esrefoglu, M., Ates, B., Yologlu, S., Taskapan, C., 2015. Amelioration of streptozotocin-induced diabetic nephropathy by melatonin, quercetin, and resveratrol in rats. Hum. Exp. Toxicol. 34 (1), 100–113.

Escande, C., Nin, V., Price, N.L., Capellini, V., Gomes, A.P., Barbosa, M.T., et al., 2013. Flavonoid apigenin is an inhibitor of the NAD+ aseCD38: implications for cellular NAD+ metabolism, protein acetylation, and treatment of metabolic syndrome. Diabetes 62 (4), 1084–1093.

Fan, J., Johnson, M.H., Lila, M.A., Yousef, G., de Mejia, E.G., 2013. Berry and citrus phenolic compounds inhibit dipeptidyl peptidase IV: implications in diabetes management. Evid. Based Complement Alternat. Med. 2013, 479505.

Fang, X.K., Gao, J., Zhu, D.N., 2008. Kaempferol and quercetin isolated from *Euonymus alatus* improve glucose uptake of 3T3-L1 cells without adipogenesis activity. Life Sci. 82 (11–12), 615–622.

Farombi, E.O., Adedara, I.A., Ajayi, B.O., Ayepola, O.R., Egbeme, E.E., 2013. Kolaviron, a natural antioxidant and anti-inflammatory phytochemical prevents dextran sulphatesodium-induced colitis in rats. Basic Clin. Pharmacol. Toxicol. 113 (1), 49–55.

Ferchichi, L., Derbré, S., Mahmood, K., Touré, K., Guilet, D., Litaudon, M., et al., 2012. Bioguided fractionation and isolation of natural inhibitors of advanced glycation end-products (AGEs) from *Calophyllum flavoramulum*. Phytochemistry 78, 98–106.

Ferreira, P.E., Lopes, C.R., Alves, A.M., Alves, É.P., Linden, D.R., Zanoni, J.N., et al., 2013. Diabetic neuropathy: an evaluation of the use of quercetin in the cecum of rats. World J. Gastroenterol. 19 (38), 6416–6426.

Fu, Y., Luo, J., Jia, Z., Zhen, W., Zhou, K., Gilbert, E., et al., 2014. Baicalein protects against type 2 diabetes via promoting Islet β-cell function in obese diabetic mice. Int. J. Endocrinol. 2014, 846742.

Fu, Z., Zhang, W., Zhen, W., Lum, H., Nadler, J., Bassaganya-Riera, J., et al., 2010. Genistein induces pancreatic-cell proliferation through activation of multiple signaling pathways and prevents insulin-deficient diabetes in mice. Endocrinology 151 (7), 3026–3037.

Garud, M.S., Kulkarni, Y.A., 2014. Hyperglycemia to nephropathy via transforming growth factor beta. Curr. Diabetes Rev. 10 (3), 182–189.

Ghaffari, M.A., Mojab, S., 2007. Influence of flavonols as in vitro on low density lipoprotein glycation. Iran. Biomed. J. 11 (3), 185–191.

Gilberta, E.R., Liu, D., 2013. Anti-diabetic functions of soy isoflavone genistein: mechanisms underlying effects on pancreatic β-cell function. Food Funct. 4 (2), 200–212.

Gomes, I.B., Porto, M.L., Santos, M.C., Campagnaro, B.P., Pereira, T.M., Meyrelles, S.S., et al., 2014. Renoprotective, anti-oxidative and anti-apoptotic effects of orallow-dose quercetin in the C57BL/6J model of diabetic nephropathy. Lipids Health Dis. 13, 184.

Gosch, C., Halbwirth, H., Stich, K., 2010. Phloridzin: biosynthesis, distribution andphysiological relevance in plants. Phytochemistry 71 (8–9), 838–843.

Guerrero-Romero, F., Rodriguez-Moran, M., 1999. Proteinuria is an independent risk factor for ischemic stroke in non-insulin dependent diabetes mellitus. Stroke 30, 1787–1791.

Guimaraes, J.F., Muzio, B.P., Rosa, C.M., Nascimento, A.F., Sugizaki, M.M., Fernandes, A.A., et al., 2015. Rutin administration attenuates myocardial dysfunction in diabetic rats. Cardiovasc. Diabetol. 14, 90.

Hao, H.H., Shao, Z.M., Tang, D.Q., Lu, Q., Chen, X., Yin, X.X., et al., 2012. Preventive effects of rutin on the development of experimental diabetic nephropathy in rats. Life Sci. 91 (19–20), 959–967.

Harding, S., 2003. Extracts from "concise clinical evidence": diabetic retinopathy. Br. Med. J. 326, 1023–1025.

Heinonen, S.M., Hoikkala, A., Wähälä, K., Adlercreutz, H., 2003. Metabolism of the soy isoflavones daidzein, genistein and glycitein in human subjects. Identification of new metabolites having an intact isoflavonoid skeleton. J. Steroid Biochem. Mol. Biol. 87, 285–299.

Hnatyszyn, O., Miño, J., Ferraro, G., Acevedo, C., 2002. The hypoglycemic effect of *Phyllanthus sellowianus* fractions in streptozotocin-induced diabetic mice. Phytomedicine 9 (6), 556–559.

Hsu, C.Y., Shih, H.Y., Chia, Y.C., Lee, C.H., Ashida, H., Lai, Y.K., et al., 2014. Rutin potentiates insulin receptor kinase to enhance insulin-dependent glucose transporter 4 translocation. Mol. Nutr. Food Res. 58 (6), 1168–1176.

Huang, H., Fu, J., Tian, H., 2005. Effects of quercetin and enalapril on amount of PDGF-B and VEGF-1 in kidney of diabetic rats. Sheng Wu Yi Xue Gong Cheng Xue Za Zhi 22 (4), 791–794.

Ibrahim, A.S., El-Shishtawy, M.M., Peña, A., Liou, G.I., 2010. Genistein attenuates retinal inflammation associated with diabetes by targeting of microglial activation. Mol. Vis. 16, 2033–2042.

IDF, 2013. IDF Diabetes Atlas, sixth ed International Diabetes Federation, Brussels.

Ijomone, O.M., Obi, A.U., 2013. Kolaviron, isolated from *Garcinia kola*, inhibits acetylcholinesterase activities in the hippocampus and striatum of wistar rats. Ann. Neurosci. 20 (2), 42–46.

Islam, M.N., Ishita, I.J., Jung, H.A., Choi, J.S., 2014. Vicenin 2 isolated from *Artemisia capillaris* exhibited potent anti-glycation properties. Food Chem. Toxicol. 69, 55–62.

Iwu, M.M., Igboko, O.A., Okunji, C.O., Tempesta, M.S., 1990. Antidiabetic and aldose reductase activities of biflavanones of *Garcinia kola*. J. Pharm. Pharmacol. 42 (4), 290–292.

Jayaprakasam, B., Vareed, S.K., Olson, L.K., Nair, M.G., 2005. Insulin secretion by bioactive anthocyanins and anthocyanidins present in fruits. J. Agric. Food Chem. 53, 28–31.

Je, H.D., Shin, C.Y., Park, S.Y., Yim, S.H., Kum, C., Huh, I.H., et al., 2002. Combination of vitamin C and rutin on neuropathy and lung damage of diabetes mellitus rats. Arch. Pharm. Res. 25 (2), 184–190.

Jeong, G.S., Lee, D.S., Song, M.Y., Park, B.H., Kang, D.G., Lee, H.S., et al., 2011. Butein from *Rhus verniciflua* protects pancreatic β cells against cytokine-induced toxicity mediated by inhibition of nitric oxide formation. Biol. Pharm. Bull. 34 (1), 97–102.

Jeong, S.M., Kang, M.J., Choi, H.N., Kim, J.H., Kim, J.I., 2012. Quercetin ameliorates hyperglycemia and dyslipidemia and improves antioxidant status in type 2 diabetic db/db mice. Nutr. Res. Pract. 6 (3), 201–207.

Jorge, A.P., Horst, H., de Sousa, E., Pizzolatti, M.G., Silva, F.R., 2004. Insulinomimetic effects of kaempferitrin on glycaemia and on 14C-glucose uptake in rat soleus muscle. Chem. Biol. Interact. 149 (2–3), 89–96.

Juan, Y.S., Chuang, S.M., Long, C.Y., Lin, R.J., Liu, K.M., Wu, W.J., et al., 2012. Protein kinase C inhibitor prevents renal apoptotic and fibrotic changes in response to partial ureteric obstruction. BJU Int. 110, 283–292.

Jung, U.J., Lee, M.K., Jeong, K.S., Choi, M.S., 2004. The hypoglycemic effects of hesperidin and naringin are partly mediated by hepatic glucose-regulating enzymes in C57BL/KsJ-db/db mice. J. Nutr. 134 (10), 2499–2503.

Kakadiya, J., Mulani, H., Shah, N., 2010. Protective effect of hesperidin on cardiovascular complication in experimentally induced myocardial infarction in diabetes in rats. J. Basic Clin. Pharm. 1 (2), 85–91.

Kamalakkannan, N., Prince, P.S., 2006. Antihyperglycaemic and antioxidant effect ofrutin, apolyphenolic flavonoid, in streptozotocin-induced diabetic wistar rats. Basic Clin. Pharmacol. Toxicol. 98 (1), 97–103.

Kamalakkannan, N., Stanely Mainzen, P.P., 2006. Rutin improves the antioxidant status in streptozotocin-induced diabetic rat tissues. Mol. Cell Biochem. 293 (1–2), 211–219.

Kang, D.G., Lee, A.S., Mun, Y.J., Woo, W.H., Kim, Y.C., Sohn, E.J., et al., 2004. Butein ameliorates renal concentrating ability in cisplatin-induced acute renal failure in rats. Biol. Pharm. Bull. 27 (3), 366–370.

Kanter, M., Aktas, C., Erboga, M., 2012. Protective effects of quercetin again stapoptosis and oxidative stress in streptozotocin-induced diabetic rat testis. Food Chem. Toxicol. 50 (3–4), 719–725.

Kappel, V.D., Zanatta, L., Postal, B.G., Silva, F.R., 2013. Rutin potentiates calcium uptake via voltage-dependent calcium channel associated with stimulation of glucose uptake in skeletal muscle. Arch. Biochem. Biophys. 532 (2), 55–60.

Kawano, A., Nakamura, H., Hata, S., Minakawa, M., Miura, Y., Yagasaki, K., 2009. Hypoglycemic effect of aspalathin, a rooibos tea component from *Aspalathus linearis*, in type 2 diabetic model db/db mice. Phytomedicine 16 (5), 437–443.

Kazama, Y., Kanemaru, Y., Noguchi, T., Onaya, T., 1987. Reevaluation of circulating prostacyclin and thromboxane in diabetes. Prostaglandins Leukot. Med. 26, 115–122.

Kerimi, A., Jailanim, F., Williamson, G., 2015. Modulation of cellular glucose metabolism in human HepG2 cells by combinations of structurally related flavonoids. Mol. Nutr. Food Res. 59 (5), 894–906.

Kim, H.J., Lee, W., Yun, J.M., 2014. Luteolin inhibits hyperglycemia-induced proinflammatory cytokine production and its epigenetic mechanism in human monocytes. Phytother. Res. 28 (9), 1383–1391.

Kobori, M., Masumoto, S., Akimoto, Y., Takahashi, Y., 2009. Dietary quercetin alleviates diabetic symptoms and reduces streptozotocin-induced disturbance of hepatic gene expression in mice. Mol. Nutr. Food Res. 53 (7), 859–868.

Krishna, K.M., Annapurna, A., Gopal, G.S., Chalam, C.R., Madan, K., Kumar, V.K., et al., 2005. Partial reversal by rutin and quercetin of impaired cardiac function instreptozotocin-induced diabetic rats. Can. J. Physiol. Pharmacol. 83 (4), 343–355.

Ku, S.K., Bae, J.S., 2015. Baicalin, baicalein and wogonin inhibits high glucose-induced vascular inflammation in vitro and in vivo. BMB Rep 48, 519–524.

Ku, S.K., Kwak, S., Kim, Y., Bae, J.S., 2015. Aspalathin and Nothofagin from Rooibos (*Aspalathus linearis*) inhibits high glucose-induced inflammation in vitro and in vivo. Inflammation 38 (1), 445–455.

Kulkarni, Y.A., Garud, M.S., 2015. Effect of *Bauhinia variegata* Linn. (Caesalpiniaceae) extract in streptozotocin induced type I diabetic rats. Orient. Pharmacy Exp. Med. 15, 191–198.

Kumar, B., Gupta, S.K., Srinivasan, B.P., Nag, T.C., Srivastava, S., Saxena, R., et al., 2013. Hesperetin rescues retinal oxidative stress, neuroinflammation and apoptosis indiabetic rats. Microvasc. Res. 87, 65–74.

Kumar, S., Alagawadi, K.R., 2013. Anti-obesity effects of galangin, a pancreatic lipase inhibitor in cafeteria diet fed female rats. Pharm. Biol. 51 (5), 607–613.

Kwon, E.Y., Jung, U.J., Park, T., Yun, J.W., Choi, M.S., 2015. Luteolin attenuates hepatic steatosis and insulin resistance through the interplay between the liver and adipose tissue in mice with diet-induced obesity. Diabetes 64 (5), 1658–1669.

Laakso, M., 1999. Hyperglycemia and cardiovascular disease in type 2 diabetes. Diabetes 48, 937–942.

Lai, P.B., Zhang, L., Yang, L.Y., 2012. Quercetin ameliorates diabetic nephropathy by reducing the expressions of transforming growth factor-β1 and connective tissue growth factor in streptozotocin-induced diabetic rats. Ren. Fail. 34 (1), 83–87.

Laishram, S., Sheikh, Y., Moirangthem, D.S., Deb, L., Pal, B.C., Talukdar, N.C., et al., 2015. Anti-diabetic molecules from *Cycas pectinata* Griff. traditionally used by the Maiba-Maibi. Phytomedicine 22 (1), 23–26.

Lakey-Beitia, J., Berrocal, R., Rao, K.S., Durant, A.A., 2014. Polyphenols as therapeutic molecules in Alzheimer's disease through modulating amyloid pathways. Mol. Neurobiol.

Lehto, S., Niskanen, L., Ronnemaa, T., Laakso, M., 1998. Serum uric acid is a strong predictor of stroke in patients with non-insulin dependent diabetes mellitus. Stroke 29, 635–639.

Li, J., Kang, S.W., Kim, J.L., Sung, H.Y., Kwun, I.S., Kang, Y.H., 2010. Isoliquiritigenin entails blockade of TGF-beta1-SMAD signaling for retarding high glucose-induced mesangial matrix accumulation. J. Agric. Food Chem. 58 (5), 3205–3212.

Li, X., Ma, H., Huang, H., Li, D., Yao, S., 2013. Natural anthocyanins from phytoresources and their chemical researches. Nat. Prod. Res. 27 (4–5), 456–469.

Liang, W., Luo, Z., Ge, S., Li, M., Du, J., Yang, M., et al., 2011. Oral administration of quercetin inhibits bone loss in rat model of diabetic osteopenia. Eur. J. Pharmacol. 670 (1), 317–324.

Liao, S., Ren, Q., Yang, C., Zhang, T., Li, J., Wang, X., et al., 2015. Liquid chromatography-tandem mass spectrometry determination and pharmacokinetic analysis of amentoflavone and its conjugated metabolites in rats. J. Agric. Food Chem. 63 (7), 1957–1966.

Lim, S.S., Jung, S.H., Ji, J., Shin, K.H., Keum, S.R., 2001. Synthesis of flavonoids and their effects on aldose reductase and sorbitol accumulation in streptozotocin-induced diabetic rat tissues. J. Pharm. Pharmacol. 53 (5), 653–668.

Lin, Y.M., Flavin, M.T., Schure, R., Chen, F.C., Sidwell, R., Barnard, D.L., et al., 1999. Antiviral activities of biflavonoids. Planta Med. 65 (2), 120–125.

Liu, D., Zhen, W., Yang, Z., Carter, J.D., Si, H., Reynolds, K.A., 2006. Genistein acutely stimulates insulin secretion in pancreatic β-cells through a cAMP-dependent protein kinase pathway. Diabetes 55, 1043–1050.

Liu, Y., Li, D., Zhang, Y., Sun, R., Xia, M., 2014. Anthocyanin increases adiponectin secretion and protects against diabetes-related endothelial dysfunction. Am. J. Physiol. Endocrinol. Metabol. 306 (8), E975–E988.

Liu, Y., Tian, X., Gou, L., Sun, L., Ling, X., Yin, X., 2013. Luteolin attenuates diabetes-associated cognitive decline in rats. Brain Res. Bull. 94, 23–29.

Lodhi, S., Singhai, A.K., 2013. Wound healing effect of flavonoid rich fraction and luteolin isolated from *Martynia annua* Linn. On streptozotocin induced diabetic rats. Asian Pac. J. Trop. Med. 6 (4), 253–259.

Lu, Q., Ji, X.J., Zhou, Y.X., Yao, X.Q., Liu, Y.Q., Zhang, F., et al., 2015. Quercetin inhibits them TORC1/p70S6K signaling-mediated renal tubular epithelial-mesenchymal transition and renal fibrosis in diabetic nephropathy. Pharmacol. Res. 99, 237–247.

Machha, A., Achike, F.I., Mustafa, A.M., Mustafa, M.R., 2007. Quercetin, a flavonoid antioxidant, modulates endothelium-derived nitric oxide bioavailability in diabetic rat aortas. Nitric Oxide 16 (4), 442–447.

Mahmoud, A.M., Ashour, M.B., Abdel-Moneim, A., Ahmed, O.M., 2012. Hesperidin and naringin attenuate hyperglycemia-mediated oxidative stress and proinflammatory cytokine production in high fat fed/streptozotocin-induced type 2 diabetic rats. J. Diabetes Complicat. 26 (6), 483–490.

Mazibuko, S.E., Muller, C.J., Joubert, E., de Beer, D., Johnson, R., Opoku, A.R., et al., 2013. Amelioration of palmitate-induced insulin resistance in C2C12 muscle cells byrooibos (*Aspalathus linearis*). Phytomedicine 20 (10), 813–819.

Middleton, E.J., 1998. Effect of plant flavonoids on immune and inflammatory cell function. Adv. Exp. Med. Biol. 439, 175–182.

Muller, C.J., Joubert, E., de Beer, D., Sanderson, M., Malherbe, C.J., Fey, S.J., et al., 2012. Acute assessment of an aspalathin-enriched green rooibos (*Aspalathus linearis*) extract with hypoglycemic potential. Phytomedicine 20 (1), 32–39.

Nabavi, S.F., Habtemariam, S., Daglia, M., Shafighi, N., Barber, A.J., Nabavi, S.M., 2015. Anthocyanins as a potential therapy for diabetic retinopathy. Curr. Med. Chem. 22 (1), 51–58.

Nagasawa, T., Tabata, N., Ito, Y., Aiba, Y., Nishizawa, N., Kitts, D.D., 2003. Dietary G-rutin suppresses glycation in tissue proteins of streptozotocin-induced diabetic rats. Mol. Cell Biochem. 252 (1–2), 141–147.

Nakamura, Y., Ishimitsu, S., Tonogai, Y., 2000. Effects of quercetin and rutin on serum and hepatic lipid concentrations, fecal steroid excretion and serum antioxidant properties. J. Health Sci. 46, 229–240.

Narayana, K.R., Reddy, S.R., Chaluvadi, M.R., Krishna, D.R., 2001. Bioflavonoids classification, pharmacological, biochemical effects and therapeutic potential. Indian J. Pharmacol. 33, 2–16.

Neveu, V., Perez-Jimenez, J., Vos, F., Crespy, V., 2010. Phenol-explorer: an online comprehensive database on polyphenol contents in foods.

Ojima, A., Ishibashi, Y., Matsui, T., Maeda, S., Nishino, Y., Takeuchi, M., et al., 2012. Glucagon-like peptide-1 receptor agonist inhibits asymmetric dimethylarginine generation in the kidney of streptozotocin-induced diabetic rats by blocking advanced glycation end product-induced protein arginine methyltranferase-1 expression. Am. J. Pathol. 182, 132–141.

Ola, M.S., Ahmed, M.M., Ahmad, R., Abuohashish, H.M., Al-Rejaie, S.S., Alhomida, A.S., 2015. Neuroprotective effects of rutin in streptozotocin-induced diabetic rat retina. J. Mol. Neurosci. 56 (2), 440–448.

Ong, K.C., Khoo, H.E., 1997. Biological effects of myricetin. Gen. Pharmacol. 29 (2), 121–126.

Ozcan, F., Ozmen, A., Akkaya, B., Aliciguzel, Y., Aslan, M., 2012. Beneficial effect ofmyricetin on renal functions in streptozotocin-induced diabetes. Clin. Exp. Med. 12 (4), 265–272.

Panayotova-Heiermann, M., Loo, D.D.R., Wright, E.M., 1995. Kinetics of steady-state currents and charge movements associated with the rat Na+ /glucose cotransporter. J. Biol. Chem. 270, 27099–27105.

Panda, S., Kar, A., 2007. Apigenin (4′,5,7-trihydroxyflavone) regulates hyperglycaemia, thyroid dysfunction and lipid peroxidation in alloxan-induced diabetic mice. J. Pharm. Pharmacol. 59 (11), 1543–1548.

Panicker, S.R., Sreenivas, P., Babu, M.S., Karunagaran, D., Kartha, C.C., 2010. Quercetin attenuates Monocyte Chemoattractant Protein-1 gene expression in glucose primedaortic endothelial cells through NF-kappaB and AP-1. Pharmacol. Res. 62 (4), 328–336.

Prasad, S., Phromnoi, K., Yadav, V.R., et al., 2010. Targeting inflammatory pathways by flavonoids for prevention andtreatment of cancer. Planta Med. 76, 1044–1063.

Qi, Z., Xu, Y., Liang, Z., Li, S., Wang, J., Wei, Y., et al., 2015. Baicalein alters PI3K/Akt/GSK3β signaling pathway in rats with diabetes-associated cognitive deficits. Int. J. Clin. Exp. Med. 8 (2), 1993–2000.

Qian, L.B., Wang, H.P., Chen, Y., Chen, F.X., Ma, Y.Y., Bruce, I.C., et al., 2010. Luteolin reduces high glucose-mediated impairment of endothelium-dependent relaxation in rat aorta by reducing oxidative stress. Pharmacol. Res. 61 (4), 281–287.

Rajendran, P., Rengarajan, T., Nandakumar, N., Palaniswami, R., Nishigaki, Y., Nishigaki, I., 2014. Kaempferol, a potential cytostatic and cure for inflammatory disorders. Eur. J. Med. Chem. 30 (86), 103–112.

Rauter, A.P., Martins, A., Borges, C., Mota-Filipe, H., Pinto, R., Sepodes, B., et al., 2010. Antihyperglycaemic and protective effects of flavonoids on streptozotocin-induced-diabetic rats. Phytother. Res. 2, S133–S134.

Riedl, E., Pfister, F., Braunagel, M., Brinkkötter, P., Sternik, P., Deinzer, M., et al., 2011. Carnosine prevents apoptosis of glomerular cells and podocyte loss in STZ diabetic rats. Cell Physiol. Biochem. 28, 279–288.

Saifudin, A., Kadota, S., Tezuka, Y., 2013. Protein tyrosine phosphatase 1B inhibitory activity of Indonesian herbal medicines and constituents of *Cinnamomum burmannii* and *Zingiber aromaticum*. J. Nat. Med. 67 (2), 264–270.

Sasaki, A., Horiuchi, N., Hasegawa, K., Uehara, M., 1995. Mortality from coronary heart disease and cerebrovascular disease and associated risk factors in diabetic patients in Osaka District, Japan. Diabetes Res. Clin. Pract. 27, 77–83.

Sheetz, M.J., King, G.L., 2002. Molecular understanding of hyperglycemia's adverse effects for diabetic complications. JAMA 288, 2579–2588.

Sheu, J.R., Hsiao, G., Chou, P.H., Shen, M.Y., Chou, D.S., 2004. Mechanisms involved in the antiplatelet activity of rutin, a glycoside of the flavonol quercetin, in human platelets. J. Agric. Food Chem. 52, 4414–4418.

Shi, X., Liao, S., Mi, H., Guo, C., Qi, D., Li, F., et al., 2012. Hesperidin prevents retinal and plasma abnormalities in streptozotocin-induced diabetic rats. Molecules 17 (11), 12868–12881.

Shindo, H., Tawata, M., Aida, K., Onaya, T., 1992. The role of cyclic adenosine 3′,5′-monophosphate and polyol metabolism in diabetic neuropathy. J. Clin. Endocrinol. Metab. 74 (2), 393–398.

Singh, R., Singh, A.K., Alavi, N., Leehey, D.J., 2003. Mechanism of increased angiotensin II levels in glomerular mesangial cells cultured in high glucose. J. Am. Soc. Nephrol. 14, 873–880.

Son, M.J., Minakawa, M., Miura, Y., Yagasaki, K., 2013. Aspalathin improves hyperglycemia and glucose intolerance in obese diabetic ob/ob mice. Eur. J. Nutr. 52 (6), 1607–1619.

Stanley Mainzen, P.P., Kamalakkannan, N., 2006. Rutin improves glucose homeostasis in streptozotocin diabetic tissues by altering glycolytic and gluconeogenic enzymes. J. Biochem. Mol. Toxicol. 20, 96–102.

Stanely Mainzen, P.P., Kannan, N.K., 2006. Protective effect of rutin on lipids, lipoproteins, lipid metabolizing enzymes and glycoproteins in streptozotocin-induced diabetic rats. J. Pharm. Pharmacol. 58 (10), 1373–1383.

Suh, K.S., Choi, E.M., Kwon, M., Chon, S., Oh, S., Woo, J.T., et al., 2009. Kaempferol attenuates 2-deoxy-d-ribose-induced oxidative cell damage in MC3T3-E1 osteoblastic cells. Biol. Pharm. Bull. 32 (4), 746–749.

Suh, K.S., Oh, S., Woo, J.T., Kim, S.W., Kim, J.W., Kim, Y.S., et al., 2012. Apigenin attenuates 2-deoxy-D-ribose-induced oxidative cell damage in HIT-T15 pancreatic β-cells. Biol. Pharm. Bull. 35 (1), 121–126.

Sumbul, S., Ahmad, M.A., Mohd, A., 2011. Role of phenolic compounds in pepticulcer: an overview. J. Pharm. Bioallied Sci. 3 (3), 361–367.

Sun, D., Huang, J., Zhang, Z., Gao, H., Li, J., Shen, M., et al., 2012. Luteolin limits infarct size and improves cardiac function after myocardium ischemia/reperfusion injury in diabetic rats. PLoS One 7 (3), e33491.

Tang, D.Q., Wei, Y.Q., Gao, Y.Y., Yin, X.X., Yang, D.Z., Mou, J., et al., 2011a. Protective effects of rutin on rat glomerular mesangial cells cultured in high glucose conditions. Phytother. Res. 25 (11), 1640–1647.

Tang, D.Q., Wei, Y.Q., Yin, X.X., Lu, Q., Hao, H.H., Zhai, Y.P., et al., 2011b. In vitro suppression of quercetin on hypertrophy and extracellular matrix accumulation in rat glomerular mesangial cells cultured by high glucose. Fitoterapia 82 (6), 920–926.

Thapa, A., Chi, E.Y., 2015. Biflavonoids as potential small molecule therapeutics for Alzheimer's disease. Adv. Exp. Med. Biol. 863, 55–77.

Tolleson, W.H., Doerge, D.R., Churchwell, M.I., Marques, M.M., Roberts, D.W., 2002. Metabolism of biochanin A and formononetin by human liver microsomes in vitro. J. Agric. Food Chem. 50, 4783–4790.

Trumbeckaite, S., Bernatoniene, J., Majiene, D., Jakstas, V., Savickas, A., Toleikis, A., 2006. The effect of flavonoids on rat heart mitochondrial function. Biomed. Pharmacother. 60, 245–248.

Tsuchiya, H., 2010. Structure-dependent membrane interaction of flavonoids associated with their bioactivity. Food Chem. 120, 1089–1096.

Tsukasa, I., 2000. The structure and distribution of the flavonoids in plants. J. Plant Res. 113 (3), 287–299.

Urios, P., Grigorova-Borsos, A.M., Sternberg, M., 2007. Flavonoids inhibit the formation of the cross-inking AGE pentosidine in collagen incubated with glucose, according to their structure. Eur. J. Nutr. 46 (3), 139–146.

Van Dijk, C., Berl, T., 2004. Pathogenesis of diabetic nephropathy. Rev. Endocr. Metab. Disord. 5, 237–248.

Vessal, M., Hemmati, M., Vasei, M., 2003. Antidiabetic effects of quercetin in streptozocin-induced diabetic rats. Comp. Biochem. Physiol. C Toxicol. Pharmacol. 135C (3), 357–364.

Vinik, A.I., Maser, R.E., Mitchell, B.D., Freeman, R., 2003. Diabetic autonomic neuropathy. Diabetes Care 26, 1553–1579.

Wakasugi, M., Noguchi, T., Inoue, M., Tawata, M., Shindo, H., Onaya, T., 1991. Effects of aldose reductase inhibitors on prostacyclin (PGI2) synthesis by aortic rings from rats with streptozotocin-induced diabetes. Prostaglandins Leukot. Essent. Fatty Acids 44 (4), 233–236.

Wang, C., Pan, Y., Zhang, Q.Y., Wang, F.M., Kong, L.D., 2012a. Quercetin and allopurinol ameliorate kidney injury in STZ-treated rats with regulation of renal NLRP3 inflammasome activation and lipid accumulation. PLoS One 7 (6), e38285.

Wang, G., Li, W., Lu, X., Bao, P., Zhao, X., 2012b. Luteolin ameliorates cardiac failure in type I diabetic cardiomyopathy. J. Diabetes Complicat. 26 (4), 259–265.

Wang, G.G., Lu, X.H., Li, W., Zhao, X., Zhang, C., 2011. Protective effects of luteolin on diabetic nephropathy in STZ-induced diabetic rats. Evid. Based Complement Alternat. Med., 323171.

Wang, Y.B., Ge, Z.M., Kang, W.Q., Lian, Z.X., Yao, J., Zhou, C.Y., 2015. Rutin alleviates diabetic cardiomyopathy in a rat model of type 2 diabetes. Exp. Ther. Med. 9 (2), 451–455.

Wang, Z., Lee, Y., Eun, J.S., Bae, E.J., 2014. Inhibition of adipocyte inflammation and macrophage chemotaxis by butein. Eur. J. Pharmacol. 738, 40–48.

Woo, E.R., Lee, J.Y., Cho, I.J., Kim, S.G., Kang, K.W., 2005. Amentoflavone inhibits the induction of nitric oxide synthase by inhibiting NF-kappaB activation in macrophages. Pharmacol. Res. 51, 539–546.

Wu, C.H., Lin, J.A., Hsieh, W.C., Yen, G.C., 2009. Low-density-lipoprotein (LDL)-bound flavonoids increase the resistance of LDL to oxidation and glycation under pathophysiological concentrations of glucose in vitro. J. Agric. Food Chem. 57 (11), 5058–5064.

Yadav, V.R., Prasad, S., Sung, B., Aggarwal, B.B., 2011. The role of chalcones in suppression of NF-κB-mediated inflammation and cancer. Int. Immunopharmacol. 11 (3), 295–309.

Yamagata, K., Miyashita, A., Matsufuji, H., Chino, M., 2010. Dietary flavonoid apigenin inhibits high glucose and tumor necrosis factor alpha-induced adhesion molecule expression in human endothelial cells. J. Nutr. Biochem. 21 (2), 116–124.

Yang, L.P., Sun, H.L., Wu, L.M., Guo, X.J., Dou, H.L., Tso, M.O., et al., 2009. Baicalein reduces inflammatory process in a rodent model of diabetic retinopathy. Invest. Ophthalmol. Vis. Sci. 50 (5), 2319–2327.

Yorek, M.A., 2011. Treatment of diabetic neuropathy with baicalein: intervention at multiple sites. Exp. Neurol. 232 (2), 105–109.

Yu, S.M., Cheng, Z.J., Kuo, S.C., 1995. Endothelium-dependent relaxation of rat aorta bybutein, a novel cyclic AMP-specific phosphodiesterase inhibitor. Eur. J. Pharmacol. 280 (1), 69–77.

Zang, Y., Zhang, L., Igarashi, K., Yu, C., 2015. The anti-obesity and anti-diabetic effects of kaempferol glycosides from unripe soybean leaves in high-fat-diet mice. Food Funct. 6 (3), 834–841.

Zarzuelo, A., Jiménez, I., Gámez, M.J., Utrilla, P., Fernadez, I., Torres, M.I., et al., 1996. Effects of luteolin 5-O-beta-rutinoside in streptozotocin-induced diabetic rats. Life Sci. 58 (25), 2311–2316.

Zhang, Y., Liu, D., 2011. Flavonol kaempferol improves chronic hyperglycemia-impaired pancreatic beta-cell viability and insulin secretory function. Eur. J. Pharmacol. 670 (1), 325–332.

Zhang, Y., Zhen, W., Maechler, P., Liu, D., 2013. Small molecule kaempferol modulates PDX-1 protein expression and subsequently promotes pancreatic β-cell survival and function via CREB. J. Nutr. Biochem. 24 (4), 638–646.

Zhao, C., Liu, Y., Cong, D., Zhang, H., Yu, J., Jiang, Y., et al., 2013. Screening and determination for potential α-glucosidase inhibitory constituents from *Dalbergia odorifera* T. Chen using ultrafiltration-LC/ESI-Ms(n). Biomed. Chromatogr. 27 (12), 1621–1629.

Zhao, L.R., Du, Y.J., Chen, L., Liu, Z.G., Pan, Y.H., Liu, J.F., et al., 2014. Quercetin protects against high glucose-induced damage in bone marrow-derived endothelial progenitor cells. Int. J. Mol. Med. 34 (4), 1025–1031.

Zhou, Y., Liao, Q., Luo, Y., Qing, Z., Zhang, Q., He, G., 2012. Renal protective effect of *Rosa laevigata* Michx. by the inhibition of oxidative stress in streptozotocin induced diabetic rats. Mol. Med. Rep. 5, 1548–1554.

Chapter 6

Curcumin: the epigenetic therapy

Anuradha Pandey[1], Yogesh A. Kulkarni[2] and Anil B. Gaikwad[1]
[1]*Birla Institute of Technology and Science, Pilani, Rajasthan, India*
[2]*Shobhaben Pratapbhai Patel School of Pharmacy & Technology Management, SVKM's NMIMS, Mumbai, Maharashtra, India*

CHAPTER OUTLINE

INTRODUCTION

The nutritional factors have been known to play an important role in maintaining human health since the time immemorial. An array of evidences proves that nutrients play a significant role in altering epigenetic modifications and associated metabolic traits. The cellular homeostasis is tightly regulated by the numerous interactions among food components and the genetic components in our cells which control the cellular phenotype. Nutritional epigenetics involves the study of effects of nutrition on gene expression and how it affects the regulation of genes whose expression is linked to the pathogenesis of various diseases including cancer, metabolic syndrome, obesity, and diabetes (Landecker, 2011). The role of epigenetics in the development of diseases was first identified by Feinberg and Vogelstein, who distinguished human cancer from normal tissues based on DNA methylation levels (Feinberg and Vogelstein, 1983). The important features of diseases which can have an epigenetic basis include increasing susceptibility with

Fruits, Vegetables, and Herbs.
DOI: http://dx.doi.org/10.1016/B978-0-12-802972-5.00006-8

age or heritability patterns that remain incompletely explained by genetics or which show the impact of imprinting due to maternal or in utero exposure (Choi and Friso, 2010). The reversibility of epigenetic alterations is much higher than those of the genetic ones, thus giving an edge to epigenetic therapy, a relatively new and potential intervention to treat epigenetic defects associated with pathogenesis of various diseases (Muñoz-Najar and Sedivy, 2011). Nowadays, several epigenetics-targeting drugs have reached advanced stages of drug delivery, that is, preclinical and clinical stages, especially for cancer treatment. Turmeric, one of the most commonly used spices, remedies, and dyes in Asian continent has demonstrated desirable therapeutic efficiency in a large number of diseases, and to some extent its pharmacological activity could be attributed to its capacity to reverse the epigenetic alterations associated with the pathogenesis. A rigorous research going on globally suggests the need to understand the epigenetic component associated with the therapeutic activity of the golden, turmeric.

TURMERIC: THE GOLDEN SPICE

Turmeric, a widely used component in traditional Indian and Chinese medicine (*Curcuma domestica, Curcuma aromatica, Curcuma Xanthorrhiza;* sobriquets: Indian saffron, turmeric root, yellow root, golden spice, haldi) is a perennial herb belonging to family *Zingiberaceae*. The part of this monocotyledonous plant used most commonly as spices, remedies, and dyes is the rhizome, which shows an intense yellow coloration and fleshy appearance (Jacob et al., 2007). The Latin name *Curcuma* is derived from the Arabic term, *Kourkoum*, the original name of saffron. This herbaceous perennial plant bears 6–10 distichous elliptical leaves that can grow up to 1 m length. The 10–15 cm long yellow flowers bloom from late autumn to mid-summer, and the petals are arranged in a spiral whorl along a spike-like stalk (Jacob et al., 2007). Curcuma does not bear fruit. Curcuma has emerged from continuous crossbreeding and selection. Today, there are some 120 known species of Curcuma. Its cultivation requires a hot and humid climate, along with abundant water supply, thus making the tropical and subtropical regions, particularly in India, China, and South East Asia (Indonesia, Thailand, Vietnam, and the Philippines) suitable for its plantation. India is the largest worldwide producer, consumer, and exporter of Curcuma. The production of Curcuma in India has grown by approximately 40% in the last 10 years, and annual production in 2008–09 was about 900,000 tons (Esatbeyoglu et al., 2012).

The major chemical constituents found in Curcuma are 3–5% curcuminoids (50–60% curcumin) and up to 5% essential oils and resins.

The species credited with the maximum curcuminoid content is *Curcuma zedoaria*. Turmeric owes its yellow color to curcumin, the main curcuminoid, the diarylheptanoids-demethoxycurcumin (4-hydroxycinnamoyl-(feruloyl)methane), and bisdemethoxycurcumin (bis(4-hydroxycinnamoyl) methane), which can be extracted from the rhizomes by employing solvent extraction followed by crystallization. Commercially available curcumin is generally composed of about 77% curcumin, 17% demethoxycurcumin, and 3% bisdemethoxycurcumin. Chemically, curcumin is a bis-α,β-unsaturated diketone of two ferulic acid units, connected through a methylene group (Esatbeyoglu et al., 2012). Though curcumin was isolated from turmeric as early as in 1842 by Vogel, its actual structure was first described by Lampe and Milobedeska in 1910 and along with other curcuminoids which have the main onus of its characteristic yellow color (Shishodia et al., 2005).

The first evidences of usefulness of curcumin are derived from Marco Polo's accounts of Indian and African travels. However, the first scientific article on the treatment of biliary disorders with turmeric was published in 1937 (Jefferson, 2015). Curcumin has been found to show a protective effect in various diseases including cardiovascular diseases (Dikshit et al., 1995; Nirmala and Puvanakrishnan, 1996a,b), neurodegenerative disorders (Frautschy et al., 2001; Lim et al., 2001), metabolic disorders (Arun and Nalini, 2002; Babu and Srinivasan, 1995; Srinivasan, 1972), stomach ache, postpartum abdominal and menstrual pain, wound healing (Phan et al., 2001), and liver injury (Morikawa et al., 2002) to name a few. When given orally, curcumin possesses emmenagogue, antidiuretic, and carminative properties, whereas topical application combats bruises, pains, sprains, boils, swelling, sinusitis, pemphigus, and various skin disorders, and it is inhaled for treatment of coryza (Ringman et al., 2005; Kumar et al., 2015). Curcumin has widely been studied for its capacity to treat different types of cancers such as breast cancer, oral cancer, lung cancer, brain tumor, colorectal cancer, multiple myeloma, osteosarcoma, and many others (Kunnumakkara et al., 2008).

MOLECULAR TARGETS OF CURCUMIN

The capability to regulate cell cycle becomes an important property while dealing with the treatment of cancer. A number of studies demonstrated the role of curcumin in inducing G0/G1 and/or G2/M phase cell cycle arrest by upregulating CDK inhibitors, p21/WAF/CIPI, and p53 (Basile et al., 2009) and by downregulating cyclin B and cdc-2. Many studies disclosed that curcumin induces cell cycle arrest in G2 phase of cell cycle, thus altering the cyclin D expression in mammary epithelial carcinoma cells. On the other hand, G2/M phase arrest renders cells more vulnerable to the cytotoxic effect of radiations which implies that curcumin may also act as a radio sensitizer (Wilken et al., 2011; Sharma et al., 2005; Yang et al., 2007). Apoptosis helps to maintain a balance between the cell birth and cell death, by wiping out the damaged or defective cells. The balance is tipped off under cancerous conditions. A large number of studies show that curcumin promotes apoptosis in cancer cells by caspases—caspase-8 and caspase-9, which trigger the downstream pathways and lead to increased expression of proapoptotic and reduced expression of antiapoptotic proteins (Aggarwal et al, 2003). NF-κB, a ubiquitous eukaryotic major transcription factor instrumental in the regulation of oncogenesis is suppressed by curcumin by blocking phosphorylation of inhibitory factor IκB (Shishodia et al., 2005; Irving et al., 2011) which in turn lowers down the levels of numerous inflammatory cytokines like TNF-α, IL-2, IL-6, IL-8, and migration of the inhibitory protein throughout the body; additionally, it also interferes with production of advanced glycation end products which could lead to cancerous mutation by triggering inflammation. It also downregulates the cyclooxygenase, lipoxygenase, inducible nitric oxide synthase enzymes, and suppresses MAPK kinase (Jurenka, 2009; Shishodia et al., 2007). The tumor development is marked by enhanced expression of various markers, including metalloproteases, STATs, β-catenin, EGFR, and C-src (Irving et al., 2011). Curcumin inhibits multiple networks of proliferation by promoting caspase-3–mediated cleavage of β-catenin and impedes activation of EGFR, C-src (Goel et al., 2008; Jaiswal et al., 2002). The metastasized malignant cells migrate away from the primary loci to the distant regions of the body.

Curcumin inhibits the production of proinflammatory chemokines and cytokines, which are involved in promotion of cell migration (Banerji et al., 2004) along with an increase in the expression of antimetastatic proteins like TIMP-2, NM-23, and E-cadherin (Johnson and Mukhtar, 2007; Hatcher et al., 2008). Curcumin, owing to its lipophilic nature inhibits 12 o-tetradecanoylphorbol acetate, which has tumor-promoting activity along with ornithine decarboxylase (Campbell and Collett, 2005). It also inhibits lipid peroxidation and arachidonic acid metabolism by inhibiting linoleate and cyclooxygenase, respectively (Campbell and Collett, 2005). Moreover, it also elevates the levels of various antioxidant enzymes like superoxide dismutase, glutathione peroxidase, and catalase to enhance curcumin's anticancer property. Another process associated with development of cancer is angiogenesis, which is assisted by an increased expression of proangiogenic factors like vascular endothelial growth factor, fibroblast growth factor, and endothelial growth factor. The treatment with curcumin has been known to control angiogenesis as well the matrix metalloproteases which digest the extracellular matrix to make way for the migration of cells from one part to another (Irving et al., 2011; Hatcher et al., 2008; Jang et al., 2008). Additionally, curcumin has antiangiogenic assets due to its inhibitory activity against serine proteinase family urokinase plasminogen activator which is one of the key mediators of angiogenesis (Goel et al., 2008). Curcumin interferes with tumor invasiveness and blocks molecules that would otherwise serve as an open pathway of dissemination to tissue. The ability of curcumin to target at more than one level helps in blocking a range of pathways of mammary gland cancer pathogenesis. Curcumin has been reported to inhibit directly the cell proliferation and migration by downregulating fibronectin, vitronectin, and collagen IV (Ioachim et al., 2002; Jia et al., 2004).

CURCUMIN AND EPIGENETICS

What is epigenetics?

The chromatin configuration is a dynamic feature being controlled by a myriad of signals and inputs which modulate the covalent modifications so as to facilitate or hinder the binding of promoters to the binding site by opening or closing the chromatin network to alter the gene expression without any change in the nucleotide sequences. These modifications were termed as epigenetic modifications (Greek: *επί*- over, above), which as per Conrad Waddington explains the interactions of genes with their environment and leads to the heritable changes in the pattern of gene expression by mechanisms other than alterations in the primary nucleotide sequence of genes (Waddington, 1957). Epigenetics modifications including DNA methylation as well as histone modifications last through cell divisions for the duration of the cell's life and sometimes even may last for multiple generations, thus providing a mechanism that allows the stable propagation of gene expression from one generation of cells to the next (Bird, 2007). The epigenetic processes have also been termed as the buffers of genetic variation, pending an epigenetic (or mutational) change of state that leads an identical combination of genes to produce a different developmental outcome. The pace and the pattern of epigenetics and associated gene expression are significantly influenced by the external as well as the internal environmental factors, which makes its' understanding critical in order to unravel the etiologies of various metabolic, neurodegenerative, inflammatory, and immunity-related diseases (Egger et al., 2004).

The expression of genetic information is regulated by the chromosomal arrangement, which is constituted by euchromatin and heterochromatin domains which denote transcriptionally active and silent domains, respectively. The process of transcription is modulated by the accessibility of chromatin through the wrapping of the DNA around octamural globular histone proteins to form "nucleosomes." Histone octamer is wrapped by 147 bp of DNA which further forms the chromatin and constitutes the nucleosomes. Two copies of each of the following core histones are present: H2A, H2B, H3, and H4 (Luger et al., 1997). All of them have a globular C-terminal domain and an unstructured N-terminal tail. The accessibility of chromatin is reversibly regulated by the epigenetic status of DNA methylation and histone modifications. The transcriptionally active regions of DNA are highly unmethylated, rich in acetylated histones, and accessible to transcription factors, whereas the inactive regions comprised methylated DNA, deacetylated histones with compacted nucleosomes, and unfavorable configuration to transcriptional machinery. This inactivation of DNA is linked to histone deacetylation through binding of methyl–CpG-binding proteins to methylated promoter regions. The methylation of lysine 9 on the N-terminus of histone protein H-3 is also a characteristic of inactive DNA, whereas methylation of lysine 4 on H-3 is a feature of activated DNA, and constitute some of the more well-characterized components of the increasingly complicated "histone code" that regulates gene expression. The heterochromatic state is epigenetically inherited and changes in heterochromatin state allow a transition from DNA sequence-specific genetic control to an adaptive sequence-independent dynamic epigenetic control. The evolutionarily conserved histone modifications include methylation of arginine and lysine residues, phosphorylation of threonine and serine residues, monoubiquitination, sumoylation, acetylation of lysine, and proline isomerization. The overall modification of the chromatin and different combinations of histone modifications work together at histone code, and it either activates or silences the gene (Jenuwein and Allis, 2001).

The epigenetic modifications are inclined by the developmental stage or stress phase in cell cycle and other environmental factors. A host of enzymes are tangled in the regulation of these histone modifications like histone deacetylases (HDACs), histone acetyl transferases (HATs), histone methyl transferases, histone demethylases, and sirtuins have been described in human (Wang et al., 2007). Each of these enzymes is responsible for a specific epigenetic mark on a specific histone location. There also appears to be some kind of combinatorial code which is frequently known as the histone code (Jenuwein and Allis, 2001).

MODULATION OF EPIGENETICS WITH CURCUMIN

Epidemiological evidences show that people who incorporate high doses of curcumin in their diets demonstrate a lower incidence of several common cancers such as breast, colorectal, and prostate cancer. A large number of studies demonstrated the anticancer property of curcumin by acted through induction of apoptosis or sensitization of cancer cells to other anticancer agents. Phase 1 clinical trial has shown that curcumin could be safely administered at an oral dose of up to 8 g/day. Another study which used pancreatic cancer patients as target subjects demonstrated that curcumin was able to reduce tumor growth by about 73% (Gupta et al., 2013). However, the major drawbacks associated with the administration of curcumin is its low oral bioavailability (Prasad et al., 2014), but the probable mechanisms through which it deciphers the pharmacologically beneficial actions involve its accumulation in the cell due to its hydrophobic nature and also because the epigenetic modifications occur at very low curcumin concentration (Reuter et al., 2011).

DNA methylation is involved in the regulation of gene activity and forms the basis of chromatin structure. In the mammalian genome, DNA methylation, a heritable epigenetic modification occurs by covalent modification of the fifth carbon (C5) in the cytosine base. 5-methyl cytosine (Me5C) constitutes around 1% of total DNA bases and is estimated to represent 70–80% of all CpG dinucleotide in the genome (Ehrlich et al., 1982). The covalent addition of methyl moiety to the cytosine base of CpG dinucleotide cluster-rich mammalian gene promoters regions has been known to be associated with the loss of the associated gene expression, which could be attributed to the stearic hindrance to the transcriptional machinery, recruitment of repressors, or alteration in chromatin configuration. This process is catalyzed by DNA methyl transferases (DNMTs) enzymes, which transfer a methyl group from S-adenosyl-L-methionine (a methyl group donor) onto the 5-position of cytosine (Robertson, 2005). Three major isoforms of DNMT are involved in establishing and maintaining the DNA methylation patterns shown in human and also interact directly with HDACs to recruit them to gene promoters. Among the three isoforms, DNMT3A and DNMT3B are primarily responsible for de novo methylation of specific DNA sites, whereas DNMT1 maintains the DNA methylation patterns. In general, activation of DNMTs is frequently associated with hypermethylation at gene promoter which resulted in a silencing of the related gene. Any mutation at 5′ methyl cytosine site in the DNA sequence converts it into uracil; so, it is hard to be identified and repaired. When the methylation occurs at the promoter site, the transcription process gets repressed. Methylation is important for silencing transcription, X chromosome inactivation, protecting the genome from transposition, tissue-specific gene expression and its regulation, heterochromatin, developmental controls, cancer therapy, and genomic imprinting. The defects in the DNA methylation has been known to be associated with diseases such as systemic lupus erythematosus (Ballestar et al., 2006), immunodeficiency, and facial anomalies syndrome (Ehrlich et al., 2006). The demethylation of promoter sequences has been increased chemosensitivity, immunogenicity, as well as response to interferon. Also it helps to decrease growth of cancerous cells. DNA hypermethylation plays a significant role in inactivation of genes such as E-cadherin, p16, MDR1, and glutathione S-transferase, whereas its hypomethylation allows the activation of several tumor-promoting genes (http://www.biotecharticles.com/DNA-Article/Mechanism-of-Epigenetics-744.html).

Two patterns of DNA methylation have been observed in cancer cells: global hypomethylation across the genome, and localized hypermethylation at specific CpG islands within the gene promoter regions of specific genes. Decreased methylation because of global hypomethylation could facilitate the expression of previously quiescent proto-oncogenes and prometastatic genes and promote tumor progression (Ehrlich, 2009). Alternatively, an aberrant increase in methylation patterns at previously unmethylated sites, such as the promoter regions of tumor suppressor genes, could result in transcriptional silencing and inability to control tumorigenesis (Sánchez-Carbayo, 2014). DNA hypomethylating agents which have already been approved by the US Food and Drug Administration include azacitidine and decitabine, which showed a potent chemotherapeutic activity for treating myelodysplastic syndrome both preclinically as well as clinically. Since, curcumin also possesses a DNA hypomethylating property, it induces cancer cell chemosensitization (Fu and Kurzrock, 2010).

In 2009, Liu et al. demonstrated for the first time that curcumin could inhibit a DNMT1 analogue which has also been supported by the computer-based modeling studies. The in silico studies to analyze the interactions between curcumin and DNMT1 showed that curcumin produces an inhibitory effect by reacting covalently with thiolate group of C1226 of DNMT1. These data show that curcumin is a potent DNA hypomethylating agent, which is consistent with its broad activity in inflammation, cancer, and many other diseases, while remaining relatively safe in normal healthy cells (Fu and Kurzrock, 2010).

CURCUMIN AND HISTONE ACETYLATION

The reversible process of histone acetylation occurs at the amino group of lysine residues in the N-terminal tails of core histones, mediates conformational changes in nucleosomes, and is controlled by the opposite actions of HATs and HDACs. HDAC enzymes do not bind to DNA directly but rather interact with DNA through multiprotein complexes that include corepressors and coactivators. HATs acetylate lysine residues on histones by transferring acetyl groups from acetyl-CoA onto lysine. On the basis of their primary sequence homology, nuclear HATs have been classified as: Gcn5/PCAF (general control nonrepressed protein 5 and p300-associated and CBP-associated factor), MYST (which stands for the founding members of this class: MOZ, Ybf2/Sas3, Sas2, and Tip60), p300/CBP (300kDa protein and CREB-binding protein), and Rtt109 (regulator of Ty1 transposition gene product) (Kim et al., 2010). The anticancer effects of HDAC inhibitors are well known and have been proved by the clinical trials as well, but the chemotherapeutic potential of HAT inhibitors has not yet been established completely. The role of HATs in cancer is complex because maintaining histones in acetylated state is crucial to various cell functions such as cell cycle progression, DNA repair, cell proliferation and differentiation, mutations, and/or chromosomal translocations. The activities of HATs and HDACs are intimately related because a complexed form of the two leads to their interaction with other regulators. Thus, modulation of histone acetylation leads to an altered activity of various downstream pathways. Thus, curcumin, which has HDAC inhibitory as well as HAT inhibitory activity may affect multiple intracellular signal transduction pathways and other target proteins.

The p300/CBP complex appears to exert both tumor suppressor and tumor promoter properties, depending on the specific cellular context. Loss of p300 heterozygosity and p300 mutation is associated with development of glioblastoma and colorectal cancer as it was evidenced by CBP knockout mice which presented an increased incidence of cancers along with improper cell proliferation. Curcumin has been identified as a specific inhibitor of p300/CBP HAT activity both in vitro and in vivo, but not of p300/CBP-associated factor, a HAT that associates with p300/CBP, which was confirmed by filter binding and gel HAT assays. Thus, curcumin was found to be a specific inhibitor for p300/CBP HAT activity, but not for other enzymes that have histone substrates and then it was also determined that a covalent interaction culminating into a conformational change in the enzyme structure had been responsible for the inhibitory activity. Through these epigenetic modifications, curcumin helped in the prevention of weakening of systolic function and heart failure–induced increases in both myocardial wall thickness and diameter. Thus, it was concluded that curcumin-mediated inhibition of p300 HAT activity could come up as a novel therapeutic strategy for heart failure in humans (Morimoto et al., 2008).

The HDAC inhibitor, Trichostatin A (TSA), and curcumin combination was found to show a better antiproliferative and apoptotic effects than their monotherapy in SkBr3 and 435eB breast cancer cells. This alteration prevailed due to decreased phosphorylation of ERK and Akt and increased phosphorylation of JNK and p38 accompanied by an increased p21 and p27, and decreased Cyclin D1 protein expression. The combination-induced cleavage of caspase 3 and poly(ADP-ribose) polymerase-1, suggesting that cell death occurred by apoptosis. It was concluded that that p53-independent apoptosis was induced by combined therapy with curcumin and TSA involves JNK activation. These findings highlight the need to study curcumin as an adjuvant to treat breast cancer (Yan et al., 2013).

At least 18 HDACs have been identified in humans, primarily occupying four classes based on homology with yeast deacetylases (Xu et al., 2007). In an in vitro study using HeLa cells' nuclear extracts, involving 33 carboxylic acid derivatives, curcumin was found to be the most effective HDAC inhibitor, ranking even higher than the known HDAC inhibitors (valproic acid and sodium butyrate) (Bora-Tatar et al., 2009). The in silico studies for human HDAC8 showed that curcumin showed a free binding energy and inhibition constant comparable to TSA and vorinostat, which proved that its potency was more as compared valproic acid and sodium butyrate (Reuter et al., 2011). Chen et al. (2007) showed that curcumin presented striking dose-dependent antiproliferative potency on Raji cells, which was accompanied by a significant reduction in p300, HDAC1, and HDAC3 expression. The protection degradation of HDAC1 and p300 by MG132 could be partially reversed by curcumin. The inflammation was also found to have reduced by the curcumin treatment as was evidenced by reduction in IκB-α and Notch-1 expression and lowered nuclear translocation of the NF-κB/p65 subunits (Chen et al., 2007).

HDAC2 plays central patients with chronic obstructive pulmonary disease (COPD), who are reported to have reduced HDAC2 activity, and this loss in activity correlates with the severity of the disease (Roche et al., 2011). The oxidative stress induced by cigarette smoke extract (CSE) was found to reduce the expression of HDAC2. The treatment with curcumin was found to improve the HDAC2 activity as well as the efficacy of corticosteroid at even nanomolar concentrations and also in the presence of protein synthesis inhibitor like cyclohexamide. MG132, a proteasomal inhibitor also blocked CSE-induced HDAC2 degradation by increasing the levels of ubiquitination at HDAC2. The results from biochemical and gene chip analysis showed that curcumin at concentrations up to 1 μM shows its effect via antioxidant-independent mechanisms associated with the phosphorylation–ubiquitin–proteasome pathway. Thus curcumin acts at a post-translational level by maintaining both HDAC2 activity and expression, thereby reversing steroid insensitivity induced by either CSE or oxidative stress in monocytes. Curcumin may therefore have potential to reverse steroid resistance, which is common in patients with COPD and asthma (Meja et al., 2008).

High glucose induces proinflammatory cytokines which are associated with the underlying epigenetic changes. In a study, aimed to analyze the effect of curcumin on histone acetylation and proinflammatory cytokine secretion under high glucose conditions in human monocytes, it was found that curcumin administration could lower the NF-κB–mediated production of cytokines by modifying the chromatin conformation. The human monocytic (THP1) cells, cultured in the presence of mannitol (osmolar control, mannitol), normoglycemic (5.5 mmol/L glucose), or hyperglycemic (25 mmol/L glucose) conditions in the presence of curcumin (1.512.5 μM) for 72 hours showed a decline in the cytokine level (IL-6, TNF-α, and MCP1), NF-κB transactivation, HDAC activity, and HATs activity. These alterations in protein expression were measured by Western blots, quantitative real-time polymerase chain reaction, enzyme-linked immunosorbent assay, and immunofluorescence staining. Curcumin treatment also significantly reduced HAT activity, level of p300 and acetylated CBP/p300 gene expression, and induced HDAC2 expression. These results indicate that curcumin decreases hyperglycemia-induced cytokine production in monocytes via epigenetic mechanisms (Yun et al., 2011). An increase in phosphorylation of JNK in the renal tissue is an important feature of diabetes and its associated complications. The administration of a curcumin analogue (C66) was found to control the upregulation of phosphorylation of JNK in diabetic rats' kidney. C66 and JNK inhibitor, both the treatments also significantly prevented diabetes-induced renal fibrosis and dysfunction. Diabetes-related increases in histone acetylation, HATs activity, and the p300/CBP HAT expression were also significantly attenuated by C66 or JNK inhibitor treatment. Chromatin immunoprecipitation assays showed that C66 and JNK inhibitor treatments decreased H3-lysine 9/14 acetylation (H3K9/14ac) level and p300/CBP occupancy at the CTGF, PAI-1, and FN-1 gene promoters. Thus, C66 may prevent renal injury and dysfunction in diabetic mice via downregulation of diabetes-related JNK activation and consequent suppression of the diabetes-related increases in HAT activity, p300/CBP expression, and histone acetylation (Wang et al., 2015).

FUTURE DIRECTIONS

The epigenetic modulations play a significant role in the progression and pathogenesis of various diseases like cancer, developmental disorders, metabolic and respiratory disorders. The nutrients being consumed regularly have a potential to accumulate in the cells and help in promoting the process of posttranslational modifications, which may reverse the pathological features. Curcumin, being one of such widely used components with desirable pharmacological activities and epigenetics altering capacity, emerges as a promising molecule which could be developed as an epigenetic drug to combat an array of diseases. This paves way for the development of novel formulations as well as analogues of curcumin which could be used to gain benefits out of this epigenetic drug with natural origin.

REFERENCES

Aggarwal, B.B., Kumar, A., Bharti, A.C., 2003. Anticancer potential of curcumin: preclinical and clinical studies. Anticancer Res. 23, 363–398.

Arun, N., Nalini, N., 2002. Efficacy of turmeric on blood sugar and polyol pathway in diabetic albino rats. Plant Foods Hum. Nutr. 57, 41–52.

Babu, P.S., Srinivasan, K., 1995. Influence of dietary curcumin and cholesterol on the progression of experimentally induced diabetes in albino rat. Mol. Cell Biochem. 152, 13–21.

Ballestar, E., Esteller, M., Richardson, B.C., 2006. The epigenetic face of systemic lupus erythematosus. J. Immunol. 176, 7143–7147.

Banerji, A., Chakrabarti, J., Mitra, A., Chatterjee, A., 2004. Effect of curcumin on gelatinase A (MMP-2) activity in B16F10 melanoma cells. Cancer Lett. 211, 235–242.

Basile, V., Ferrari, E., Lazzari, S., Belluti, S., Pignedoli, F., Imbriano, C., 2009. Curcumin derivatives: molecular basis of their anti-cancer activity. Biochem. Pharmacol. 78, 1305–1315.

Bird, A., 2007. Perceptions of epigenetics. Nature 447, 396–398.

Bora-Tatar, G., Dayangaç-Erden, D., Demir, A.S., Dalkara, S., Yelekçi, K., Erdem-Yurter, H., 2009. Molecular modifications on carboxylic acid derivatives as potent histone deacetylase inhibitors: activity and docking studies. Bioorg. Med. Chem. 17, 5219–5228.

Campbell, F.C., Collett, G.P., 2005. Chemopreventive properties of curcumin. Future Oncol. 1, 405–414.

Chen, Y., Shu, W., Chen, W., Wu, Q., Liu, H., Cui, G., 2007. Curcumin, both histone deacetylase and p300/CBP-specific inhibitor, represses the activity of nuclear factor kappa B and notch 1 in raji cells. Basic Clin. Pharmacol. Toxicol. 101, 427–433.

Choi, S.-W., Friso, S., 2010. Epigenetics: a new bridge between nutrition and health. Adv. Nutr. 1, 8–16.

Dikshit, M., Rastogi, L., Shukla, R., Srimal, R.C., 1995. Prevention of ischaemia-induced biochemical changes by curcumin & quinidine in the cat heart. Indian J. Med. Res. 101, 31–35.

Egger, G., Liang, G., Aparicio, A., Jones, P.A., 2004. Epigenetics in human disease and prospects for epigenetic therapy. Nature 429, 457–463.

Ehrlich, M., 2009. DNA hypomethylation in cancer cells. Epigenomics 1, 239–259.

Ehrlich, M., Gama-Sosa, M.A., Huang, L.-H., Midgett, R.M., Kuo, K.C., McCune, R.A., et al., 1982. Amount and distribution of 5-methylcytosine in human DNA from different types of tissues or cells. Nucleic Acids Res. 10, 2709–2721.

Ehrlich, M., Jackson, K., Weemaes, C., 2006. Immunodeficiency, centromeric region instability, facial anomalies syndrome (ICF). Orphanet J. Rare Dis. 1, 1–9.

Esatbeyoglu, T., Huebbe, P., Ernst, I., Chin, D., Wagner, A.E., Rimbach, G., 2012. Curcumin—from molecule to biological function. Angew. Chem. Int. Ed. Engl. 51, 5308–5332.

Feinberg, A.P., Vogelstein, B., 1983. Hypomethylation distinguishes genes of some human cancers from their normal counterparts. Nature 301, 89–92.

Frautschy, S.A., Hu, W., Kim, P., Miller, S.A., Chu, T., Harris-White, M.E., et al., 2001. Phenolic anti-inflammatory antioxidant reversal of Abeta-induced cognitive deficits and neuropathology. Neurobiol. Aging. 22, 993–1005.

Fu, S., Kurzrock, R., 2010. Development of curcumin as an epigenetic agent. Cancer 116, 4670–4676.

Goel, A., Kunnumakkara, A.B., Aggarwal, B.B., 2008. Curcumin as "Curcumin": from kitchen to clinic. Biochem. Pharmacol. 75, 787–809.

Gupta, S.C., Patchva, S., Aggarwal, B.B., 2013. Therapeutic roles of curcumin: lessons learned from clinical trials. AAPS J. 15, 195–218.

Hatcher, H., Planalp, R., Cho, J., Torti, F.M., Torti, S.V., 2008. Curcumin: from ancient medicine to current clinical trials. Cell Mol. Life Sci. 65, 1631–1652.

Ioachim, E., Charchanti, A., Briasoulis, E., Karavasilis, V., Tsanou, H., Arvanitis, D.L., et al., 2002. Immunohistochemical expression of extracellular matrix components tenascin, fibronectin, collagen type IV and laminin in breast cancer: their prognostic value and role in tumour invasion and progression. Eur. J. Cancer 38, 2362–2370.

Irving, G.R., Karmokar, A., Berry, D.P., Brown, K., Steward, W.P., 2011. Curcumin: the potential for efficacy in gastrointestinal diseases. Best Pract. Res. Clin. Gastroenterol. 25, 519–534.

Jacob, A., Wu, R., Zhou, M., Wang, P., 2007. Mechanism of the anti-inflammatory effect of curcumin: PPAR-gamma activation. PPAR Res. 2007, 89369.

Jaiswal, A.S., Marlow, B.P., Gupta, N., Narayan, S., 2002. Beta-catenin-mediated transactivation and cell–cell adhesion pathways are important in curcumin (diferuylmethane)-induced growth arrest and apoptosis in colon cancer cells. Oncogene 21, 8414–8427.

Jang, Y.H., Namkoong, S., Kim, Y.M., Lee, S.J., Park, B.J., Min, D.S., 2008. Cleavage of phospholipase D1 by caspase promotes apoptosis via modulation of the p53-dependent cell death pathway. Cell Death Differ. 15, 1782–1793.

Jefferson, W., 2015. The Healing Power of Turmeric. Healthy Living Publications, Summertown, United States of America.

Jenuwein, T., Allis, C.D., 2001. Translating the histone code. Science 293, 1074–1080.

Jia, Y., Zeng, Z.Z., Markwart, S.M., Rockwood, K.F., Ignatoski, K.M., Ethier, S.P., et al., 2004. Integrin fibronectin receptors in matrix metalloproteinase-1-dependent invasion by breast cancer and mammary epithelial cells. Cancer Res. 64, 8674–8681.

Johnson, J.J., Mukhtar, H., 2007. Curcumin for chemoprevention of colon cancer. Cancer Lett. 255, 170–181.

Jurenka, J.S., 2009. Anti-inflammatory properties of curcumin, a major constituent of Curcuma longa: a review of preclinical and clinical research. Altern. Med. Rev. 14, 141–153.

Kim, G.-W., Gocevski, G., Wu, C.-J., Yang, X.-J., 2010. Dietary, metabolic, and potentially environmental modulation of the lysine acetylation machinery. Int. J. Cell Biol. 2010, 632739.

Kumar, P., Kadakol, A., Krishna Shasthrula, P., Arunrao Mundhe, N., Sudhir Jamdade, V., C Barua, C., et al., 2015. Curcumin as an adjuvant to breast cancer treatment. AntiCancer Agents Med. Chem. 15, 647–656.

Kunnumakkara, A.B., Anand, P., Aggarwal, B.B., 2008. Curcumin inhibits proliferation, invasion, angiogenesis and metastasis of different cancers through interaction with multiple cell signaling proteins. Cancer Lett. 269, 199–225.

Landecker, H., 2011. Food as exposure: nutritional epigenetics and the new metabolism. Biosocieties 6, 167–194.

Lim, G.P., Chu, T., Yang, F., Beech, W., Frautschy, S.A., Cole, G.M., 2001. The curry spice curcumin reduces oxidative damage and amyloid pathology in an Alzheimer transgenic mouse. J. Neurosci. 21, 8370–8377.

Luger, K., Mäder, A.W., Richmond, R.K., Sargent, D.F., Richmond, T.J., 1997. Crystal structure of the nucleosome core particle at 2.8 Å resolution. Nature 389, 251–260.

Meja, K.K., Rajendrasozhan, S., Adenuga, D., Biswas, S.K., Sundar, I.K., Spooner, G., et al., 2008. Curcumin restores corticosteroid function in monocytes exposed to oxidants by maintaining HDAC2. Am. J. Respir. Cell Mol. Biol. 39, 312–323.

Morikawa, T., Matsuda, H., Ninomiya, K., Yoshikawa, M., 2002. Medicinal foodstuffs. XXIX. Potent protective effects of sesquiterpenes and curcumin from Zedoariae Rhizoma on liver injury induced by D-galactosamine/lipopolysaccharide or tumor necrosis factor-alpha. Biol. Pharm. Bull. 25, 627–631.

Morimoto, T., Sunagawa, Y., Kawamura, T., Takaya, T., Wada, H., Nagasawa, A., et al., 2008. The dietary compound curcumin inhibits p300 histone acetyltransferase activity and prevents heart failure in rats. J. Clin. Invest. 118, 868–878.

Muñoz-Najar, U., Sedivy, J.M., 2011. Epigenetic control of aging. Antioxid. Redox. Signal. 14, 241–259.

Nirmala, C., Puvanakrishnan, R., 1996a. Effect of curcumin on certain lysosomal hydrolases in isoproterenol-induced myocardial infarction in rats. Biochem. Pharmacol. 51, 47–51.

Nirmala, C., Puvanakrishnan, R., 1996b. Protective role of curcumin against isoproterenol induced myocardial infarction in rats. Mol. Cell. Biochem. 159, 85–93.

Phan, T.T., See, P., Lee, S.T., Chan, S.Y., 2001. Protective effects of curcumin against oxidative damage on skin cells in vitro: its implication for wound healing. J. Trauma. 51, 927–931.

Prasad, S., Tyagi, A.K., Aggarwal, B.B., 2014. Recent developments in delivery, bioavailability, absorption and metabolism of curcumin: the golden pigment from golden spice. Cancer Res. Treat. 46, 2–18.

Reuter, S., Gupta, S.C., Park, B., Goel, A., Aggarwal, B.B., 2011. Epigenetic changes induced by curcumin and other natural compounds. Genes Nutr. 6, 93–108.

Ringman, J.M., Frautschy, S.A., Cole, G.M., Masterman, D.L., Cummings, J.L., 2005. A potential role of the curry spice curcumin in Alzheimer's disease. Curr. Alzheimer Res. 2, 131–136.

Robertson, K.D., 2005. Epigenetic mechanisms of gene regulation DNA Methylation and Cancer Therapy. Springer, Heidelberg, New York, 13–30.

Roche, N., Marthan, R., Berger, P., Chambellan, A., Chanez, P., Aguilaniu, B., et al., 2011. Beyond corticosteroids: future prospects in the management of inflammation in COPD. Eur. Respir. Rev. 20, 175–182.

Sánchez-Carbayo, M., 2014. Hypermethylation in cancer. In: Poptsova, M.S. (Ed.), Genome Analysis: Current Procedures and Applications, Caister Academic Press, Norfolk, United Kingdom, 151.

Sharma, R.A., Gescher, A.J., Steward, W.P., 2005. Curcumin: the story so far. Eur. J. Cancer 41, 1955–1968.

Shishodia, S., Chaturvedi, M.M., Aggarwal, B.B., 2007. Role of curcumin in cancer therapy. Curr. Probl. Cancer 31, 243–305.

Shishodia, S., Sethi, G., Aggarwal, B.B., 2005. Curcumin: getting back to the roots. Ann. N. Y. Acad. Sci. 1056, 206–217.

Srinivasan, M., 1972. Effect of curcumin on blood sugar as seen in a diabetic subject. Indian J. Med. Sci. 26, 269–270.

Waddington, C.H., 1957. The strategy of the genes. A discussion of some aspects of theoretical biology. With an appendix by H. Kacser. The strategy of the genes. A discussion of some aspects of theoretical biology. With an appendix by H. Kacser., pp. 256–262.

Wang, G.G., Allis, C.D., Chi, P., 2007. Chromatin remodeling and cancer, part I: covalent histone modifications. Trends Mol. Med. 13, 363–372.

Wang, Y., Wang, Y., Luo, M., Wu, H., Kong, L., Xin, Y., et al., 2015. Novel curcumin analog C66 prevents diabetic nephropathy via JNK pathway with the involvement of p300/CBP-mediated histone acetylation. Biochim. Biophys. Acta 1852, 34–46.

Wilken, R., Veena, M.S., Wang, M.B., Srivatsan, E.S., 2011. Curcumin: a review of anticancer properties and therapeutic activity in head and neck squamous cell carcinoma. Mol. Cancer. 10, 12.

Xu, W.S., Parmigiani, R.B., Marks, P.A., 2007. Histone deacetylase inhibitors: molecular mechanisms of action. Oncogene 26, 5541–5552.

Yan, G., Graham, K., Lanza-Jacoby, S., 2013. Curcumin enhances the anticancer effects of trichostatin a in breast cancer cells. Mol. Carcinog. 52, 404–411.

Yang, L., Wu, S., Zhang, Q., Liu, F., Wu, P., 2007. 23,24-Dihydrocucurbitacin B induces G2/M cell-cycle arrest and mitochondria-dependent apoptosis in human breast cancer cells (Bcap37). Cancer Lett. 256, 267–278.

Yun, J.-M., Jialal, I., Devaraj, S., 2011. Epigenetic regulation of high glucose-induced proinflammatory cytokine productionin monocytes by curcumin. J. Nutr. Biochem. 22, 450–458.

Chapter 7

Nutraceuticals as therapeutic agents for inflammation

Kalyani H. Barve[1], Yogesh A. Kulkarni[1] and Anil B. Gaikwad[2]

[1]*Shobhaben Pratapbhai Patel School of Pharmacy & Technology Management, SVKM's NMIMS, Mumbai, Maharashtra, India*

[2]*Birla Institute of Technology and Science, Pilani, Rajasthan, India*

CHAPTER OUTLINE

Fruits, Vegetables, and Herbs.
DOI: http://dx.doi.org/10.1016/B978-0-12-802972-5.00007-X

INTRODUCTION

Nutraceutical is a term coined by Stefane De Felice, who defined it as a food, or parts of a food, that provides medical or health benefits, including the prevention and treatment of disease. Nutraceuticals are legally not classified as medicines, with a few exceptions in some countries. They are obtained from a large number of sources that include human, mammalian, and plant metabolites, dietary sources of plant and animal origin, and a few, which are produced by microbial fermentation. Of all these sources, most of the nutraceuticals are derived from plants either as whole plant foods, for example, soya and tea, multicomponent products such as grape seed extract and pycnogenol or purified components such as lycopene and resveratrol. The therapeutic applications of nutraceuticals encompass many areas providing symptomatic as well as curative effect (Evans, 2009). The advantages of using nutraceuticals as a part of therapy are it helps in lowering the cost of therapy and has a lower toxicity in the range of normal diet. Nutraceuticals need a thorough investigation in order to understand the mechanism of action/clinical applications. In this chapter we would be focusing on use of nutraceuticals as antiinflammatory agents. Plant products rich in phenolics, carotenoids, and terpenoids display antioxidant properties by the virtue of which it may show antiinflammatory effect.

Conventional antiinflammatory agents include the nonsteroidal antiinflammatory drugs'/selective cox II inhibitors both of which have severe side effects which necessitate the search for newer and safe approaches. Since these nutraceuticals have antiinflammatory properties, they can be used to delay, prevent, or treat many chronic inflammatory diseases like rheumatoid arthritis (RA), cardiovascular diseases (CVD), obesity, diabetes, atherosclerosis, etc.

Inflammation is a protective response intended to eliminate the initial cause of cell injury as well as the necrotic cells and tissues resulting from the original insult (Kumar et al., 2007). Although inflammation helps clear infections and other noxious stimuli and initiates repair, the inflammatory reaction and the subsequent repair process can cause considerable harm. Acute inflammation is a protective mechanism against infections, trauma, and physical and chemical agents while facilitating wound repair. If the inflammatory process remains persistent and prolongs, it takes the shape of chronic inflammation which increases the risk of developing associated degenerative diseases like RA, inflammatory bowel disease, atherosclerosis, heart disease, diabetes, cancer, and Alzheimer's disease.

During either type of inflammation, tissue injury stimulates the release of inflammatory mediators which include proinflammatory cytokines, tumor necrosis factor α (TNF-α), and interleukin 1 (IL-1) which further stimulate the release of cell adhesion molecules (CAM), selectins, integrins, and immunoglobulins. A simultaneous increase in the expression of phospholipase A2 stimulates the generation of arachidonic acid metabolites: prostaglandins (PGs) and leukotrienes (LTs). Reactive oxygen species (ROS) are also released from the activated neutrophils and macrophages. There is an increased expression of ROS-generating enzymes such as NADPH oxidase, xanthine oxidase, and myeloperoxidase. Ultimately, the activation of the transcription factor NF-κB appears to play a pivotal role in the regulation of inducible enzymes, inflammatory cytokines, CAMs, and other substances that are initiators or enhancers of the inflammatory process (Huang et al., 2004).

Nutraceuticals may function as antiinflammatory agents by regulating the activity of any one or multiple inflammatory markers. Nutraceuticals may have the potential to inhibit or reduce the inflammatory process via the following mechanisms:

Inhibition of the activation of NF-κB

NF-κB is a protein complex that activates gene transcription and hence affects the expression of proinflammatory cytokines, chemokines, CAMs, and many enzymes like phospholipase A2, lipoxygenase, COX-2, inducible nitric oxide synthase (iNOS), and myeloperoxidase (Baldwin 1996; Pahl 1999). Activation of NF-κB is involved in the progression of a number of chronic inflammatory diseases like asthma, atherosclerosis, and Alzheimer's. Some examples of nutraceuticals which act by inhibiting the expression of NF-κB are green tea polyphenols, curcumin, and resveratrol.

Blocking the overexpression of proinflammatory cytokines

The major proinflammatory cytokines involved in inflammation are TNF and IL-1, as well as a group of chemoattractant cytokines called chemokines. TNF and IL-1 are majorly involved in endothelial activation, and they also increase the release of chemokines and eicosanoids. Apart from this, TNF increases the thrombogenecity of the endothelium and IL-1 increases the production of extracellular matrix, both of which are detrimental to the tissue. Natural flavonoids such as quercetin and catechin have shown to possess TNF-α inhibitory activity.

Downregulation of the overexpression of CAMs and inhibiting enzyme activity (phospholipase A2, COX-2, 5-LOX, iNOS, and myeloperoxidase)

CAMs can be divided into three: selectins, integrins, and immunoglobulins. Each one of this plays an important role in rolling, adhesion, transmigration, and chemotaxis of leukocytes. Any product be it from plants or synthetic drug which helps to downregulate the overexpression of CAM will definitely suppress the inflammation.

COX inhibitors are the most common targets for antiinflammatory activity. Overexpression of cyclooxygenase increases the synthesis of PGs. Selective COX-2 inhibition can target inflammation and pain with reduced risk of chronic ulceration and acute injury. A classic example of COX inhibition is treatment of pain with an ancient Greek remedy which uses willow bark extract (now known as a rich source of salicylic acid).

Lipoxygenase is an enzyme involved in formation of LTs which function as chemoattractants. Thus, LOX inhibitors have been identified to be useful in treatment of inflammation. 5-LOX inhibitors have been identified to potentially counteract the gastric damage associated with the COX-1 inhibitors.

As seen earlier, phospholipase A2 is the enzyme involved in hydrolysis of phospholipids to arachidonic acid, a precursor for proinflammatory mediators: prostaglandins, LTs, and platelet-activating factor. Phospholipase A2 inhibitors definitely have a role in inflammation treatment since these would inhibit the formation of eicosanoids, which are strong chemotactic agents.

Inhibit ROS-generating enzyme activity/increasing ability to scavenge ROS

ROS are synthesized via the NADPH oxidase pathway within neutrophils and macrophages activated by tumor promoters or foreign bodies. At lower concentration they destroy phagocytosed microbes and necrotic cells. During the process of phagocytosis they release superoxide anion (O_2^-), hydrogen peroxide (H_2O_2), and hydroxyl radicals (HO) as well as other oxygen-related, more toxic substances such as HOCl. These ROS help to amplify the cascade of inflammatory mediators and are responsible for tissue injury. Thus if ROS are inhibited or the defense mechanism of the body against free radicals is improved, by supplying plant-derived antioxidants, inflammation may be taken care of.

Nutraceuticals used in their extracted/isolated constituents from foods which have antiinflammatory activity have been reviewed in this section.

FLAVONOIDS

Flavonoids are water-soluble phenolic compounds. They contain conjugated aromatic systems and thus show intense absorption band in the UV and visible regions of the spectrum. They have a wide distribution in all vascular plants. Flavonoids show antiinflammatory effect by inhibiting the enzymes responsible for generation of eicosanoids specifically phospholipase A2, cyclooxygenase, and lipoxygenase. It also inhibits the proinflammatory gene expression including iNOS and cytokines (Kim et al., 2004; Yuan et al., 2006) (Fig. 7.1).

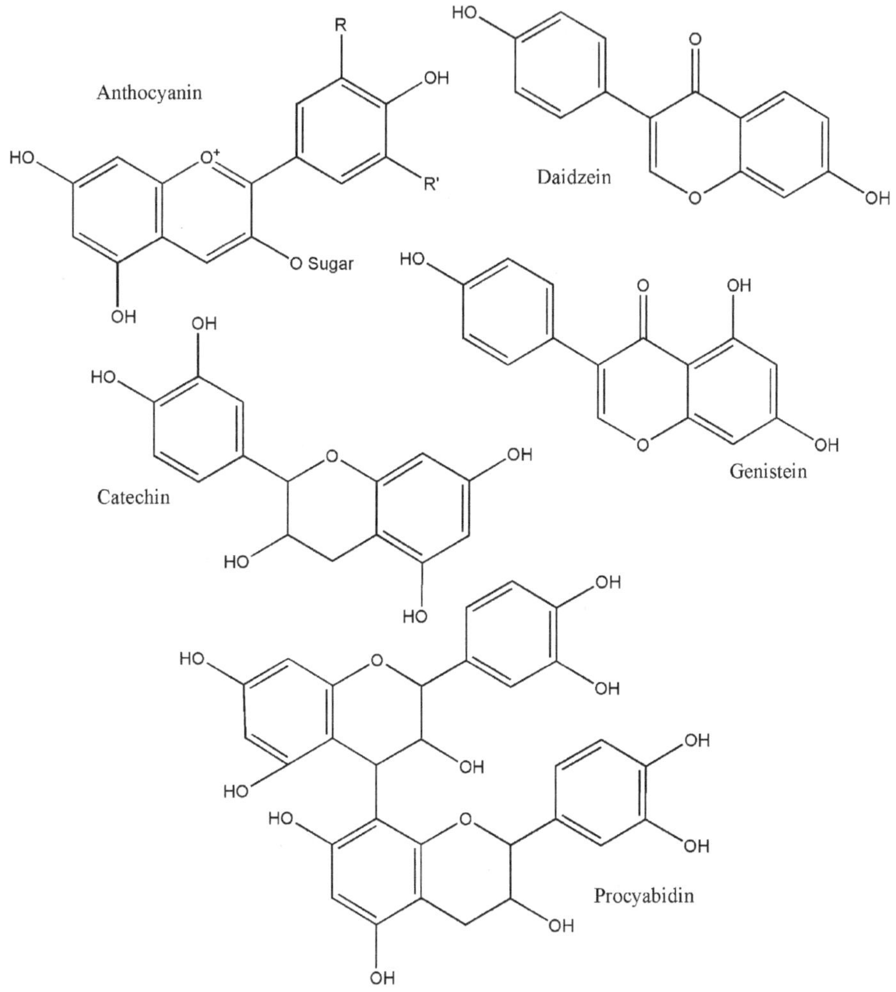

■ **FIGURE 7.1** Structures of phytoconstituents belonging to the flavonoid group.

Some 10 classes of flavonoids are recognized. There are four major classes of flavonoids: flavones (isoflavones), flavanones, catechins, and anthocyanins.

Majority of the studies involving antiinflammatory effect of flavonoids are done in vitro. Flavonoids undergo the process of metabolism to molecules with a different chemical structure. Moreover the amount of flavonoids ingested as nutraceutical may not be sufficient to achieve a plasma concentration which may produce antiinflammatory effect. Hence, it is necessary not only to get these studies done in vivo but also to establish a correlation between the amount of intact flavonoid in the plasma and the activity.

Some of the isolated flavonoids having reported antiinflammatory uses are quercetin, hesperidin, and apigenin.

Soy isoflavones

Soy isoflavones include genistein, daidzein, biochanin, and glycetein which are in the form of glycosides, come under the special class of phytoestrogens and are considered as potential alternatives to the synthetic selective estrogen receptor modulators. The content of isoflavones may vary from 0.4 to 2.4 mg/g depending on climatic conditions and crop variety. Soy isoflavones are extracted from pods of *Glycine max*, belonging to the family Fabaceae.

Soy isoflavones have been used to reduce the risk of cardiovascular heart disease and cancer. It has also been targeted as a safe and effective alternative therapy for treatment of postmenopausal syndrome. They have been investigated for their effect on modulation of IL-6 gene expression levels and are projected as agents useful for treatment of inflammation, and thereby prevent cancer progression, ageing discomforts and restore immune homeostasis (Dijsselbloem et al., 2004).

Another study reports the use of isoflavone for the treatment of airway inflammatory disease as it reduces the mRNA expression of eotaxin, IL-5, IL-4, and matrix metalloproteinase-9, and increased mRNA expression of interferon (IFN)-γ and tissue inhibitor of metalloproteinase-1. It is also found to inhibit the lung tissue eosinophil infiltration, airway mucus production, and collagen deposition in lung tissues (Bao et al., 2011). They are also being projected to be used in treatment of cutaneous inflammation by the virtue of inhibiting the proinflammatory cytokines, attenuation of oxidative stress, expression of COX-2, inhibiting NF-κB activation, and also reducing the formation of 5-hydroxymethyl-2′-deoxyuridine (5-OHmdU), a marker for oxidative DNA damage (Khan et al., 2012; Davis et al., 2001). They are further found to be useful in reducing insulin resistance and hence may be considered as a complimentary therapy for control of diabetes. It prevented the secretion of the inflammatory factors prostaglandin E2 and IL-6. Isoflavones reduced inflammation in 3T3-L1 adipocytes and were also capable of downregulating the cytokine gene expression and inflammatory factors (Pinent et al., 2011; Mahesha et al., 2007). Another interesting study indicates that soy isoflavones are not helpful in reducing the IL-6 levels in postmenopausal women probably because of the lack of enzyme for the formation of equol, a metabolic product of isoflavones (Mangano et al., 2013). Despite the applications mentioned above for soy isoflavones, their bioavailability seems to be a problem. All these isoflavones are present in their bound form with a sugar moiety. It has been found that these isoflavones are not absorbed intact and their bioavailability requires initial hydrolysis of sugar moiety for peripheral circulation (Setchell et al., 2002). Now, whether the unbound form is active or not needs to be understood. Soy isoflavones are available in a range of formulations either alone or in combination with other ingredients.

Catechins

Green tea is the main source for this flavonoid. Four principle catechins found in tea include epicatechin, epicatechin gallate, epigallocatechin, and epigallocatechin gallate. The healing activity of catechins is attributed to their polyphenolic nature. These polyphenols have been reported to have antiplatelet, antiinflammatory, and antithrombotic activity, thereby reducing the risk of congestive heart disease. It is also shown to produce chemopreventive effect. Catechin is reported to be beneficial for cardiovascular disorders and is found to inhibit the NF-κB initiated production of cytokines and adhesion molecules (Bhardwaj and Khanna, 2013). Catechin is further investigated for its role in reducing the incidence of coronary artery disease and has been found to be effective in reducing atherosclerosis by affecting inflammatory cell recruitment and expression in the vascular wall (Norata et al., 2007). Another interesting report suggests the use of green tea catechin in treatment of periodontal inflammation for the same reason as quoted above and also because it reduces the gingival oxidative stress (Maruyama et al., 2011). It inhibits the signal transduction pathway activated by the Toll-like receptor 1 (TLR-1), thereby markedly reducing the levels of proinflammatory mediators (Hirao et al., 2010). Another report suggests that catechins are useful as antiinflammatory agent in treating liver dysfunction (Saito et al., 2011). *Acacia catechu*, another rich source of catechins, is also found to exhibit significant antiinflammatory activity in osteoarthritis (Stohs and Bagchi, 2015).

There are about 60 formulations containing green tea extract; few of them have been enlisted in the Table 7.1.

Table 7.1 List of Formulations for Respective Nutraceuticals

Product Name	Quantity of the Nutraceutical Present	Indication
Soyisoflavones		
Alfaflavon	Soy isoflavones 40% 30 mg	Used as dietary supplements
Bio-d3 fem-macleods	Soy isoflavones 40% 50 mg	Agents affecting bone metabolism
Bonex 1	40	Calcium with vitamins
Caldec pm	60	Calcium with vitamins
Calmcare	100	Vitamins and/or minerals
Calmquest	60	Vitamins and/or minerals
Celol-xt	60	Agents affecting bone metabolism
Dairical plus	30	Vitamins and/or minerals
Ease-pms	75	Supplement and adjuvant therapy
Estovon	75	Supplement and adjuvant therapy
Estovon-xt	60	Supplement and adjuvant therapy
Evepearl-mp	75	Drugs acting on uterus
Gynacea	75	Supplement and adjuvant therapy
Isoflav-cr	Pure	Supplement and adjuvant therapy
Isovon	75	Enteral/nutritional products
Melaglow	0.1% (w/w)	Dermatologicals
Menoease	75	Vitamins and/or minerals
Menopace-iso	100	Vitamins and/or minerals
Menosoft	40	Vitamins and/or minerals
Menosoy		Vitamins and/or minerals
Moxafav	40	Vitamins and/or minerals
Mumbels	50	Vitamins and/or minerals
Soyace	40	Agents affecting bone metabolism
Soycal-d	60 mg	Calcium with vitamins
Catechins		
R & D—weight loss formula/fats burner		Antiobesity agents
Fame green tea capsules		Supplement and adjuvant therapy
Absolut-3g	10	Supplement and adjuvant therapy
Acteva	10	Enteral/nutritional product
Becospecial	10	Vitamins and/or minerals
Bonefit	100	Vitamins and/or minerals
Colred	300 mg	Dyslipidemia and cholestrol associated cardiac complications

(*Continued*)

Table 7.1 List of Formulations for Respective Nutraceuticals (Continued)

Product Name	Quantity of the Nutraceutical Present	Indication
Dayvital	10	Enteral/nutritional product
Depiderm	0.1	Dermatologicals
Exgreen	20% 200 mg	Vitamins and/or minerals
F-gam	100	Supplement and adjuvant therapy
Gardian	250 mg	Vitamins and/or minerals
Jubiglow-h	Polyphenols 10 mg	Supplement and adjuvant therapy
Keraglo-men	10	Vitamins and/or minerals
Morvit	10	Supplement and adjuvant therapy
Neuroage-og	10	Nootropics/neurotonic/ neurotrophics
Obedeuce	200	Antiobesity
Tissot	100	Vitamins and/or minerals
Xplode sf	100	Vitamins and/or minerals
Pycnogenol		
A–Z ns	10	Enteral/nutritional products
Axbex-ns	4	Supplement and adjuvant therapy
B-colen	2	Vitamins and/or minerals
Cosglo	2% (w/w)	Dermatologicals
Enlarge	5	Supplement and adjuvant therapy
Glambak	2% (w/w)	Dermatologicals
Gloeye	–	Enteral/nutritional product
Jwell	10	Vitamins and/or minerals
Kojiglo	2% (w/w)	Dermatologicals
Purelite	0.4%	Dermatologicals
Radiance	20	Supplement and adjuvant therapy
Rqual-gold	25	Supplement and adjuvant therapy
Stamina-od	10	Vitamins and/or minerals
Tgia plus	10	Vitamins and/or minerals
Zemin-pb	50	Vitamins and/or minerals
Resveratrol		
Lecitrol liquid-filled cap	50 mg	Supplements and adjuvant therapy
Harty cap	5 g	Supplements and adjuvant therapy
Resmep softgel	30% 5 mg	Cardiac drug

(Continued)

Table 7.1 List of Formulations for Respective Nutraceuticals (Continued)

Product Name	Quantity of the Nutraceutical Present	Indication
Lipoic acid (thioctic acid)		
Agemax-g cap	100 mg	Neuropathic pain
Alcrin-m cap	270 mg	Nootropics and neurotonics/neurotrophics
Alfacure tab	100 mg	Vitamin B complex with C
Aluno-a tab	100 mg	Hyperuricemia and gout preparations
Beminal forte film-coated tab	100 mg	Nutritional supplement during pregnancy and lactation, for growing children, old patients, and during convalescence
		Vitamins and minerals (pre- and postnatal)/antianemics
Benfo forte cap	100 mg	Neuropathy
Bigvin plus soft-gelatin cap	100 mg	Diabetes, cataract, CAD, IHD, cancer, arthritis, and obesity
L-Nit cap	100 mg	Enteral/nutritional products
Fotia plus tab	50 mg	Diabetic neuropathy, diabetic nephropathy, diabetic retinopathy, cardiovascular disease, sciatica, fibromyalgia, Alzheimer disease, alcoholic polyneuropathy
Me plus-od cap	300 mg	Diabetic neuropathy and hyperhomocysteinemia
Metmin-a tab	200 mg	Antidiabetic agent
Nervup forte cap	200 mg	Chronic diabetic neuropathy
Neuro-od cap	100 mg	Peripheral neuropathy
Renewliv forte soft-gelatin cap	50 mg	Cholagogues, cholelitholytics, and hepatic protectors
Biolite cream		Emollients, cleansers, and skin protectives
Reviz cap	300 mg	Maintains peripheral circulation, promoting general health, improving metabolic function
Optica softgel cap	250 mg	Ophthalmic preparation
R & D—weight loss formula/fats burner cap 470 mg	60 mg	Dietary supplement

(*Continued*)

Table 7.1 List of Formulations for Respective Nutraceuticals (Continued)

Product Name	Quantity of the Nutraceutical Present	Indication
R & D—super ALA cap 600 mg	600 mg	Restores and protects nerve functioning, supports healthy blood glucose metabolism, defends against free radical damage, maintains radiant complexion
R & D—skin whitening supplement (202) cap 500 mg		Promotes skin whitening, elasticity, and collagen production
R & D—botanical (nano) stem cells essence topical liquid		Rejuvenates skin and helps fight ageing. Smoothes away fine lines, wrinkles, dark spots, and pigmentation. Excellent use (for doctors) pre- and posttreatment by laser/IPL/RF
Olivenol livin' youthful cap	50 mg	Supplements and adjuvant therapy
Alanerv softgel cap	300 mg	Food supplement w/antioxidant effect on free radicals, w/action on cell trophism and helps protect the nervous cells
Linolenic acid		
Prime e cap	γ-Linolenic acid 100 mg	Supplements and adjuvant therapy
Abipro-DHA	γ-Linolenic acid 25 mg	Enteral/nutritional product
Alphaneuron	γ-Linolenic acid 180 mg	Nootropics and neurotonics/neurotrophic
GLA-120		Supplements and adjuvant therapy
GLA-AD	γ-Linolenic acid 0.5% (w/w)	Emollients and skin protective
GMAB-Plus	γ-Linolenic acid 100 mg	Nootropics and neurotonics/neurotrophic
Matilda-AF	γ-Linolenic acid 60 mg	Vitamins and/or minerals
Nutriright-mom	γ-Linolenic acid 25 mg	Enteral/nutritional products
Rejunex plus	γ-Linolenic acid 100 mg	Nootropics and neurotonics/neurotrophic

(Continued)

Table 7.1 List of Formulations for Respective Nutraceuticals (Continued)

Product Name	Quantity of the Nutraceutical Present	Indication
Trinerve	γ-Linolenic acid 60 mg	Supplements and adjuvant therapy
Extraa-P	α-Linolenic acid 858 mg	Enteral/nutritional products
Farex-2	α-Linolenic acid 250 mg	Enteral/nutritional products
Lacotdex-3	α-Linolenic acid 110 mg	Enteral/nutritional products
Lactogen-1	α-Linolenic acid 250 mg	Infant nutritional product
Maxoflam gel	α-Linolenic acid 3% (w/w)	Nonsteroidal antiinflammatory drugs
Moistures-AF	α-Linolenic acid 10% (w/w)	Emollients and skin protectives
Neurovit-MC	α-Linolenic acid 50 mg	Vitamins and/or minerals
Pediasure	α-Linolenic acid 0.4 g	Enteral/nutritional product
Lupeol		
Mustela 9-month stretch marks double action topical cream		Emollients, cleansers, and skin protectives
Mustela 9-month stretch marks intensive actions topical cream		Helps reduce stretch marks that formed during pregnancy or after giving birth
Astaxanthin		
Astador cap	1 mg,	Vitamins and/or minerals
Bestage softgel	10% 4 mg	Supplements and adjuvant therapy
Hi-q 300 film-coated tab	8 mg	Oligospermia and asthenospermia Drugs for erectile dysfunction
Lycofact plus cap	1 mg	Enteral/nutritional products
Ovaa shield combi-kit	4 mg	Trophic hormones and related synthetic drugs
Astaplus fc caplet	4 mg	Supplements and adjuvant therapy

(*Continued*)

Table 7.1 List of Formulations for Respective Nutraceuticals (Continued)

Product Name	Quantity of the Nutraceutical Present	Indication
Astatin soft-gelatin cap 4 mg		Helps maintain the immune system
Asthin force topical gel	0.02%	Antioxidant and moisturizer for the skin health
Nutrivision cap	125 µm	Dietary supplement for healthy vision; antioxidant
Nuvit regenesis sachet 7.5 g		Supplements and adjuvant therapy
Armolipid tab		Helps support healthy cholesterol levels in association with a suitable diet
Optamin cap	2 mg	Nutritional supplement for vision and eye. Helps to reduce risk of age-associated macular degeneration

Pycnogenol

Pycnogenol is a mixture of flavonoids isolated from the pine tree bark. It is a registered name of a standardized extract of the bark of *Pinus pinaster*, Pinaceae. The pine bark extracts have been used since many centuries for the treatment of wounds, and history says that it was an instant cure to a crew in Canada dying from scurvy (Ince et al., 2009). Pycnogenol is a mixture of procyanidins and phenolic acids. The procyanidins range from monomeric catechin to oligomers with seven or more flavonoid subunit. Benzoic acid and cinnamic acid derivatives form the phenolic acid part (Rohdewald, 2002). Supplementation with pycnogenol in humans is able to modulate the arachidonic acid pathway, blocking both the COX-2 and 5-LOX pathways (Canali et al., 2009). Studies have proven that pycnogenol is highly bioavailable and the mixture is more effective than individual components due to synergistic effect.

Pretreatment with pycnogenol ameliorates lung inflammation and reduces airway inflammation by reducing the formation of major proinflammatory cytokines like TNF-α, IL-6, IL-1β via inhibiting the activation of NF-κB (Xia et al., 2015) and by reducing inflammatory cell count and the levels of IL-4, IL-5, IL-13 (Shin et al., 2013), respectively.

Being polyphenolic in nature, it is attributed to have antioxidant activity and has also been reported to be useful in the treatment of neurodegenerative disorders as it not only ameliorates oxidative stress and protects the dopaminergic neurons but also significantly reduces neuroinflammation (Khan et al., 2013).

Pycnogenol has been further found to be effective in animal model of gouty arthritis again by reducing the inflammatory cell infiltration, decreasing the expression of COX-2 and iNOS in the synovial fluid and articular cartilage (Peng et al., 2011). Pycnogenol is also tested clinically and has shown to be effective in treating inflammatory conditions like arthritis, diabetes, and hypertension (Cordova et al., 2013). Pycnogenol was found to have antiapoptic activity due to its potential to inhibit inflammation by modulating the inflammatory markers like iNOS and COX-2, and NF-κB nuclear translocation. Due to this effect observed in the renal tubular cells, it is proposed that pycnogenol may be explored further for the treatment of diabetic nephropathy (Kim et al., 2011b). Pycnogenol is reported to affect the cardiovascular system by exerting vasorelaxant activity, angiotensin-converting enzyme inhibiting activity, and the ability to enhance the microcirculation by increasing capillary permeability (Packer et al., 1999).

One of the studies conducted on macrophages, an important inflammatory cell, suggests that the antiinflammatory effect of pycnogenol may be due to its ability to modulate the gluthathione redox cycle and activities of catalase and superoxide dismutase (Bayeta and Lau, 2000). Diabetes increases the expression of endothelial cell adhesion molecule ICAM-1 (intercellular adhesion molecule-1) and its counterpart on the leukocyte CD-18. Pycnogenol inhibits the NF-κB–mediated expression of adhesion molecules like ICAM-1, vascular cell adhesion molecule-1 (VCAM-1), and cytokines. Due to this inhibition, it prevents the retinal leukocyte adhesion and blood–retinal barrier breakdown (Schönlau and Rohdewald, 2001). Pycnogenol can also be used as a second-line therapy to reduce inflammation associated with systemic lupus erythematosus (Stefanescu et al., 2001). There are around 18 formulations available in the market, which incorporate *P. pinaster* extract either as a single ingredient or in combination with other. Few important ones are highlighted in Table 7.1.

ANTHOCYANINS

Anthocyanins are coloring pigments belonging to the flavonoid class, which have raised interest due to their beneficial health effects and range of colors. They are responsible for intense colors like pink, scarlet, red, mauve, violet, and blue. They are found to be distributed in flowers, fruits, and vegetables. Anthocyanins are nearly universal in all vascular plants; they may be replaced with similar group of pigments like betacyanins in higher plants, the Centrospermae (Harborne, 1998). Anthocyanins reduce the inflammatory cell infiltration and the proinflammatory mediators. A review reports that anthocyanins exert their antiinflammatory effect by downregulating the redox-sensitive NF-κB signaling pathway and the mitogen-activated protein kinase (MAPK) pathway (Vendrame and Klimis-Zacas, 2015).

A clinical study done in the United States reports that higher intake of anthocyanins reduces the risk of certain chronic diseases probably by exerting antiinflammatory effects (Cassidy et al., 2015). A mixture of anthocyanins reduced the inflammation in hypercholesterolemic individuals, thereby greatly halting the progression of atherosclerosis (Zhu et al., 2013). It was found to protect against inflammatory and oxidative damages induced by demyelination (Carvalho et al., 2015). Berry anthocyanins isolated from blueberry, blackberry, and blackcurrant were found to exert antiinflammatory effect in macrophages due to inhibition of translocation of NF-κB (Lee et al., 2014), whereas those from tart cherries inhibited the enzymes involved in the biosynthesis of PGs in vitro (Wang et al., 1999). It has also been proved in vivo in carrageenan-induced model of inflammation that these tart cherry anthocyanins do exhibit antiinflammatory properties (Tall et al., 2004). Anthocyanins isolated from the blue flower petals of *Clitoria ternatae* are reported to suppress the production of proinflammatory mediators by inhibiting NF-κB translocation and hence can be proposed as an ingredient in developing nutraceuticals (Nair et al., 2015). Another berry called as black chokeberry is reported to exert antiinflammatory effect by inhibiting the release of TNF, IL-6, and IL-8 in the peripheral monocytes and activation of NF-κB in the macrophages (Appel et al., 2015).

This class of flavonoids may also play a protective role in the development of asthma by downregulating Th2 cytokines (IL-4, IL-13, IL-13R1α, IL-13R2α), proinflammatory cytokines, and COX-2 (Park et al., 2007).

Resveratrol

Resveratrol is a phytoalexin polyphenolic stilbene derivative. It is found in the leaves, skins, and petals of *Vitis vinifera*, wines, and grape juice. It is also found in peanut butter and berries. It is reported to have a range of biological activities like antioxidant, chemopreventive, and antiinflammatory activity. It is well documented for its beneficial effects on the cardiovascular system. Its antiinflammatory effects are attributed to its regulation of NF-κB signaling pathway (Kang et al., 2009). This effect may also be beneficial in treating diabetes-associated macrovascular complications like coronary heart disease (Zheng et al., 2013). This NF-κB modulation also contributes to the neuroprotective effects of resveratrol (Tiwari and Chopra, 2013). Moreover neuroinflammation due to microglial activation is a contributing factor for neurodegenerative diseases like Alzheimer's, Parkinson's, and Huntington's disease; since resveratrol can cross the blood–brain barrier easily, it is a promising candidate for treatment of these diseases (Zhang et al., 2010). The protective effect of resveratrol against neuroinflammation may also be due to modulation of the expression of neurotropic factor in the brain and reducing the levels of proinflammatory cytokines in circulation (Yazir et al., 2015). The antiinflammatory effect of resveratrol is not just due to reduced expression of proinflammatory cytokines but also due to increased expression of antiinflammatory IL-10 and modulation of the JAk-STAT-3 signaling pathway in the microglial cells (Cianciulli et al., 2015) and IFN-γ–activated macrophages (Chung et al., 2011). This pathway is a component of many cytokine receptor systems, wherein it activates the genes that promotes inflammatory response. Ulcerative colitis is an inflammatory condition, and reducing inflammation is the main stay of therapy for this disease. A clinical study reports the beneficial effect of resveratrol in reducing inflammation (Samsami-kor et al., 2015). It also reduces the mRNA expression of proinflammatory cytokines as well as COX-2, thus improving the inflammatory condition of the aged liver (Tung et al., 2015). The hepatic inflammation observed in diabetic patients may be reversed by the administration of resveratrol as it reduces the inflammatory response (Sadi et al., 2015). The antiinflammatory effect of resveratrol on bone marrow-derived mesenchymal stem cells makes it useful in the treatment of inflammation-associated bone disease. It reverses the effect of TNF-α and inhibits the NF-κB signaling (Zhang et al., 2015). It can also be used for respiratory conditions arising due to persistent inflammation as it reduces the levels of nerve growth factor, a neurotropin mediator of persistent pain associated with inflammation (Zang et al., 2015). It may be used in controlling obesity and metainflammation since it is reported to downregulate the levels of proinflammatory cytokines in adipose tissue and their upstream signaling molecules like TLR-2 and TLR-4. The stimulation of these receptors results in activation of the proinflammatory processes, at the same time they are also involved in innate immune response (Kim et al., 2011a). There are many reports which suggest antiinflammatory effect of resveratrol in vitro or in vivo in animal models, but human trials to prove the same are very limited. One such clinical study indicates that long-term supplementation with resveratrol either in its pure form or as an extract downregulates the formation of proinflammatory cytokines in type 2 diabetes mellitus hypertensive patients (Kang et al., 2009). The marketed formulations for resveratrol are enlisted in Table 7.1.

Lipoic acid

Also known as thioctic acid, it is a very powerful sulfur containing antioxidant. A healthy human body produces sufficient lipoic acid (LA), but in cases where an individual is suffering from a disease, supplementation with LA which is free and not bound to any protein is needed. The dietary sources of LA are yeast, spinach, broccoli, potatoes, and various meat products like heart, liver, and kidneys. It has been reported that LA downregulates the expression of redox-sensitive proinflammatory proteins including TNF and iNOS and hence may function as antiinflammatory agent (Maczurekb et al., 2008). It can also modify the cyclic AMP/protein kinase A signaling cascade and inhibit the formation of proinflammatory cytokines thus exerting antiinflammatory activity (Salinthone et al., 2010). LA is reported to reduce the neurovascular inflammation and thereby protect the blood–brain barrier from the degenerative effects of inflammation (Takechi et al., 2013). Increased activity of microglial cells plays an important role in the immune and inflammatory response and thus in the progression of neurodegenerative diseases. The exact mechanism of LA in the microglia is not known; however, it is proposed to modulate the activity of Akt/glycogen synthase kinase 3β (Koriyama et al., 2013). It also may inhibit the activation of NF-κB and expression of proinflammatory cytokines in microglia (Li et al., 2015). Alpha LA increases the expression of brain-derived neurotropic factor, thereby reversing the neuroinflammation (Miao et al., 2013). Moreover LA is also reported to increase the glutathione biosynthesis, inhibit the proinflammatory molecule expression in glial cells, and also modulate the extracellular signal-regulated kinases and heme-oxygenase 1 pathways (Santos et al., 2015). The HO-1 plays a role in inflammation-induced lung injury, thus LA also has a protective role in acute lung injury (Lin et al., 2013).

A clinical study has shown its efficacy in reducing the expression of cell adhesion molecules, VCAM-1 and ICAM-1, in gestational diabetes women and thereby be able to counter the adverse inflammatory effects of chronic hyperglycemia on the endothelial cells (Di Tomo et al., 2015). LA may also be beneficial in the treatment of endometriosis, one of the chronic inflammatory conditions as it is capable of modulating the inflammatory process (Agostinis et al., 2015) and may also be beneficial to counter the inflammation associated with acute kidney injury as it attenuates the inflammatory response in mesangial cells by inhibiting NF-κB signaling pathway (Li et al., 2014). The same antiinflammatory activity is useful in preventing the glomerular injury in type 2 diabetes patients (Bao et al., 2014). LA administration during cardiac surgery may help to reduce the cytokine level and the oxidative stress which is usually enhanced due to extracorporeal circulation of blood (Uya et al., 2013). Some of the known formulations are listed in Table 7.1.

Linolenic acid

It is a tri-unsaturated fatty acid. α-Linolenic acid (ALA) is Ω-3 fatty acid whereas γ-linolenic acid is Ω-6 fatty acid. γ-Linolenic acid is found in *Oenthera* spp. Borage oil contains around 25% of this acid. It is also present in starflower oil, evening primrose oil, and blackcurrant seed oil. It is not usually purified and used as it is. It is most commonly used for the treatment of atopic eczema and premenstrual syndrome (Evans, 2009). ALA is found in vegetable oils, nuts (walnut), and seeds like chia, flaxseed, and linseed. Linolenic acid can be converted to eicosapentaenoic acid and docosahexaenoic acid (DHA) which have been shown to have an array of protective role against, cardiovascular, neuronal, osteoporotic, and inflammatory diseases, but being lipoidal in nature may undergo lipid peroxidation increasing the risk for diseases like macular degeneration and prostate cancer. Linolenic acid is known to directly suppress proinflammatory cytokines like TNF-α and IL-6/IL-8, and regulate the expression of NF-κB (Kim et al., 2014). Diabetic patients over a period of time suffer from myocardial dysfunction which may be in the form of myocardial ischemia/reperfusion injury. ALA consumption over a long period of time provides cardioprotection due to its antiinflammatory and antioxidant effects possibly through phosphatidylinositol-3-kinase (PI3K)/Akt-dependent mechanism (Xie et al., 2011). Colitis is a type of inflammatory bowel disease. It was found that ALA-rich diet reduces the expression of CAM like ICAM-1, VCAM-1, and vascular endothelial growth factor A receptor-2. It also reduces the expression of HO-1 (Ibrahim et al., 2012). Atopic dermatitis is a chronic inflammatory condition with pruritic symptoms. Dihomo-gamma-linolenic acid upregulates the formation of prostaglandin D1 (PGD1) which in turn suppresses the gene expression of thymic stromal lymphopoietin in keratinocytes and prevents atopic dermatitis in mice (Amagai et al., 2015). Conjugated forms of linolenic acid, namely α-eleostearic acid and punicic acid, found in bitter gourd and snake gourd oil, respectively, show a synergistic antiinflammatory and antioxidant activity (Saha et al., 2012). It is reported that increasing the supplementation of linolenic acid shifts the metabolic balance from arachidonic acid to eicosapentanoic acid resulting into production of less inflammatory profile. Moreover it can directly alter the functioning of inflammatory cells: endothelial cells and leukocytes (Yates et al., 2014).

The formulations containing either of the isomers of linolenic acid are enlisted in Table 7.1.

Thymoquinone

Thymoquinone is the active ingredient of black cumin (*Nigella sativa*), and is responsible for therapeutic effects such as asthma, arthritis, and neurodegenerative disorders all of which are chronic inflammatory conditions. It has a number of pharmacological actions like antioxidant, antiinflammatory, immunomodulatory, antihistaminic, antimicrobial, antitumor effects, gastroprotective, hepatoprotective, nephroprotective, and neuroprotective activities. It has proven beneficial effects in bone complications, cardiovascular disorders, diabetes, reproductive and respiratory disorders (Darakhshan et al., 2015). Thymoquinone administration reduces the expression of proinflammatory cytokines like IL-6 in the microglial cells and hence can delay the onset of inflammation-induced neurodegeneration (Taka et al., 2015). It downregulates the COX and LOX enzymes and thus reduces the formation of eicosanoids. It reduces the serum levels of proinflammatory cytokines: IL-6, TNF-α, and IL-1β. It further has antioxidant activity as it inhibits the formation of ROS, lipid peroxidation, and nitric oxide production and also increases the activity of antioxidant enzymes (Majdalawieh and Fayyad, 2015). It has been projected as a therapy for bone lytic disorders as it prevents NF-κB ligand Receptor activator of nuclear factor kappa-B ligand (RANKL) induced osteoclastogenesis via inhibition of MAPK and NF-κβ (Thummuri et al., 2015). Thymoquinone also has its beneficial effects in the treatment of RA, a chronic inflammatory condition. TNF-α-activated apoptosis signaling kinase-1 plays an important role in the pathology of RA. It acts as an inhibitor in the TNF-α-induced signaling pathway decreasing the formation of proinflammatory cytokines and the subsequent tissue destruction (Umar et al., 2015) (Fig. 7.2).

Lupeol

There has been a lot of interest in triterpenes being used for beneficial health effects. One such triterpene is lupeol found in white cabbage, green pepper, strawberry, olive, mangoes, and grapes and in many medicinal plants. It targets multiple sites to have antiinflammatory effect such as NF-κB, cFLIP, Fas, Kras, PI3K/Akt and Wnt/β-catenin in a variety of cells (Mohammad, 2009). There are very few reports of lupeol showing an activity as an antiinflammatory. One such article states that it inhibits the phosphorylation of P38 MAPK and c-Jun N-terminal kinase in the microglia and thus may be used in the treatment of neuroinflammatory disorders (Badshah et al., 2015). The formulations have been enlisted in Table 7.1.

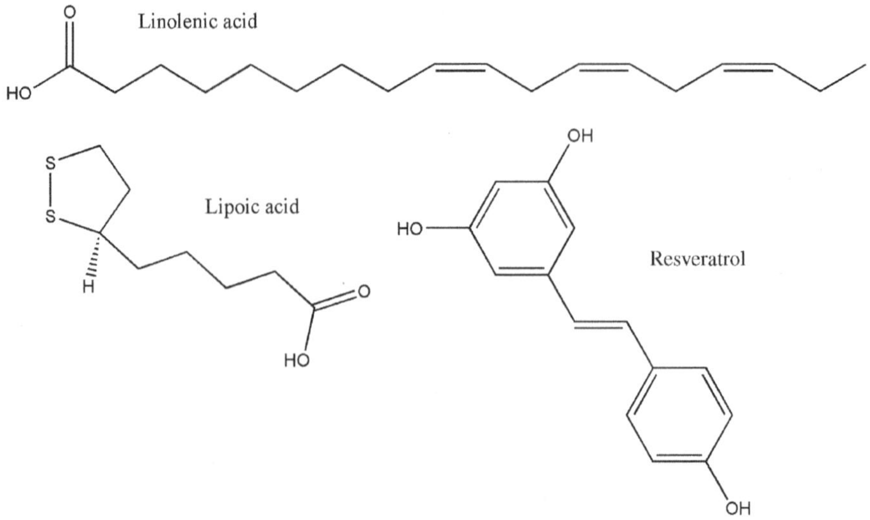

■ FIGURE 7.2 Structures for linolenic acid, lipoic acid, and resveratrol.

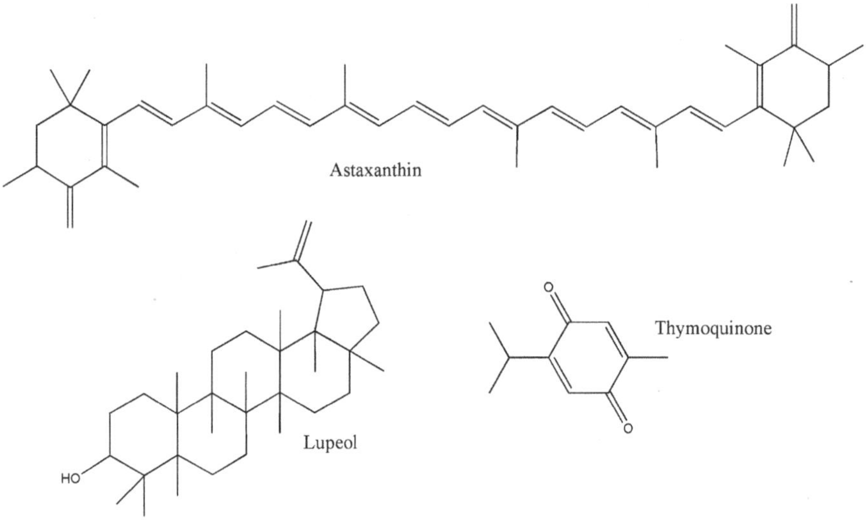

■ FIGURE 7.3 Structures of phytoconstituents belonging to the terpenoid group.

Astaxanthin

Haematococcus pluvialis is the richest source of natural astaxanthin (Guerin et al., 2003). Astaxanthin is a carotenoid showing promising antiinflammatory activity. It possesses antioxidant activity due to which it is capable of inhibiting the production of inflammatory mediators by blocking NF-κB activation and as a consequence suppression of IkB kinase activity and IkB-α degradation (Lee et al., 2003). It also inhibits the production of inflammatory mediators by blocking iNOS and COX-2 activation or by the suppression of iNOS and COX-2 degradation (Choi et al., 2008). Further to this, it also suppresses NO, PGE2, and TNF-α production, through directly blocking NOS enzyme activity (Ohgami et al., 2003). Table 7.1 gives the list of important formulations of astaxanthin (Fig. 7.3).

Phosphopeptides

There is just one report which states that phosphopeptides (PPPs) isolated from hen egg yolk may serve as nutraceutical compounds with antiinflammatory properties as it downregulates some key proinflammatory markers like TNF-α, IL-1β, IL-6, iNOS, IL-8, MCP-1, and IL-12 (Xu et al., 2012). A precaution needs to be taken while considering PPPs as antiinflammatory since they may act as antigens and invoke an immune response.

REFERENCES

Agostinis, C., Zorzet, S., De Leo, R., Zauli, G., De Seta, F., Bulla, R., 2015. The combination of N-acetyl cysteine, alpha-lipoic acid, and bromelain shows high anti-inflammatory properties in novel in vivo and in vitro models of endometriosis. Mediators Inflamm. 2015, 9180–9189.

Amagai, Y., Oida, K., Matsuda, A., Jung, K., Kakutani, S., Tanaka, T., et al., 2015. Dihomo-γ-linolenic acid prevents the development of atopic dermatitis through prostaglandin D1 production in NC/Tnd mice. J. Dermatol. Sci. 79, 30–37.

Appel, K., Meiser, P., Millán, E., Collado, J.A., Rose, T., Gras, C.C., et al., 2015. Chokeberry (*Aronia melanocarpa* (Michx.) Elliot) concentrate inhibits NF-κB and synergizes with selenium to inhibit the release of pro-inflammatory mediators in macrophages. Fitoterapia 105, 73–82.

Badshah, H., Ali, T., Rehman, S.U., Amin, F.U., Ullah, F., Kim, T.H., et al., 2015. Protective effect of lupeol against lipopolysaccharide-induced neuroinflammation via the p38/c-Jun N-terminal kinase pathway in the adult mouse brain. J. Neuroimmune Pharmacol. 2015 Jul 3.

Baldwin, A.S., 1996. The NF-_B and I_B proteins: new discoveries and insights. Ann. Rev. Immunol. 14, 649–681.

Bao, X.H., Xu, J., Chen, Y., Yang, C.L., Ye, S.D., 2014. Alleviation of podocyte injury: the possible pathway implicated in anti-inflammation of alpha-lipoic acid in type 2 diabetics. Aging Clin. Exp. Res. 26, 483–489.

Bao, Z.S., Hong, L., Guan, Y., Dong, X.W., Zheng, H.S., Tan, G.L., et al., 2011. Inhibition of airway inflammation, hyperresponsiveness and remodeling by soy isoflavone in a murine model of allergic asthma. Int. Immunopharmacol. 11, 899 906.

Bayeta, E., Lau, B.H.S., 2000. Pycnogenol inhibits generation of inflammatory mediators in macrophages. Nutr. Res. 20, 249–259.

Bhardwaj, P., Khanna, D., 2013. Green tea catechins: defensive role in cardiovascular disorders. Chin. J. Nat. Med. 11, 345–353.

Canali, R., Comitato, R., Schonlau, F., Virgil, F., 2009. The anti-inflammatory pharmacology of Pycnogenol® in humans involves COX-2 and 5-LOX mRNA expression in leukocytes. Int. Immunopharmacol. 9, 1145–1149.

Carvalho, F.B., Gutierres, J.M., Bohnert, C., Zago, A.M., Abdalla, F.H., Vieira, J.M., et al., 2015. Anthocyanins suppress the secretion of proinflammatory mediators and oxidative stress, and restore ion pump activities in demyelination. J. Nutr. Biochem. 26, 378–390.

Cassidy, A., Rogers, G., Peterson, J.J., Dwyer, J.T., Lin, H., Jacques, P.F., 2015. Higher dietary anthocyanin and flavonol intakes are associated with anti-inflammatory effects in a population of US adults. Am. J. Clin. Nutr. 102, 172–181.

Choi, S.K., Park, Y.S., Choi, D.K., Chang, H.I., 2008. Effects of astaxanthin on the production of NO and the expression of COX-2 and iNOS in LPS-stimulated BV2 microglial cells. J. Microbiol. Biotechnol. 18, 1990–1996.

Chung, E.Y., Kim, B.H., Hong, J.T., Lee, C.K., Ahn, B., Nam, S.Y., et al., 2011. Resveratrol down-regulates interferon-γ-inducible inflammatory genes in macrophages: molecular mechanism via decreased STAT-1 activation. J. Nutr. Biochem. 22, 902–909.

Cianciulli, A., Dragone, T., Calvello, R., Porro, C., Trotta, T., Lofrumento, D.D., et al., 2015. IL-10 plays a pivotal role in anti-inflammatory effects of resveratrol in activated microglia cells. Int. Immunopharmacol. 24, 369–376.

Cordova, F.M., Marks, M.B.F., Watson, R.R., 2013. Anti-inflammatory actions of pycnogenol: diabetes and arthritis Bioactive Food as Dietary Interventions for Diabetes. Elsevier, Boston, MA.495–501

Darakhshan, S., Pour, A.B., Colagar, A.H., Sisakhtnezhad, S., 2015. Thymoquinone and its therapeutic potentials. Pharmacol. Res. 95–96, 138–158.

Davis, J.N., Kucuk, O., Djuric, Z., Sarkar, F.H., 2001. Soy isoflavone supplementation in healthy men prevents NF-κB activation by TNF-α in blood lymphocytes. Free Radic. Biol. Med. 30, 1293–1302.

Dijsselbloem, N., Berghe, W.V., Naeyer, A.D., Haegeman, G., 2004. Soy isoflavone phyto-pharmaceuticals in interleukin-6 affections: multi-purpose nutraceuticals at the crossroad of hormone replacement, anti-cancer and anti-inflammatory therapy. Biochem. Pharmacol. 68, 1171–1185.

Di Tomo, P., Di Silvestre, S., Cordone, V.G., Giardinelli, A., Faricelli, B., Pipino, C., et al., 2015. *Centella asiatica* and lipoic acid, or a combination thereof, inhibit monocyte adhesion to endothelial cells from umbilical cords of gestational diabetic women. Nutr. Metab. Cardiovasc. Dis. 25, 659–666.

Evans, W.C., 2009. Trease and Evans' Pharmacognosy, sixteenth ed. Elsevier, Amsterdam, pp. 459–468.

Guerin, M., Huntley, M.E., Olaizola, M., 2003. *Haematococcus* astaxanthin: applications for human health and nutrition. Trends Biotechnol. 21, 210–216.

Harborne, J.B., 1998. Phytochemical Methods, third ed. Springer (India) Pvt. Ltd., New Delhi.66–68

Hirao, K., Yumoto, H., Nakanishi, T., Mukai, K., Takahashi, K., Takegawa, D., et al., 2010. Tea catechins reduce inflammatory reactions via mitogen-activated protein kinase pathways in toll-like receptor 2 ligand-stimulated dental pulp cells. Life Sci. 86, 654–660.

Huang, M.T., Ghai, G., Ho, C.T., 2004. Inflammatory process and targets for anti-inflammatory nutraceuticals. Compr. Rev. Food Sci. Food Saf. 3, 127–139.

Ibrahim, A., Aziz, M., Hassan, A., Mbodji, K., Collasse, E., Coëffier, M., et al., 2012. Dietary α-linolenic acid-rich formula reduces adhesion molecules in rats with experimental colitis. Nutrition 28, 799–802.

Ince, I., Celiktas, Y., Yavasoglu, N.U.K., Elgin, G., 2009. Effects of *Pinus brutia* bark extract and Pycnogenol® in a rat model of carrageenan induced inflammation. Phytomedicine 16, 1101–1104.

Kang, O.H., Jang, H.J., Chae, H.S., Oh, Y.C., Choi, J.G., Lee, Y.S., et al., 2009. Anti-inflammatory mechanisms of resveratrol in activated HMC-1 cells: pivotal roles of NF-κB and MAPK. Pharmacol. Res. 59, 330–337.

Khan, A.Q., Khan, R., Rehman, M.U., Lateef, A., Tahir, M., Ali, F., et al., 2012. Soy isoflavones (daidzein & genistein) inhibit 12-O-tetradecanoylphorbol-13-acetate (TPA)-induced cutaneous inflammation via modulation of COX-2 and NF-κB in Swiss albino mice. Toxicology 302, 266–274.

Khan, M.M., Kempuraj, D., Thangavel, R., Zaheer, A., 2013. Protection of MPTP-induced neuroinflammation and neurodegeneration by pycnogenol. Neurochem. Int. 2, 379–388.

Kim, H.P., Son, K.H., Chang, H.W., Kang, S.S., 2004. Anti inflammatory plant flavonoids and cellular action mechanisms. J. Pharmacol. Sci. 96, 229–245.

Kim, K.B., Nam, Y.A., Kim, H.S., Hayes, A.W., Lee, B.M., 2014. α-Linolenic acid: nutraceutical, pharmacological and toxicological evaluation. Food Chem. Toxicol. 70, 163–178.

Kim, S., Jin, Y., Choi, Y., Park, T., 2011a. Resveratrol exerts anti-obesity effects via mechanisms involving down-regulation of adipogenic and inflammatory processes in mice. Biochem. Pharmacol. 81, 1343–1351.

Kim, Y.J., Kim, Y.A., Yokozawa, T., 2011b. Pycnogenol modulates apoptosis by suppressing oxidative stress and inflammation in high glucose-treated renal tubular cells. Food Chem. Toxicol. 49, 2196–2201.

Koriyama, Y., Nakayama, Y., Matsugo, S., Sugitani, K., Ogai, K., Takadera, T., et al., 2013. Anti-inflammatory effects of lipoic acid through inhibition of GSK-3β in lipopolysaccharide-induced BV-2 microglial cells. Neurosci. Res. 77, 87–96.

Kumar, V., Abbas, A.K., Fausto, N., Mitchell, R., 2007. Robbins Basic Pathophysiology, eighth ed. Elsevier, pp. 31–57.

Lee, S.G., Kim, B., Yang, Y., Pham, T.X., Park, Y.K., Manatou, J., et al., 2014. Berry anthocyanins suppress the expression and secretion of proinflammatory mediators in macrophages by inhibiting nuclear translocation of NF-κB independent of NRF2-mediated mechanism. J. Nutr. Biochem. 25, 404–411.

Lee, S.J., Bai, S.K., Lee, K.S., Namkoong, S., Na, H.J., Ha, K.S., et al., 2003. Astaxanthin inhibits nitric oxide production and inflammatory gene expression by suppressing I(kappa)B kinase-dependent NF-kappaB activation. Mol. Cells 16, 97–105.

Li, G., Gao, L., Jia, J., Gong, X., Zang, B., Chen, W., 2014. α-Lipoic acid prolongs survival and attenuates acute kidney injury in a rat model of sepsis. Clin. Exp. Pharmacol. Physiol. 41, 459–468.

Li, Y.H., He, Q., Yu, J.Z., Liu, C.Y., Feng, L., Chai, Z., et al., 2015. Lipoic acid protects dopaminergic neurons in LPS-induced Parkinson's disease model. Metab. Brain Dis. Jun 19.

Lin, Y.C., Lai, Y.S., Chou, T.C., 2013. The protective effect of alpha-lipoic acid in lipopolysaccharide-induced acute lung injury is mediated by heme oxygenase-1. Evid. Based Complement Alternat. Med. http://dx.doi.org/10.1155/2013/590363.

Maczurekb, A., Hagera, K., Kenkliesa, M., Sharmand, M., Martinsd, R., Engele, J., et al., 2008. Lipoic acid as an anti-inflammatory and neuroprotective treatment for Alzheimer's disease. Adv. Drug Deliv. Rev. 60, 1463–1470.

Mahesha, H.G., Singh, S.A., Rao, A.G.A., 2007. Inhibition of lipoxygenase by soy isoflavones: evidence of isoflavones as redox inhibitors. Arch. Biochem. Biophys. 461, 176–185.

Majdalawieh, A.F., Fayyad, M.W., 2015. Immunomodulatory and anti-inflammatory action of *Nigella sativa* and thymoquinone: a comprehensive review. Int. Immunopharmacol. 28, 295–304.

Mangano, K.M., Hutchins-Wiese, H.L., Kenny, A.M., Walsh, S.J., Abourizk, R.H., Bruno, R.S., et al., 2013. Soy proteins and isoflavones reduce interleukin-6 but not serum lipids in older women: a randomized controlled trial. Nutr. Res. 33, 1026–1033.

Maruyama, T., Tomofuji, T., Endo, Y., Irie, K., Azuma, T., 2011. Supplementation of green tea catechins in dentifrices suppresses gingival oxidative stress and periodontal inflammation. Arch. Oral Biol. 56, 48–53.

Miao, Y., Ren, J., Jiang, L., Liu, J., Jiang, B., Zhang, X., 2013. α-Lipoic acid attenuates obesity-associated hippocampal neuroinflammation and increases the levels of brain-derived neurotrophic factor in ovariectomized rats fed a high-fat diet. Int. J. Mol. Med. 32, 1179–1186.

Mohammad, S., 2009. Lupeol, a novel anti-inflammatory and anti-cancer dietary triterpene. Cancer Lett. 285, 109–115.

Nair, V., Bang, W.Y., Schreckinger, E., Andarwulan, N., Cisneros-Zevallos, L., 2015. The protective role of ternatin anthocyanins and quercetin glycosides from butterfly pea (*Clitoria ternatea* Leguminosae) blue flower petals against LPS-induced inflammation in macrophage cells. J. Agric. Food Chem. 2015 Jun 29.

Norata, G.D., Marchesi, P., Passamonti, S., Pirillo, A., Violi, F., 2007. Anti-inflammatory and anti-atherogenic effects of cathechin, caffeic acid and trans-resveratrol in apolipoprotein E deficient mice. Atherosclerosis 191, 265–271.

Ohgami, K., Shiratori, K., Kotake, S., Nishida, T., Mizuki, N., Yazawa, K., et al., 2003. Effects of astaxanthin on lipopolysaccharide-induced inflammation in vitro and in vivo. Invest. Ophthalmol. Vis. Sci. 44, 2694–2701.

Packer, L., Rimbach, G., Virgili, F., 1999. Antioxidant activity and biologic properties of a procyanidin-rich extract from pine (*Pinus maritima*) bark, pycnogenol. Free Radic. Biol. Med. 27, 704–724.

Pahl, H.L., 1999. Activators and target genes of Rel/NF-_B transcription factors. Oncogene. 18, 6853–6866.

Park, S.J., Shin, W.H., Seo, J.W., Kim, E.J., 2007. Anthocyanins inhibit airway inflammation and hyperresponsiveness in a murine asthma model. Food Chem. Toxicol. 45, 1459–1467.

Peng, Y.J., Lee, C.H., Wang, C.C., Salter, D.M., Lee, H.S., 2011. Pycnogenol attenuates the inflammatory and nitrosative stress on joint inflammation induced by urate crystals. Free Radic. Biol. Med. 52, 765–774.

Pinent, M., Espinel, A.E., Delgado, M.A., Baiges, I., Bladé, C., Arola, L., 2011. Soy isoflavones are also known to inhibit the lipoxygenase and cyclooxygenase enzymes and also function as antioxidants thereby exhibiting anti inflammatory effects. Food Chem. 125, 513–520.

Rohdewald, P., 2002. A review of the French maritime pine bark extract (pycnogenol), a herbal medication with a diverse clinical pharmacology. Int. J. Clin. Pharmacol. Ther. 40, 158–168.

Sadi, G., Pektaş, M.B., Koca, H.B., Tosun, M., Koca, T., 2015. Resveratrol improves hepatic insulin signaling and reduces the inflammatory response in streptozotocin-induced diabetes. Gene In Press, Corrected Proof, Available online 10 June 2015.

Saha, S.S., Dasgupta, P., Sengupta (Bandyopadhyay), S., Ghosh, M., 2012. Synergistic effect of conjugated linolenic acid isomers against induced oxidative stress, inflammation and erythrocyte membrane disintegrity in rat model. Biochim. Biophys. Acta Gen. Subj. 1820, 1951–1970.

Saito, Y., Shimada, M., Utsunomiya, T., Imura, S., Morine, Y., Ikemoto, T., et al., 2011. Green tea catechins improve liver dysfunction following massive hepatectomy through anti-oxidative and anti inflammatory activities in rats. Gastroenterology 140, S928.

Salinthone, S., Yadav, V., Schillace, R.V., Bourdette, D.N., Carr, D.W., 2010. Lipoic acid attenuates inflammation via cAMP and protein kinase A signaling. PLoS One 5, e13058.

Samsami-kor, M., Daryani, N., Asl, P.R., Hekmatdoost, A., 2015. Anti-inflammatory effects of resveratrol in patients with ulcerative colitis: a randomized, double-blind, placebo-controlled pilot study. Arch. Med. Res. 46, 280–285.

Santos, C.L., Bobermin, L.D., Souza, D.G., Bellaver, B., Bellaver, G., Arús, B.A., et al., 2015. Lipoic acid and N-acetylcysteine prevent ammonia-induced inflammatory response in C6 astroglial cells: the putative role of ERK and HO1 signaling pathways. Toxicol. In Vitro 29, 1350–1357.

Schönlau, F., Rohdewald, P., 2001. Pycnogenol® for diabetic retinopathy. Int. Ophthalmol. 24, 161–171.

Setchell, K.D.R., Brown, N.M., Zimmer-Nechemias, L., Brashear, W.T., Wolfe, B.E., Kirschner, A.S., et al., 2002. Evidence for lack of absorption of soy isoflavone glycosides in humans, supporting the crucial role of intestinal metabolism for bioavailability. Am. J. Clin. Nutr. 2002, 447–453.

Shin, I.S., Shin, N.R., Jeon, C.M., Hong, J.M., Kwon, O.K., Kim, J.C., et al., 2013. Inhibitory effects of Pycnogenol® (French maritime pine bark extract) on airway inflammation in ovalbumin-induced allergic asthma. Food Chem. Toxicol. 62, 681–686.

Stefanescu, M., Matache, C., Onu, A., Tanaseanu, S., Dragomir, C., Constantinescu, I., et al., 2001. Pycnogenol® efficacy in the treatment of systemic lupus erythematosus patients. Phytother. Res. 15, 698–704.

Stohs, S.J., Bagchi, D., 2015. Antioxidant, anti-inflammatory, and chemoprotective properties of *Acacia catechu* heartwood extracts. Phytother. Res. 29, 818–824. Epub 2015 Mar 20.

Taka, E., Mazzio, E.A., Goodman, C.B., Redmon, N., Flores-Rozas, H., Reams, R., et al., 2015. Anti-inflammatory effects of thymoquinone in activated BV-2 microglial cells. J. Neuroimmunol. 286, 5–12.

Takechi, R., Pallebage-Gamarallage, M.M., Lam, V., Giles, C., Mamo, J.C., 2013. Nutraceutical agents with anti-inflammatory properties prevent dietary saturated-fat induced disturbances in blood-brain barrier function in wild-type mice. J. Neuroinflammation 1, 73.

Tall, J.M., Seeram, N.P., Zhao, C., Nair, M.G., Meye, R.A., Raja, S.N., 2004. Tart cherry anthocyanins suppress inflammation-induced pain behavior in rat. Behav. Brain Res. 153, 1181–1188.

Thummuri, D., Jeengar, M.K., Shrivastava, S., Nemani, H., Ramavat, R.N., Chaudhari, P., et al., 2015. Thymoquinone prevents RANKL-induced osteoclastogenesis activation and osteolysis in an in vivo model of inflammation by suppressing NF-KB and MAPK signalling. Pharmacol. Res. 99, 63–73.

Tiwari, V., Chopra, K., 2013. Resveratrol abrogates alcohol-induced cognitive deficits by attenuating oxidative–nitrosative stress and inflammatory cascade in the adult rat brain. Neurochem. Int. 62, 861–869.

Tung, B.T., Rodrĺguez-Bies, E., Talero, E., Gamero-Estévez, E., Motilva, V., Navas, P., et al., 2015. Anti-inflammatory effect of resveratrol in old mice liver. Exp. Gerontol. 64, 1–7.

Umar, S., Hedaya, O., Singh, A.K., Ahmed, S., 2015. Thymoquinone inhibits TNF-α-induced inflammation and cell adhesion in rheumatoid arthritis synovial fibroblasts by ASK1 regulation. Toxicol. Appl. Pharmacol. In Press, Uncorrected Proof, Available online 29 June 2015.

Uya, I.S., Onal, S., Akpinar, M.B., Gonen, I., Sahin, V., Uguz, A.C., et al., 2013. Alpha lipoic acid attenuates inflammatory response during extracorporeal circulation. Cardiovasc. J. Afr. 24, 322–326.

Vendrame, S., Klimis-Zacas, D., 2015. Anti-inflammatory effect of anthocyanins via modulation of nuclear factor-κB and mitogen-activated protein kinase signaling cascades. Nutr. Rev. 73, 348–358.

Wang, H., Nair, M.G., Strasburg, G.M., Chang, Y.C., Booren, A.M., Gray, J.I., et al., 1999. Antioxidant and antiinflammatory activities of anthocyanins and their aglycon, cyanidin, from tart cherries. J. Nat. Prod. 1999, 294–296.

Xia, Y.F., Zhang, J.H., Xu, Z.F., Deng, X.M., 2015. Pycnogenol, a compound isolated from the bark of pinus maritime mill, attenuates ventilator-induced lung injury through inhibiting NF-κB-mediated inflammatory response. Int. J. Clin. Exp. Med. 8, 1824–1833. eCollection 2015.

Xie, N., Zhang, W., Li, J., Liang, H., Zhou, H., Duan, W., et al., 2011. α-Linolenic acid intake attenuates myocardial ischemia/reperfusion injury through anti-inflammatory and anti-oxidative stress effects in diabetic but not normal rats. Arch. Med. Res. 42, 171–181.

Xu, C., Yang, C., Yin, Y., Liu, J., Mine, Y., 2012. Phosphopeptides (PPPs) from hen egg yolk phosvitin exert anti-inflammatory activity via modulation of cytokine expression. J. Funct. Foods 4, 4718–4726.

Yates, C.M., Calder, P.C., Rainger, G.E., 2014. Pharmacology and therapeutics of omega-3 polyunsaturated fatty acids in chronic inflammatory disease. Pharmacol. Ther. 141, 272–282.

Yazir, Y., Utkan, T., Gacar, N., Aricioglu, F., 2015. Resveratrol exerts anti-inflammatory and neuroprotective effects to prevent memory deficits in rats exposed to chronic unpredictable mild stress. Physiol. Behav. 138, 297–304.

Yuan, G., Wahlqvist, M.L., He, G., Yang, M., Li, D., 2006. Natural products and anti-inflammatory activity. Asia Pac. J. Clin. Nutr. 15, 143–152.

Zang, N., Li, S., Li, W., Xie, X., Ren, L., Long, X., et al., 2015. Resveratrol suppresses persistent airway inflammation and hyperresponsivess might partially via nerve growth factor in respiratory syncytial virus-infected mice. Int. Immunopharmacol. 28, 121–128.

Zhang, A., Zhang, X., Tan, X., Cai, B., Ge, W., Dai, G., et al., 2015. Resveratrol rescued the TNF-α-induced impairments of osteogenesis of bone-marrow derived mesenchymal stem cells and inhibited the TNF-α-activated NF-κB signaling pathway. Int. Immunopharmacol. 26, 409–415.

Zhang, F., Liu, J., Shi, J.S., 2010. Anti-inflammatory activities of resveratrol in the brain: role of resveratrol in microglial activation. Eur. J. Pharmacol. 636, 1–7.

Zheng, X., Zhu, S., Chang, S., Cao, Y., Dong, J., Li, J., et al., 2013. Protective effects of chronic resveratrol treatment on vascular inflammatory injury in streptozotocin-induced type 2 diabetic rats: role of NF-kappa B signaling. Eur. J. Pharmacol. 720, 147–157.

Zhu, Y., Ling, W., Guo, H., Song, F., Ye, Q., Zou, T., et al., 2013. Anti-inflammatory effect of purified dietary anthocyanin in adults with hypercholesterolemia: a randomized controlled trial. Nutr. Metab. Cardiovasc. Dis. 23, 843–849.

Chapter 8

Vegetarian diets and disease outcomes

Ming-Chin Yeh and Marian Glick-Bauer
City University of New York, New York, NY, United States

CHAPTER OUTLINE

INTRODUCTION

The relationship between diet and health is a rapidly expanding field of study, and increasingly, attention has turned to the role of vegetarian diets in health and disease prevention. The Academy of Nutrition and Dietetics (formerly the American Dietetic Association) position paper on vegetarian diets (Craig and Mangels, 2009) asserts that vegetarian diets may provide health benefits in the treatment of some diseases including cardiovascular disease, hypertension, diabetes, obesity, cancer, osteoporosis, renal disease, dementia, diverticulitis, gall stones, and rheumatoid arthritis (RA). Many foods that form the basis of a vegetarian diet may directly contribute to these purported benefits, including an increased intake of fruits, vegetables, fiber, whole grains, nuts, soy products, and phytochemicals,

Fruits, Vegetables, and Herbs.
DOI: http://dx.doi.org/10.1016/B978-0-12-802972-5.00008-1

and a reduced intake of saturated fat and high calorie foods. The Dietary Guidelines for Americans, 2010, supported this position by stating that "vegetarian-style eating patterns have been associated with improved health outcomes, lower levels of obesity, a reduced risk of cardiovascular disease, and lower total mortality" (U.S.D.A. and U.S.D.H.H.S., 2010).

As such, population studies are increasingly focusing on vegetarian diets as a variable to help explain rates of disease and all-cause mortality (Chiang et al., 2013; Lee et al., 2014; Chauveau et al., 2013; Agrawal et al., 2014; Orlich and Fraser, 2014; Le and Sabaté, 2014). Similarly, clinical trials are exploring the use of vegetarian diets in treating or preventing disease conditions (McDougall et al., 2014; Kahleova et al., 2011; Barnard et al., 2009a). These population studies and clinical trials are examined below for multiple health conditions, including obesity and weight loss, cardiovascular disease, hypertension, metabolic syndrome, diabetes, cancer, and kidney disease.

Many of the studies focusing on vegetarian diets utilize naturally occurring vegetarian populations, such as Buddhists in Asia (Chiang et al., 2013; Lee et al., 2014; Chauveau et al., 2013; Agrawal et al., 2014) or Seventh Day Adventists in the United States (Orlich and Fraser, 2014; Le and Sabaté, 2014), which have adopted vegetarian diets for religious and/or cultural reasons. The Adventist Health Study-2 (AHS-2) provides a unique opportunity to study and compare adherents of four distinct types of vegetarian diets: vegan, lacto-ovo vegetarian, pesco-vegetarian, and semivegetarian. Overall findings from the Adventist population studies suggest that vegetarian diets are associated with a reduced prevalence of hypertension, metabolic syndrome, diabetes mellitus, all-cause mortality, and are linked to lower BMI values, and reduced rates of some cancers (Orlich and Fraser, 2014; Le and Sabaté, 2014). It should be noted that Buddhists in Asia tend to be strict vegetarians or lacto-ovo vegetarians, while the AHS-2 also includes semivegetarians and pesco-vegetarians, and thus direct comparisons between vegetarian populations in Asia and the West may be misleading (Chiang et al., 2013).

The purported medical benefits of a vegetarian diet may be attributed to any number of components including increased intake of fruit and vegetables, fiber, phytochemicals, antioxidants, vitamins C and E, ferric iron, and folic acid along with a reduced consumption of sodium, cholesterol, total fat, and saturated fat (Li, 2014; Clarys et al., 2014). It should be noted, however, that the more restrictive vegetarian diets may be found lacking in zinc, vitamins A, B12, and D, n-3 polyunsaturated fatty acids, calcium, and the more bioavailable ferrous iron (Li, 2014; Clarys et al., 2014). Thus, the diet as a whole must be examined relative to health outcomes and disease risk.

Tools such as the Healthy Eating Index 2010 (HEI-2010) and the Mediterranean diet score (MDS) can be utilized to relate diet quality with positive health outcomes in a general population. For example, a recent survey utilizing a food frequency questionnaire from 1475 participants found that a vegan diet received the highest diet quality scores on both the HEI-2010 and MDS, while unrestricted omnivores received the lowest (Clarys et al., 2014). Diets deemed "prudent," including vegetarian, semi-vegetarian, and pesco-vegetarian, obtained scores in between the restricted (vegan) and unrestricted (omnivore) groups.

It is likely that vegetarian diets can be evaluated on a continuum, with vegans being the most distinct from omnivores, while other less-restrictive vegetarian diets fall somewhere in the middle. For example, while vegetarian diets in general have been labeled beneficial when compared to omnivore diets, vegan diets appear to confer a particular advantage in lowering odds ratios for developing type 2 diabetes (Tonstad et al., 2013; Tonstad et al., 2009) and for all-cause mortality (Orlich et al., 2013). Similarly, while vegetarian diets in the Adventist cohort conferred protection against cardiovascular diseases, cardiometabolic risk factors, some cancers, and total mortality, vegan diets in particular provided additional protection against obesity, hypertension, type 2 diabetes, and cardiovascular mortality (Le and Sabaté, 2014). However, less-restrictive "low-meat" diets, which allow small intakes of meat, fish, and dairy products may confer similar benefits as a vegetarian diet, while avoiding deficiencies in iron, vitamin B12, vitamin D, and n-3 fatty acids (McEvoy et al., 2012).

VEGETARIAN DIETS AND HEALTH OUTCOMES

Cardiovascular disease/hypertension

Population studies indicate that a vegetarian diet may have cardioprotective benefits; however, this positive association is more evident in some populations than others. The EPIC-Oxford study followed 44,561 participants in England and Scotland, of which 34% were vegetarians. After 11.6 years the vegetarians were found to have a 32% lower risk of ischemic heart disease than did nonvegetarians, even when factors of sex, age, BMI, and smoking were taken into account. The vegetarian participants had lower mean BMI and non-high-density lipoprotein cholesterol (HDL-C) and systolic blood pressure (Crowe et al., 2013). The Indian Migration Study on 6555 volunteers found that vegetarian subjects had a better lipid profile than the nonvegetarians and slightly reduced blood pressure, though the populations did not differ in BMI or rates of hypertension or diabetes, partially because of the relatively low meat consumption among the omnivorous subjects (Shridhar et al., 2014). This suggests again that a prudent diet with only modest meat consumption may provide similar health benefits as a vegetarian diet.

Vegetarian diets may be associated with a reduction in both systolic and diastolic blood pressure when compared to omnivorous diets (Yokoyama et al., 2014a). An analysis of 500 white subjects from the AHS-2 found that vegetarians, and especially vegans, had lower systolic and diastolic blood pressure and less hypertension than the omnivores in the cohort (Pettersen et al., 2012). Correspondingly, among the 592 black participants in the AHS-2, the vegetarians and vegans had significantly lower odds of hypertension than the nonvegetarians in the black cohort (Fraser et al., 2015). Black vegans and lacto-ovo vegetarians had significantly lower overall CVD risk factors including lower low-density lipoprotein cholesterol (LDL-C), lower total cholesterol, and reduced risk for obesity and diabetes.

While the Seventh Day Adventist studies and others suggest that a vegetarian diet may have benefits in reducing ischemic heart disease, the evidence from some populations may not be as strong (Kwok et al., 2014). Conflicting results have been found regarding the impact of a vegetarian diet on HDL and LDL cholesterol. For example, a meta-analysis of studies comparing vegetarian and omnivorous diets found no difference in plasma HDL-C levels between the two diet groups (Zhang et al., 2014). A study of vegetarian Buddhists found lower total cholesterol and LDL-C in the study population, but also lower HDL-C (Chiang et al., 2013).

Multiple studies have found this association between vegetarian diets and lower HDL-C levels, calling into question the cardioprotective benefits of a meat-free diet. A study of vegan, lacto-ovo vegetarian, and omnivorous participants in the Taiwanese Survey on the Prevalence of Hyperglycemia, Hyperlipidemia and Hypertension found that a vegan diet was associated with lower levels of HDL-C in both males and females, while both vegan and lacto-ovo vegetarian diets lowered LDL-C in men (Jian et al., 2014). Thus, the benefit of reduced LDL-C may be more evident in men following a vegetarian diet than in women and may occur with a corresponding disadvantageous reduction in HDL-C levels. Another study focusing on 3551 women from the Taiwanese Survey suggests that a vegan diet in particular is not optimal for premenopausal women (Huang et al., 2014). The authors found that premenopausal vegans had significantly lower HDL-C, higher LDL-C/HDL-C, total cholesterol, and higher triglycerides than omnivores.

Clinical trials generally support the finding that a vegetarian diet may reduce the risk for heart disease. A dietary intervention with 1615 participants found that 7 days on an *ad libitum* plant-based diet was sufficient to produce a significant reduction in biomarkers used to predict future risk for cardiovascular and metabolic diseases (McDougall et al., 2014). These included a decrease in total cholesterol, blood pressure, and blood glucose. Similarly, a study of 171 vegetarians and 129 matched omnivores in China found that the vegetarian subjects consumed less energy, protein, and fat, and displayed a decrease in cardiovascular risk factors including BMI, blood pressure, and lipid profile (Yang et al., 2011). A study of 169 Chinese lacto-vegetarian males and 126 omnivore males found that the lacto-vegetarians had lower cardiovascular disease risk as indicated by lower BMI, blood pressure, serum triglycerides, total cholesterol, LDL-C, and thinner carotid intima media thickness (Yang et al., 2012). Long-term vegetarians in Korea were also found to have lower percent body fat and lower oxidative stress, as well as lower total cholesterol and LDL-C (Kim et al., 2012). Thus it appears overall that a vegetarian diet may reduce heart disease risk factors, though the benefits may differ by gender or population.

Metabolic syndrome and diabetes

Numerous population studies have uncovered a correlation between vegetarian diets and a reduced risk for metabolic syndrome, obesity, and type 2 diabetes. Characteristics of a vegetarian diet which may contribute to this reduced risk include reduced intake of energy, saturated fat, heme iron, and red and processed meat, with a corresponding greater intake of fruits, vegetables, and fiber (Turner-Mc-Grievy and Harris, 2014, Yokoyama et al., 2014b). A study comparing 391 female vegetarian Buddhists (80% of whom were lacto-ovo vegetarians) to 315 nonvegetarians found better metabolic profiles, and lower risk for metabolic syndrome and insulin resistance among the vegetarian subjects (Chiang et al., 2013). The vegetarian Buddhists had significantly lower BMI, obesity, and central obesity, as well as lower systolic blood pressure, fasting plasma glucose, serum insulin level, total cholesterol, and LDL-C. However, the vegetarian sample also had lower HDL-C.

Similarly, a study of 4384 Buddhist volunteers found that the 1484 vegetarian subjects had lower odds for impaired fasting glucose and diabetes, compared to the 2900 omnivores (Chiu et al., 2014). Even though the vegetarians had higher intakes of carbohydrates and similar or higher energy consumption than the omnivores, the vegetarians had lower BMI.

The authors attribute the lower incidence of diabetes in the vegetarian volunteers with lower consumption of heme iron and greater intake of green leafy vegetables and magnesium, both of which may be protective against diabetes.

An analysis 156,317 adults from India's third National Family Health Survey found that lacto-vegetarian, lacto-ovo vegetarian, and semivegetarian diets were associated with lower likelihood of diabetes than a nonvegetarian diet, even after adjusting for socioeconomic and lifestyle factors, and BMI (Agrawal et al., 2014). A survey of 97 vegetarians in Jordan, and an equal number of controls who consumed meat and poultry, found a lower incidence of diabetes and obesity, as well as hypertension, among the vegetarian respondents (Alrabadi, 2013).

Experimental trials provide support for the use of a vegetarian diet as adjuvant therapy for treating type 2 diabetes, and clinical studies suggest that the acceptability of vegan and vegetarian diets is comparable to other therapeutic treatments (Barnard et al., 2009b). A 24-week trial on patients with type 2 diabetes found that the 37 patients assigned to a calorie-restricted vegetarian diet showed improved insulin sensitivity and greater loss of both visceral and subcutaneous fat than the 37 patients assigned to a conventional diabetes diet. The vegetarian diet also led to an improvement in oxidative stress markers (Kahleova et al., 2011). A 74-week study on type 2 diabetes patients found that both a vegan and a conventional diabetes diet produced significant weight loss as well as reductions in Hemoglobin A1c levels. However, when medication changes were taken into account, the 49 vegan subjects showed significantly improved glycemia and plasma lipids compared to the 50 subjects assigned to an omnivorous conventional diabetes diet (Barnard et al., 2009a).

Again, there may be challenges evaluating studies in which "vegetarians" are compared to meat eaters, as variation may exist even among different types of vegetarian diets. For example, a retrospective cohort study utilizing a Taiwan longitudinal health checkup database of 93,209 participants (of which 1116 were vegan) found a decrease in metabolic syndrome with pesco-vegetarian, lacto-vegetarian, and nonvegetarian diets, but not with vegan diets. The authors propose that vegan diets, which exclude fish among other animal products, lack the n-3 fatty acids that play a role in reducing risk for metabolic syndrome and cardiovascular disease (Shang et al., 2011). Nonetheless, low-fat vegetarian diets should be explored further as a therapeutic strategy for lowering glycemia, improving weight control, and reducing cardiovascular risk in patients at risk for metabolic syndrome(Trapp and Barnard, 2010).

Cancer

Diets with high intakes of meat and animal products have been linked to higher rates of colorectal and prostate cancer, as well as breast, endometrial, pancreatic, and gallbladder cancers (Key et al., 2014; Lanou and Svenson, 2010). Vegetarian diets in contrast may be cancer preventive, either due to the absence of animal products (and the potentially carcinogenic heterocyclic amines produced by cooking meats at high temperatures) or to the greater proportion of whole plant foods in the diet, including fruits, vegetables, legumes, whole grains, spices, nuts, and seeds. Several constituents of a vegetarian diet, and whole foods in particular, have been proposed as cancer preventive, including antioxidants, phytochemicals, and soluble fiber, with some studies pointing more specifically to carotenoids, indoles, and soy isoflavones as cancer protective (Lanou and Svenson, 2010; Tantamango-Bartley et al., 2013). In addition, vegetarian diets may protect against cancers associated with obesity, insulin resistance and diabetes, and elevated IGF-I levels. Plant-based diets are characterized by both high consumption of fiber, which promotes insulin sensitivity, and lower circulating levels of insulin-like growth factor-I (IGF-I). The downregulation of insulin and IGF-I, both of which act as promoters, may contribute to reduced cancer rates among vegetarians (Tantamango-Bartley et al., 2013).

A study of the dietary habits of 69,120 participants in the AHS-2 found a significant association between vegetarian diet and reduced cancer risk. Although vegetarian diets overall showed a reduced cancer risk, vegan diets showed the greatest protection overall for both genders and for female-specific cancers, while lacto-ovo vegetarians were associated with decreased risk for cancers of the gastrointestinal tract (Tantamango-Bartley et al., 2013). However, there were age, gender, and race differences that distinguished the vegetarians from the nonvegetarians in the sample. Lifestyle factors also distinguished the two groups. For example, the nonvegetarians tended to be less educated, more likely to have consumed alcohol and smoked cigarettes, and had higher BMI than the vegetarians.

A British study of diet association and cancer risk in 61,647 subjects found an 11% lower overall cancer risk in vegetarians, a 12% lower risk in pesco-vegetarians, and a 19% lower risk in vegans compared to meat eaters (Key et al., 2014). For some cancers the distinction was greater; for example, stomach cancer risk in vegetarians and vegans combined was 63% lower than in meat eaters. Interestingly, this study found a reduced risk for colorectal cancer among fish eaters compared to meat eaters, although this benefit did not extend to other vegetarians. Similarly, pesco-vegetarians in the AHS-2 were found to have the lowest incidence of colorectal cancers, although all vegetarian diets were associated with reduced risk compared with meat eaters (Orlich et al., 2015). Similarly, vegetarian Buddhist priests in Korea were found to have lower incidence of colorectal adenoma and advanced adenoma than nonvegetarian-matched controls (Lee et al., 2014). Thus although plant-based diets are associated with reduced cancer risk overall, the protective effects may vary both by the type of vegetarian diet and the type of cancer in question.

Kidney disease

Vegetarian diets may prove beneficial as medical nutrition therapy in patients with chronic kidney disease (CKD), due to the benefits of a plant-based diet, which include improved phosphate balance, insulin sensitivity, and control of metabolic acidosis (Chauveau et al., 2013). A diet that favors plant versus meat-based proteins may contribute to improvements in proteinuria, hyperfiltration, renal perfusion, and decreased renal injury, (Lin et al., 2010). For example, a 74-week clinical trial comparing a low-fat vegan diet ($n = 49$) and a conventional diabetes diet ($n = 50$) found a significant reduction in urinary albumin in the vegan group compared to the group following an omnivorous diabetic diet (Barnard et al., 2009a).

However, it is not evident whether a vegetarian diet can protect renal function. A study comparing 102 vegetarian Buddhist nuns with an equal number of matched omnivore controls found no difference in renal functions between the vegetarian and omnivorous subjects. Even though the vegetarian subjects had lower systolic blood pressure, blood urea nitrogen (BUN), BUN/creatinine ratio, sodium, total cholesterol, and fasting plasma glucose, no significant difference was found in estimated glomerular filtration rate (GFR) between the two groups (Lin et al., 2010).

Several considerations must be weighed before recommending a vegetarian diet as therapy for CKD patients (Chauveau et al., 2013). Vegetarian diets may protect against hyperphosphatemia, as the bioavailability of dietary phosphorous from vegetarian sources is considerably less than that from meat sources. A diet high in fruits and vegetables may also reduce risk for metabolic acidosis, as plant foods yield an alkaline load, whereas a high consumption of meat worsens acidosis. However, a vegetarian diet may be high in potassium, and thus may pose a risk for a patient with a low GFR. Finally, protein-energy malnutrition is a serious concern in CKD patients, and as such, any vegetarian diet must be carefully designed to provide adequate nutritional status.

Weight loss

Observational studies suggest that vegetarians have lower BMI and reduced caloric intake compared to nonvegetarians, and thus vegetarian diets may be an effective prescription for weight loss (Farmer, 2014; Barnard et al., 2015). A meta-analysis of studies, in which vegetarian diets were prescribed within the context of clinical trials, found an associated mean weight loss (Barnard et al., 2015). A 6-month weight loss trial in which 50 overweight adults were assigned to a vegan, vegetarian, pesco-vegetarian, semivegetarian, or omnivorous diet found that vegans lost significantly more weight than the omnivorous, semivegetarian, or pesco-vegetarian groups (Turner-Mc-Grievy et al., 2015a).

Nutritional adequacy may be a concern when prescribing a calorie-reduced vegetarian diet for weight loss, given that effective weight management requires long-term diet adherence (Farmer, 2014). For example, vegans in the AHS-2 had the lowest BMI of any dietary group, yet inadequate nutrient intake was noted for those following this strictest of vegetarian diets (Rizzo et al., 2013). An evaluation of NHANES data suggests that vegetarians have lower mean intakes of vitamin B12, protein, and zinc than do nonvegetarians, which may have a detrimental effect on diet quality when combined with calorie restriction for weight loss (Farmer, 2014).

VEGETARIAN DIETS, INFLAMMATION, AND THE GUT MICROBIOTA CONNECTION

Chronic inflammation has been linked to numerous adverse health conditions including obesity, metabolic syndrome, cancer, and cardiovascular disease. Elevated levels of inflammatory factors, including C-reactive protein (CRP), and the inflammatory cytokines IL-6 and tumor necrosis factor-α, are associated with cardiovascular disease, obesity, elevated BMI and metabolic syndrome (Cavicchia et al., 2009).

Diet is known to impact and modulate inflammation, as diets high in red meat and high-fat dairy, refined grains, and simple carbohydrates are associated with elevated CRP and IL-6, while plant-based diets are associated with lower CRP levels (Cavicchia et al., 2009). As such, studies are increasingly examining the relationship between diet, inflammation, health, and disease. A 7-year study of 557 participants at increased CVD risk examined plasma biomarkers of endothelial dysfunction and low-grade inflammation. The study found that diets with higher consumption of fish, raw vegetables, fresh fruit, poultry, wine, and limited high-fat dairy products were associated with less endothelial dysfunction and less low-grade inflammation (van Bussel et al., 2015). In clinical trials, patients with type 2 diabetes assigned to a vegetarian diet displayed reduced plasma oxidative stress markers along with reduced insulin resistance and a reduction in visceral fat (Kahleova et al., 2011). Similarly, switching to a vegan, vegetarian, or pesco-vegetarian diet for 2 months was shown to improve the Dietary Inflammatory Index score of overweight and obese adults at least in the short term (Turner-Mc-Grievy et al., 2015b).

The gut microbiota is thought to be the key link between dietary intake patterns and inflammatory response, such that it may be possible to modify microbial communities with plant-based diets for the purpose of managing and treating chronic disease (Wong, 2014). The role of the gut microbiota in influencing inflammation and disease state is discussed below, with closer examination of metabolic disease and obesity, cardiovascular disease, and autoimmune diseases. Vegetarian diets are of particular interest for their role in reducing inflammation and impacting health outcomes. Most importantly, the relationship between diet and the intestinal microbial profile appears to follow a continuum, with vegans displaying a gut microbiota most distinct from that of omnivores but not always significantly different from that of other vegetarians (Glick-Bauer and Yeh, 2014). Thus, a patient's personal taste and cultural traditions may need to dictate which type of vegetarian diet is the best choice for medical nutrition therapy (Khazrai et al., 2014).

Metabolic disease and obesity

Obesity is associated with an altered gut bacterial profile and a state of chronic low-grade inflammation. This inflammation, in turn, can interfere with insulin signaling and contribute to the metabolic dysfunction found in obesity and type 2 diabetes (Requena et al., 2013; Sanz and Moya-Pérez, 2014). Obesity has been linked to a decreased prevalence of Bacteroidetes, which includes enterotypes associated with low-calorie and vegetarian diets, and an increase in Firmicutes and Actinobacteria which have been associated with Western diets (Jeffery and O'Toole, 2013; Musso et al., 2010). For example, one study found that the microbiota of obese subjects was characterized by a reduced bacterial diversity, a decreased ratio of Bacteroidetes to Firmicutes, and an increased abundance of potentially inflammatory proteobacteria (Verdam et al., 2013).

A vegan diet in particular may be associated with a decrease in pathobionts such as *Enterobacteriaceae*, a family of bacteria implicated in triggering low-grade inflammation. A study of six obese subjects with diabetes and/or hypertension who followed a vegan diet for 1 month found improved blood glucose levels and reduced body weight, a decrease in *Enterobacteriaceae*, and a reduction in the abundance of Firmicutes with a significant increase in Bacteroidetes (Kim et al., 2013). A study of 144 vegetarians, 105 vegans, and an equal number of matched omnivores found that vegan and vegetarian diets produced a significant shift in the gut microbiota, with a significant reduction in *Enterobacteriaceae* in the vegan subjects (Zimmer et al., 2012). Dietary fiber in plant-based diets may play a key role in this process, as short-chain fatty acids generated by gut microbiota can act as signaling molecules, modulating the host's inflammatory response (Chiu et al., 2014). The high level of fiber in vegan and vegetarian diets may thus contribute toward reduced levels of inflammation and decreased risk for metabolic disease and obesity.

Cardiovascular disease

Those who adhere to a plant-based diet, or a "prudent" diet with low meat intake, exhibit a reduced risk for cardiovascular disease along with a corresponding modulation of the gut microbiota (Wong, 2014). The link between dietary patterns and risk of cardiovascular disease may be the presence of low-grade inflammation (van Bussel et al., 2015). Inflammation at the vascular level is thought to be involved in the development of atherosclerosis, leading to plaque rupture and thrombosis (Cavicchia et al., 2009).

The most direct evidence that a vegetarian diet promotes a gut microbiota that directly reduces metabolic disease risk is the research linking dietary patterns to L-carnitine metabolism and atherosclerosis risk. Microbial metabolism of dietary L-carnitine, a trimethylamine found in red meat, produces trimethylamine-*N*-oxide (TMAO), which has been shown to promote atherosclerosis. Clinical trials have shown that fasting baseline TMAO levels were significantly lower in 23 vegan and vegetarian subjects when compared to 51omnivores. Long-term (>1 year) vegans and vegetarians displayed a reduced capacity to produce TMAO from dietary carnitine (Koeth et al., 2013). Thus dietary patterns may directly influence gut microbiota, plasma TMAO levels, and ultimately, the associated risk for atherosclerosis. This research supports the premise that diets can be evaluated along a continuum. While a vegan diet may be the best option to reduce proatherosclerotic TMAO and thus reduce CVD risk, similar benefits can be attained by a less-restrictive vegetarian diet as well.

Autoimmune disease

Plant-based diets may provide some level of protection against autoimmune diseases such as thyroid disorders and RA. Vegan diet adherence in the AHS-2 was associated with reduced risk for hypothyroidism while vegan, lacto-ovo, and pesco-vegetarian diets were associated with lower risk for hyperthyroidism, when compared to omnivores (Tonstad et al., 2013; Tonstad et al., 2014). However, the factor of dietary influence and associated modifications of the gut microbiota has been studied in greater depth for RA than for other autoimmune disorders. The raw vegan diet (the Living Food movement) in particular has been examined as a promising treatment for RA.

Many features of a vegan diet have been credited with alleviating RA symptoms among vegan diet adherents. These include an increase in fruit, vegetable, and fiber intake; a reduction in saturated fat and caloric intake, altered antioxidant levels, and weight loss; and a reduction in food allergies and intolerances (Smedslund et al., 2010; Hafström et al., 2001). The probiotic component of a raw vegan diet may be helpful to RA patients as well, as a raw vegan diet rich in *lactobacilli* and fiber has been shown to decrease symptoms of RA (Nenonen et al., 1998; Hänninen et al., 1999; Hänninen et al., 2000). A further possibility is that plant-based diets may induce modifications in intestinal flora with a corresponding reduction in inflammation severity ultimately leading to a reduction in symptoms of RA sufferers.

A study of 53 RA patients found a significant change in intestinal flora after the subjects were transitioned from a conventional diet to a vegan diet and then subsequently to a lacto-vegetarian diet (Peltonen et al., 1994). The fecal flora of test subjects in the high improvement group was significantly different from that of the low improvement group, suggesting a direct connection between diet, gut profiles, and levels of disease activity. The role of fecal flora in diet-induced levels of RA activity was further tested with 43 RA patients randomly assigned to either a raw vegan diet rich in *lactobacilli* or an omnivorous diet. After 1 month, there was a significant change in the fecal flora of the 18 subjects in the vegan diet group who completed the study, along with a decrease in disease activity in some of these RA patients; no such change was found in the omnivore control group (Peltonen et al., 1997). In a subsequent study, RA patients were put on a fast, then a 3.5-month vegan diet, followed by a 9-month lacto-vegetarian diet (Kjeldsen-Kragh, 1999). Subjects in the vegan/vegetarian diet group improved significantly over those maintained on an omnivorous diet. Moreover, subjects' fecal flora during times of clinical improvement differed significantly from times of no or minor improvements. Thus there appears to be a measurable impact of vegetarian and vegan diets on both the fecal flora of RA patients and their corresponding level of disease activity.

CONCLUSION

Vegetarian diets may provide health benefits in the treatment of diseases including cardiovascular disease and hypertension, metabolic syndrome and diabetes, obesity, cancer, renal disease, and RA, among others. Vegetarian diets are associated with lower levels of obesity, improved weight loss, a reduced risk of cardiovascular disease, and lower total mortality. Given the increasing evidence for the health benefits of plant-based diets, vegetarian diets may hold promise as adjuvant therapy in disease management. Research is increasingly looking into the role of vegetarian diets in influencing the gut microbiota, which in turn modulates the inflammatory response and impacts disease states. More research is needed to understand the mechanisms that link diet and health and whether short-term diet therapy can confer long-term health benefits.

REFERENCES

Agrawal, S., et al., 2014. Type of vegetarian diet, obesity and diabetes in adult Indian population. Nutr. J. 13, 89.

Alrabadi, N.I., 2013. The effect of lifestyle food on chronic disease: a comparison between vegetarians and non-vegetarians in Jordan. Global J. Health Sci. 5 (1), 65–69.

Barnard, N.D., et al., 2009a. A low-fat vegan diet and a conventional diabetes diet in the treatment of type 2 diabetes: a randomized, controlled, 74-wk clinical trial. Am. J. Clin. Nutr. 89 (5), 1588S–1596S.

Barnard, N.D., et al., 2009b. Vegetarian and vegan diets in type 2 diabetes management. Nutr. Rev. 67 (5), 255–263.

Barnard, N.D., Levin, S.M., Yokoyama, Y., 2015. A systematic review and meta-analysis of changes in body weight in clinical trials of vegetarian diets. J. Acad. Nutr. Diet 115 (6), 954–969.

Cavicchia, P.P., et al., 2009. A new dietary inflammatory index predicts interval changes in serum high-sensitivity C-reactive protein. J. Nutr. 139 (12), 2365–2372.

Chauveau, P., et al., 2013. Vegetarianism: advantages and drawbacks in patients with chronic kidney diseases. J. Ren. Nutr. 23 (6), 399–405.

Chiang, J.K., et al., 2013. Reduced risk for metabolic syndrome and insulin resistance associated with ovo-lacto-vegetarian behavior in female Buddhists: a case-control study. PLoS One 8 (8), e771799.

Chiu, T.H.T., et al., 2014. Taiwanese vegetarians and onmivores: dietary composition, prevalence and diabetes and IFG. PLoS One 9 (2), e88547.

Clarys, P., et al., 2014. Comparison of nutritional quality of the vegan, vegetarian, semi-vegetarian, pesco-vegetarian and omnivorous diet. Nutrients 6 (3), 1318–1332.

Craig, W.J., Mangels, A.R., 2009. Position paper of the American Dietetic Association: vegetarian diets. J. Am. Diet. Assoc. 109 (7), 1266–1282.

Crowe, F.L., et al., 2013. Risk of hospitalization or death from ischemic heart disease among British vegetarians and nonvegetarians: results from the EPIC-Oxford cohort study. Am. J. Clin. Nutr. 97, 597–603.

Farmer, B., 2014. Nutritional adequacy of plant-based diets for weight management: observations from the NHANES. Am. J. Clin. Nutr. 100 (Suppl. 1), 365S–368S.

Fraser, G., et al., 2015. Vegetarian diets and cardiovascular risk factors in black members of the Adventist Health Study-2. Public Health Nutr. 18 (3), 537–545.

Glick-Bauer, M., Yeh, M.-C., 2014. The health advantage of a vegan diet: exploring the gut microbiota connection. Nutrients 6, 4822–4838.

Hafström, I., et al., 2001. A vegan diet free of gluten improves the signs and symptoms of rheumatoid arthritis: the effects on arthritis correlate with a reduction in antibodies to food antigens. Rheumatology 40, 1175–1179.

Hänninen, O., et al., 1999. Vegan diet in physiological health promotion. Acta Physiol. Hung. 86 (3–4), 171–180.

Hänninen, O., et al., 2000. Antioxidants in vegan diet and rheumatic disorders. Toxicology 155 (1–3), 45–53.

Huang, Y.-W., et al., 2014. Vegan diet and blood lipid profiles: a cross-sectional study of pre and postmenopausal women. BMC Women's Health 14, 55.

Jeffery, I.B., O'Toole, P.W., 2013. Diet-microbiota interactions and their implications for healthy living. Nutrients 5 (1), 234–252.

Jian, Z.-H., et al., 2014. Vegetarian diet and cholesterol and TAG levels by gender. Public Health Nutr. 18 (4), 721–726.

Kahleova, H., et al., 2011. Vegetarian diet improves insulin resistance and oxidative stress markers more than conventional diet in subjects with type 2 diabetes. Diabet. Med. 28 (5), 549–559.

Key, T.J., et al., 2014. Cancer in British vegetarians: updated analyses of 4998 incident cancers in a cohort of 32,491 meat eaters, 8612 fish eaters, 18,298 vegetarians, and 2246 vegans. Am. J. Clin. Nutr. 100 (1), 378S–385S.

Khazrai, Y.M., Defeudis, G., Pozzilli, P., 2014. Effect of diet on type 2 diabetes mellitus: a review. Diabetes Metab. Res. Rev. 30 (Suppl. 1), 24–33.

Kim, M.-S., et al., 2013. Strict vegetarian diet improves the risk factors associated with metabolic diseases by modulating gut microbiota and reducing intestinal inflammation. Environ. Microbiol. Rep. 5 (5), 765–775.

Kim, M.K., Cho, S.W., Park, Y.K., 2012. Long-term vegetarians have low oxidative stress, body fat, and cholesterol levels. Nutr. Res. Pract. 6 (2), 155–161.

Kjeldsen-Kragh, J., 1999. Rheumatoid arthritis treated with vegetarian diets. Am. J. Clin. Nutr. 70 (3 Suppl.), 594S–600S.

Koeth, R.A., et al., 2013. Intestinal microbiota metabolism of L-carnitine, a nutrient in red meat, promotes atherosclerosis. Nat. Med 19 (5), 576–585.

Kwok, C.S., et al., 2014. Vegetarian diet, sevenths day adventists and risk of cardiovasculr mortality: a systematic review and meta-analysis. Int. J. Cardiol. 176, 680–686.

Lanou, A.J., Svenson, B., 2010. Reduced cancer risk in vegetarians: analysis of recent reports. Cancer Manag. Res. 3, 1–8.

Le, L.T., Sabaté, J., 2014. Beyond meatless, the health effects of vegan diets: findings from the adventist cohorts. Nutrients 6 (6), 2131–2147.

Lee, C.G., et al., 2014. Vegetarianism as a protective factor for colorectal adenoma and advanced adenoma in Asians. Dig. Dis. Sci. 59, 1025–1035.

Li, D., 2014. Effect of the vegetarian diet on non-communicable diseases. J. Sci. Food Agric. 94, 169–173.

Lin, C.K., et al., 2010. Comparison of renal function and other health outcomes in vegetarians versus omnivores in Taiwan. J. Health Popul. Nutr. 28 (5), 470–475.

McDougall, J., et al., 2014. Effects of 7 days on an ad libitum low-fat vegan diet: the McDougall Program cohort. Nutr. J. 13.

McEvoy, C.T., Temple, N., Woodside, J.V., 2012. Vegetarian diets, low-meat diets and health: a review. Public Health Nutr. 15 (12), 2287–2294.

Musso, G., Gambino, R., Cassader, M., 2010. Obesity, diabetes, and gut microbiota: The hygiene hypothesis expanded. Diabetes Care 33 (10), 2277–2284.

Nenonen, M.T., et al., 1998. Uncooked, lactobacilli-rich, vegan food and rheumatoid arthritis. Br. J. Rheumatol. 37 (3), 274–281.

Orlich, M.J., Fraser, G.E., 2014. Vegetarian diets in the Adventist Health Study 2: a review of initial published findings. Am. J. Clin. Nutr. 100 (suppl.), 353S–358S.

Orlich, M.J., et al., 2013. Vegetarian dietary patterns and mortality in Adventist Health Study 2. JAMA Intern. Med. 173 (13), 1230–1238.

Orlich, M.J., et al., 2015. Vegetarian dietary patterns and the risk of colorectal cancers. JAMA Intern. Med.

Peltonen, R., et al., 1994. Changes of faecal flora in rheumatoid arthritis during fasting and one-year vegetarian diet. Br. J. Rheumatol. 33 (7), 638–643.

Peltonen, R., et al., 1997. Faecal microbial flora and disease activity in rheumatoid arthritis during a vegan diet. Br. J. Rheumatol. 36, 64–68.

Pettersen, B.J., et al., 2012. Vegetarian diets and blood pressure among white subjects: results from the Adventist Health Study-2 (AHS-2). Public Health Nutr. 15 (10), 1909–1916.

Requena, T., et al., 2013. Interactions between gut microbiota, food and the obese host. Trends Food Sci. Technol. 34, 44–53.

Rizzo, N.S., et al., 2013. Nutrient profiles of vegetarian an nonvegetarian dietary patterns. J. Acad. Nutr. Diet. 113 (12), 1610–1619.

Sanz, Y., Moya-Pérez, A., 2014. Chapter 14: microbiota, inflammation and obesity. In: Lyte, M., Cryan, J.F. (Eds.), Microbial Endocrinology: The Microbiota-Gut-Brain in Health and Disease Springer, New York, pp. 291–317.

Shang, S., et al., 2011. Veganism does not reduce the risk of the metabolic syndrome in a Taiwanese cohort. Asia Pac. J. Clin. Nutr. 20 (3), 404–410.

Shridhar, K., et al., 2014. The association between a vegetarian diet and cardiovascular disease (CVD) risk factors in India: the Indian Migration Study. PLoS One 9, 10.

Smedslund, G., et al., 2010. Effectiveness and safety fo dietary interventions for rheumatoid arthritis: a systematic review of randomized controlled trials. J. Am. Diet. Assoc. 110, 727–735.

Tantamango-Bartley, Y., et al., 2013. Vegetarian diets and the incidence of cancer in a low-risk population. Cancer Epidemiol. Biomarkers Prev. 22 (2), 286–294.

Tonstad, S., et al., 2009. Type of vegetarian diet, body weight, and prevalence of type 2 diabetes. Diabetes Care 32 (5), 791–796.

Tonstad, S., et al., 2013. Vegetarian diets and the incidence of diabetes in the Adventist Health Styudy-2. Nutr. Metab. Cardiovasc. Dis. 23 (4), 292–299.

Tonstad, S., et al., 2013. Vegan diets and hypothyroidism. Nutrients 5 (11), 4642–4652.

Tonstad, S., et al., 2014. Prevalence of hyperthyroidism according to type of vegetarian diet. Public Health Nutr. 29, 1–6.

Trapp, C.B., Barnard, N.D., 2010. Usefulness of vegetarian and vegan diets for treating type 2 diabetes. Curr. Diab. Rep. 10, 152–158.

Turner-McGrievy, G., Harris, M., 2014. Key elements of plant-based diets associated with reduced risk of metabolic syndrome. Curr. Diab. Rep. 14 (9), 524.

Turner-Mc-Grievy, G.M., et al., 2015a. Comparative effectiveness of plant-based diets for weight loss: a randomized controlled trial of five different diets. Nutrition 31 (2), 350–358.

Turner-Mc-Grievy, G.M., et al., 2015b. Randomization to plant-based dietary approaches leads to larger short-term improvements in dietary inflammatory Index scores and macronutrient intake compared with diets that contain meat. Nutr. Res. 35 (2), 97–106.

U.S.D.A., U.S.D.H.H.S., 2010. Dietary Guildelines for Americans. In: U.S.D.o. Agriculture and U.S.D.o.H.a.H. Services, U.S. Government Printing Office, Washington, DC.

van Bussel, B.C., et al., 2015. A healthy diet is associated with less endothelial dysfunction and less low-grade inflammation over a 7-year period in adults at risk of cardiovascular disease. J. Nutr. 145 (3), 532–540.

Verdam, F.J., et al., 2013. Human intestinal microbiota composition is associated with local and systemic inflammation in obesity. Obesity 21 (12), E607–E615.

Wong, J.M., 2014. Gut microbiota and cardiometabolic outcomes: influence of dietary patterns and their associated components. Am. J. Clin. Nutr. 100 (Suppl. 1), 369S–377S.

Yang, S.-Y., et al., 2011. Relationship of carotid intima-media thickness and duration of vegetarian diet in Chinese male vegetarians. Nutr. Metab., 8.

Yang, S.-Y., et al., 2012. Chinese lacto-vegetarian diet exerts favorable effects on metabolic parameters, intima-media thickness, and cardiovascular risks in healthy men. Nutr Clin Pract. 27 (3), 392–398.

Yokoyama, Y., et al., 2014a. Vegetarian diets and glycemic control in diabetes: a systematic review and meta-analysis. Cardiovasc. Diagn. Ther. 4 (5), 373–382.

Yokoyama, Y., et al., 2014b. Vegetarian diets and blood pressure: a meta analysis. JAMA Intern. Med. 174 (4), 577–587.

Zhang, Z., et al., 2014. Comparison of vegetarian diets and omnivorous diets on plasma level of HDL-c: a meta-analysis. PLoS One 9 (3), e92609.

Zimmer, J., et al., 2012. A vegan or vegetarian diet substantially alters the human colonic faecal microbiota. Eur. J. Clin. Nutr. 66, 53–60.

Chapter 9

Diet and nutrition role in prostate health

Akram Elembaby and Ronald Ross Watson
University of Arizona, Tucson, AZ, United States

CHAPTER OUTLINE

INTRODUCTION

Interest in diet and nutrition role in diseases and alternative therapies continues to grow in the United States and the world. In 2012, 68% of American adults took nutritional or dietary supplements, says the Council for Responsible Nutrition, based on data released from its annual consumer survey (Council for Responsible Nutrition, n.d.). Prostate diseases are one of the most self-treated conditions with diet modification and over-the-counter supplements in the United States (Avins and Bent, 2006). This chapter will provide a general background on the anatomy of the prostate, primary pathologic conditions affecting the prostate, and risk factors and treatments

Fruits, Vegetables, and Herbs.
DOI: http://dx.doi.org/10.1016/B978-0-12-802972-5.00009-3

of each condition. However, the chief focus will be on the epidemiological evidence concerning the role of different food, herbs, and supplements in maintaining the health of the prostate health and treating prostate diseases.

The male reproductive system consists of the testes, genital ducts, accessory glands, and penis. The accessory genital glands are the seminal glands (or vesicles), the prostate gland, and the bulbourethral glands. The walnut-sized prostate gland is located between the bladder and the penis in front of the rectum. It surrounds the urethra, which runs through the center of the prostate and carries the urine out of the body. The prostate gland produces fluid that contains various glycoproteins, enzymes, and small molecules and is stored until ejaculation. This fluid nourishes and protects sperm, and during ejaculation, the prostate secretes this fluid into the urethra, and it is ejaculated with sperm as semen (Mescher, 2013).

The two primary pathologic conditions affecting the prostate are benign prostatic hyperplasia (BPH), also called benign prostatic hypertrophy (BPH) and prostatic cancer. Each condition will be discussed in a separate section (Kemp et al., 2008).

The first condition to address is the fourth most common diagnosis in older men (Lee, 2014). As a result of the enlargement of the prostate gland, it presses against the urethra, resulting in narrowing the urethral tube. Consequently, various lower urinary tract symptoms (LUTS) could arise (Kellogg Parsons et al., 2006) such as frequent urination, the urgency to urinate, nocturia, weak urinary stream, incomplete bladder emptying, straining to void, an intermittent stream, and urinary retention. The latest could increase the risk of recurrent urinary tract infections, bladder calculi, and occasionally renal insufficiency.

Pharmacological management options for BPH include 5α-reductase inhibitors such as Finasteride, which decrease the prostate size, increase urine flow rates, and improve symptoms (Scher and Eastham, 2015). Also, data show that Finasteride could slow the progression of the disease. Another option would be α-adrenergic blockers such as tamsulosin, doxazosin, and terazosin. These medications act by relaxing the smooth muscle of the bladder neck and increasing peak urinary flow rates. However, these drugs only improve symptoms and have no influence on the progression of the disease. If pharmacological options fail, surgical approaches to remove or reduce the size of the gland could be the last line.

There are nonmodifiable and modifiable risk factors associated with an increase in risk to develop BPH.

NONMODIFIABLE RISK FACTORS

Age is the first nonmodifiable risk factor in developing BPH. Unfortunately, as a man grows in age, the prostate tends to increase in size. Benign prostatic hyperplasia affects nearly half of all men over age 50 years, and 80–90% of men in their 80s. Genetics also could play a role in developing BPH. Approximately 50% of men under age 60 years who undergo surgery for benign prostatic hyperplasia may have a heritable form of the disease (Meng et al., 2014). This form is most likely an autosomal dominant trait, and first-degree male relatives of such patients carry an increased relative risk of approximately fourfold. In addition to age and genetics, race and ethnicity could play a role in developing BPH. African-Americans and Hispanics might have a greater chance of developing BPH compared to white men. Risks for total benign prostatic hyperplasia were 41% higher for black ($P < 0.03$) and Hispanic men ($P < 0.06$) compared to white men, and for severe benign prostatic hyperplasia these increases were 68% ($P < 0.01$) and 59% ($P < 0.03$), respectively (Kristal et al., 2007).

MODIFIABLE RISK FACTORS

Epidemiological and clinical data indicate that modifiable lifestyle factors, including obesity, physical activity, and diet, significantly influence the risks of symptomatic benign prostatic hyperplasia (BPH) and LUTS (Raheem and Parsons, 2014). Physically active men who exercise regularly have been associated with decreased risks of BPH and LUTS. On the contrary, living a sedentary lifestyle has been associated with increased risk of BPH and LUTS. Also, increased body weight, body mass index (BMI), and waist circumference are associated with increased prostate volume, and consequently higher risk of developing BPH and LUTS. Another important factors that affect the risk of symptomatic BPH and LUTS are nutrition, diet, and alcohol intake.

DIET

There are indications that both macronutrients and micronutrients may affect the risk of BPH and LUTS.

Macronutrients

For macronutrients, increased total energy intake, energy-adjusted total protein intake, red meat, fat, milk and dairy products, cereals, bread, poultry, and starch potentially increase the risks of symptomatic BPH and BPH surgery (Bravi et al., 2006). In contrast, vegetables (particularly carotenoids such as tomatoes and carrots) and fruits potentially decrease the risks of BPH. One potential explanation is that vegetables and fruits contain high levels of antioxidants, polyphenols, vitamins, minerals, and fiber that may play important roles in altering inflammatory pathways associated with the pathogenesis of BPH (Parsons, 2007).

Micronutrients

For micronutrients, higher circulating concentrations of vitamin E, lycopene, selenium, and carotene have been inversely associated with symptomatic BPH and LUTS; zinc and vitamin C have been associated with both increased and decreased risk; and polyunsaturated fatty acids, linoleic acid, vitamin A, and vitamin D have been associated with decreased risk (Raheem and Parsons, 2014).

Alcohol

Surprisingly, moderate alcohol intake appears to be protective against BPH (Parsons, 2010). In a metaanalysis of 19 studies that incorporated 120,091 men and divided total alcohol intake (grams per day) into six strata, alcohol intake was associated with a significantly or marginally significantly decreased likelihood of BPH in all six strata (P values 0.08, 0.01, < 0.001). However, alcohol's protective effects against BPH do not seem to apply to LUTS. Of the four studies that used LUTS as the primary outcome, three demonstrated a significantly increased likelihood of LUTS with alcohol consumption (Raheem and Parsons, 2014).

Herbs and supplements

Saw palmetto

Saw palmetto (also known as *Serenoa repens*) is commonly used to treat symptoms of benign prostatic hypertrophy (BPH) by inhibiting the 5α-reductase enzyme that converts testosterone to 5-dehydrotestosterone, prostaglandin synthesis, and growth factor actions. Early Cochrane systematic reviews and metaanalyses of randomized clinical trials of the herb *S. repens* for the treatment of BPH and LUTS in 2000 and 2002 concluded that it diminished LUTS and improved urinary flow parameters (Wilt et al., 1998). However, updated reviews in 2009 and 2012, which included more randomized trials and higher quality clinical evidence, concluded that *S. repens* did not decrease LUTS, diminish nocturia, improve urinary flow parameters, or reduce prostate size (Raheem and Parsons, 2014).

β-Sitosterol

In a systematic review by Wilt et al., four double-blind clinical trials were reported with lasting around 4–26 weeks (Wilt et al., 1999). They concluded that β-sitosterol could improve the urinary symptom and flow in comparison of placebo and did not decrease prostate size. In only trial with pure daucosterol, no improvement in urinary flow was observed. Moreover, men who consumed β-sitosterol alone did not show different withdrawal rates from placebo. However, the duration of those studies was short and for this reason, probably effect of β-sitosterol in elongated period, its safety and capacity to prevent the complications of BPH are still in doubt (Saeidnia et al., 2014).

Pygeum

Pygeum (*Pygeum africanum* bark extract) has been observed to moderately improve urinary symptoms associated with enlargement of the prostate gland or prostate inflammation (Wilt and Ishani, 2011). Numerous human studies report that pygeum significantly reduces urinary hesitancy, urinary frequency, the number of times patients need to wake up at night to urinate, and pain with urination in men who experience mild-to-moderate symptoms. However, pygeum does not appear to reduce the size of the prostate gland or reverse the process of benign prostatic hypertrophy. Avoid if allergic or hypersensitive to pygeum (Kim et al., 2012).

Another condition, that is a common age-related disease, that occurs primarily in older men is prostate cancer. The Centers for Disease Control and Prevention (CDC) has classified prostate cancer as the most common cancer among men of all races, aside from nonmelanoma skin cancer. Also, it is the second most common cancer in men (behind skin cancer) and the second leading cause of cancer death (behind lung cancer) (Corn and Logothetis, 2011). In 2009 it is estimated that 192,280 men will be newly diagnosed with prostate cancer and 27,360 men will die from prostate cancer. There are a number of unique clinical features of prostate cancer that distinguish it from other solid tumor types (Corn and Logothetis, 2011):

1. Prostate cancer has high prevalence; however, it progresses slowly. Consequently, over the course of a normal lifetime, most men will develop "clinically occult" prostate cancer. The majority of patients eventually die from other causes before experiencing symptoms or requiring treatments for prostate cancer. Contrarily, other aggressive cancers such as lung cancer leads to death after the majority of patients diagnose with the disease.

2. Androgens, such as testosterone, are a major driving force in normal prostate development and are related in developing prostate cancer.
3. Prostate cancers have a predictable rate and pattern of progression.
4. Bone-forming metastases dominate the clinical progression in the majority of patients with advanced disease.

Similar to BPH, there are nonmodifiable and modifiable risk factors associated with an increase in risk to develop prostate cancer.

NONMODIFIABLE RISK FACTORS

Aging

It has long been recognized that prostate cancer is a disease of the elderly, and epidemiologic data demonstrate that rates of prostate cancer incidence and mortality increase with age (Gann, 2002). While prostate-specific antigen (PSA) screening has led to an earlier average age at diagnosis, mortality is still largely seen in patients 70 years of age or older (Patel and Klein, 2009). As the longevity of populations increases worldwide, the burden of prostate cancer creates a significant health-care challenge. This has generated a sense of urgency among physicians to refine our ability to predict cancer virulence and apply therapy to those patients who need it (Corn and Logothetis, 2011).

Endocrine

Androgens are central to the normal growth, differentiation, and function of the prostate gland, although the role of androgen receptor (AR) signaling in prostate carcinogenesis and progression has not been fully elucidated (Scher and Sawyers, 2005). Even in the clinically castrate state (serum testosterone <50 ng/mL), there is growing evidence that prostate cancer cells continue to rely on AR signaling for proliferation. Potential mechanisms accounting for this include intratumoral amplification of the AR, mutations of the AR, changes in levels of AR cofactors, ligand-independent activation of the AR, upregulation of enzymes involved in androgen synthesis, and conversion of testosterone to dihydrotestosterone. Thus during prostate cancer progression, there is a gradual shift from endocrine sources of androgens (ie, from the testes and adrenal glands) to paracrine/autocrine/intracrine sources. All these events can occur in the setting of a low serum testosterone (Scher and Sawyers, 2005).

Race and Ethnicity

African-Americans have a higher frequency of death from prostate cancer compared to Caucasian and Hispanic Americans. This has variably been attributed to differences in steroid metabolism, genetics, environmental effects, or social factors. There is a reduced incidence of prostate cancer among Chinese and Japanese Americans, but their incidence is higher than that reported in native Chinese or Japanese persons. Of interest is the fact that northern European males have a higher frequency of prostate cancer than males from southern Europe. A similar finding has been reported in the United States, suggesting that the incidence of prostate cancer is inversely related to sun exposure. These findings have epidemiologically linked prostate cancer to vitamin D metabolism (Corn and Logothetis, 2011).

Genetic Predisposition

As with breast and colon cancer, familial clustering of prostate cancer has been reported. Unlike with breast and colon cancer, specific genetic lesions have not been identified to merit the routine use of genetic screening for prostate cancer (Smith et al., 1996; Corn and Logothetis, 2011). The search for "prostate cancer genes" has identified candidate genetic events implicated in tumorigenesis, but these findings have been more useful in understanding the underlying etiology of prostate cancer than in screening. For example, a major hereditary prostate cancer susceptibility locus resides at 1q24, though the responsible gene(s) remains under investigation (Xu et al., 2003). More recently, men carrying BRCA1/BRCA2 mutations have been shown to be at increased risk of developing prostate cancer (Gayther et al., 2000). However, it has not been established that familial cases of prostate cancer are more virulent than nonfamilial cases; so it is unclear how this information will influence management decisions for individual patients (Ford et al., 1994; Corn and Logothetis, 2011).

MODIFIABLE RISK FACTORS

Clinical prostate cancer is more prevalent in Western than Eastern societies, although incidence rates increase for men from China and Japan who immigrate to the United States. This observation implicates environmental factors (diet, lifestyle, etc.) in prostate cancer development.

Diet and obesity

Conflicting data

A research in 2008 did not provide any evidence for the role of diet in prostate cancer survival (Bekkering et al., 2008). In a small-scale study (n = 43), reliant on self-report for broadly defined dietary changes, men in the intervention group consumed significantly more vegetables and had significantly higher serum levels of carotenoids, as confirmed by increases in serum carotenoids (Parsons et al., 2008). However, the intervention produced a nonsignificant increase in PSA; there was a nonsignificant change in mean PSA levels of +2.28 in the intervention group versus −0.06 in the control group ($P = 0.29$). Another prospective study of the association between postdiagnostic consumption of processed and unprocessed red meat, fish, poultry, and eggs and the risk of prostate cancer recurrence or progression ($n = 1294$) in 2010 was conducted (Richman et al., 2010). They found that intakes of processed and unprocessed red meat, fish, total poultry, and skinless poultry were not associated with recurrence or progression. Greater consumption of eggs and poultry with skin was associated with twofold increases in risk in a comparison of extreme quantiles: eggs (hazard ratio (HR) = 2.02; 95% confidence interval (CI) = 1.10–3.72; P for trend = 0.05) and poultry with skin (HR = 2.26; 95% CI = 1.36–3.76; P for trend = 0.003). The overall findings suggest that the consumption of processed or unprocessed red meat, fish, or skinless poultry postdiagnosis may not be associated with prostate cancer recurrence or progression, whereas postdiagnosis consumption of eggs and poultry with the skin may increase the risk.

However, several lines of clinical and experimental evidence support a central role for diet, caloric intake, and obesity in the development of prostate cancer with lethal potential. A recent prospective, randomized intervention by Aronson et al. (2010) examined a 4-week low-fat diet compared with a Western diet in newly diagnosed prostate cancer patients ($n = 18$) (Aronson et al., 2010). Findings suggest that a low-fat diet might inhibit the growth rate of hormonally responsive prostate cancer cells. A recent review conducted by Hori et al. (2011) highlights that there is some evidence suggesting that green tea, isoflavone, lycopene, cruciferous vegetable, and omega-3 polyunsaturated fatty acid intake is beneficial in the prevention and/or progression of prostate cancer (Hori et al., 2011). They also found evidence to suggest that a high total fat, meat (especially well cooked), and multivitamin intake may be associated with an increased risk of developing prostate cancer, but more research is required to establish its effect on progression.

Obesity, defined as BMI above 30, is manifested by overgrowth of white adipose tissue (WAT). Recently, obesity has been associated with progression of a number of different cancer types, including prostate cancer. For example, obese patients with prostate cancer are more likely to develop a recurrence following radical prostatectomy or radiation therapy for localized disease. The mechanism for the association between obesity and prostate cancer progression is poorly understood. Current models suggest that predetermined genetic traits associated with both obesity and cancers are influenced by lifestyle components such as diet and physical activity. However, epidemiological studies show that cancer can be accelerated in obese patients irrespective of their lifestyle. Thus it has been proposed that WAT itself may have a direct effect on cancer progression.

One hypothesis is that WAT acts as a potent endocrine organ that secretes numerous soluble growth and inflammatory factors (such as leptin, adiponectin, insulin-like growth factor (IGF-1), and hepatocyte growth factor (HGF)) that stimulate tumor growth. In support of this, abdominal adiposity causes a metabolic syndrome characterized by insulin resistance and hyperinsulinemia. Previous research efforts have focused on measuring adipokine levels to explain a functional link between obesity and cancer. Results, however, have been inconsistent, suggesting alternate mechanisms account for the association between obesity and cancer. Ongoing clinical trials will test many of these hypotheses (eg, by targeting the IGF-1 signaling axis as a therapy strategy).

Recommendations for diet comprise guidance on limiting consumption of energy-dense foods with a high sugar or fat content (Davies et al., 2011).

REFERENCES

Aronson, W.J., Barnard, R.J., Freedland, S.J., Henning, S., Elashoff, D., Jardack, P.M., et al., 2010. Growth inhibitory effect of low fat diet on prostate cancer cells: results of a prospective, randomized dietary intervention trial in men with prostate cancer. J. Urol. 183 (1), 345–350.

Avins, A.L., Bent, S., 2006. Saw palmetto and lower urinary tract symptoms: what is the latest evidence? Curr. Urol. Rep. 7 (4), 260–265.

Bekkering, G.E., Harris, R.J., Thomas, S., Mayer, A.M.B., Beynon, R., Ness, A.R., et al., 2008. How much of the data published in observational studies of the association between diet and prostate or bladder cancer is usable for meta-analysis? Am. J. Epidemiol. 167 (9), 1017–1026.

Bravi, F., Bosetti, C., Dal Maso, L., Talamini, R., Montella, M., Negri, E., et al., 2006. Macronutrients, fatty acids, cholesterol, and risk of benign prostatic hyperplasia. Urology 67, 1205–1211.

Corn, P., Logothetis, C., 2011. Prostate cancer (Chapter 34). In: Kantarjian, H.M., Wolff, R.A., Koller, C.A. (Eds.), The MD Anderson Manual of Medical Oncology, 2e McGraw-Hill, New York, NY.

Council for Responsible Nutrition-The Science Behind the Supplements. (n.d.). Retrieved from: <http://www.crnusa.org/CRNPR12-SurveyFindingsUsage031312.html> (accessed 14.07.15.).

Davies, N.J., Batehup, L., Thomas, R., 2011. The role of diet and physical activity in breast, colorectal, and prostate cancer survivorship: a review of the literature. British journal of cancer 105, S52–S73.

Ford, D., Easton, D.F., Bishop, D.T., et al., 1994. Risks of cancer in BRCA1-mutation carriers. Breast Cancer Linkage Consortium. Lancet 343 (8899), 692–695.

Gann, P.H., 2002. Risk factors for prostate cancer. Rev. Urol. 4 (Suppl. 5), S3–S10.

Gayther, S.A., de Foy, K.A., Harrington, P., et al., 2000. The frequency of germ-line mutations in the breast cancer predisposition genes BRCA1 and BRCA2 in familial prostate cancer. The Cancer Research Campaign/British Prostate Group United Kingdom Familial Prostate Cancer Study Collaborators. Cancer Res. 60 (16), 4513–4518.

Hori, S., Butler, E., McLoughlin, J., 2011. Prostate cancer and diet: food for thought? BJU Int. 107 (9), 1348–1359.

Kellogg Parsons, J., Ballentine Carter, H., Partin, A.W., Gwen Windham, B., Jeffrey Metter, E., Ferrucci, L., et al., 2006. Metabolic factors associated with benign prostatic hyperplasia. J. Clin. Endocrinol. Metab. 91, 2562–2568.

Kemp, W.L., Burns, D.K., Brown, T.G., 2008. Chapter 17. Pathology of the male and female reproductive tract and breast. In: Kemp, W.L., Burns, D.K., Brown, T.G. (Eds.), Pathology: The Big Picture

Kim, T.H., Lim, H.J., Kim, M.S., Lee, M.S., 2012. Dietary supplements for benign prostatic hyperplasia: an overview of systematic reviews. Maturitas 73 (3), 180–185.

Kristal, A.R., Arnold, K.B., Schenk, J.M., Neuhouser, M.L., Weiss, N., Goodman, P., et al., 2007. Race/ethnicity, obesity, health related behaviors and the risk of symptomatic benign prostatic hyperplasia: results from the prostate cancer prevention trial. J. Urol. 177 (4), 1395–1400.

Lee, M., 2014. Chapter 67. Benign prostatic hyperplasia. In: DiPiro, J.T., Talbert, R.L., Yee, G.C., Matzke, G.R., Wells, B.G., Posey, L. (Eds.), Pharmacotherapy: A Pathophysiologic Approach, ninth ed.

Meng, M.V., Walsh, T.J., Chi, T.D., 2014. Urologic disorders. In: Papadakis, M.A., McPhee, S.J., Rabow, M.W. (Eds.), *Current Medical Diagnosis & Treatment* 2015 McGraw-Hill

Mescher, A.L., 2013. Chapter 21. The male reproductive system. In: Mescher, A.L. (Ed.), Junqueira's Basic Histology: Text & Atlas, thirteenth ed.

Parsons, J.K., 2007. Modifiable risk factors for benign prostatic hyperplasia and lower urinary tract symptoms: new approaches to old problems. J. Urol. 178, 395–401.

Parsons, J.K., 2010. Benign prostatic hyperplasia and male lower urinary tract symptoms: epidemiology and risk factors. Curr. Bladder Dysfunct. Rep. 5 (4), 212–218.

Parsons, J.K., Newman, V.A., Mohler, J.L., Pierce, J.P., Flatt, S., Marshall, J., 2008. Dietary modification in patients with prostate cancer on active surveillance: a randomized, multicentre feasibility study. BJU Int. 101 (10), 1227–1231.

Patel, A.R., Klein, E.A., 2009. Risk factors for prostate cancer. Nat. Clin. Pract. Urol. 6 (2), 87–95.

Raheem, O.A., Parsons, J.K., 2014. Associations of obesity, physical activity and diet with benign prostatic hyperplasia and lower urinary tract symptoms. Curr. Opin. Urol. 24 (1), 10–14.

Richman, E.L., Stampfer, M.J., Paciorek, A., Broering, J.M., Carroll, P.R., Chan, J.M., 2010. Intakes of meat, fish, poultry, and eggs and risk of prostate cancer progression. Am. J. Clin. Nutr. 91 (3), 712–721.

Saeidnia, S., Manayi, A., Gohari, A.R., Abdollahi, M., 2014. The story of beta-sitosterol-a review. Eur. J. Med. Plants 4 (5), 590–609.

Scher, H.I., Eastham, J.A., 2015. Benign and malignant diseases of the prostate. In: Kasper, D., Fauci, A., Hauser, S., Longo, D., Jameson, J., Loscalzo, J. (Eds.), Harrison's Principles of Internal Medicine, 19e McGraw-Hill, New York, NY.

Scher, H.I., Sawyers, C.L., 2005. Biology of progressive, castration-resistant prostate cancer: directed therapies targeting the androgen-receptor signaling axis. J. Clin. Oncol. 23 (32), 8253–8261.

Smith, J.R., Freije, D., Carpten, J.D., et al., 1996. Major susceptibility locus for prostate cancer on chromosome 1 suggested by a genome-wide search. Science 274 (5291), 1371–1374.

Wilt, T.J., MacDonald, R., Ishani, A., 1999. Beta-sitosterol for the treatment of benign prostatic hyperplasia: a systematic review. BJU Int. 83, 976–983.

Wilt, T.J., & Ishani, A. (2011). Extracts from the African prune tree (*Pygeum africanum*) may be able to help relieve urinary symptoms caused by enlarged prostate (benign prostatic hyperplasia). Cochrane Database Syst. Rev.

Wilt, T.J., Ishani, A., Stark, G., MacDonald, R., Lau, J., Mulrow, C., 1998. Saw palmetto extracts for treatment of benign prostatic hyperplasia: a systematic review. JAMA 280 (18), 1604–1609.

Xu, J., Gillanders, E.M., Isaacs, S.D., et al., 2003. Genome-wide scan for prostate cancer susceptibility genes in the Johns Hopkins hereditary prostate cancer families. Prostate 57 (4), 320–325.

Section 2

Fruit and Health and Diseases

Chapter 10

Advances in the study of the health benefits and mechanisms of action of the pulp and seed of the Amazonian palm fruit, *Euterpe oleracea* Mart., known as "Açai"

Alexander G. Schauss[1,2]
[1]*AIBMR Life Sciences, Puyallup, WA, United States*
[2]*University of Arizona, Tucson, AZ, United States*

CHAPTER OUTLINE

Fruits, Vegetables, and Herbs.
DOI: http://dx.doi.org/10.1016/B978-0-12-802972-5.00010-X

INTRODUCTION

Since 2005, *Euterpe oleracea* Mart., a member of the palm family, *Arecaceae*, has attracted considerable attention since the discovery of the fruit mesocarp's potent antioxidant and antiinflammatory properties (Lichtenthaler et al., 2005; Schauss et al., 2006a,b). Beverages and dietary supplements have appeared around the world containing açai pulp. The intent of the author is to review the nearly 200 papers that have appeared in recent years that investigated açai's pulp and seed to determine its chemistry, properties, attributes, and bioactivities.

BOTANY OF FRUIT

Euterpe oleracea is a multistemmed hydrophytic and monoecious plant that is, a mass of epigeous roots reaching a height of 8–30m, with pneumatophores that grow to above the surface to facilitate aeration essential for root respiration, especially given its predominance in the Amazonian floodplains.

The plant is straight, cylindrical, and 12–60cm in width depending on age. Pinnate leaves are 50–100cm in length. The inflorescence produces reddish-blue to purple flowers ~2mm in diameter in threes, a central female and two lateral males, bearing 80–130 rachilla. The fruit is globose, ranging in size from 1.25 to 1.5cm. At immaturity, the fruit is green eventually turning dark purple-black at maturity when ready for harvesting. A single seed accounts for 82–85% of the fruit, covered by a thin fibrous and fleshy mesocarp (the "pulp") ~1.0–1.5mm. Flowering and fruiting occurs for most of the year. However, fruit only appears in the floodplains in late June when the rainy season ends and continue to produce fruit in four cycles that end in December. During this second half of the year most commercial harvesting for domestic consumption and export occurs (Schauss, 2011).

Each palm tree can yield up to hundreds of fruit per rachilla, weighing between 0.5 and 1.5kg/rachilla. Upon maturity, most palms can produce around 1000kg or more of fruit in a 5-year period. As palms can continue to produce fruit for more than 25years, and given their abundance of *E. oleracea* amidst over 11 million hectares in the floodplains of the Amazon, the quantity of açai fruit available annually for harvesting and consumption domestically and for export seems limitless.

AÇAI SEED

Toward the end of the first decade of the 21st century research began on the chemistry, nutritional composition, and particularly, the bioactivity of the açai fruit's seed.

The seed is globose and occupies most of the fruit. It has only one germination pore and a voluminous, homogeneous, solid, and hard endosperm (Henderson and Scariot, 1993). Nascimento and Da Silva (2005) studied the germination of seed and determined that loss-of-moisture affects the ability of the seed to germinate. While a moisture content of 39% did not affect the seed, further drying to ~33% of water content reduced seed vigor and germination rates; seeds did not germinate when moisture content is reduced to 15%.

Roche and colleagues were among the first investigators to study the bioactivities of açai seed in vivo (Rocha et al., 2007a). They undertook experiments to determine whether a hydroalcoholic extract of açai seed induced vasodilator effects in rat mesenteric vascular bed preconditioned with norepinephrine to elucidate its mechanism of action. In cultured endothelial cells they demonstrated that the vasodilator effect was dependent on activation of the nitric oxide-cyclic guanosine monophosphate (cGMP) pathway, but did not involve prostanoids release, receptors activated by acetylcholine (ACh), histamine, adrenaline, bradykinin, or opening of either potassium$_{atp}$ (K_{atp}) or $K_{voltage\text{-}gated}$ channels, while possibly involving endothelium-derived hyperpolarizing factor (EDHF) release.

Açai fruit is very rich in polyphenols, including anthocyanins and proanthocyanidins, as well as flavonoids, as shown in Table 10.1 (Odendaal and Schauss, 2014) and Table 10.2, adapted from Gallori et al. (2004), Schauss et al. (2006a), Kang et al. (2010), Kang et al. (2011).

Polyphenol compounds have been shown to have significant vasodilatory effects in vitro (Stoclet et al., 2004). The protective effect of a lyophilized hydroalcoholic extract of açai seeds was studied in experiments undertaken in female Wistar rats to: (1) determine the extracts effect on

Table 10.1 Anthocyanins Detected in Mesocarp of Açai

Major Anthocyanins
Cyanidin 3-glucoside
Cyanidin 3-rutinoside
Minor Anthocyanins
Cyanidin 3-arabinoside
Cyanidin 3-sambubiosides
Cyanidin 3-(acetyl) hexose
Cyanidin 3,5-hexose pentose
Penoidin 3-glucoside
Peonidin 3-rutinoside

Table 10.2 Polyphenolic Flavonoids in Mature Açai Pulp

Major Anthocyanins
Cyanidin-3-*O*-glucoside Cyanidin 3-*O*-rutinoside
Minor Anthocyanins
Cyanidin 3-*O*-arabinoside Cyanidin 3-*O*-arabinosylarabinoside Cyanidin 3-*O*-sambubioside Peonidin 3-*O*-glucoside Peonidin 3-*O*-rutinoside
Other Flavonoids
Flavan-3-ols (Flavanols):
Catechin Epi-catechin
Flavanonols:
Dihydrokaempferol (2R, 3R)-Dihydrokaempferol-3-*O*-β-D-glucoside (2S, 3S)-Dihydrokaempferol-3-*O*-β-D-glucoside
Flavones:
5,4′-Dihydroxy-7,3′,5′-trimethoxyflavone Apigenin Chrysoeriol Homoorientin Isovitexin Luteolin Orientin Taxifolin deoxyhexose Velutin Vitexin
Flavonol:
Quercetin
Phenolic Acids:
Catechin Ferulic acid Epi-catechin p-Hydroxybenzoic acid Protocatechuic acid Syringic acid Vanillic acid

Adapted from Gallori et al. (2004), Schauss et al. (2006a), Kang et al. (2010), Kang et al. (2011), Dias et al. (2012), Gordon et al. (2012), Dias et al. (2013), Odendaal and Schauss, 2014.

cardiovascular, endothelial, and renal functioning, blood pressure, and oxidative status; and (2) test whether the beneficial effects of the extract on cardiovascular control of dams would pass on to male offspring exposed to maternal protein restriction during gestation. Earlier, the same investigators had reported that açai seed extract had potent endothelium-dependent vasodilator effects and nitric oxide induction from endothelial cells in culture (Rocha et al., 2007a). In separate experiments, the same extract had an antihypertensive effect, attributed by the authors to its antioxidant bioactivities (Rocha et al., 2008).

To determine if chronic administration of the açai seed extract has antihypertensive effects in the prevention of hypertension-induced vascular dysfunction, oxidative damage, and structural vascular changes, da Costa and colleagues (2012) used a 2K-1C hypertension animal model associated with impaired vascular function and morphological changes in vasculature leading to hypertension. As there had been no report on the effect of oral administration of açai seed in 2K-1C hypertension on vascular function and morphological changes, the investigators sought to evaluate whether chronic treatment with the extract produced antihypertensive effects, or mitigated the oxidative damage and vascular structural changes associated with hypertension. The study included sham-operated control rats, and animals were treated either with or without açai seed extract. The primary finding was that the extract prevented the development of hypertension and endothelial dysfunction and medial thickening of the aortic and mesenteric arteries, otherwise seen in untreated 2K-1C hypertension. The effects observed is also associated with a reduction in matrix metalloproteinase-2 (MMP-2) levels and oxidative stress.

These earlier findings raised questions as to whether açai seed might protect offspring from hypertension later in life. To test the hypothesis, de Bem and colleagues (2014) used a maternal protein restriction-during-gestation animal model to determine if treatment with the extract would provide protection of offspring in developing hypertension. That protein restriction in pregnancy would result in hypertension has been demonstrated in some studies. Brawley and colleagues (2003) showed impaired maternal hemodynamic adaptation due to protein restriction in pregnancy adversely affecting systemic vasodilation, which contributes to hypertension and endothelial dysfunction of adult offspring later in life.

De Bem and coworkers (2014) study demonstrated multiple preventive actions of açai seed extract on cardiovascular and renal function, as well as favorable structural changes in offspring of dams. Treatment with seed extract increased both malondialdehyde (MDA) and carbonyl protein levels associated with a decrease in nitrite levels and antioxidant activity in plasma and kidney. In addition, the extract when given during pregnancy improved adult offspring's renal structure (and improved nephrogenesis), normalized body weight, renal function, serum albumin, urea, and creatinine levels, the percent fractional sodium excretion (%FENa$^+$), while increasing renin levels, all of which was attributed to the extract's antioxidant bioactivities. The results of the study suggest that administration of açai seed extract, when added to the diet early in pregnancy, may confer protection against the long-term adverse effects a low-protein diet has on offspring later in life.

Another line of investigation has examined the effect of açai seed on pulmonary function and the prevention of respiratory diseases, such as emphysema and chronic obstructive pulmonary disease (COPD). The term COPD includes two different respiratory conditions, chronic bronchitis and emphysema. Dome and colleagues (2014) have pointed out that in the respiratory system, reactive oxygen species (ROS), and reactive nitrogen species (RNS) may be "either exogenous from more or less inhalative gaseous or particulate agents such as air pollutants, cigarette smoke, ambient high-altitude hypoxia, and some occupational dusts, or endogenously generated in the context of defense mechanism against such infectious pathogens as bacteria, viruses, or fungi." Considerable evidence has shown the degree of damage to the respiratory system depends on the duration of exposure, which if prolonged triggers further ROS generation released by the immune system (eg, eosinophilic peroxidase from eosinophilic leukocytes, or myeloperoxidase (MPO) from neutrophils) resulting in inflammation.

A free radical is defined as a reactive molecule with one or more unpaired electrons that can exist independently. ROS is a collective term that includes both oxygen radicals, such as the hydroxyl, peroxyl, and superoxide radicals, and nonradical oxidizing agents, such as hydrogen peroxide. During the process of human metabolism, ROS is continuously generated during cell metabolism. When present in excess these reactive species can cause oxidative damage of macromolecules such as lipids, proteins, and DNA, that can lead to the development of a wide range of pathologies, including cancer and cardiovascular diseases, and facilitate the process of aging.

There is compelling evidence that consumption of antioxidant compounds from dietary plant sources, such as fruits and vegetables may prevent these pathologies attributed to ROS (Schumacker, 2006; Bazzano et al., 2002). Thus, from a nutritional and disease prevention perspective, it is important to evaluate the antioxidant potential of phytochemicals in antioxidant-rich fruits and vegetables that might produce an epigenetic effect to attenuate the damaging effects of ROS and resultant endogenously generated free radicals.

Dietary antioxidant strategies to treat respiratory diseases such as emphysema and COPD have drawn recent attention (Biswas et al., 2013). ROS induced by tobacco smoke stimulates inflammatory responses in the lungs that is associated with expression of proinflammatory mediator genes, signal transduction, chromatin remodeling, and histone acetylation and expression, as well as, activation of nuclear factor kappa-B (NF-κB) and activator protein-1 (AP-1).

Cigarette smoke also triggers macrophage adhesion and activation due to posttranslational modifications of histone deacetylase and macrophages (Kirkham, et al., 2003; Yang et al., 2006).

In a review of the most promising dietary approaches to improve lung antioxidant levels to treat or intervene in the progression of COPD to modulate the adverse effects of cigarette smoke-induced oxidative and aldehyde/carbonyl stress, açai has been suggested as a promising candidate, along with thiol molecules and compounds found in foods rich in polyphenols (Biswas et al., 2013).

de Moura et al. (2011) studied the protective effect of açai seed in mitigating the development of emphysema in a novel experiment in mice exposed to chronic secondhand cigarette smoke. Emphysema is a disease that damages the air sacs and also the small airways in the lungs. The study exposed one group of mice to 60-days of chronic inhalation of cigarette smoke, and compared them to another group exposed to the same amount of smoke that contained 100 mg of a hydroalcoholic extract of açai seed incorporated into the tobacco of the cigarette. Mice exposed to sham smoke served as controls. At the end of the study, mice were sacrificed and histopathological and biochemical investigations carried out, including bronchoalveolar lavage. The açai seed extract + tobacco cigarette inhaling group (ASTC) experienced a remarkable protective effect against emphysema, compared to the cigarette smoke group (CS). Unlike the ASTC group, which experienced some enlarged areas and some leukocytes in the alveoli in the lung parenchyma, the alveolar space in all of the CS group were found enlarged. The CS group also had higher leukocytes and reduced antioxidative enzymes (eg, MPO, glutathione, and 4-hydroxynonenal). By comparison, the CS + açai seed group had elevated antioxidant enzyme levels, and reduced macrophage and neutrophil elastase levels.

In understanding the protective mechanism of the açai seed extract against emphysema, the investigators observed a significant reduction in the level of metalloelastase (MMP-12 or macrophage elastase), an enzyme that breaks down lung extracellular matrix during its development. This finding suggests that the seed contains antiproteinase activity that protects mouse lungs by reacting directly with MMP-12. Similarly, it was determined that neutrophil elastase was reduced in the lungs of the ASTC group. This elastase is a potent proteolytic enzyme that also breaks down extracellular matrix. MPO was significantly lower in the ASTC group than the CS group ($P < 0.022$). Reduced levels of the MPO enzyme in lungs is a biomarker of neutrophil influx and acute lung injury often associated with pulmonary leukostasis. Interestingly, since 2003, MPO has been found to be a sensitive predictor for myocardial infarction in patients presenting with chest pain (Brennan et al., 2003). Individuals treated for myocardial infarction and stroke are the highest risk group to experience subsequent coronary and cerebral events, according to the World Health Organization (WHO) (Mendis et al., 2011). Since myocardial infarction remains a leading cause of morbidity and mortality in the United States and worldwide, it is only fitting that a study would look at whether açai seed might improve cardiac function to reduce risk of the disease, particularly as açai pulp demonstrates such benefits in vivo, as will be discussed later.

The recent interest in the bioactivity and potential health benefits of the seed of açai is encouraging. As more research is performed with the seed, a byproduct in the production of açai pulp, it may no longer be seen as a waste disposal problem, but rather as a value-added component of the fruit with demonstrated health promoting benefits. Of particular interest is the finding of da Moura and colleagues of the seeds' ability to mitigate the seriously damaging effects caused by cigarette smoking and exposure to secondhand cigarette smoke. Hopefully, studies are envisioned by researchers to see what effect the seed would have or its components in attenuating chronic bronchitis associated with COPD.

Efforts to characterize the compounds in açai seed that might someday help to attribute which ones are responsible for the observed health benefits. A recent effort by a collegium of chemists and natural products researchers has begun this work. Led by Smith with the U.S. FDA, Wycoff at the University of Missouri, two medical schools in Brazil, and AIBMR Life Sciences in the United States, the chemical and nutrition analysis of the seeds of both the purple and while variety was carried out (Wycoff et al., 2015). It determined that the seeds primarily contain glycosidic carbons due to their cellulose and hemicellulose content, as well as, aliphatic carbons, and a mixture of saturated and unsaturated fats, and fatty acids not previously reported in the fruit, by using solid state 1H-decoupled 13C CPMAS and MAS NMR, NMR, and LC-MS/MS. Unlike the pulp, neither of the major anthocyanidins, cyanidin 3-*O*-glucoside, or cyanidin 3-*O*-rutinoside, were detected in the seed. In light of the potential life-saving benefits of the seed, further characterization work should be carried out using bioassay-guided fractionation to unravel the bioactivity of specific compounds or classes of compounds in the seed capable of potentially preventing, mitigating, or treating diseases. Others have reported using nondestructive near infrared (NIR) spectroscopy to determine total anthocyanin levels in intact fruit to monitor quality (Inacio et al. (2013); de Almeida Teixeira et al. (2015)), as well as, a new validated method for analysis of β-sitosterol and total phytosterol content (Cheng et al., 2014).

AÇAI PULP OF THE FRUIT

Oxidative stress from overproduction of ROS is implicated in a wide range of conditions such as atherosclerosis, diabetes, malignant diseases, chronic inflammation, and ischemia-reperfusion. In recent years, studies have examined particular foods, including the pulp of açai, shown to exhibit potent antioxidant and antiinflammatory capacities and bioactivities. Açai pulp is also rich in polyphenols. Consumption of foods rich in polyphenols has been inversely correlated with the incidence of chronic diseases such as cardiovascular disease (Manach et al., 2005). As research progressed during the last two decades, near unanimity has been reached that antioxidant intake from exogenous sources (supplements and diet) and endogenous antioxidant defenses are critical factors in disease prevention and maintenance of health. Nevertheless, there has been critics who argue that the benefits of antioxidants are overrated and insignificant (Bast and Haenen, 2013). Acceptance of the benefits has been a driving force in studying the pulp given its extraordinary high antioxidant capacity against ROS compared to the vast majority of other foods, including those touted for similar attributes.

Well-designed investigations into the characterization of both the pulp's chemistry and its nutritional composition has been a focus of interest in the last two decades, particularly with the revelations reported in two papers published in 2006 by a larger collaboration of investigators (Schauss et al., 2006a,b). Eight years later a thorough review of açai pulp's nutritional and phytochemical composition was published to assist additional analytical efforts to perform characterization studies given its complex chemistry (Odendaal and Schauss, 2014).

Research has been trying to determine which phytochemicals in açai pulp is responsible for any of its health-giving properties. Blueberries and strawberries, for example, are among the foods that contain high levels of anthocyanins, as determined in two *Vaccinium* species (cranberry and bilberry), as well as Rubus berries (blackberry, black raspberry, red raspberry, black and red currant, cherry), and certain vegetables (black rice, red cabbage, purple corn, and eggplant peel) (Wu et al., 2006). Current evidence suggests that just three portions a week of such foods can reduce the risk of heart disease, type 2 diabetes, Parkinson's disease, prevent cognitive decline, and reduce mortality from all causes, including cardiovascular disease and cancer (Wang et al., 2014). Anthocyanins, which are found in abundance in açai pulp, seem to work by helping to dilate arteries and by countering the buildup of plaque along with other cardiovascular benefits such as lowering blood pressure and improving cholesterol and the lipid profile. Long-term clinical trials to understand more clearly what the optimal dose of anthocyanins is for health benefits so that we can refine dietary guidelines and give consumers clear dietary advice to optimize health must be achieved. Nevertheless, these foods are readily incorporated into the diet, and simple dietary change could have a significant impact in reducing the risk of chronic disease.

By mid-2015, over 200 papers had been published on the açai pulp, with a near majority focusing on its potential health benefits. Many of the studies reported are discussed below.

In 2008, a cell-based antioxidant protection assay, using fresh human red blood cells and polymorphonuclear cells, demonstrated that following consumption of açai pulp, the pulp protected cells during oxidative stress within minutes of ingestion, continuing to provide this function for nearly 4 h. This study was noteworthy in that it abandoned reliance on chemical-based assays which by then had been found to poorly correlate with in vivo outcomes, and instead employed a new approach, namely, cell-based assays, that found growing support within the research community, as in vitro results have been shown to correspond well with subsequent in vivo observations.

A pilot study and small randomized, double-blind, placebo-controlled, crossover study demonstrated that consumption of an açai-rich fruit and berry juice blend increased serum antioxidant levels, protected cells from oxidative damage, reduced formation of ROS, and down-regulated production of proinflammatory cytokines and chemokines (Jensen et al., 2008). Oral administration of the same açai-enriched juice blend, twice daily, was given to 48- to 84-year-olds daily for 12 weeks, who complained of reduced range-of-motion associated with joint pain. Within 4 weeks of ingestion of the beverage blend a significant reduction in pain was reported by subjects along with a significant improvement in range-of-motion

(Jensen et al., 2011). Monitoring of serum antioxidant status at periodic intervals during the study showed that starting in just 2 weeks after the start of the study, and continuing through to the end, various biomarkers had improved, such as C-reactive protein (CRP) associated with lipid peroxidation and inflammation.

The incidence of inflammatory bowel disease (IBD), which can lead to functional disability and a decreased quality of life, is increasing worldwide. IBD primarily includes Crohn's disease and ulcerative colitis. Both are inflammatory diseases, the former involving long-lasting inflammation and ulcers in the colon and rectum, the latter, the small intestine and/or large intestine. Other less common forms of IBD include Behçet's disease, collagenous colitis, diversion colitis, lymphocytic colitis, and indeterminate colitis.

The antiinflammatory activity of açai in intestinal myofibroblasts CCD-18Co cells subjected to LPS-stimulation was evaluated by Dias et al. (2015). The investigation focused on measuring changes in ROS scavenging activity, proinflammatory biomarkers, and involved signaling pathways, and mRNA protein expression of inflammatory proteins, with potential relevance to the prevention and mitigation of IBD. Açai was found to downregulate the expression of proinflammatory genes and proteins in CCD-18Co cells involved in inflammation of the GI tract. Inhibition of toll-life receptor-4 (TLR-4) and NF-κB, was found to be accountable for açai's antiinflammatory effects. The authors report that açai down-regulated LPS-induced mRNA expression of tumor necrosis factor-alpha (TNF-α), cyclooxygenase 2 (COX-2), TLR-4, TNF receptor-associated factor 6 (TRAF-6), nuclear factor kappa B (NF-κB), vascular cell adhesion molecule 1 (VCAM-1), and intercellular adhesion molecule 1 (ICAM-1), in a dose-dependent manner. This finding that açai down-regulates COX-2, TLR-4, TNF-α, and TRAF-6, is critical to decreasing inflammation, and provides preliminary evidence for the potential of açai to play a role in the prevention of IBD and other conditions involving intestinal inflammation.

The ability of açai pulp to reduce inflammation may be due to a class of flavones identified by Kang and colleagues (2010). Among the flavones identified by the authors was the flavone, velutin, shown to have exceptionally potent antiinflammatory capacity in mouse macrophages, a more potent antiinflammatory than any flavonoid found in nature at the time of its discovery. Velutin demonstrated an ability to inhibit the expression of proinflammatory cytokines such as TNF-α and interleukin-6 (IL-6) at very low micromole levels. Further work determined that it did this by inhibiting NF-κB activation, and c-Jun N-terminal kinase (JNK), a stress-activated protein kinase involved in a variety of disease processes (Cui et al., 2007), as well as, p38 mitogen-activated protein kinase (MAPK) phosphorylation. IL-6 and TNF-α perform important roles in production of vascular inflammation that underlies, is characterized by, and serves as predictive biomarkers of cardiovascular disease and related mortality, while JNK inhibitors can serve in controlling certain arthroses, such as rheumatoid arthritis (Johnson and Lapadat, 2002).

Açai pulp is also surprisingly rich in monounsaturated and polyunsaturated fatty acids, similar to or exceeding that of levels found in olives or avocadoes. It has been shown that phospholipids promote the absorption of polyphenols, especially anthocyanins, thereby enhancing their bioavailability and availability in the bloodstream (Miyazawa et al., 1999). A pharmacokinetic study in healthy humans observed a significant increase in the antioxidant capacity of plasma, which supports the potential of açai as an antioxidant, or to stimulate endogenous antioxidant production. Absorption of total anthocyanins, following acute consumption of an clarified açai juice, was found to be nearly 8–10 times greater than in that found in other fruits and berries rich in anthocyanins, which has been attributed to the pulp's high fatty acid content. A Caco-2 cell monolayer model system was studied to evaluate the role of phospholipids and terpenes and their role in transepithelial transport (Cardona et al., 2015). The model can demonstrate whether phospholipids can promote the transport of anthocyanins through the intestinal barrier by fusing with membrane lipids. Using clarified açai pulp concentrate the authors reported observing the enhanced absorption of anthocyanins using soy lecithin to demonstrated the effect. Having potential health giving polyphenols and flavonoids in foods reach the bloodstream to contribute to the prevention and mitigation of diseases is essential.

CARDIOVASCULAR AND LIPID PROFILE STUDIES

Atherosclerosis is a disorder of lipid metabolism, characterized by an accumulation of lipids and fiber-like elements found in large arteries. It is also an inflammatory disease. The pathogenesis of atherosclerosis can eventually cause a heart attack, angina pectoris, or, in the case of cerebrovascular disease, manifested itself as a stroke.

Oxidative damage to the arterial wall is implicated in the pathogenesis of atherosclerosis. Given açai pulp's antioxidant and antiinflammatory bioactivities, it should mitigate the development of atherosclerosis or cerebrovascular disease, if given at an effective dose, as part of the diet, during the early progressive stages of the disease. To test this theory, the athero-protective effects of an açai-rich juice blend was studied by Xie and colleagues at the USDA Arkansas Children's Nutrition Center in two feeding studies using hyperlipidemic ApoE-deficient ($ApoE^{-/-}$) mice (Xie et al., 2011). $ApoE^{-/-}$ mice were fed a high-fat diet with or without 5% of the açai juice blend (AJB) for 20-weeks. At the end of the study, mean lesion areas in the aorta of the AJB fed mice were found to be 58% lower compared to control animals fed a calorically identical diet. Biomarkers of lipid peroxidation were measured and found significantly lower in the serum and liver of the AJB-fed animals. Expression of two antioxidant enzyme genes, glutathione reductase (GR) and glutathione peroxidase (GPX), that protect cells against oxidative stress and injury, and counteract oxidative stress, were significantly up-regulated in the AJB-fed animals but not in the control group. Levels of TNF-α were significantly lower, as were interleukin-6 (IL-6) levels in resident macrophages. TNF-α, during an inflammatory response, has been shown to initiate and stimulate the expression of chemokines and cytokines, as well as, endothelial adhesion molecules (Terzic et al., 2010).

Previous studies have shown that the proinflammatory cytokines IL-6 and TNF-α amplify an inflammatory response in atherosclerotic lesions (Libby, 2002), and can serve as predictors of the severity of coronary arterial disease (Gotsman et al., 2008; Szekanecz, 2008).

Macrophages play an important role in inflammation and lipid metabolism in the pathogenesis of atherosclerosis. In the USDA study, the supernatant of cultured resident macrophages was used in the SEAP reporter assay taken from AJB fed mice. A reduction in the ability to activate the NF-κB pathway was demonstrated in the assay. Previously, it had been shown that endothelial oxidant stress and the activation of the NF-κB family of transcription factors is associated with the initiation of atherosclerotic lesion formation (Collins, 1993), and its presence in atherosclerotic lesions (Brand et al., 1996).

Only the AJB group developed significantly less atherosclerotic lesions, despite a significant increase in weight in both groups of animals due to the diet's high-fat composition. Both epidemiological and clinical studies have reported an inverse and independent association between serum HDL cholesterol levels and coronary heart disease (CHD) risk (Tabet and Rye, 2009).

The rise in HDL cholesterol in the AJB group is of interest, as the authors speculated that a contributing mechanism associated with açai's athero-protective effect was the observed increase in HDL cholesterol.

To measure other plausible contributing factors to explain the significant reduction in the formation of atherosclerotic lesions, the investigators performed a second study using the same $ApoE^{-/-}$ mice using the same diet for a 5-week period. Surprisingly, the second study demonstrated an identical 58% reduction in the formation of atherosclerotic lesions in the AJB group. Also, the second study revealed recruitment and activation of macrophages in the vascular system's major cell types that was attenuated in the early stages of atherosclerotic lesion formation. Although macrophages play a central role in innate immunity, NF-κB is the central transcriptional regulator of the innate immune response. Whether açai affects liver X receptors (LXRs), established as mediators of lipid-inducible gene expression, was not determined. The LXR ligand is known to inhibit expression of inflammatory mediators (eg, IL-6 and cyclooxygenase-2 (COX-2)). The likelihood that it might be supported by earlier work using a COX assay that showed açai pulp could potentially inhibit both COX-1 and COX-2. Based on the IC_{50} ratio between the two the assay found the pulp inhibited the COX-1 enzyme more efficiently than the COX-2 enzyme (Schauss et al., 2006b).

In a study by de Souza et al. (2012), they investigated the effect of feeding rats for 6 weeks with a hypercholesterolemic diet. Half of the animals received the hypercholesterolemic diet while the other half received the same diet supplemented with 2% açai pulp. After 6 weeks, the dietary-induced hypercholesterolemia group experienced a decrease in high-density lipoprotein (HDL) cholesterol and an increase in total cholesterol and LDL cholesterol. The group that consumed the same diet supplemented with açai pulp had a reduction in both total and LDL cholesterol levels. Total, free, and protein sulfhydryl concentration is also reduced in the açai pulp group, along with a significant decrease in serum triacylglycerol levels. It is suggested by the authors that the ingestion of the monounsaturated oleic acid, polyunsaturated alpha-linolenic, and linoleic acid, found in the pulp accounted for the animal's improved lipid profile. The presence of phytosterols in açai is also proposed as playing a role since this class of compounds have been shown to reduce the absorption of biliary and dietary cholesterol from the intestinal tract.

In addressing the possible molecular mechanisms involved in improving the lipid profile by administration of açai pulp, de Souza and colleagues also focused on the hypocholesterolemic activity exerted by the pulp on gene expression. They reported that the hypocholesterolemic effect observed is primarily attributed to the enhanced expression of the ABCG5 and ABCG8 transporters. Previous work by Yu and colleagues (2002) showed that increased expression of these two transporters cause profound alterations in the liver and small intestine, characterized by increased biliary cholesterol secretion and reduced cholesterol absorption in the gut. Based on this knowledge (Jakulj et al., 2010), and the observed secretion of cholesterol into the bile via these transporters, the authors concluded that supplementation of the diet with açai pulp in hypercholesterolemic rats, increased the mRNA levels of the ATP-binding cassette (ABCG)G5/ABCG8 transporters, while "up-regulation of the transporters is the likely mechanism underlying the decreased concentration of serum cholesterol and increased fecal cholesterol excretion."

An association was also found between the concentrations of plasma and intracellular cholesterol regulated by the nuclear transcription factor that binds to the membranes of the endoplasmic reticulum, sterol regulatory element-binding protein-2 (SREBP-2), and hepatic cholesterol metabolism, by supplementing açai in a hypercholesterolemic diet. Hypercholesterolemic rats exhibit a lower expression of SREBP-2, a key regulator of cholesterol (Miserez et al., 2002). In the rats fed the same diet but supplemented with açai pulp in their study, cholesterol concentration was decreased which in turn led to an up-regulation in the expression of SREBP-2. This increase in expression of SREBP-2 in turn activates the promoters of the low-density lipoprotein receptor (LDL-R) and the 3-hydroxy-3-methylglutaryl CoA reductase receptor (HMG CoA-R) genes. The result is the increased clearance of plasma LDL cholesterol, strongly associated with a decreased risk of cardiovascular disease in humans (Ansell et al., 1999).

In separate studies, de Souza and colleagues (2012) evaluated the gene expression of apolipoprotein B100 (ApoB 100), which is synthesized by the liver. This lipoprotein is the most important apolipoprotein transporting cholesterol and triglycerides in blood in terms of atherosclerosis and cardiovascular disease risk factors. ApoB 100 is found in chylomicrons, very-low density lipoprotein (VLDL), low-density lipoprotein (LDL), and lipoprotein(a) (LP(a)) particles, each of which contains a single ApoB molecule, and all of which are atherogenic. Studies have shown that ApoB 100 levels in the blood are a better predictor of cardiovascular disease risk than LDL cholesterol (Lamarche et al., 1996). A large prospective study in humans showed that ApoB may be elevated despite low or normal concentrations of LDL cholesterol (Walldius et al., 2001). de Souza and coworkers also found that açai supplementation decreases mRNA levels of ApoB 100, which would explain the reduction seen in VLDL cholesterol and LDL cholesterol observed in the animals fed with hypercholesterolemic diet.

Using a classic rabbit model of diet-induced atherosclerosis, Feio and colleagues (2012) added açai pulp to the diet to see if it would attenuate atherosclerosis. They found while investigating the phytosterol content in açai pulp that 15 mg of a 100 g extract, of which β-sitosterol was the most abundant, confirmed earlier reports that reported on the nutritional composition of açai pulp (Schauss et al., 2006a). Following the feeding portion of the study, Feio and coworkers concluded that the reduction in atherosclerosis observed in the animals was due to decreased ratios of markers of cholesterol synthesis and absorption, increased expression of LDL receptors, reduced oxidative modification of lipoproteins, and improved endothelial function.

Feio and coworkers cited a study by Noratto and colleagues (2011) that reported açai pulp exerted a protective effect in human umbilical vascular endothelial cells (HUVEC) during inflammatory stress. The study showed açai pulp protected HUVEC against glucose-induced oxidative stress and inflammation, and down-regulated protein expression of IL-6 and interleukin-8 (IL-8) cytokines at the mRNA level. The pulp also inhibited gene expression of adhesion molecules and activation of the inducible transcription factor NF-κB involved in the pathogenesis of atherosclerosis, while also decreasing production of platelet endothelial cell adhesion molecule 1 (PECAM-1) and intracellular adhesion molecule 1 (ICAM-1) protein. Gene and protein expression of vascular cell adhesion protein 1 (VCAM-1) was also inhibited by açai, associated with mRNA-126 expression. Up-regulation and production of ICAM-1 and VCAM-1 is associated with sites of atherosclerotic lesions (Nakaskima et al., 1998) while PECAM-1 has been reported to contribute to atherosclerotic lesion formation.

These animal studies support the position that açai pulp benefits endothelial function, the maintenance of vascular homeostasis, and reduces atherogenic processes necessary for the development of atherosclerosis. But what is the evidence for such benefits in humans?

Gale and colleagues (2014) reported on a small randomized, double blind, placebo-controlled, crossover study that evaluated the hemodynamic and electrocardiographic (ECG) effects of açai pulp in 18 healthy volunteers. Subjects were administered either a 500 mg gel capsule of açai pulp powder or matching placebo. After a washout period of 7 days, participants returned for the second phase of the trial to receive the opposite treatment. During 1, 2, 4, and 6-h postingestion periods, electrocardiographic (ECG) and hemodynamic measurements were performed and compared to treatment or placebo. Endpoints measured any ECG changes between groups at baseline, 1- and 2-h postingestion. Co-primary hemodynamic endpoints included changes in seated systolic blood pressure (SBP); secondary hemodynamic endpoints measured changes in seated diastolic blood pressure (DBP).

The study found no significant differences in baseline ECG or blood pressure between the açai and placebo groups, nor significant differences in any of the primary or secondary ECG endpoints between groups, with the exception of a significant lower standing blood pressure difference between açai and placebo at 6h. Subjects reported no adverse effects during the study.

The question was raised as to what the long-term benefits might be of the pulp on blood pressure or hypertension, as an earlier study in animals suggested long-term benefits for açai seed (da Costa et al., 2012), whereas any beneficial effect in humans for the pulp was unknown.

Udani and colleagues (2011) included recordings of blood pressure and heart rate in an open-label study of overweight healthy adult subjects given 100g of açai pulp product twice daily for a month. The study evaluated the effect of açai pulp on risk factors associated with metabolic disorders in 10 overweight subjects with a body mass index (BMI) between $\geq$25 and $\leq$30kg/m^2. Endpoints measured at baseline and following 30-days of açai pulp ingestion included fasting plasma glucose, insulin, cholesterol, triglycerides, exhaled nitric oxide metabolites (eNO), and plasma levels of high-sensitivity C-reactive protein (hs-CRP). The study observed significant reductions in fasting glucose and insulin, along with a significant reduction in total cholesterol, borderline reductions in total cholesterol to HDL cholesterol ratios, and LDL cholesterol.

At the conclusion of the study, treatment with açai ameliorated the postprandial increase in plasma glucose following consumption of the standardized meal, compared to baseline. No significant changes were seen in blood pressure or nitric oxide metabolites, which stayed within the normal range, or in hs-CRP. No adverse events or changes in vital signs in subjects were reported.

In that açai pulp reduced levels of selected markers associated with metabolic disease risk in overweight adults, Udani and coworkers recommended that further studies be carried out.

Sadowska-Krepa and colleagues (2015) evaluated the effects of daily consumption of an açai-enriched berry juice blend for 6 weeks on antioxidant status, lipid profile, and athletic performance, in seven 16- to 19-year-old track athletes specializing in hurdling. The athletic performance included an examination of the effects of the açai juice blend on anaerobic exercise-induced changes in blood antioxidant defense systems. Although consumption of the juice had no effect on 300m dash performance, a marked increase in total antioxidant capacity of plasma, attenuation of exercise-induced muscle damage, and a significant improvement in the serum lipid profile was observed, including a reduction in total cholesterol, LDL cholesterol, and triglycerides, along with an increase in HDL cholesterol, improved lipid ratios, and decline in the atherogenic index of plasma. The improvements in the lipid profile were found positively associated with an increased concentration of plasma total polyphenols and in blood nonenzymatic antioxidant levels.

Whether cholesterol levels play a significant role in the pathogenesis of atherosclerosis has been increasingly challenged upon closer scrutiny of the evidence. Some critics of the cholesterol-heart disease theory argue that atherosclerosis is an inflammatory disease initiated by endothelial dysfunction mediated by T-lymphocytes and macrophages (Ross, 1999). Others have pointed out that the inflammatory response promotes migration and proliferation of smooth muscle cells that act together to create a fibroproliferative process culminating in atherosclerosis independent of cholesterol levels (Ravnskov, 2002; Taubes, 2008) (Miller, 2015). If it is primarily an inflammatory disease, as the evidence has been pointing to for well over a decade, then given the demonstrated antiinflammatory properties of açai pulp, it bodes well for the pulp when it is eventually tested in controlled clinical trials. That inflammation is central to the disease's pathogenesis becomes even more likely when examining the pulp's epigenetic effect on gene expression related to its antiinflammatory properties as discussed below.

EPIGENETIC EFFECTS OF AÇAI PULP ON LIFE SPAN EXTENSION

Given the results of both $ApoE^{-/-}$ mice/atherosclerosis study outcomes, Sun and colleagues decided to evaluate the effect of açai pulp on modulating life span in the fruit fly (*Drosophila melanogaster*) as this would provide information on the effect açai had on transcript levels for over a dozen genes known to be associated with aging, metabolic diseases, and various disease processes (Sun et al., 2010). They also knew that oxidative damage tends to accumulate in the cell with increasing age, and would over time contribute to degenerative diseases including atherosclerosis and cerebrovascular disease as the flies aged. Prior to this study, it had been shown that a high intake of polyphenolics would reduce some of the damaging effects associated with aging over time. However, it had never been directly tested.

The study looked at changes in cell signaling and gene expression affected by a standard diet supplemented with açai pulp. *D. melanogaster* received either 0.25%, 0.5%, 1%, or 2% lyophilized açai pulp powder added to the diet. To determine the effect of certain fats on life span and aging, saturated fat and palmitic acid was added to the standard diet, emulsified with Tween-80, to improve palatability. The study showed the 2% added palmitic acid diet caused a significant decrease in mean life span by approximately 19%, or from 32.6 to 26.4 days, compared to a diet without the added fat. Essentially, the high-fat diet was found to be detrimental to flies life span. Whether this is the case for humans is controversial. Much depends on what fats are consumed and in what proportion to other caloric sources, such as simple carbohydrates, and/or macro- and micronutrients. What is of interest particular interest was the discovery that flies fed the high-fat diet containing 2% palmitic acid, supplemented with 2% açai pulp, experienced significantly prolonged mean life spans of ~22% compared to controls on just a high-fat diet. When analyzing the data for the 0.1% and 0.5% açai supplemented high-fat groups they also experienced a significant mean increase in life span. However, when the data was analyzed by sex, life extension was only seen in the 2% male group.

By measuring changes in the transcript levels, the study also found açai pulp supplementation activated a subset of JNK and insulin-life signaling pathways, including phosphoenolpyruvate carboxykinase (*Pepck*) an enzyme in the metabolic pathway that generates glucose from substrates, partially transcriptionally regulated by *dFoxo*, a forkhead transcription factor that regulates the protein phosphorylation level by insulin and insulin-like signaling pathways involved in regulating aging and metabolism. The investigators observed significantly suppressed *Pepck* expression, without altering the transcript level of *dFoxo*, which suggests the açai prolongevity effect when consuming a high-fat diet is partially mediated by suppression of *Pepck* expression and activation of stress response pathways. Supporting this conclusion was the finding that *Lethal(2) essential for life* (*l(2)efl*) encoded a heat shock response protein that affects the stress response that is regulated by *dFoxo* and *JNK*. Overexpression of (*l(2)efl*) extends life span, whereas a high-fat diet decreases transcription of (*l(2)efl*) by nearly twofold compared to what is seen with a normal diet. Açai supplementation increased the (*l(2)efl*) transcript level by twofold in the high-fat diet groups, to nearly the same level observed in flies fed with normal diet. Finally, when comparing the groups to two downstream genes, glutathione S-transferase (*GstD1*) and metallothionein A (*MtnA*) involved in antioxidant functions, both significantly increased transcript levels.

The investigators opined that given the reduction in the transcript level of *Pepck* by more than fourfold compared to the nonsupplemented diet group, açai pulp might be effective in the prevention and control of type-2 diabetes, not just life span prolongation. Certain types of high-fat diets can result in insulin resistance and ultimately diabetes for which drugs are used to treat the condition by suppressing *Pepck* expression and in turn gluconeogenesis and glyconeogenesis (Srivastava, 2009). By lowering glucose levels and improving the lipid profile, animals and patients with type-2 diabetes one is able to resolve diabetic symptoms (Quinn and Yeagley, 2005).

Bonomo and colleagues (2013) studied the mechanisms of action of açai in modulating oxidative stress in the nematode, *Caenorhabditis elegans*. An increase in stress after which an aqueous extract of açai was administered resulted in an increase in stress resistance that correlated with a reduction in production of ROS. As observed in *D. melanogaster* by Sun and colleagues (2010) in *C. elegans*, the downstream target of insulin-like signaling was the Fork head transcription (DAF-16), required for life span regulation and stress resistance (Kenyon, 2010). DAF-16 functions as a transcription factor that acts in the insulin/IGF-1-mediated signaling pathway that regulates dauer formation (Wang et al., 2009), longevity, fat metabolism, stress response, and innate immunity (Ogg et al., 1997). Nuclear translocation of DAF-16/Foxo is regulated by JNK along with insulin-like signaling. The increase in oxidative stress resistance observed in *C. elegans* fed açai extract was attributed to DAF-16/Foxo, independent of JNK-1. JNK-1, which has four isoforms, directly interacts with and phosphorylates DAF-16 (Cui et al., 2007).

The results of these studies showed that açai pulp increases oxidative stress resistance by activating the antioxidant genes via DAF-16. Increased oxidative stress resistance was found in these studies associated with MAPK signaling, and osmotic stress resistance protein (OSR-1), a secreted protein that couples with stress-activated protein kinase (SAPK)/stress-activated Erk kinase-1 (SEK-1) to activate the MAPK homologues, SAPK, and JNK, in response to various cellular stresses and inflammatory cytokines (Nishina et al., 2004), while also regulating behavioral as well as physiological responses (Solomon et al., 2004), and two of its downstream effectors: a gain-of-function-43 (UNC-43) and SEK-1 (Reiner et al., 1999). UNC-43 is the gene for calcium/calmodulin-dependent serine/threonine kinase type II (CaMKII), one of the most abundant proteins in the human brain, where it is thought to regulate synaptic plasticity and other processes.

The findings of these studies also address the question of whether açai removes ROS directly or indirectly. Based on the data, particularly the work of Bonomo and colleagues, the evidence supports the position that açai removes ROS directly, while at the same time improving antioxidant status, which protects against damage caused by oxidative stress.

AÇAI PULP, TRANSCRIPTION AND MODULATION OF IMMUNE FUNCTION

Mast cells contribute to chronic inflammation in response to allergens. These specialized cells enhance recruitment of numerous inflammatory cells including eosinophils, natural killer cells, IL-8, and TNF-α. Activation of mast cells perform a major role in defense against pathogens and in mediating allergic diseases (Urb and Sheppard, 2012). Both leukocytes and mast cells circulate in the blood in tissues particularly in areas where contact occurs with the external environment, such as the airways, intestines, and skin.

In response to an allergen or pathogen, mast cells go through a series of transformations upon activation that stimulate components of the immune system, including TNF-α and interleukin-4 (IL-4), and transcriptional upregulation of a host of cytokines and chemokines. Following initiation to an external threat, mast cells produce eicosanoids, such as prostaglandin D2 and leukotriene C4 (LTC4), resulting in the release of any combination of agents. In humans, allergic reactions to inhaled soluble small-proteins elicit an immunoglobulin E (IgE) antibody response to even the minutest dose of an allergen. Chronic symptoms such as a constant runny nose, watery eyes, and an increase in periods of severe fatigue, when unrelieved, are typical symptoms people experience.

Horiguchi and colleagues (2011) studied the effect of açai pulp on IgE-mediated mast cell activation, using mouse bone marrow-derived mast cells (BMMC) pretreated with açai pulp and then stimulated with an antigen at different concentrations. Cells pretreated with açai pulp inhibited IgE-mediated degranulation of mast cells in a dose-dependent manner. Using a cultured mast cell line of rat basophilic leukemia (RBL)-2H3 cells, the transcription of cytokine genes were found to be suppressed in a dose-dependent manner, demonstrating that açai pulp is a potent inhibitor of IgE-mediated mast cell activation in vitro. However, when an extract of açai is prepared with ethanol, no such benefit was observed. This suggests that agents that facilitated the response seen in BMMC cells earlier after the addition of pulp were removed using ethanol extraction.

Using the nuclease protection (RNase) assay, a sensitive method for transcription site location, Horiguchi and colleagues used rat basophilic leukemic-2H3 cells (RBL-2H3) pretreated with or without açai pulp then stimulated the cells with an antigen, which led to the discovery that pretreatment of the cells inhibited the transcription of cytokine genes, including TNF-α, IL-2, and INF-gamma (INF γ). To determine how açai pulp affects IgE-mediated cellular signaling pathways that lead to mast cell degranulation and production of cytokines, the investigators used antigen-presented BMMC cells. This led to the discovery that açai pulp inhibited tyrosine phosphorylation of cellular proteins which "dramatically suppressed" the antigen-induced tyrosine phosphorylation of high affinity IgE receptors (FcεRI) on mast cells. This demonstrated that açai pulp inhibits cellular signaling pathways upon initiation when antigen-induced degranulation and production of numerous cytokines occurs. To confirm this, IgE-mediated activation of downstream protein kinases was tested using açai pulp. These protein kinases regulate the production of cytokines. It turned out that açai pulp selectively inhibits downstream signaling of these pathways by extracellular signal-regulated kinases, including ERK, the classic mitogen-activated protein (MAP) kinase.

As understanding the mechanisms of action is important, biofractionation studies are still needed to identify what compounds account for the observed inhibitory properties of the pulp. Horiguchi's study did start work in this direction by extracting different components of the pulp. They determined that the fat-soluble fraction of açai pulp does not suppress IgE-mediated mast cell activation, leaving open the question of what does unanswered.

The answers are found in the work of Holderness and colleagues (2011) and others who have studied the polysaccharide fractions in the pulp. They observed gamma delta (γδ) T cell agonist activity in the polysaccharides created from the pulp but not by polyphenol fractions. To work this out, the investigators examined cytokine production in açai-treated human peripheral blood mononuclear cells (PBMCs). Among 12 samples analyzed, six are consistently induced by 100 μg/mL of açai polysaccharide fractions, including interleukin-1a (IL-1a), IL-1-β, IL-6, IL-10, TNF-α, and the hematopoietic cytokine, granulocyte-macrophage colony-stimulating factor (GM-CSF), compared to control cells. The polysaccharide fractions induced immune recruitment and activation responses in mice, demonstrating that previously observed in vitro immune-stimulatory responses were preserved in vivo, evidence that the polysaccharides in açai pulp contributes in some way to its potent immunomodulatory activities. The investigators concluded that the responses seen in the mouse, bovine, and human cells correlate with in vivo responses observed in animals; the polysaccharides contain a distinct innate immune agonist. What that mechanism is remains unknown.

Holderness and colleagues line of investigation is promising in terms of fractions in the pulp as γδ T cells represent a subset of T cells that possess distinctive T-cell receptors on their surface that conserve the population of lymphocytes that have been the subject of increasing research interest owing to their involvement in the immune systems response associated with immunopathologies (Vantourout and Hayday, 2013). γδ T cells are now believed to play a vital role in the initiation phase of immune reactions to pathogens where they contribute to an effective innate immune response against a variety of infectious agents, while modulating the inflammatory response. Preliminary indications are that some fruits, such as açai, and vegetables, affect γδ T cells (Nantz et al., 2006; Percival et al., 2008), exerting a beneficial effect on the innate immune system. Whether açai's pulp is able to affect desirable innate immune responses against infectious agents in vivo is warranted, especially against drug-resistant pathogens. Fortunately, the results of such studies are beginning to appear in the literature.

Francisella tularensis and *Burkholderia pseudomallei* are two highly lethal pathogens that cause serious pulmonary infections that have been the subject of study by Skyberg and coworkers to determine their activity against these pathogens using açai pulp polysaccharides (Skyberg et al., 2012).

To appreciate the results, it would be useful to understand why their findings are important. Current antibiotic treatments (eg, tetracycline, chloramphenicol) are not always effective against pathogens such as *B. pseudomallei* and *F. tularensis*. Should a large-scale infection occur, antibiotics such as streptomycin, gentamicin, doxycycline, or ciprofloxacin would be used. While *B. pseudomallei* is less resistant to treatment by a host of antibiotics, it has developed resistance to numerous antibiotics, including β-lactams, aminoglycosides, and polymyxins. Vaccines to prevent or treat infections of these pathogens have been under development for some time but progress challenged due to their resistance (Silva and Dow, 2013).

Francisella tularensis, in particular, is so resistant to antibiotic therapy that it has been proposed as a biological weapon using airborne tularemia to cause a severe outbreak that can cause widespread respiratory failure, shock, and death (Dennis et al., 2001). Use of *F. tularensis*, in biological warfare, goes back to 1320–1318 BC (Gurcan, 2014), and more recently has been studied by Japanese germ warfare research units before and during WWII, as well as, former Soviet Union biological weapons scientists. The United States terminated its biological weapons development program in 1973, including *F. tularensis* research. Nevertheless, periodic natural occurrences of inhalation tularemia are reported around the world, since ticks, which can carry the bacteria by both *trans*-ovarial and *trans*-stadial transmission, flies, and mosquitoes, are vectors of tularemia transmission to mammals.

Skyberg's group has demonstrated that açai polysaccharides are potent innate immune agonists able to resolve *B. pseudomallei* and *F. tularensis* infections. Mice infected with *F. Tularensis* experienced up to an 80% survival rate when açai polysaccharide treatment was administered nasally. Nasal açai polysaccharide treatment also conferred protection in vivo against pulmonary infection caused by *B. pseudomallei* strain-1026b. Repeated experiments in animals by this group showed that açai polysaccharide treatment "dramatically" reduced the ability of *B. pseudomallei* to reproduce in the lung while at the same time blocking the spread of the bacteria to either the spleen or liver. It was also discovered that the polysaccharides enhance IFN-γ response by natural killer (NK) cells and $\gamma\delta$ T cells in the lungs, which provides some insight as to the polysaccharide's mechanism of action.

That açai polysaccharides works against such virulent pathogens suggests that compounds in açai may have broad-spectrum activity against virulent intracellular pathogens, including those that have developed drug resistance.

The immune system also plays an essential role in preventing carcinogenesis. An ever growing number of epidemiological and experimental studies report on the role of fruits, berries, and vegetables, in preventing the incidence of certain cancers, particularly by those foods rich in antioxidants, as chronically increased levels of ROS have been shown to damage DNA and promote mutations that initiate tumor growth (Wiseman and Halliwell, 1996). That antioxidant rich foods may play a role in suppressing carcinogenesis by affecting ROS scavenging and tempering free radical reactions that increase the production of malignant cells is proposed for years since ROS and oxidative stress influence cellular processes, such as proliferation, apoptosis, senescence, each of which is implicated in the development of cancer (Mates and Sanchez-Jimenez, 2000; Waris and Ahsan, 2006).

A study investigated the antiproliferative and antioxidant properties of an oil-free açai pulp extract for its effects on proliferation of C-6 rat brain glioma cells and MDA-468 human breast cancer cells (Hogan et al., 2010). The extract was compared to other anthocyanin-rich extracts for potential antiproliferative activity, including blackberry, blueberry, raspberry, strawberry, and wolfberry. It was discovered that açai extract possessed strong antioxidant activities and antiproliferative activity against C-6 brain glioma cells, while none of the other anthocyanin-rich extracts exhibited similar inhibitory activity, which suggests that açai's antiproliferative activity may not be due to its anthocyanin content.

By comparison, the açai extract exhibited no inhibitory activity against MDA-468 human breast cancer cells. The authors suggest something in the extract specifically targets C-6 glioma cells, but is ineffective against the breast cancer cell line. In contrast to these results, Silva and colleagues observed that a hydroalcoholic extract of açai pulp showed significant antitumorigenic potential in a human breast MCF-7cell line (Silva et al., 2014). In açai extract-treated MCF-7 cells, a significant reduction in cell viability was observed along with altered cell morphological features caused by an increase in autophagy, rather than by apoptosis. Further work on determining the mechanism that affects autophagy activation and regulation against cancer cells is needed.

The difference in outcomes reported by Hogan et al. and that of Silva et al. may be due to the nature of the breast cells studied. MCF-7 cells have an estrogen receptor that is absent in MDA-468 cells, although both are derived from breast cancers. Silva and colleagues speculate that the reason MCF-7 cells experienced morphological changes due to an increase in autophagy is that açai contains lignans that act as phytoestrogens with cytotoxic activity related to estrogen receptors in the MCF-7 cells. How the stimulation and increased autophagic activity inhibits the growth of MCF-7 cells is unknown. A 2006 report reported antiproliferative effects by açai pulp against HL-60 human leukemia cells (Pozo-Insfran et al., 2006). Induction of apoptosis of cells is observed through activation of caspase-3 in a dose- and time-dependent manner.

CENTRAL NERVOUS SYSTEM (CNS) AND BRAIN FUNCTION

Açai pulp has been the subject of numerous studies on its effects on brain function and prevention, mitigation, and possible treatment of neurodegenerative diseases, as oxidative stress has been associated with early onset of Alzheimer's disease and dopaminergic cell degeneration in Parkinson's disease (Barja, 2004). Whether ROS is the cause or a consequence of other etiologies in the development of neurological and neurodegenerative diseases is debatable (Andersen, 2004).

Excessive production of oxidative stress has been implicated in recent years in the initiation and progression of convulsions and seizures in the brain, as this organ utilizes the highest quantity of oxygen of any order in the body (Shin et al., 2011). The brain is also rich in lipids and iron that are prone to lipid oxidation and iron oxidation, respectively. An inability to control excessive ROS production and maintain low ROS levels, critical to normal cell function, increases the risk of neurodegeneration in conditions such as epilepsy. Abnormalities in biochemical and physiological traits have been linked to oxidative stress (Shin et al., 2008).

Since the 1980s, epilepsy-prone mice have been used as models of generalized tonic/clonic epilepsy to understand its mechanisms in human epilepsy. Their availability has encouraged finding therapeutic interventions with antioxidant components that might of beneficial among strategies to attenuate and minimize neurodegeneration in neuronal targets damaged by overproduction of ROS. Recently, Souza-Monteiro and collaborators studied the neuroprotective and anticonvulsant effects of an açai-pulp juice (containing >1400 mg gallic acid equivalents, with anthocyanins representing the major part of the phenolic compounds) in mice. They reported that the juice provided significant protection against seizures and seizure-related oxidative stress that might have implications for humans (Souza-Monteiro et al., 2015). In one experiment, for example, electrocortical alterations provided by pentylenetetrazole were administered to the mice. Pentylenetetrazole is a central nervous system (CNS) stimulant with epileptogenic properties used to study seizure phenomenon and in identifying agents that may control seizures. Açai juice did prevent and significantly diminished the amplitude and frequency discharges associated with seizures. The group also reported that different doses of the juice were able "to increase latencies to both first myoclonic jerk and first generalized tonic-clonic seizure and significantly decrease the total duration of tonic-clonic seizures caused by pentylenetetrazole administration." Further, the juice was able to "completely prevent lipid peroxidation in the cerebral cortex," thereby demonstrating a potent and direct scavenging property of the açai juice in vivo.

Studies of antioxidant-rich foods have also reported attenuation of oxidative stress and inflammation in the brain resulting in improved motor function, cognition, and/or other behavioral benefits (Lau et al., 2005; Shukitt-Hale et al., 2008; Devore et al., 2012; Poulose et al., 2014a).

Poulose and collaborators (2012) examined the effects of açai pulp on oxidative stress and inflammation in mouse brain microglial cells to understand the effect of the pulp on neuronal signaling. At the molecular level, microglial cells in the brain respond to pathogens and injury by becoming activated and migrating to the site of injury or infection, where they phagocytose to destroy the pathogen, followed by removal of damaged cells, a process known as autophagy. Chronic activation of microglial cells will ultimately lead to brain pathology through repeated release of proinflammatory cytokines, ROS and its intermediates, proteinases, and complement proteins (Dheen et al., 2007). Microglial cells are also able to resolve inflammation in the brain following response to injury or infection through signaling and up-regulation of antiinflammatory cytokines. Since the inflammatory response in the brain to injury or infection is mediated by activated microglial substances that can dampen its pro-inflammatory bioactivities while maintaining its other beneficial functions are of tantamount value.

An initial investigation to determine whether açai pulp can suppress microglial-mediated inflammation and facilitate autophagy, studied its suppressive effect on inflammation in microglia, and mice BV-2 microglial cells, pretreated with açai pulp alcohol (ETOH), methanol (MEOH), acetone (ACE), and ethyl acetate (ETAC) fractions. The ETOH and MEOH fractions were found to be the richest in anthocyanins, including cyanidin, delphinidin, malvidin, pelargonidin, and peonidin, whereas the ACE was richest in other phenolics, including catechin, ferulic acid, quercetin, resveratrol, synergic, and vanillic acids.

The study discovered that the ETOH and MEOH fractions significantly reduced the production of nitrite leading to a decrease in inducible nitric oxide synthase (iNOS) expression, and a significant dose-dependent reduction in TNF-α, NF-κB, COX-2, and p38-MAPK. iNOS expression in the brain has been linked to neurotoxicity in Alzheimer's disease (Heneka et al., 2000). Pretreatment of microglial with each fraction significantly attenuated lipopolysaccharide (LPS)-induced NO production, with the MEOH anthocyanin-rich fraction the most effective at inhibiting ROS release. iNOS produces NO. LPS-induced expression of iNOS significantly decreased following pretreatment in a dose-dependent manner with all fractions of açai pulp.

Proinflammatory biomarkers and ROS and RNS production suppression has been found to significantly affect key signaling proteins involved in regulating inflammation in the brain. All açai fractions in the study had significant inhibitory effects on p38-MAPK activation. P38 inhibitors are sought for their therapeutic effects in treating autoimmune diseases and other diseases characterized by chronic inflammation (Goldstein and Gabriel, 2005). Except for the ETAC fraction, all other fractions reduced phosphorylation of NFκB in a dose-dependent manner. Phosphorylation of NFκB leads to expression or activation of many inflammatory genes. The study found that the MEOH and ETOH fractions were highly significant in phosphorylating NFκB even at concentrations as low as 50 and 25 μg/mL, which correlated with levels of cyanidin, delphidin, malvidin, pelargonidin and peonidin, anthocyanins. In evaluating the effect of the açai fractions on expression of COX-2, the ETOH fraction that contained the most polyphenolics per unit of weight in the pulp and the highest concentration of anthocyanins had the most significant effect in inhibiting COX-2 at concentrations as low as 10 μg/mL.

That açai fractions affect p38-MAPK signaling that down-regulates phosphorylation of NF-κB, thereby transcriptionally suppressing production of COX-2 and iNOS, in BV-2 microglial cells, is significant, and reflected in the authors conclusion that açai pulp may contribute to extending "health span" in aging, "as it is able to combat some of the inflammatory and oxidative mediators of aging at the cellular level," in that an "effective reduction in oxidative damage and inflammation in brain cells is likely to be an effective intervention to reduce the incidence of age-related neurodegenerative disorders."

A second study by Poulose and coworkers carried out further molecular studies to evaluate the putative health effects of açai pulp on brain cells, to investigate the specific effects on restoring stressor-induced calcium dysregulation, stunted growth of basal dendrites, and autophagy inhibition using embryonic hippocampal and HT22 hippocampal neurons (Poulose et al., 2014b). Dysregulation of intracellular calcium (Ca^{2+}) in hippocampal and cortical neurons in the brain leads to impairment of mitochondrial function, and irreversible neuronal cell damage and death, which is why it is implicated in age-associated neurodegenerative disorders and changes in the aging brain.

The study observed that primary hippocampal neurons pretreated with açai pulp at exceedingly low concentrations significantly mitigated the toxic effect of excess Ca^{2+}, and calcium sequestration. Pretreatment of cells also resulted in a dose-dependent inhibition of the mechanistic target of rapamycin (mTOR), a master growth regulator that senses and integrates diverse nutritional and environmental cues, including amino acids, growth factors, cellular stress, and energy levels (Dowling et al., 2010). It couples these signals to the promotion of cellular growth by phosphorylating substrates that potentiate anabolic processes such as autophagy, which in the brain can affect synaptic changes in higher order brain function, including long-term memory (Hoeffer and Klann, 2010). Abnormal mTOR signaling is associated with numerous degenerative diseases, including atherosclerosis, cancer, and diabetes (LaPlante and Sabatini, 2012).

The dose-dependent inhibition of mTOR suggests açai pulp has a neuroprotective benefit, confirmed by testing the effect of adding wortmannin, a compound that inhibits neurite/dendrite outgrowth in the brain essential to synaptic plasticity needed to maintain functional memory. Pretreatment with açai pulp was able to negate the effects of wortmannin on basal neuritic outgrowth. Other studies have shown that this inhibitory effect, observed for açai pulp, contributes to the development of basal neuritis and dendritic trees, leading to synaptic plasticity and enhanced brain function (Shehata et al., 2012).

Spada and colleagues studied the antioxidant and antimutagenic activity of açai pulp to evaluate the effects of açai pulp on brain tissues in vivo (Spada et al., 2009), based on earlier results that found it had antioxidant and antimutagenic activity in vitro (Spada et al., 2008). The brain is especially susceptible to oxidative stress since it consumes ~20% of the oxygen used by the body, as it contains endogenous iron that creates regional susceptibility in the brain to oxidative damage as iron is a catalyst that facilitates lipid peroxidation (Zaleska and Floyd, 1985). Lipid peroxidation in the brain is associated with the loss of membrane permeability and cellular damage leading to progressive neurodegeneration.

Therefore, Spada and colleagues investigated the effects of açai pulp to reduce oxidative stress and inhibit lipid peroxidation in brain tissues. Pretreatment of animals with açai pulp was discovered to attenuate hydrogen peroxide (H_2O_2)-induced damage of proteins and lipids in brain tissues, and reduce lipid damage, as measured by the formation of thiobarbituric acid-reaction species (TBARS), by 72% in the cerebellum, 64% in the hippocampus, and 48% in the cerebral cortex, of adult rats. Reduction of protein damage was 55% in the cerebral cortex, 42% in the cerebellum, and 36% in the hippocampus. These results led the authors to speculate that açai pulp might slow down the progression or possibly prevent the development of some neurodegenerative diseases. However, to test their hypothesis, chronic feeding studies are needed.

It did not take long for such studies to report promising results. The first of such studies was reported in 2013, to determine if açai pulp can reverse or delay the progression of age-related cognitive or motor deficits commonly observed in neurodegenerative diseases (Miller et al., 2013). In the study, old (19–21 months) rats were either fed a diet supplemented with 2% açai pulp or a nonsupplemented control diet for 7 weeks prior to initiating 4 days of cognitive testing twice a day to measure changes in working memory and spatial learning between groups. Serum was collected from all animals and brain cell cultures taken from euthanized animals. Production of NO, extracellular release of NO_2 was measured, along with ELISA testing to quantify TNF-α, and Western blots to measure levels of iNOS and COX-2. The study showed that the açai-supplemented animals showed improved working and reference memory compared to controls. Açai-fed rats had lower levels of NO_2, TNF-α, and iNOS, versus control animals, but showed no difference in COX-2. The enhancement in working memory was discovered to be associated with decreased levels of NO_2 and TNF-α.

The açai pulp has neuroprotective properties acting via multiple pathways, the ability of the pulp to attenuate the formation of beta-amyloid (Aβ) in the brain, has been investigated. There is compelling evidence that the neurotoxicity seen in Alzheimer's disease (AD) is associated with elevated levels of Aß (Mattson, 2004) and chronic inflammation that damages neurons. Wong and coworkers (2013) evaluated whether açai pulp might inhibit human Aβ aggregation in vitro, and exhibit antifibrillar activity able to protect against Aβ-mediated loss of cell viability and oxidative stress and inflammation associated with the disease.

Pretreatment of açai pulp was shown to exert neuroprotection against the major neurotoxic Aβ alloform, $A\beta_{1-42}$. A significant reduction was seen in both microscopic and biochemical indices associated with Aβ fibril formation suggesting that açai has antiaggregative properties. The authors suggested that the suppression of proinflammatory microglial activation by açai could provide a basis to support the neuroprotection afforded by açai. Whatever the cause(s) is for the reported neuroprotective effects against Aβ formation and pathology by açai pulp, "further studies into its antifibrillar and neuroprotective effects are warranted," as stated by the authors. Unfortunately, the Toll-like receptor-2 (TLR-2) protein was not measured, as it plays an important role in recognizing foreign substances and then passing on signals to the cells of the immune system to respond.

To evaluate the protective effect of frozen açai pulp, rat brain tissue exposed to carbon tetrachloride (CCl_4)-induced damage was studied (de Souza Machado et al., 2015). The investigators measured changes in levels of anti- and proinflammatory cytokines in the cerebral cortex, hippocampus, and cerebellum, in animals that had been treated via daily oral (gavage) with açai. While CCl_4 increased TNF-α, IL-1β, and IL-18 levels in all brain tissues studied, 15 days after intraperitoneal injection of CCl_4, açai prevented an increase, while IL-6 and IL-10 remained unchanged. The authors report that further work is underway to elucidate the mechanism by which açai is able to modulate proinflammatory cytokine production in the brain. Carey and colleagues (2015) have demonstrated in vivo that the protection of memory by açai during aging may be due to its ability to modulate antioxidant and anti-inflammatory signaling, such as the response of microglia to inflammatory stimulus.

ANTIPROLIFERATIVE EFFECTS

Reactive oxygen species have been shown to damage DNA and promote mutations that can grow into tumors (Wiseman and Halliwell, 1996). Chronic overproduction of ROS and the resulting oxidative stress has also been implicated in the development of cancer (Mates and Sancheze-Jimenez, 2000; Waris and Ahsan, 2006).

Antiproliferative properties of an oil-free açai pulp were studied for its effects on the proliferation of C-6 rat brain glioma cells and MDA-468 human breast cancer cells (Hogan et al., 2010). The açai extract was compared to other anthocyanin-rich extracts including blueberry, strawberry, raspberry, blackberry, and wolfberry, all rich in anthocyanins, for antiproliferative activity. Açai extract was found to possess both antioxidant activities and strong antiproliferative activity against C-6 brain glioma cells, whereas none of the other anthocyanin-rich berry extracts exhibited similar inhibitory activity. However, the study did not identify the active constituents in the açai extract that induced C-6 glioma cell apoptosis. What is particularly interesting, given the results, implies that it may be unlikely that anthocyanins are responsible for the observed antiproliferative bioactivity. Or it may be that something in açai has selective properties against cancerous glioma cells, in that other berries have shown antiproliferative activity against other cancer cells, including: bilberry extract against HL-60 human leukemia cells; blueberry and cranberry against HT-29 colon carcinoma cells and MCF-7 human breast cancer cells; and, raspberry and strawberries and against CaCo-2 human colon cancer cells.

The possibility of selective antiproliferative and anticancer properties is supported by the observation that the extract has no effect against MDA-468 human breast cancer cells. By studying the fragmentation of DNA, in agarose gels, an indication of programmed cell death (apoptosis), the açai extract was found to induce apoptosis of C-6 glioma cells, but not in MDA-468 breast cells.

Further evidence of the extracts selectively is suggested by Hogan and colleagues and Silva and coworkers who reported that a hydroalcoholic extract of açai possessed significant antitumorigenic potential against the human breast MCF-7 cell line (Silva et al., 2014) They found that in açai-treated MCF-7 cells a significant reduction in cell viability along with altered cell morphological features occurred by increased autophagic activity, not by apoptosis. The difference in outcomes reported by these two investigators may be due to the characteristics of the breast cells studied. Whereas MCF-7 cells have an estrogen receptor, these are absent in MDA-468 cells. Silva and colleagues speculate that MCF-7 cells experience morphological changes associated with increased autophagy because açai contains lignans that act as phytoestrogens with the cytotoxic activity that would affect MCF-7 estrogen receptors. Unknown is how increased autophagic activity and its stimulation inhibits the growth of MCF-7 cells.

Further work is needed to determine what enzymes affect autophagy activation and regulation of cancer cells, along with a determination of which phytochemicals in açai pulp accounts for its observed anticancer activity. Interestingly, an earlier study also demonstrated antiproliferative effects and induction of apoptosis in HL-60 human leukemia cells by açai pulp in 2006, but no follow up work was carried out by the investigators in vivo (Pozo-Insfran et al., 2006).

In a study of urinary bladder carcinogenesis using açai pulp, Fragoso and coworkers described feeding a standard diet or the same diet supplemented with either 2.5% or 5% açai pulp to mice for 10 weeks in mice chemically-induced to develop urothelial bladder cancer (Fragoso et al., 2012). The study also determined the incidence of simple and nodular hyperplasia and incidence and number of transitional cell carcinoma. In a second study, mice were fed either a standard diet or diet supplemented with 5% açai pulp for three weeks and various antigenotoxicity screenings performer, which showed açai pulp exhibited significant anticancer and antiproliferative against urothelial bladder carcinogenesis. The authors concluded that "induction of endogenous antioxidant/repair enzymes and antiinflammatory events by açai pulp intake are potential mechanisms for future investigations."

HEPATIC, RENAL FUNCTION, AND LIVER STUDIES

The earlier discussion on the demonstrated antiatherosclerotic effects of açai pulp in vivo (Xie et al., 2011), suggests that açai might play a role in inhibiting the pathogenesis associated with renovascular disease. Atherosclerosis is the most common cause of renovascular disease. It develops at the renal artery ostium on the luminal surface of the proximal renal artery where the formation of atheroma obstructs renal blood flow leading to chronic renal ischemia. Chronic oxidative stress and resultant inflammation and vascular rarefication all play a role in renovascular disease. Textor and Lerman (2015) have pointed out that the "classic paradigms for simply restoring blood flow are shifting to implementation of therapy targeting mitochondria and cell-based functions to allow regeneration of vascular, glomerular, and tubular structures sufficient to recover, or at least stabilize, renal function. These developments offer exciting possibilities of repair and regeneration of kidney tissue that may limit progressive chronic kidney disease (CKD) in atherosclerotic renovascular disease and may apply to other conditions in which inflammatory injury is a major common pathway."

The protective effect of an açai extract (20:1 w/v) in a rat renal ischemic/reperfusion model was studied (El Morsy et al., 2015). Administration of the açai extract at a dose of 1000 mg/kg before induction of renal injury/reperfusion modulated the level of the renal prooxidant enzyme, MPO, as well as, interferon-gamma (IFN-γ) and interleukin-10 (IL-10). IL-10 suppresses the innate immune system following injury which helps in promoting functional recovery (Moore et al., 2001). The study also found that the extract inhibited renal injury/reperfusion renal endothelin-1 (ET-1) in a dose-dependent manner. In light of these findings, the study authors strongly encouraged further study of this extract in the prevention of renal ischemia/reperfusion injury during shock and renal transplantation to see whether it contribute to the prevention of either acute renal failure and/or graft dysfunction.

Similar results were reported by Qu and colleagues (2014). They studied the mechanism of action and protective effect of açai on chronic alcoholic hepatic injury in rats. Their investigation included random groups of alcoholic hepatic injury-induced Wistar rats fed various doses of açai which showed it not only had a protective effect against alcoholic hepatic injury but it also significantly reduced serum ALT and AST, MDA, triglyceride, and serum TNF-α and IL-6, while significantly increasing glutathione and superoxide dismutase levels.

Acute renal failure has a high mortality rate. Although the pathogenesis of the condition is not fully understood, it has been shown to involve oxidative stress and diminished renal blood flow. One study explored the oral administration of an açai pulp and skin extract (ABE) on glycerol-induced acute renal failure in rats (Unis, 2015). Relying on earlier studies by de Souza et al. and Spada et al. that showed açai pulp significantly improved biomarkers of oxidative stress in hypercholesterolemic animals resulting in protection against H_2O_2-mediated damage to lipids and proteins, various groups of animals were given either 100 or 200mg/kg/day ABE for 7 days or served as controls, where after acute renal failure was induced. This resulted in a significant deterioration in renal oxidative stress biomarkers compared to controls. By comparison, both the 100 and 200mg ABE açai groups experienced significant improvement in renal oxidative stress markers, with the 200mg ABE administered group showing the most improvement in renal oxidative stress markers. The induction of acute renal failure also showed significant renal histopathological damage as compared to the controls, as the ABE prophylactic and treated animals experienced much less damage, with the high dose group experiencing the least damage. Administration of the ABE extract resulted in significant improvement in kidney function tests, particularly more pronounced in the high dose group, along with a significant decrease in serum urea, serum creatinine, and BUN. This study demonstrated that oral administration of the açai pulp and skin protected animals from induced renal failure and impairment of renal functions.

Further studies demonstrating açai's renoprotective properties in humans are needed to both show its clinical benefit in protecting and treating acute renal failure and in elucidating the precise cellular mechanism for its protective effects.

Nonalcoholic fatty liver disease (NAFLD) is the most common liver disease in the world. NAFLD leads to hepatocellular injury, an increased risk of developing cardiovascular disease, and diabetes (Paredes et al., 2012). In collaboration with Efrat Broide and colleagues at the Institute of Gastroenterology, Liver Diseases and Nutrition, affiliated with the Sackler Faculty of Medicine at Tel Aviv University, and this author, the effect of açai pulp powder supplementation to a fructose-enriched diet (FED) on steatosis, hepatic lipid content, and oxidative stress, was studied in non-obese rats. A FED diet given to rats is characterized by many components of the metabolic syndrome (Ackerman et al., 2005; Kawasaki et al., 2009). In this study, rats were divided into five groups given either: a standard rat chow diet (SRCD); SRCD and 3% açai; FED; FED and 3% açai from day-1; or, FED and 3% açai starting on day-21. After 6 weeks, the rats were sacrificed and lipid profile, ADT, ALT, ALP, bilirubin, liver cholesterol, triglycerides, and serum glucose determined. Liver sections were performed using a modified Brunt scoring system for grading and staging of non-alcoholic steatohepatitis. In addition, α-tocopherol, paraoxonase (Px), glutathione (GSH), and lipid peroxidation, were assessed. As was expected, the FED fed animals had a higher grade of steatosis compared to the SRCD group. The group given FED with 3% açai, experienced a higher antioxidant profile, along with decreased MDA level in the liver. No significant differences were found in ballooning, portal inflammation, intra-acinar inflammation, and hepatic fibrosis between groups.

Of particular interest was the observed increase in serum and hepatic triglyceride profile, despite no significant reduction in steatosis, suggesting an antiobesity effect, an effect previously suggested to be mediated by an induction of adiponectin gene expression by high polyphenol intake (Tsuda, 2008; de Oliveira et al., 2010). Further, supplementation of FED with 3% açai substantially increased the activity of both GSH and GSH-Px, which is significant as GSH-Px catalyzes the reduction of hydrogen peroxide and organic hydroperoxides by using glutathione. Overall, this study found that açai can improve NAFLD in rats by increasing antioxidant production thereby decreasing oxidative stress, while decreasing intra-hepatic trigylceride levels.

It is only a matter of time for more human clinical trials to determine the degree to which açai pulp plays a role in preventing, mitigating and/or treating neurodegenerative diseases, and promoting healthy brain aging, in addition to its renoprotective, cardiovascular protective, and antiproliferative (anticancer) effects.

REFERENCES

Ackerman, Z., Oron-Herman, M., Grozovski, M., Rosenthal, T., Pappo, O., Link, G., et al., 2005. Fructose-induced fatty liver disease: hepatic effects of blood pressure and plasma triglyceride reduction. Hypertension 45, 1012–1018.

Andersen, J.K., 2004. Oxidative stress in neurodegeneration: cause or consequence? Nat. Rev. Neurosci. (Suppl. 10), 18–25.

Ansell, B.J., Watson, K.E., Fogelman, A.M., 1999. An evidence-based assessment of the NCEP Adult Treatment Panel II guidelines. National cholesterol education program. J. Am. Med. Assoc. 282, 2051–2057.

Barja, G., 2004. Free radicals and aging. Trends Neurosci. 27, 595–600.

Bast, A., Haenen, G.R.M.M., 2013. Ten misconceptions about antioxidants. Trends. Pharmacol. Sci. 34, 430–436.

Bazzano, L.A., He, J., Ogden, L.G., Loria, C.M., Vupputuri, S., Myers, L., et al., 2002. Fruit and vegetable intake and risk of cardiovascular disease in US adults: the first National Health and Nutrition Examination Survey Epidemiologic Follow-up Study. Am. J. Clin. Nutr. 76, 93–99.

Biswas, S., Hwang, J.W., Kirkham, P.A., Rahman, I., 2013. Pharmacological and dietary antioxidant therapies for chronic obstructive pulmonary disease. Curr. Med. Chem. 20, 1496–1530.

Bonomo, L., Silva, D.N., Boasquivis, P.F., Paiva, F.A., Guerrra, J.F.C., Martins, T.A., et al., 2013. Açai (*Euterpe oleracea* Mart.) modulates oxidative stress resistance in *Caenorhabditis elegans* by direct and indirect mechanisms. PLoS One 9, e89933.

Brand, K., Page, S., Rogler, G., Bartsch, A., Brandl, R., Knuechel, R., et al., 1996. Activated transcription factor nuclear factor-kappa B is present in the atherosclerotic lesion. J. Clin. Investig. 97, 1715–1722.

Brawley, L., Poston, L., Hanson, M.A., 2003. Mechanisms underlying the programming of small artery dysfunction: review of the model using low protein diet in pregnancy in the rat. Arch. Physiol. Biochem. 111, 23–35.

Brennan, M.L., Penn, M.S., Van Lente, F., Nambi, V., Shishehbor, M.H., Aviles, R.J., et al., 2003. Prognostic value of myeloperoxidase in patients with chest pain. N. Engl. J. Med. 349 (17), 1595–1604.

Cardona, J.A., Mertens-Talcott, S.U., Talcott, S.T., 2015. Phospholipids and terpenes modulate Caco-2 transport of açai anthocyanins. Food Chem. 175, 267–272.

Carey, A.N., Miller, M.G., Fisher, D.R., Bielinski, D.F., Gilman, C.K., Poulose, S.M., et al., 2015. Dietary supplementation with the polyphenol-rich açaí pulps (*Euterpe oleracea* Mart. and *Euterpe precatoria* Mart.) improves cognition in aged rats and attenuates inflammatory signaling in BV-2 microglial cells. Nutr. Neurosci. (Epub ahead of print) <http://www.ncbi.nlm.nih.gov/pubmed/26618555>.

Cheng, H.E., Wei, L., Zhang, J.-J., Qu, S.-S., Li, J.-J., Wang, L.-Y., 2014. Determination of β-sitosterol and total sterols content and antioxidant activity of oil in açai (*Euterpe oleracea*). China J. Chin. Mater. Med. 39, 4620–4624.

Collins, T., 1993. Endothelial nuclear factor-kappa B and the initiation of the atherosclerotic lesion. Lab. Investig. 68, 499–508.

Cui, J., Zhang, M., Zhang, Y., Xu, Z., 2007. JNK pathway, diseases and therapeutic potential. Acta Pharmacol. Sin. 28, 601–608.

da Costa, C.A., de Oliveira, P.R., de Bem, G.F., de Cavalho, L.C., Ognibene, D.T., da Silva, A.F., et al., 2012. *Euterpe oleracea* Mart.-derived polyphenols prevent endothelial dysfunction and vascular structural changes in renovascular hypertensive rats: role of oxidative stress. Naunyn Schmiedebergs Arch. Pharmacol. 385, 1199–1209.

de Almeida Teixeira, G.H., Lopes, V.G., Cunha Júnior, L.C., Pessoa, J.D.C., 2015. Total anthocyanin content in intact acai (*Euterpe oleracea* Mart.) and jucara (*Euterpe edulis* Mart.) fruit predicted by near infrared spectroscopy. HortScience 50, 1218–1223.

de Bem, F.G., da Costa, A.A., de Oliveira, P.R.B., Cordeiro, V.S.C., Santos, I.B., de Carvalho, L.C., et al., 2014. Protective effect of *Euterpe oleracea* Mart (açai) extract on programmed changes in the adult rat offspring caused by maternal protein restriction during pregnancy. J. Pharm. Pharmacol. 2014 (66), 1328–1338.

de Moura, R.S., Pires, K.M., Santos Ferreira, T., Lopes, A.A., Nesi, R.T., Resende, A.C., et al., 2011. Addition of açai (*Euterpe oleracea*) to cigarettes has a protective effect against emphysema in mice. Food Chem. Toxicol. 49, 855–863.

de Oliveira, P.R., da Costa, C.A., de Bem, G.F., de Cavalho, L.C., de Souza, M.A., de Lemos Neto, M., et al., 2010. Effects of an extract obtained from fruits of *Euterpe oleracea* Mart. in the components of metabolic syndrome in C57BL/6J mice fed a high-fat diet. J. Cardiovasc. Pharmacol. 56, 619–626.

de Souza, M., Silva, L.S., Magalhaes, C.L., de Figueiredo, B.B., Costa, D.C., Silva, M.E., et al., 2012. The hypocholesterolemic activity of açaí (*Euterpe oleracea* Mart.) is mediated by the enhanced expression of the ATP-binding cassette, subfamily G transporters 5 and 8 and low-density lipoprotein receptor genes in the rat. Nutr. Res. 32, 976–984.

de Souza Machado, F., Marinho, J.P., Abujamra, A.L., Quincozes-Santos, A., Funchal, C., 2015. Carbon tetrachloride increases the pro-inflammatory cytokines levels in different brain areas of Wistar rats: the protective effect of acai frozen pulp. Neurochem. Res. 40, 1976–1983.

Dennis, D.T., Inglesby, T.V., Henderson, D.A., Bartlett, J.G., Ascher, M.S., Eitzen, E., et al., 2001. Tularemia as a biological weapon: medical and public health management. J. Am. Med. Assoc. 285, 2763–2773.

Devaraj, S., Jialal, I., 2006. The role of dietary supplementation with plant sterols and stanols in the prevention of cardiovascular disease. Nutr. Rev. 64, 348–354.

Devore, E.E., Kang, J.H., Breteler, M.M., Grodstein, F., 2012. Dietary intakes of berries and flavonoids in relations to cognitive decline. Ann. Neurol. 72, 135–143.

Dheen, S.T., Kaur, C., Ling, E.A., 2007. Microglial activation and its implications in the brain diseases. Curr. Med. Chem. 14, 1189–1197.

Dias, A.L.S., Rozet, E., Chataigné, G., Oliveira, A.C., Rabelo, C.A., Hubert, P., et al., 2012. A rapid validated UHPLC–PDA method for anthocyanins quantification from *Euterpe oleracea* fruits. J. Chromatogr. B 907, 108–116.

Dias, A.L.S., Rozet, E., Larondelle, Y., Hubert, P., Rogez, H., Quetin-Leclercq, J., 2013. Development and validation of an UHPLC-LTQ-Orbitrap method for non-anthocyanin flavonoids quantification in *Euterpe oleracea* juice. Anal. Bioanal. Chem. 405, 9235–9249.

Dias, M., Martino, H.S., Noratto, G., Roque-Andrade, A., Stringheta, P.C., Talcott, S., et al., 2015. Anti-inflammatory activity of polyphenolics from acai (*Euterpe oleracea* Martius) in intestinal myofibroblasts CCD-18Co cells. Food Funct. 6, 3249–3256.

do Nascimento, W.M.O., Da Silva, W.R., 2005. Comportamento fisiológico de sementes de açaì (*Euterpe oleracea* Mart.) submetidas à desidratação. Rev. Frutica Jaboticabal 27, 349–351.

Dome, W., Oettl, K., Renner, W., 2014. Oxidative stress and free radicals in COPD – implications and relevance for treatment. Int. J. COPD 9, 1207–1224.

Dowling, R.J., Topisirovic, I., Fonseca, B.D., Sonenberg, N., 2010. Dissecting the role of mTOR: lessons from mTOR inhibitors. Biochim. Biophys. Acta 1804, 433–439.

El-Bahr, S.M., 2013. Biochemistry of free radicals and oxidative stress. Sci. Int. 1, 111–117.

El Morsy, E.M., Ahmed, M.A., Ahmed, A.A., 2015. Attenuation of renal ischemia/reperfusion injury by açai extract preconditioning in a rat model. Life. Sci. 123, 35–42.

Evans, D., 2012. Cholesterol and Saturated Fats Prevent Heart Disease: Evidence from 1010 Scientific Studies. Grosvenor House Publishing, Guildford, UK.

Feio, C.A., Izar, M.C., Ihara, S.S., Kasmas, S.H., Martins, C.M., Feio, M.N., et al., 2012. *Euterpe oleracea* (açai) modifies sterol metabolism and attenuates experimentally-induced atherosclerosis. J. Atheroscler. Thromb. 19, 237–245.

Fragoso, M.E., Prado, M.G., Barbosa, L., et al., 2012. Inhibition of mouse urinary bladder carcinogenesis by açai fruit (*Euterpe oleracea* Martius) intake. Plant Food Hum. Nutr. 67, 235–241.

Gale, A.M., Kaur, R., Baker, W.L., 2014. Hemodynamic and electrocardiographic effects of açai berry in healthy volunteers: a randomized controlled trial. Int. J. Cardiol. 174, 421–423.

Gallori, S., Bilia, A.R., Bergonzi, M.C., Barbosa, W.L.R., Vincieri, F.F., 2004. Polyphenolic constituents of fruit pulp of *Euterpe oleracea* Mart. (Açai palm). Chromatographia 59, 739–743.

Goldstein, D.M., Gabriel, T., 2005. Pathway to the clinic: inhibition of P38 MAP kinase. A review of ten chemotypes selected for development. Curr. Top. Med. Chem. 5, 1017–1029.

Gordon, A., Cruz, A.P.G., Cabral, L.M.C., de Freitas, S.C., Taxi, C.M., Donangelo, C.M., et al., 2012. Chemical characterization and evaluation of antioxidant properties of Açai fruits (*Euterpe oleraceae* Mart.) during ripening. Food Chem. 133, 256–263.

Gotsman, I., Stabholz, A., Planer, D., Pugatsch, T., Lapidus, L., Novikov, Y., et al., 2008. Serum cytokine tumor necrosis factor-α and interleukin-6 associated with the severity of coronary artery disease: indicators of an active inflammatory burden? Israeli Med. Assoc. J. 10, 494–498.

Gurcan, S., 2014. Epidemiology of tularemia. Balkan Med. J. 31, 3–10.

Harry, B.L., Sanders, J.M., Feaver, R.E., Lansey, M., Deem, T.L., Zarbock, A., et al., 2008. Endothelial cell PECAM-1 promotes atherosclerotic lesions in areas of disturbed flow in ApoE-deficient mice. Arterioscler. Thromb. Vasc. Biol. 28, 2003–2008.

Henderson, A., Scariot, A., 1993. A florula da Reserva Ducke, i: Palmae (Arecacea). Acta Amazonica 23, 349–369.

Heneka, M.T., Klockgether, T., Feinstein, D.L., 2000. Peroxisome proliferator-activated receptor-γ ligans reduce neuronal inducible nitric oxide synthase expression and cell death in vivo. J. Neurosci. 20, 6862–6867.

Hoeffer, C.A., Klann, E., 2010. mTOR signaling: at the crossroads of plasticity, memory, and disease. Trends Neurosci. 33, 67–75.

Hogan, S., Chung, H., Zhang, L., Li, J., Lee, Y., Dai, Y., et al., 2010. Antiproliferative and antioxidant properties of anthocyanin-rich extract from açai. Food Chem. 118, 208–214.

Holderness, J., Schepetkin, I.A., Freedman, B., Kirpotina, L.N., Quinn, M.T., Hedges, J.F., et al., 2011. Polysaccharides isolated from açai fruit induce innate immune responses. PLoS One 6, e17301.

Horiguchi, T., Ishiguro, N., Chihara, K., Ogi, K., Nakashima, K., Sada, K., et al., 2011. Inhibitory effect of açai (*Euterpe oleracea* Mart.) pulp on IgE-mediated mast cell activation. J. Agric. Food Chem. 59, 5595–5601.

Inacio, M.R., de Lima, K.M., Lopes, V.G., Pessoa, J.D., de Almeida Teixeira, G.H., 2013. Total anthocyanin content determination in intact açaí (*Euterpe oleracea* Mart.) and palmitero-juçara (*Euterpe edulis* Mart.) fruit using near infrared spectroscopy (NIR) and multivariate calibration. Food Chem. 136, 1160–1164.

Jakulj, L., Visses, M.N., Tanck, M.W.T., Hutten, B.A., Stellard, F., Kastelein, J.J.P., et al., 2010. ABCG5/G8 polymorphisms and markers of cholesterol metabolism: systematic review and meta-analysis. J. Lipid. Res. 51, 3016–3023.

Jensen, G.S., Ager, D.M., Redman, K.A., Mitzner, M.A., Benson, K.F., Schauss, A.G., 2011. Pain reduction and improvement in range of motion after daily consumption of an açai (*Euterpe oleracea* Mart.) pulp-fortified polyphenolic-rich fruit and berry juice bland. J. Med. Food. 14, 702–711.

Jensen, G.S., Wu, X., Patterson, K.M., Carter, S.G., Wu, X., Scherwitz, L., et al., 2008. In vitro and in vivo antioxidant and anti-inflammatory capacities of an antioxidant-rich fruit and berry juice blend. Results of a pilot and randomized, double-blinded, placebo-controlled crossover study. J. Agric. Food Chem. 56, 8326–8333.

Johnson, G.L., Lapadat, R., 2002. Mitogen-activated protein kinase pathways mediated by ERK, JNK, and p38 protein kinases. Science 298, 1911–1912.

Kang, J., Li, Z., Wu, T., Jensen, G.S., Schauss, A.G., Wu, X., 2010. Antioxidant capacities and anti-inflammatory effects of flavonoid compounds from açai pulp (*Euterpe oleracea* Mart.). Food Chem. 122, 610–617.

Kang, J., Xie, C., Li, Z., Wu, T., Nagarajan, S., Schauss, A.G., et al., 2011. Flavonoids from açai (*Euterpe oleracea* Mart.) pulp and their antioxidant and anti-inflammatory activities. Food Chem. 128, 152–157.

Kawasaki, T., Igarashi, K., Koeda, T., Sugimoto, K., Nakagawa, K., Hayashi, S., et al., 2009. Rats fed fructose-enriched diets have characteristics of nonalcoholic hepatic steatosis. J. Nutr. 139, 2067–2071.

Kenyon, C., 2010. The first long-lived mutants: discovery of the insulin/IG-1 pathway for ageing. Philos. Trans. R. Soc. B Biol. Sci. 366, 9–16.

Kirkham, P.A., Spooner, G., Foulkes-Jones, C., Calvez, R., 2003. Cigarette smoke triggers macrophage adhesion and activation: role of lipid peroxidation products and scavenger receptor. Free Radic. Biol. Med. 35, 697–710.

Lamarche, B., Moorjani, S., Lupien, P.J., Cantin, B., Bernard, P.M., Dagenais, G.R., et al., 1996. Apolipoprotein A-1 and B levels and the risk of ischemic heart disease during a five-year follow up of men in the Quebec cardiovascular study. Circulation 94, 273–278.

LaPlante, M., Sabatini, D.M., 2012. mTOR signaling in growth control and disease. Cell 149, 274–293.

Lau, F.C., Shukitt-Hale, B., Joseph, J.A., 2005. The beneficial effects of fruit polyphenols on brain aging. Neurobiol. Aging. 26S, S128–S132.

Libby, P., 2002. Inflammation in atherosclerosis. Nature 420, 868–874.

Lichtenthaler, R., Rodrigues, R.B., Maia, J.G., Papagiannopoulos, M., Fabricius, H., Marx, F., 2005. Total oxidant scavenging capacities of *Euterpe oleracea* Mart. (Açai) fruits. Int. J. Food Sci. Nutr. 56, 53–64.

Manach, C., Mazur, A., Scalbert, A., 2005. Polyphenols and prevention of cardiovascular diseases. Curr. Opin. Lipidol. 16, 77–84.

Mates, J.M., Sanchez-Jimenez, F.M., 2000. Role of reactive oxygen species in apoptosis: implications for cancer therapy. Int. J. Biochem. Cell Biol. 32, 157–170.

Mattson, M.P., 2004. Pathways towards and away from Alzheimer's disease. Nature 430, 631–639.

Mendis, S., Thygesen, K., Kuulasmaa, K., Giampaoli, S., Mähönen, M., Ngu Blackett, K., et al., 2011. Writing group on behalf of the participating experts of the WHO consultation for revision of WHO definition of myocardial infarction. Int. J. Epidemiol. 40, 139–146.

Miller, M.G., Fisher, D.R., Bieliski, D.F., Poulose, S.M., 2013. Dietary açai fruit improves cognition in aged rats Neuroscience Meeting Planner. Society for Neuroscience, San Diego, CA, 252.04, online.

Miller, D.W., 2015. Fallacies in modern medicine: statins and the cholesterol-heart hypothesis. J. Am. Phys. Surg. 20, 54–56.

Miserez, A.R., Muller, P.Y., Barella, L., Barella, S., Staehelin, H.B., Leitersdorf, E., et al., 2002. Sterol-regulatory elements binding protein (SREBP)-2 contributes to polygenic hypercholesterolaemia. Atherosclerosis 164, 15–26.

Miyazawa, T., Nakagawa, K., Kudo, M., Muraishi, K., Someya, K., 1999. Direct intestinal absorption of cyanidin-3-glucoside and cyanidin-3,5-diglucoside, into rats and humans. J. Agric. Food Chem. 47, 1083–1091.

Moore, K.W., de Waal Malefyt, R., Coffman, R.L., O'Garra, A., 2001. Interleukin-10 and the interleukin-10 receptor. Annu. Rev. Immuol. 19, 683–765.

Nakaskima, Y., Raines, E.W., Plump, A.S., Breslow, J.L., Ross, R., 1998. Upregulation of VCAM-1 and ICAM-1 at atherosclerotic-prone sites on the endothelium in the ApoE-deficient mouse. Arterioscler. Thromb. Vasc. Biol. 18, 842–851.

Nantz, M.P., Rowe, C.A., Nieves Jr., C., Percival, S.S., 2006. Immunity and antioxidant capacity in humans is enhanced by consumption of a dried, encapsulated fruit and vegetable juice concentrate. J. Nutr. 136, 2606–2610.

Nishina, H., Wada, T., Katada, T., 2004. Physiological roles of SAPK/JNK signaling pathway. J. Biochem. 136, 123–126.

Noratto, G.D., Angel-Morales, G., Talcott, S.T., Mertens-Talcott, S.U., 2011. Polyphenolics from açai (*Euterpe oleracea* Mart.) and red muscadine grape (*Vitis rotundifolia*) protect human umbilical vascular endothelial cells (HUVEC) from glucose- and lipopolysaccharide (PS)-induced inflammation and target microRNA-126. J. Agric. Food Chem. 59, 7999–8012.

Odendaal, A.Y., Schauss, A.G., 2014. Potent antioxidant and anti-inflammatory flavonoids in the nutrient-rich Amazonian palm fruit, açaí (*Euterpe* spp.). In: Watson, R.R., Reedy, V.R., Zibadi, S. (Eds.), Polyphenols in Human Health and Disease Academic Press, San Diego, pp. 219–239.

Ogg, S., Paradis, S., Gottlieb, S., Patterson, G.I., Lee, L., Tissenbaum, H.A., et al., 1997. The Fork head transcription factor DAF-16 transduces insulin-like metabolic and longevity signals in *C. elegans*. Nature 389, 994–999.

Paredes, A.H., Torres, D.M., Harrison, S.A., 2012. Nonalcoholic fatty liver disease. Clin. Liver Dis. 16, 397–419.

Percival, S.S., Bukowski, J.F., Milner, J., 2008. Bioactive food components that enhance gamma delta T cell function may play a role in cancer prevention. J. Nutr. 138, 1–4.

Poulose, S.M., Bielinski, D.F., Carrihill-Knoll, K.L., Rabin, B.M., Shukitt-Hale, B., 2014a. Protective effects of blueberry- and straberry diets on neuronal stress following exposure to ^{56}Fe particles. Brain. Res. 1593, 9–18.

Poulose, S.M., Fischer, D.R., Bielinski, D.F., Gomes, S.M., Rimando, A.M., Schauss, A.G., et al., 2014b. Restoration of stressor-induced calcium dysregulation and autophagy inhibition by polyphenol-rich açai (*Euterpe* spp.) fruit pulp extracts in rodent brain cells in vitro. Nutrition 30, 853–862.

Poulose, S.M., Fisher, D.R., Larson, J., Bielinski, D.F., Rimando, A.M., Carey, A.N., et al., 2012. Anthocyanin-rich açai (*Euterpe oleracea* Mart.) fruit pulp fractions attenuate inflammatory stress signaling in mouse brain BV-2 microglial cells. J. Agric. Food Chem. 60, 1084–1093.

Pozo-Insfran, D.D., Percival, S.S., Talcott, S.T., 2006. Açai (*Euterpe oleracea* Mart.) polyphenolics in their glycoside and aglycone forms induce apoptosis of HL-60 leukemia cells. J. Agric. Food Chem. 54, 1222–1229.

Qu, S.S., Zhang, J.J., Li, Y.X., Zheng, Y., Zhu, Y.L., Wang, L.Y., 2014. Protective effect of açai berries on chronic alcoholic hepatic injury in rats and their effect on inflammatory cytokines. Zhonggue Zhong Yao Za Zhi 39, 4869–4872.

Quinn, P.G., Yeagley, D., 2005. Insulin regulation of PEPCK gene expression: a model for rapid and reversible modulation. Curr. Drug Targets Immune Endocr. Metabol. Disord. 5, 424–437.

Ravnskov, U., 2002. A hypthesis out-of-date: the diet-heart idea. J. Clin. Epidemiol. 55, 1057–1063.

Reiner, D.J., Newton, E.M., Tian, H., Thomas, J.H., 1999. Diverse behavioural defects caused by mutations in *Caenorhabditis elegans* unc-43 CaM Kinase II. Nature 402, 199–203.

Rocha, A.P.M., Carvalho, L.C.R.M., Sousa, M.A.V., Madeira, S.V.F., Sousa, P.J.C., Tano, T., et al., 2007a. Endothelium-dependent vasodilator effect of *Euterpe oleracea* Mart. (Açai) extracts in mesenteric vascular bed of the rat. Vascul. Pharmacol. 46, 97–104.

Rocha, A.P.M., Resende, A.C., Souza, M.A.V., Carvalho, L.C.R.M., Sousa, P.J.C., Tano, T., et al., 2008. Antihypertensive effects and antioxidant action of a hydro-alcoholic extract obtained from fruits of *Euterpe oleracea* Mart. (açaí). J. Pharmacol. Toxicol. 3, 435–448.

Ross, R., 1999. Atherosclerosis - an inflammatory disease. N. Engl. J. Med. 340, 115–126.

Sadowska-Krepa, E., Podgorski, T., Szade, B., Tyl, K., Hadzik, A., 2015. Effects of supplementation with açai (*Euterpe oleracea* Mart.) berry-based juice blend on the blood antioxidant defence capacity and lipid profile in junior hurdlers. A pilot study. Biol. Sport 32, 161–168.

Schauss, A.G., 2011. Açai: An Extraordinary Antioxidant-rich Palm Fruit from the Amazon, third ed. Biosocial Publications, Tacoma.33–40

Schauss, A.G., Wu, X., Prior, R.L., Ou, B., Patel, D., Huang, D., et al., 2006a. Phytochemical and nutrient composition of the freeze-dried Amazonian palm berry, *Euterpe oleracea* Mart. (Açai). J. Agric. Food Chem. 54, 8598–8603.

Schauss, A.G., Wu, X., Prior, R.L., Ou, B., Huang, D., Owens, J., et al., 2006b. Antioxidant capacity and other bioactivities of the freeze-dried Amazonian palm berry, *Euterpe oleracea* Mart. (Açai). J. Agric. Food Chem. 54, 8604–8610.

Schumacker, P.T., 2006. Reactive oxygen species in cancer cells: live by the sword, die by the sword. Cancer. Cell. 10, 175–176.

Shehata, M., Matsumura, H., Okubo-Suzuki, R., Ohkawa, N., Inokuchi, K., 2012. Neuronal stimulation induces autophagy in hippocampal neurons that is involved in AMPA receptor degradation after chemical long-term depression. J. Neurosci. 32, 10413–10422.

Shukitt-Hale, B., Lau, F.C., Carey, A.N., Galli, R.L., Spangler, E.L., Ingram, D.K., et al., 2008. Blueberry polyphenols attenuate kainic acid-induced decrements in cognitio and altern inflammatory gene expression in rat hippocampus. Nutr. Neurosci. 11, 172–182.

Shin, E.J., Ko, K.H., Kim, W.K., Chae, J.S., Yen, T.P., Kim, H.J., et al., 2008. Role of glutathione peroxidase in the ontogeny of hippocampal oxidative stress and kainate seizure sensitivity in the genetically epilepsy-prone rats. Neurochem. Int. 52, 1134–1147.

Shin, E.-J., Jeong, J.H., Chung, Y.H., Kin, W.-K., Ko, K.-H., Bach, J.-H., et al., 2011. Role of oxidative stress in epileptic seizures. Neurochem. Int. 59, 122–137.

Silva, D.F., Vidal, F.C.B., Santos, D., Costa, M.C.P., Morgado-Diaz, J.A., Nascimento, M.S.B., et al., 2014. Cytotoxic effects of *Euterpe oleracea* Mart. in malignant cell lines. BMC. Complement. Altern. Med. 14, 175.

Silva, E.B., Dow, S.W., 2013. Development of *Burkholderia mallei* and *pseudomallei* vaccines. Front. Cell Infect. Microbiol. 11, 10.

Skyberg, J.A., Rollins, M.F., Holderness, J.S., 2012. Nasal açai polysaccharides potentiate innate immunity to protect against pulmonary *Francisella tularensis* and *Burkholderia pseudomallei* infections. PLoS Pathog. 8, e1002587.

Solomon, A., Bandhavaki, S., Jabbar, S., Shah, R., Beitel, G.J., Morimoto, R.I., 2004. *Caenorhabhitis elegans* OSR-1 regulates behavioral and physiological responses to hyperosmotic environments. Genetics 167, 161–170.

Souza-Monteiro, J.R., Hamoy, M., Santana-Coelho, D., Arrifano, G.P., Paraense, R.S., Costa-Malaquias, A., et al., 2015. Anticonvulsant properties of *Euterpe oleracea* in mice. Neurochem. Int. 90, 20–27. Epub ahead of print. http://dx.doi.org/10.1016/j.neuint.2015.06.014.

Spada, P.D., Dani, C., Bortolini, G.V., Funchal, C., Henriques, J.A.P., Salvador, M., 2009. Frozen fruit pulp of *Euterpe oleracea* Mart. (açaí) prevents hydrogen peroxide-induced damage in the cerebral cortex, cerebellum, and hippocampus of rats. J. Med. Food. 12, 1084–1088.

Srivastava, R.A., 2009. Fenofibrate ameliorates diabetic and dyslipidemic profiles in KKAy mice partly via down-regulation of 11beta-HSD1, PEPCK and DGAT2. Comparison of PPARalpha, PPARgamma, and liver x receptor agonists. Eur. J. Pharmacol. 607, 258–263.

Stoclet, J.-C., Chataigneau, T., Ndjaye, M., Oak, M.-H., Bedoui, J.E., Chataigneaus, M., et al., 2004. Vascular protection by dietary polyphenols. Eur. J. Pharmacol. 500, 299–313.

Sun, X., Seeberger, J., Albericao, T., Wang, C., Wheeler, C.T., Schauss, A.G., et al., 2010. Aci plam fruit (*Euterpe oleracea* Mart.) pulp improves survival of flies on a high fat diet. Exp. Gerontol. 45, 243–251.

Szekanecz, Z., 2008. Pro-inflammatory cytokines in atherosclerosis. Israeli Med. Assoc. J. 10, 529–530.

Tabet, F., Rye, K.A., 2009. High-density lipoproteins, inflammation and oxidative stress. Clin. Sci. 116, 87–98.

Taubes, G., 2008. Good Calories, Bad Calories: Fats, Carbs, and the Controversial Science of Diet and Health. Anchor Books, New York, NY.

Terzic, J., Grivennikov, W., Karein, E., Karin, M., 2010. Inflammation and colon cancer. Gastroenterology 138, 2101–2114.

Textor, S.C., Lerman, L.O., 2015. Paradeigm shifts in atherosclerotic renovascular disease: where are we now? J. Am. Soc. Nephrol. 26, 2074–2080.

Tsuda, T., 2008. Regulation of adipocyte function by anthocyanins; possibility of preventing the metabolic syndrome. J. Agric. Food Chem. 56, 642–646.

Udani, J.K., Singh, B.B., Singh, V.J., Barrett, M.L., 2011. Effects of açaí (*Euterpe oleracea* Mart.) berry preparation on metabolic parameters in a healthy overweight population: a pilot study. Nutr. J. 10, 45.

Unis, A., 2015. Açai berry extract attenuates glycerol-induced acute renal failure in rats. Ren. Fail. 37, 310–317.

Urb, M., Sheppard, D.C., 2012. The role of mast cells in the defence against pathogens. PLoS Pathol. 8, e1002619.

Vantourout, P., Hayday, A., 2013. Six-of-the-best: unique contribution of $\gamma\delta$ T cells to immunology. Nat. Rev. Immunol. 13, 88–100.

Walldius, G., Jungner, I., Holme, I., Aastveit, A.H., Kolar, W., Steiner, E., 2001. High apolipoprotein B, low apolipoprotein A-1, and improvement in the prediction of fatal myocardial infarction (AMORS study): a prospective study. Lancet 358, 2026–2033.

Wang, X., Ouyang, Y., Liu, J., Zhu, M., Zhao, G., Bao, W., et al., 2014. Fruit and vegetable consumption and mortality from all causes, cardiovascular disease, and cancer: systematic review and dose-response meta-analysis of prospective cohort studies. BMJ 349, g4490.

Wang, Y., Ezemaduka, A.N., Tang, T., Chang, Z., 2009. Understanding the mechanism of the dormant dauer formation of *C. elegans*: from genetics to biochemistry. Life 61, 607–612.

Waris, G., Ahsan, H., 2006. Reactive oxygen species: role in the development of cancer and various chronic conditions. J. Carcinog. 5, 14.

Wiseman, H., Halliwell, B., 1996. Damage to DNA by reactive oxygen and nitrogen species: role in inflammatory disease and progression to cancer. Biochem. J. 313, 17–29.

Wong, D.Y., Musgrave, I.F., Harvey, B.S., Smid, S.D., 2013. Açai (*Euterpe oleracea* Mart.) berry extract exerts neuroprotective effects against β-amyloid exposure in vitro. Neurosci. Lett. 556, 221–226.

Wu, X., Beecher, G.R., Holden, J.M., Haytowitz, D.B., Gebhardt, S.E., Prior, R.L., 2006. Concentrations of anthocyanins in common foods in the United States and estimation of normal consumption. J. Agric. Food Chem. 54, 4069–4075.

Wycoff, W., Luo, R., Schauss, A.G., Neal-Kababick, J., Sabaa-Srur, A.U.O., Maia, J.G.S., et al., 2015. Chemical and nutritional analysis of seeds from purple and white açai (*Euterpe oleracea* Mart.). J. Food Compost. Anal. 42, 181–187.

Xie, C., Kang, J., Burris, R., Ferguson, M.E., Schauss, A.G., Nagarajan, S., et al., 2011. Açaí juice attenuates atherosclerosis in ApoE deficient mice through antioxidant and anti-inflammatory activities. Atherosclerosis 216, 327–333.

Yang, S.R., Chida, A.S., Bauter, M.R., Shafiq, N., Seweryniak, K., Maggirwar, S.B., et al., 2006. Cigarette smoke induces proinflammatory cytokine release by activation of NF-kappaB and posttranslational modifications of histone deacetylase in macrophages. Am. J. Physiol. Lung Cell. Mol. Physiol. 291, L46–L57.

Yu, L., Li-Hawkins, J., Hammer, R.E., Berge, K.E., Horton, J.D., Cohen, J.C., et al., 2002. Overexpression of ABCG5 and ABCG8 promotes biliary cholesterol secretion and reduces fractional absorption of dietary cholesterol. J. Clin. Investig. 110, 671–680.

Zaleska, M.M., Floyd, R.A., 1985. Regional lipid peroxidation in rat brain in vitro: possible role of endogenous iron. Neurochem. Res. 10, 397–410.

Chapter 11

Grape bioactives for human health

Marcello Iriti and Elena Maria Varoni
Milan State University, Milan, Italy

CHAPTER OUTLINE

INTRODUCTION

The archeological record suggests that cultivation of the domesticated grape, *Vitis vinifera* subsp. *vinifera*, began about 8000 years ago in the Near East from its wild progenitor, *Vitis vinifera* subsp. *sylvestris*. The earliest evidence for production of wine was found in the Middle East, in well-preserved ancient jars dated approximately 5000 BC (McGovern, 2013). The multitude of decorative elements on ancient coins, temples, ritual potteries, mosaics, and sculptures attested the importance of grape and its products in the development of human cultures as well as their relevance in ancient societies (McGovern, 2013) (Fig. 11.1). Nowadays, the grape is one of the most valuable crop in the world (Table 11.1), mainly produced in the European Mediterranean countries (Fig. 11.2), processed into wine and nonalcoholic juice, distilled into spirits or destined for fresh consumption as table

Fruits, Vegetables, and Herbs.
DOI: http://dx.doi.org/10.1016/B978-0-12-802972-5.00011-1

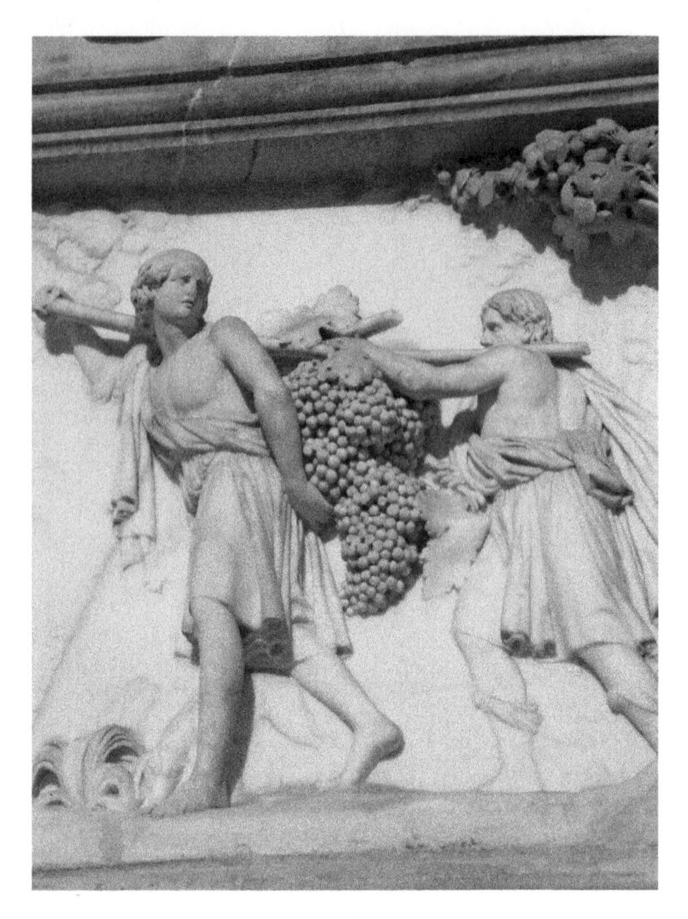

■ **FIGURE 11.1** Bas relief in the main facade of the Milan Cathedral depicting grape bunches carried by two grape pickers.

grapes or dried into raisins. The nutritional composition of grape, in terms of macronutrients and essential micronutrients (ie, minerals and vitamins), is shown in Table 11.2.

GRAPE PHYTOCHEMISTRY

Grape phytochemistry is quite complex due to hundreds of phytochemicals occurring in the berry tissues, exocarp (or epidermis or skin) and endo-mesocarp (or flesh or pulp), as well as in seeds (Fig. 11.3; Table 11.3). These compounds are low molecular weight secondary metabolites which exert a plethora of physiological, pathophysiological, and ecological roles in the plant organisms, thus improving their *fitness*. Some phytochemicals

Table 11.1 Top 20 Commodities in the World in 2013 (http://faostat.fao.org)

Rank	Commodity	Production (1000$ Int)[a]
1	Milk, whole fresh cow	198,338,449.28
2	Rice, paddy	190,576,416.11
3	Meat indigenous, pig	172,682,907.04
4	Meat indigenous, cattle	171,163,310.87
5	Meat indigenous, chicken	137,224,034.26
6	Wheat	85,942,102.55
7	Soybeans	69,476,638.75
8	Maize	67,126,425.38
9	Sugar cane	60,784,342.86
10	Tomatoes	59,884,397.37
11	Eggs, hen, in shell	56,616,155.17
12	Potatoes	49,460,870.90
13	Vegetables, fresh nes	47,565,545.39
14	Grapes	44,118,041.37
15	Cotton lint	35,077,740.59
16	Apples	33,860,008.14
17	Milk, whole fresh buffalo	31,952,941.55
18	Bananas	29,740,293.40
19	Cassava	27,212,109.63
20	Mangoes, mangosteens, guavas	25,942,441.48

[a]*International dollar: in any non US-country, it allows to buy amounts of goods and services equal to those would be bought in the United States, using US dollars.*

confer colors and aromas to flowers and fruits, thus attracting pollinators and animals responsible for the seed dispersal or, conversely, repelling noxious phytophagi. Other secondary metabolites are phytoalexins, ie, wide-spectrum antimicrobial and toxic compounds which are part of the plant defense armamentarium against microbial infections phytophagi attacks. In the soil, phytochemicals are signaling molecules involved in the symbiosis between roots and beneficial microbes such as plant growth-promoting rhizobacteria and mycorrhizal fungi (Iriti and Faoro, 2009a).

Among grape secondary metabolites, phenylpropanoids and isoprenoids are the most relevant (Fig. 11.3). Phenylpropanoids are phenylalanine derivatives including simple phenols or phenolic acids (hydroxybenzoates and hydroxycinnamates) and polyphenols (flavonoids, stilbenes, and proanthocyanidins); isoprenoids consist of many classes of compounds arising from acetyl CoA: hemiterpenes, monoterpenes, sesquiterpenes, diterpenes,

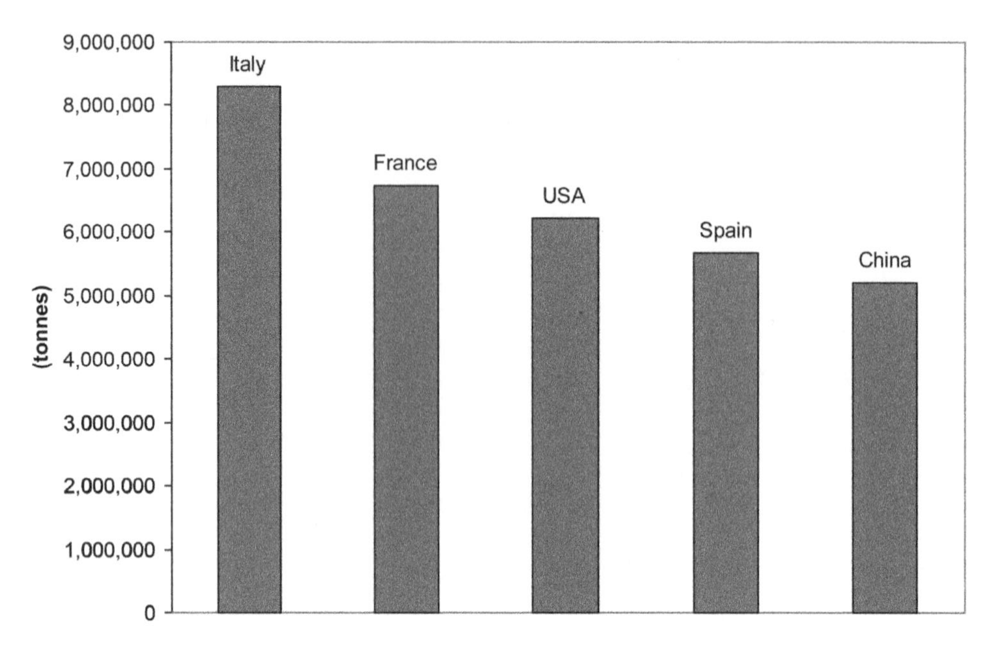

■ **FIGURE 11.2** Top five grape producer countries: average from 1993 to 2013 (http://faostat.fao.org).

triterpenes, tetraterpenes, and polyterpenes (Fig. 11.3). These compounds have a pivotal role in grapevine chemoecology. For example, anthocyanins, a class of flavonoids, are the red pigments responsible for the color of the berry exocarp. Other flavonoids and stilbenes are phytoalexins and, among stilbenes, resveratrol protects berry tissues from the harmful UV radiation. For phytophagous species, proanthocyanidines, or condensed tannins, are feeding deterrents which confer astringency to unripe fruits (Iriti and Faoro, 2009a; Iriti, 2011). Two classes of isoprenoids, monoterpenes and sesquiterpenes, both hydrocarbons and oxygenated derivatives, greatly contribute to the scent of flowers and fruits (Iriti and Faoro, 2009a,b). Therefore, from the grapes to the wine, aromatic, chromatic, and other quality traits of the most important Mediterranean alcoholic beverage strictly depend on grape chemicals. Melatonin and phytosterols (β-sitosterol, stigmasterol, and campesterol) were also recently reported in grapes and wines (Fig. 11.3) (Iriti et al., 2006; Ruggiero et al., 2013).

BIOACTIVITIES OF GRAPE CHEMICALS

In the last decades, a huge amount of preclinical (ie, *in vitro* and *in vivo*) studies has been carried out on grape, wine, and their phytochemicals, which ascribed a plethora of biological activities to these products and

Table 11.2 Nutritional Composition of Grapes[a]

Constituents	Value per 100 g
Water	80.5 g
Energy	69 kcal
Fiber	0.9 g
Nutrients	
Protein	0.72 g
Total lipids	0.16 g
Carbohydrate	18.10 g
Sugars (total)	15.50 g
Minerals	
Calcium (Ca)	10 mg
Iron (Fe)	0.36 mg
Magnesium (Mg)	7 mg
Phosphorous (P)	20 mg
Potassium (K)	191 mg
Sodium (Na)	2 mg
Zinc (Z)	0.07 mg
Vitamins	
Vitamin C (ascorbic acid)	3.2 mg
Vitamin B1 (thiamin)	0.069 mg
Vitamin B2 (riboflavin)	0.070 mg
Vitamin B3 (niacin)	0.188 mg
Vitamin B6 (piridoxine)	0.086 mg
Folate	2 μg
Vitamin A	3 μg
Vitamin E (α-tocopherol)	0.19 mg
Vitamin K (phylloquinone)	14.6 μg
Lipids	
Fatty acids (total saturated)	0.054 g
Fatty acids (total monounsaturated)	0.007 g
Fatty acids (total polyunsaturated)	0.048 g

[a]U.S. Department of Agriculture Database Nutrient Database for Standard Reference (http://nal.usda.gov, retrieved 04.05.15).

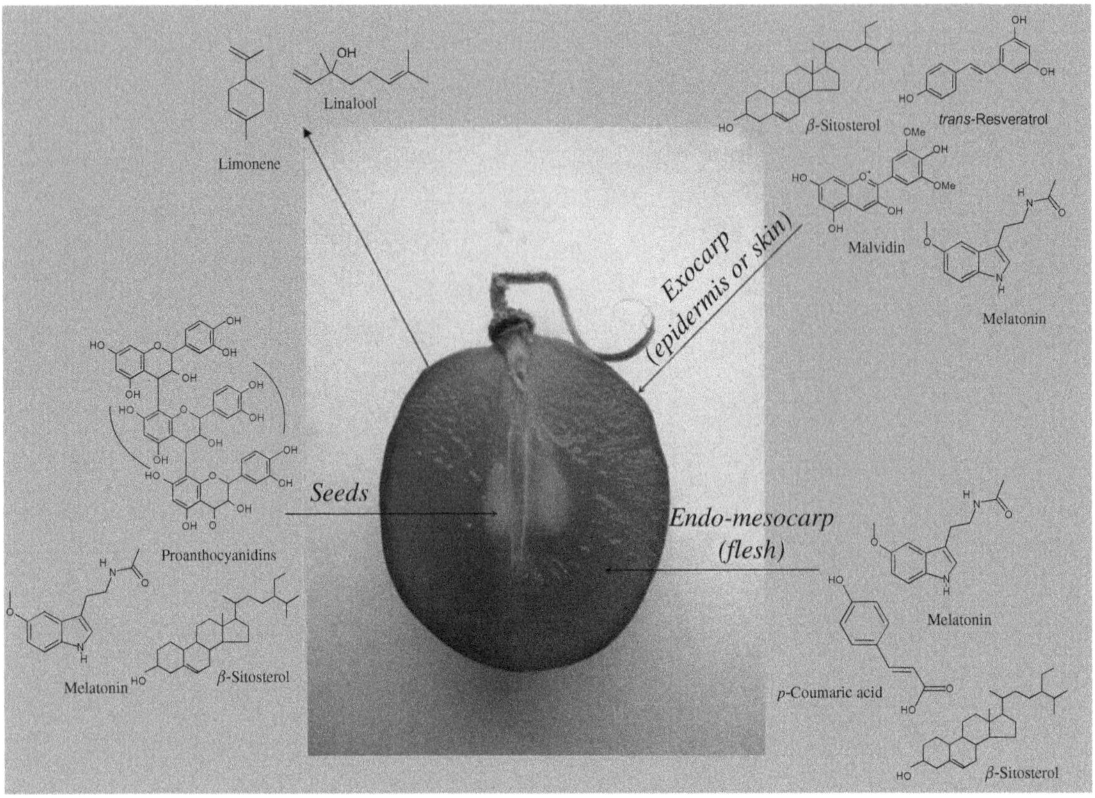

■ **FIGURE 11.3** Occurrence of main polyphenols (malvidin, an anthocyanin; *trans*-resveratrol, a stilbene; proanthocyanidins or condensed tannins), hydroxycinnamates (*p*-coumaric acid), isoprenoids (linalool and limonene, two monoterpenes), and new phytochemicals (melatonin and β-sitosterol, the latter a phytosterol) in grape berry and seed tissues.

their main components: antioxidant, anti-inflammatory, antimicrobial, anticancer, pro/antiapoptotic, antithrombotic, vasodilating, immunomodulatory, wound healing, and hormone modulatory, to name but a few. In particular, compelling evidence has pointed out the cardioprotective, cancer preventive, and neuroprotective properties of polyphenols, the most studied grape chemicals. However, high levels of polyphenols are present in many plant foods, thus supporting the association between dietary styles rich in fruits and vegetables, such as the Mediterranean diet, and a reduced risk of chronic-degenerative disorders, mainly cardiovascular diseases, certain types of cancer and neurological disorders.

Since the health promoting effects of grape products and phytochemicals have been comprehensively reviewed, until 2010, in two chapters

Table 11.3 Phenolic Composition of Red Grapes on Fresh Weight (FW) Basis[a]

Flavonoids		**Mean Content ($mg\ 100\,g^{-1}$ FW)**
Anthocyanins	Cyanidin 3-*O*-(6″-*p*-coumaroyl-glucoside)	0.10
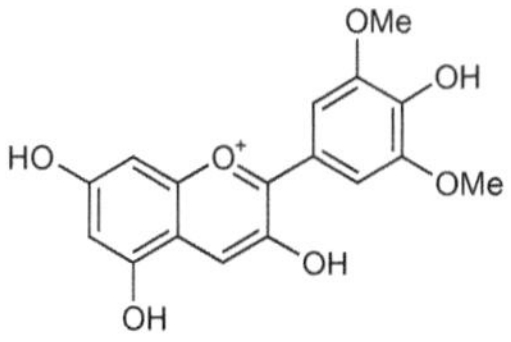	Cyanidin 3-*O*-glucoside	1.08
	Delphinidin 3-*O*-(6″-acetyl-glucoside)	0.54
	Delphinidin 3-*O*-glucoside	2.63
	Malvidin 3-*O*-(6″-acetyl-glucoside)	9.66
	Malvidin 3-*O*-(6″-*p*-coumaroyl-glucoside)	9.91
	Malvidin 3-*O*-glucoside	39.23
Malvidin	Peonidin 3-*O*-(6″-*p*-coumaroyl-glucoside)	0.34
	Peonidin 3-*O*-glucoside	5.80
	Petunidin 3-*O*-(6″-*p*-coumaroyl-glucoside)	0.05
	Petunidin 3-*O*-glucoside	2.76
Flavanols	(+)-Catechin	5.46
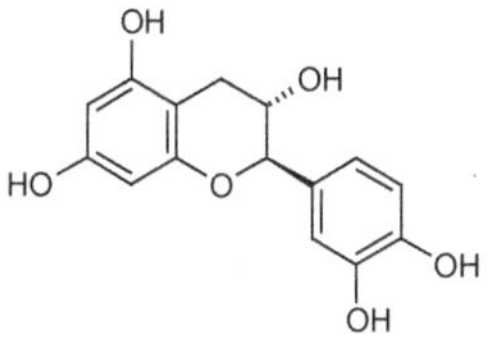	(−)-Epicatechin	5.24
	(−)-Epicatechin 3-*O*-gallate	1.68
	(−)-Epigallocatechin	0.03
	Procyanidin dimer B1	0.43
	Procyanidin dimer B2	0.36
	Procyanidin dimer B3	0.12
(–) Catechin	Procyanidin dimer B4	0.33
	Procyanidin dimer C1	0.38
Flavonols		
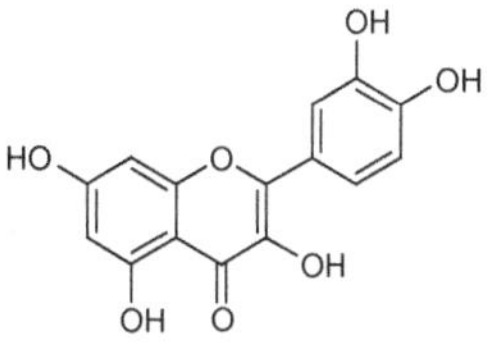		
Quercetin	Quercetin 3-*O*-galactoside	0.93
	Quercetin 3-*O*-glucuronide	2.15
Phenolic acids		
Caffeic acid 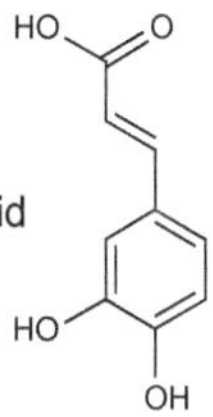	Caffeoyl tartaric acid	1.13
	p-Coumaroyl tartaric acid	0.56

(*Continued*)

Table 11.3 Phenolic Composition of Red Grapes on Fresh Weight (FW) Basis[a] (Continued)

Flavonoids		Mean Content (mg 100 g^{-1} FW)
Stilbenes		
	Piceatannol	0.005
	Resveratrol	0.15
	Resveratrol 3-*O*-glucoside	0.03
	trans-Resveratrol	0.15
Resveratrol	*trans*-Resveratrol 3-*O*-glucoside	0.01

[a]*Phenol Explorer—Database on polyphenol content in foods (http://phenol-explorer.eu, retrieved 04.05.15).*

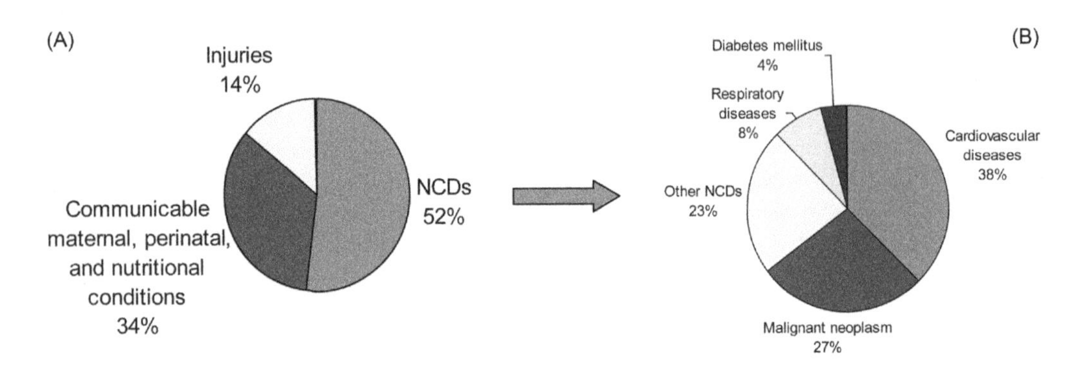

■ **FIGURE 11.4** Proportion of (A) global and (B) NCD deaths in 2012 among people under the age of 70 years. *World Health Organization, 2014. Global Health Estimates: Deaths by Cause, Age, Sex and Country, 2000–2012. WHO, Geneva.*

previously published in this book series and mainly based on preclinical evidences (Iriti and Faoro, 2009b, 2010), the herein chapter will deal with more recent clinical trials, at the top of the evidence-based nutrition pyramid (Varoni et al., 2014), focusing on cardiovascular diseases, the leading cause of noncommunicable disease (NCD) deaths under the age of 70 years, in 2012 (Fig. 11.4). Table 11.4 provides a list of not yet recruiting, recruiting, and active clinical trials on dietary supplements of grape extracts and phytochemicals. These data were obtained from http://ClinicalTrial.gov, a U.S. NIH (National Institutes of Health) registry database of publicly- and/or privately supported clinical trials all over the world: 6 out of 20 studies pertained to cardiovascular health, focusing mainly on endothelial function, hypertension. The E.U. Clinical Trials Register was also consulted to refine search, but not any study on grape products was registered in this database.

Table 11.4 Not Yet Recruiting, Recruiting, and Active Clinical Trials on Grape Consumption[a]

Title			
Condition(s)	**Intervention(s)**	**Identifier Number**	**Status**[b]
Phase 2 Study to Examine Grape Seed Extract as an Antioligomerization Agent in Alzheimer's Disease			
Alzheimer's disease	Grape seed extract, placebo	NCT02033941	NR
Resveratrol to Enhance Vitality and Vigor in Elders			
Mitochondrial function, physical function	Resveratrol, 1000–1500 mg/day	NCT02123121	NR
Impact of Polyphenols on Endothelial Function in Obstructive Sleep Apnea			
Obstructive sleep apnea	Polyphenols (600 mg/1 month), placebo	NCT01977924	NR
Physiological Effects of Grape Seed Extract in Diastolic Heart Failure			
Diastolic heart failure, hypertensive heart disease	Grape seed extract	NCT01185067	R
Effect of *Vitis vinifera* Extract on Oxidative Stress, Inflammatory Biomarkers, and Hormones in High Trained Subjects			
Athletic injuries	Grape fruit extracts (capsule, 205 mg)	NCT01875497	R
Dose-Dependent Effect of Grape Seed Extract on Glucose Control in People with Impaired Glucose Tolerance			
Impaired glucose tolerance	Grape seed extract (300–900 mg), placebo	NCT02254317	R
Edible Plant Exosome Ability to Prevent Oral Mucositis Associated with Chemoradiation Treatment of Head and Neck Cancer			
Head and neck cancer, oral mucositis	Grape extract	NCT01668849	R
Phase I Assay-Guided Trial of Anti-Inflammatory Phytochemicals in Patients with Advanced Cancer			
Solid cancers	Grape seed extract, vitamin D	NCT01820299	R
Polyphenols and Overfeeding			
Overfeeding	Grape polyphenol extract (2 g), placebo	NCT02145780	R
Effects of Chardonnay Seed Flour on Vascular Health			
Endothelial dysfunction	Chardonnay seed flour, placebo	NCT02093455	R
Resveratrol in Metabolic Syndrome			
Metabolic syndrome	Resveratrol, placebo	NCT02219906	R
Resveratrol and Cardiovascular Health in the Elderly			
Vascular resistance, aging, hypertension	Resveratrol, placebo	NCT01842399	R
Resveratrol and the Metabolic Syndrome			
Obesity, insulin resistance	Resveratrol, placebo	NCT01714102	R
Effects of Red Gape Cells Powder in Type 2 Diabetes			
Type 2 diabetes	Red grape cells (powder), placebo	NCT01938521	A
The Effect of Grape Seed Extract on Blood Pressure in People with Prehypertension			
Hypertension	Grape seed extract, placebo	NCT00979732	A
Effect of Concord Grape Juice on Endothelial Function			
Obesity, overweight	Concord grape juice 12 oz per day, placebo	NCT01775748	A
Acute Effects of Grape Seed Extract on Insulin Sensitivity and Oxidative Stress and Inflammation Markers			
Metabolism	Grape seed extract, placebo	NCT01995643	A

(*Continued*)

Table 11.4 Not Yet Recruiting, Recruiting, and Active Clinical Trials on Grape Consumption[a] (Continued)

Title			
Condition(s)	**Intervention(s)**	**Identifier Number**	**Status[b]**
Studying the Effect of Freeze-Dried Table Grape Powder on Blood Estrogen Levels in Postmenopausal Women			
Breast cancer	Standardized freeze-dried table grape powder	NCT00611104	A
Effects of Two Doses of MPX Capsules on Rising Prostate-Specific Antigen Levels in Men Following Initial Therapy for Prostate Cancer			
Prostate cancer	Muscadine plus grape skin extract	NCT01317199	A
Effect of resVida on Liver Fat Content			
Liver fat content, insulin resistance	Resveratrol, placebo	NCT01635114	A

[a]*www.clinicaltrials.gov; www.clinicaltrialsregister.eu (retrieved 04.0515).*
[b]*NR, not yet recruiting; **R**, recruiting; **A**, active.*

THE CARDIOPROTECTIVE POTENTIAL OF GRAPE PRODUCTS AND POLYPHENOLS

From a mechanistic point of view, the protective effects of grape polyphenols on cardiovascular system have been ascribed to their ability to: (1) increase the high-density lipoprotein (HDL) levels; (2) improve the endothelium-dependent vasodilation; (3) decrease the inflammatory processes occurring during atherogenesis; (4) raise the antioxidant plasmatic potential, thus reducing low-density lipoprotein (LDL) oxidation; (5) decrease the blood pressure (BP); (6) inhibit platelet aggregation and leukocyte adhesion (Wightman and Heuberger, 2015). Grape seed extracts, rich in proanthocyanidines, resveratrol and grape juice are the most extensive grape polyphenols and products investigated as cardioprotective phytochemicals, both for primary and secondary prevention of cardiovascular diseases (Wu and Hsieh, 2011; Wang et al., 2012; Tomé-Carneiro et al., 2013a).

Grape seed extracts

In a meta-analysis of randomized controlled clinical trials, the Authors analyzed the effects of grape seed extract on cardiovascular risk markers, ie, systolic and diastolic BP, heart rate, total cholesterol, LDL cholesterol and HDL cholesterol, triglycerides and C-reactive protein (CRP). Grape seed extract significantly lowered systolic BP and heart rate, whereas no significant effect was found for the other endpoints (Feringa et al., 2011).

However, data on the effects of grape seed extracts on BP are somewhat controversial. Sixty-nine treated hypertensive individuals were given 500 mg/day of vitamin C, 1000 mg/day of grape seed polyphenols, both vitamin C and polyphenols, or neither (placebo) for 6 weeks. Compared with placebo, treatment with vitamin C and polyphenols did not significantly alter BP, whereas supplementation with the vitamin C and polyphenol combination resulted in significantly increased BP in the study participants with treated hypertension (Hodgson et al., 2014). Similarly, in a study including both pre- and stage 1 subjects with arterial hypertension, Ras et al. (2013) observed no difference in 12 h ambulatory BP between placebo and the group taking grape seed extract.

The acute effects of grape polyphenols on endothelial function in adults were investigated in a further meta-analysis. Endothelial function was assessed by flow-mediated vasodilatation (FMD) of the brachial artery, a noninvasive ultrasound method. This study revealed that endothelial function can be significantly improved in the initial 2 h after the intake of grape polyphenols in healthy adults. Intriguingly, this peak was delayed in subjects with a history of smoking or coronary heart disease as compared with healthy individuals (Li et al., 2013).

The antioxidant activity and cardioprotective effects of a whole grape extract (WGE) were studied in a single-center, randomized, double-blind, placebo-controlled, 6-week pilot study conducted on 24 prehypertensive, overweight, and/or prediabetic subjects. WGE subjects had significantly lower superoxide dismutase concentrations and total cholesterol/HDL cholesterol ratios, and significantly higher HDL cholesterol levels compared to the placebo subjects after 6 weeks. The concentration of 8-isoprostane and oxidized LDL decreased by 5% and 0.5%, respectively, for WGE subjects, but increased by 50% and 5%, respectively, for the placebo subjects (Evans et al., 2014).

Resveratrol

Magyar et al. (2012) studied the effects of resveratrol supplementation in secondary prevention after myocardial infarction. They designed a two parallel arms, randomized, double-blind, placebo-controlled trial with 40 postinfarction Caucasian patients (26 men and 14 women) who were followed for 3 months. Compared to the placebo group and baseline, the daily administration of 10 mg resveratrol in capsules, in combination with standard medication, improved endothelial function (50%) and left ventricular diastolic function (2%), decreased LDL cholesterol levels (8%) and platelet aggregation, and protected from unfavorable hemorheological changes.

Tomé-Carneiro et al. (2012a) explored the effects of resveratrol on atherogenic markers, ie, serum lipid profile, apolipoprotein (Apo) B, and oxidized LDL. The authors designed a three parallel arms, randomized, triple blind, placebo-controlled trial with 75 patients under statin treatment at high risk of cardiovascular diseases, with a follow-up of 6 months. The intervention consisted in the daily administration of 350 mg placebo ($n = 25$), resveratrol-containing grape extract (GE-RES, grape phenolics + 8 mg resveratrol, $n = 25$), or conventional grape extract without resveratrol (GE), in capsules. GE-RES decreased ApoB (−9.8%) and LDLox (−20%) in patients beyond their treatment according to standard guidelines for primary prevention of cardiovascular disease. Neither drug interactions nor adverse effects on hematological profile, hepatic, thyroid, and renal functions were reported. Therefore, resveratrol complemented statins, the standard medication to lower atherogenic risk factor markers. The effects of resveratrol on the inflammatory and fibrinolytic status of patients were further investigated in the same cohort of patients (Tomé-Carneiro et al., 2012b): GE-RES decreased high-sensitivity (hs)CRP (−26%), tumor necrosis factor (TNF)α (−19.8%), plasminogen activator inhibitor (PAI)-1 (−16.8%), and interleukin (IL)-6/IL-10 ratio (−24%), and increased IL-10 (19.8%). In a similar study conducted on patients with stable coronary artery disease, the same research group reported significant improvement in the level of the anti-inflammatory molecule adiponectin (10%) along with a decrease in PAI-1 level in resveratrol-treated group (Tomé-Carneiro et al., 2013b). Furthermore, LDL cholesterol decreased significantly in both GE and GE-RES groups, and proinflammatory genes were downregulated in peripheral blood mononuclear cells (PBMCs) isolated from GE-RES group patients (Tomé-Carneiro et al., 2013b). Finally, in a subpopulation of male cardiovascular disease patients with type-2 diabetes mellitus and hypertension, 1-year supplementation with GE-RES modulated inflammatory-related transcription factors, miRNA, and cytokine expression in PBMCs (Tomé-Carneiro et al., 2013c).

A randomized, double-blinded, active-controlled, parallel clinical trial using resveratrol and calcium fructoborate (CF) was carried out on 116 patients with stable angina pectoris who received 30 and 60 days of oral supplementation with CF (112 mg/day), resveratrol (20 mg/day), and their combination. Data showed resveratrol treatment decreased inflammatory markers, hsCRP and prohormone of brain natriuretic peptide (BNP), and improved lipid profile. Moreover, a synergistic action of resveratrol and CF has been also observed (Militaru et al., 2013).

A systematic review of randomized controlled trials and meta-analysis was carried out on the effects of resveratrol supplementation on plasma lipids, among the primary outcome measures. Seven studies with a total of 282 subjects were considered according to the eligibility criteria. Overall, resveratrol supplementation showed no significant effect on the levels of any of the plasma lipid parameters assessed: total cholesterol, LDL cholesterol, HDL cholesterol, and triglycerides (Sahebkar, 2013). The author hypothesized that mechanisms other than hypolipidemic effects may account for the established cardioprotective properties of resveratrol.

Grape juice

The effects of red grape juice intake on HDL cholesterol, apoAI, apoB, and homocysteine (Hcy) were investigated in 26 healthy and nonsmoking males, aged between 25 and 60 years. Red grape juice consumption significantly increased serum HDL cholesterol and decreased Hcy levels (Khadem-Ansari et al., 2010).

Interestingly, Concorde grape juice administration significantly improved the endothelial function as measured by FMD in smokers who were otherwise considered healthy. In particular, chronic consumption of Concord grape juice prevented an immediate smoking-induced decrease in FMD (Siasos et al., 2014).

The bioavailability of grape phytochemicals in Autumn Royal grape juice was determined in 16 healthy volunteers divided into two groups: the experimental group (receiving 300 mL of juice) and the placebo group (receiving 300 mL of artificial beverage). At 30 min, in plasma, the levels of catechin and gallic acid were 3.18 ± 0.06 and 0.33 ± 0.06 nmol/mL, respectively. These levels peaked at 180 min (7.11 ± 0.53 and 1.56 ± 0.07 nmol/mL of catechin and gallic acid, respectively). After 300 min, gallic acid was not detected and only two subjects showed measurable levels of catechin. In 24 urine samples, catechin and gallic acid contents were significantly higher than the baselines (Lutz et al., 2014).

ORAL BIOAVAILABILITY OF GRAPE POLYPHENOLS

The health benefits of dietary phytochemicals strictly depend on their bioavailability, which, in turn, relies on (1) the individual biotransformation systems, (2) the chemical structure and properties of each compound, and (3) the complexity of the food matrix consisting of seeds, skin, and other plant tissues. After the food intake, bioactive compounds have to be absorbed, distributed, and metabolized before reaching the target tissues and cells; finally, the metabolites of the native compounds are excreted in urine and feces. The gastrointestinal tract, the systemic circulation, and the

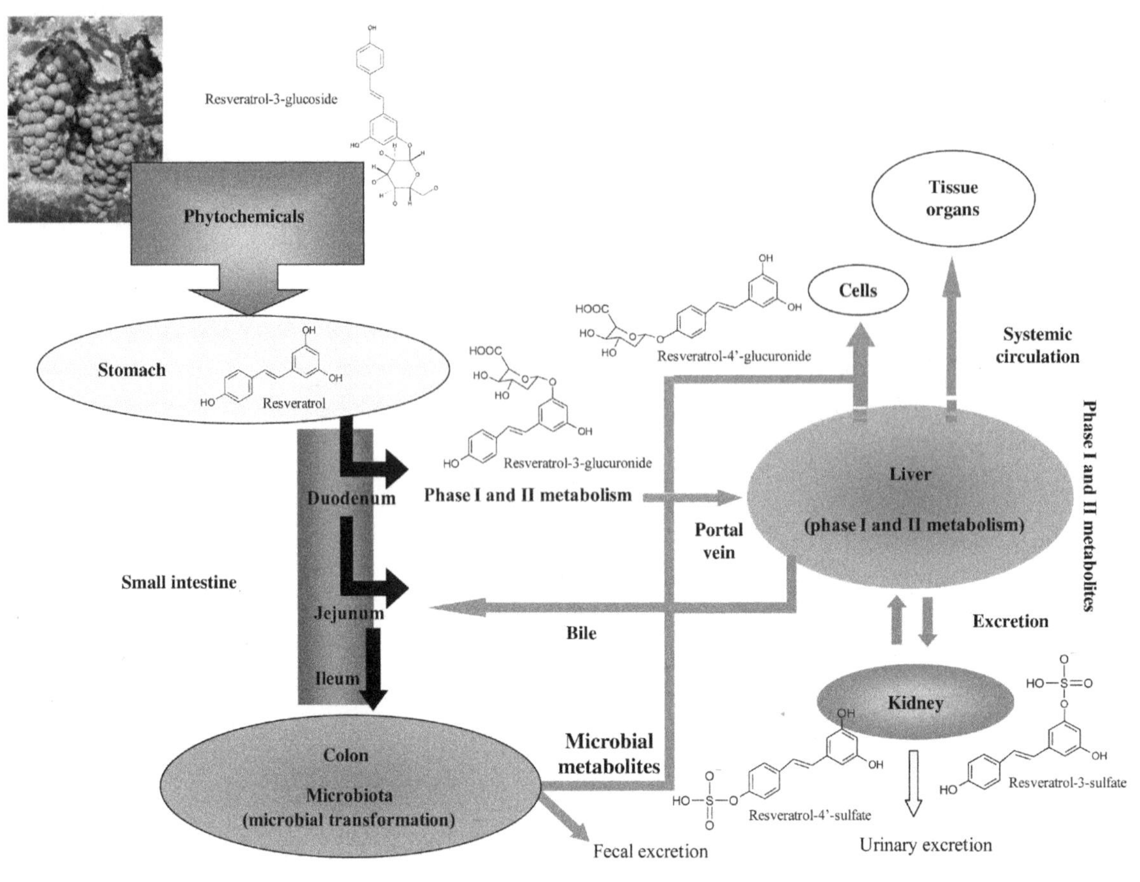

■ **FIGURE 11.5** Metabolism of resveratrol-3-glucoside (piceid), the main metabolite of resveratrol present in grapes, in human gastrointestinal tract; after piceid deconjugation, resveratrol-3-glucuronide, resveratrol-4′-glucuronide, resveratrol-3-sulfate, and resveratrol-4′-sulfate are the main Phase II metabolites of resveratrol.

urinary system are involved in these complex and coordinated biotransformation processes (Fig. 11.5).

Though they are considered "natural" products, grape polyphenols are recognized as xenobiotics by the human organism, as any other phytochemical, and, therefore, they are extensively metabolized. In grapes, polyphenols mainly occur as glycosides (flavonoids and stilbenes) and oligomers (proanthocyanidins).

Overall, only a small percentage of polyphenols (5–10% of the total intake) can be directly absorbed in the small intestine, generally aglycones, after deglycosylation, and some intact glucosides. After absorption into the small intestine, aglycones, glucosides, and monomers can be transported, via passive diffusion and membrane carriers, into the enterohepatic circulation where they are subjected to extensive Phase I (oxidation, reduction, and hydrolysis) and Phase II (conjugation) metabolisms in the enterocytes and then the hepatocytes, resulting in a series of water-soluble conjugate metabolites (methyl, glucuronide, and sulfate derivatives) rapidly liberated into the systemic circulation for further distribution to organs and excretion in urine. Alternatively, these derivatives can be returned again to the small intestine with the bile.

Polyphenols not absorbed in the small intestine (90–95% of the total intake) reach the large intestine where the microbial glucuronidases and sulfatases deconjugate the Phase II metabolites extruded via the bile throughout the enterohepatic circulation, facilitating the reuptake of aglycones. In addition, colonic microbiota can also degrade aglycones by the cleavage of their heterocyclic skeleton, releasing more simple lactones, aromatic compounds and phenolic acids, such as phenylvalerolactones, phenylvaleric acids, phenylpropionic acids, phenylacetic acids, hippuric and benzoic acids. All these microbial-derived metabolites can be absorbed or excreted by feces. When absorbed, they reach the liver through the portal vein where they can be further subjected to extensive first-pass Phase II metabolism (including glucuronidation, methylation, sulfation, or a combination of these) until they finally enter the systemic circulation and are distributed to the organs or excreted in urine (Zamora-Ros et al., 2012; Cardona et al., 2013).

CONCLUSION

Dietary styles rich in fruits and vegetables, such as the Mediterranean diet, have been recently associated to a reduced risk of cardiovascular diseases (Iriti and Vitalini, 2012). Therefore, grape, a typical component of traditional Mediterranean diet, can certainly contribute to the health promoting effects of nutritional habits rich in plant foods. Of course, the reported cardioprotective properties of grape bioactives may be due to and further maximized by additive or synergistic effects with hundreds of micronutrients (such as vitamins and minerals) and bioactive phytochemicals present in the plant foods daily introduced by diet: in these terms, grape polyphenols are part of the huge phytochemical diversity of the Mediterranean diet.

As regards the dietary supplements of grape extracts or polyphenols, it seems that their administration may exert health benefits, by reducing the levels of a number of markers of cardiovascular risk, even if controversial effects of grape seed extracts have been reported on BP. Finally, the paucity of biokinetics data on metabolism and bioavailability of grape polyphenols in healthy subjects as well as in patients at risk of or with cardiovascular diseases, after grape intake and supplement administration, represents a major drawback of the research in the field of grape bioactives for human health.

CONFLICT OF INTEREST

The authors declare no conflict of interest.

REFERENCES

Cardona, F., Andrés-Lacueva, C., Tulipani, S., Tinahones, F.J., Queipo-Ortuño, M.I., 2013. Benefits of polyphenols on gut microbiota and implications in human health. J. Nutr. Biochem. 24, 1415–1422. http://dx.doi.org/10.1016/j.jnutbio.2013.05.001.

Evans, M., Wilson, D., Guthrie, N., 2014. A randomized, double-blind, placebo-controlled, pilot study to evaluate the effect of whole grape extract on antioxidant status and lipid profile. J. Funct. Foods 7, 680–691. http://dx.doi.org/10.1016/j.jff.2013.12.017.

Feringa, H.H.H., Laskey, D.A., Dickson, J.E., Coleman, C.I., 2011. The effect of grape seed extract on cardiovascular risk markers: a meta-analysis of randomized controlled trials. J. Am. Diet. Assoc 111, 1173–1181. http://dx.doi.org/10.1016/j.jada.2011.05.015.

Hodgson, J.M., Croft, K.D., Woodman, R.J., Puddey, I.B., Bondonno, C.P., Wu, J.H.Y., et al., 2014. Effects of vitamin E, vitamin C and polyphenols on the rate of blood pressure variation: results of two randomised controlled trials. Br. J. Nutr. 112, 1551–1561. http://dx.doi.org/10.1017/S0007114514002542.

Iriti, M., 2011. Editorial: introduction to polyphenols, plant chemicals for human health. Mini Rev. Med. Chem. 11, 1183–1185.

Iriti, M., Faoro, F., 2009a. Bioactivity of grape chemicals for human health. Nat. Prod. Commun. 4, 611–634.

Iriti, M., Faoro, F., 2009b. Chemical diversity and defence metabolism: how plants cope with pathogens and ozone pollution. Int. J. Mol. Sci. 10, 3371–3399. http://dx.doi.org/10.3390/ijms10083371.

Iriti, M., Faoro, F., 2010. Bioactive chemicals and health benefits of grapevine products. In: Watson, R.R., Preedy, V.R. (Eds.), Bioactive Foods in Promoting Health: Fruits and Vegetables, Amsterdam, Academic Press.

Iriti, M., Vitalini, S., 2012. Health-promoting effects of traditional mediterranean diets—a review. Pol. J. Food Nutr. Sci. 62, 71–76.

Iriti, M., Rossoni, M., Faoro, F., 2006. Melatonin content in grape: myth or panacea? J Sci Food Agric 86, 1432–1438. http://dx.doi.org/10.1002/jsfa.2537.

Khadem-Ansari, M.H., Rasmi, Y., Ramezani, F., 2010. Effects of red grape juice consumption on high density lipoprotein-cholesterol, apolipoprotein AI, apolipoprotein B and homocysteine in healthy human volunteers. Open. Biochem. J. 4, 96–99. http://dx.doi.org/10.2174/1874091X01004010096.

Li, S.-H., Tian, H.-B., Zhao, H.-J., Chen, L.-H., Cui, L.-Q., 2013. The acute effects of grape polyphenols supplementation on endothelial function in adults: meta-analyses of controlled trials. PLoS One 8, e69818. http://dx.doi.org/10.1371/journal.pone.0069818.

Lutz, M., Castro, E., García, L., Henríquez, C., 2014. Bioavailability of phenolic compounds in grape juice cv. Autumn Royal. CyTA J. Food. 12, 48–54. http://dx.doi.org/10.1080/19476337.2013.793213.

Magyar K., Halmosi R., Palfi A., Feher G., Czopf L., Fulop A., et al. Cardioprotection by resveratrol: a human clinical trial in patients with stable coronary artery disease. Clin. Hemorheol. Microcirc. 2012;50:179–187. http://dx.doi.org/10.3233/CH-2011-1424.

McGovern, P.F., 2013. Ancient Wine: the Search for the Origins of Viniculture. Princeton University Press.

Militaru, C., Donoiu, I., Craciun, A., Scorei, I.D., Bulearca, A.M., Scorei, R.I., 2013. Oral resveratrol and calcium fructoborate supplementation in subjects with stable angina pectoris: effects on lipid profiles, inflammation markers, and quality of life. Nutr. Burbank Los Angel Cty Calif 29, 178–183. http://dx.doi.org/10.1016/j.nut.2012.07.006.

Ras, R.T., Zock, P.L., Zebregs, Y.E.M.P., Johnston, N.R., Webb, D.J., Draijer, R., 2013. Effect of polyphenol-rich grape seed extract on ambulatory blood pressure in subjects with pre- and stage I hypertension. Br. J. Nutr. 110, 2234–2241. http://dx.doi.org/10.1017/S000711451300161X.

Ruggiero, A., Vitalini, S., Burlini, N., Bernasconi, S., Iriti, M., 2013. Phytosterols in grapes and wine, and effects of agrochemicals on their levels. Food. Chem. 141, 3473–3479. http://dx.doi.org/10.1016/j.foodchem.2013.05.153.

Sahebkar, A., 2013. Effects of resveratrol supplementation on plasma lipids: a systematic review and meta-analysis of randomized controlled trials. Nutr. Rev. 71, 822–835. http://dx.doi.org/10.1111/nure.12081.

Siasos, G., Tousoulis, D., Kokkou, E., Oikonomou, E., Kollia, M.-E., Verveniotis, A., et al., 2014. Favorable effects of concord grape juice on endothelial function and arterial stiffness in healthy smokers. Am. J. Hypertens. 27, 38–45. http://dx.doi.org/10.1093/ajh/hpt176.

Tomé-Carneiro, J., Gonzálvez, M., Larrosa, M., Yáñez-Gascón, M.J., García-Almagro, F.J., Ruiz-Ros, J.A., et al., 2012a. One-year consumption of a grape nutraceutical containing resveratrol improves the inflammatory and fibrinolytic status of patients in primary prevention of cardiovascular disease. Am. J. Cardiol. 110, 356–363. http://dx.doi.org/10.1016/j.amjcard.2012.03.030.

Tomé-Carneiro, J., Gonzálvez, M., Larrosa, M., García-Almagro, F.J., Avilés-Plaza, F., Parra, S., et al., 2012b. Consumption of a grape extract supplement containing resveratrol decreases oxidized LDL and ApoB in patients undergoing primary prevention of cardiovascular disease: a triple-blind, 6-month follow-up, placebo-controlled, randomized trial. Mol. Nutr. Food Res. 56, 810–821. http://dx.doi.org/10.1002/mnfr.201100673.

Tomé-Carneiro, J., Gonzálvez, M., Larrosa, M., Yáñez-Gascón, M.J., García-Almagro, F.J., Ruiz-Ros, J.A., et al., 2013a. Grape resveratrol increases serum adiponectin and downregulates inflammatory genes in peripheral blood mononuclear cells: a triple-blind, placebo-controlled, one-year clinical trial in patients with stable coronary artery disease. Cardiovasc. Drugs. Ther. 27, 37–48. http://dx.doi.org/10.1007/s10557-012-6427-8.

Tomé-Carneiro, J., Larrosa, M., Yáñez-Gascón, M.J., Dávalos, A., Gil-Zamorano, J., González, M., et al., 2013b. One-year supplementation with a grape extract containing resveratrol modulates inflammatory-related microRNAs and cytokines expression in peripheral blood mononuclear cells of type 2 diabetes and hypertensive patients with coronary artery disease. Pharmacol. Res. Off. J. Ital. Pharmacol. Soc. 72, 69–82. http://dx.doi.org/10.1016/j.phrs.2013.03.011.

Tomé-Carneiro, J., Gonzálvez, M., Larrosa, M., Yáñez-Gascón, M.J., García-Almagro, F.J., Ruiz-Ros, J.A., et al., 2013c. Resveratrol in primary and secondary prevention of cardiovascular disease: a dietary and clinical perspective. Ann. N. Y. Acad. Sci. 1290, 37–51. http://dx.doi.org/10.1111/nyas.12150.

Varoni, E., Lodi, G., Iriti, M., 2014. Efficacy behind activity—Phytotherapeutics are not different from pharmaceuticals. Pharm. Biol. http://dx.doi.org/10.3109/13880209.2014.923000.

Wang, H., Yang, Y.-J., Qian, H.-Y., Zhang, Q., Xu, H., Li, J.-J., 2012. Resveratrol in cardiovascular disease: what is known from current research? Heart Fail. Rev. 17, 437–448. http://dx.doi.org/10.1007/s10741-011-9260-4.

Wightman, J.D., Heuberger, R.A., 2015. Effect of grape and other berries on cardiovascular health. J. Sci. Food Agric. 95, 1584–1597. http://dx.doi.org/10.1002/jsfa.6890.

Wu, J.M., Hsieh, T., 2011. Resveratrol: a cardioprotective substance: cardioprotection by resveratrol. Ann. N. Y. Acad. Sci. 1215, 16–21. http://dx.doi.org/10.1111/j.1749-6632.2010.05854.x.

Zamora-Ros, R., Urpi-Sarda, M., Lamuela-Raventós, R.M., Martínez-González, M.Á., Salas-Salvadó, J., Arós, F., et al., 2012. High urinary levels of resveratrol metabolites are associated with a reduction in the prevalence of cardiovascular risk factors in high-risk patients. Pharmacol Res Off. J. Ital. Pharmacol. Soc. 65, 615–620. http://dx.doi.org/10.1016/j.phrs.2012.03.009.

Chapter 12

Kiwifruit and health

Denise C. Hunter[1], Margot A. Skinner[2] and A. Ross Ferguson[1]
[1]*The New Zealand Institute for Plant & Food Research Limited, New Zealand*
[2]*The University of Auckland, Auckland, New Zealand*

CHAPTER OUTLINE

INTRODUCTION

The word "kiwifruit" is generally used for plants in the genus *Actinidia* Lindl. and the fruit they produce. *Actinidia* species come predominantly from south-western China, but a small number occur in countries adjoining China (Ferguson and Huang, 2007). Although more than 50 species are currently recognized (Li et al., 2007), only three have been domesticated, and this only in the past century. The fruit available commercially are usually of *A. chinensis* Planch., mainly with yellow-fleshed fruit, sometimes with a red ring around the core, or of *A. deliciosa* (A. Chev.) C.F. Liang et A.R. Ferguson, which has a green-fleshed fruit. These two species are closely related and are increasingly treated as varieties of the one species: *A. chinensis* var. *chinensis* and *A chinensis* var. *deliciosa* (Li et al., 2007). Very small quantities of a third species, *A. arguta* (Sieb. et Zucc.) Planch. ex Miq. ("hardy" kiwifruit, "baby kiwi," or now, more commonly, "kiwiberries"), are also produced. There is also some interest in cultivating *A. eriantha* Benth. and *A. kolomikta* (Maxim. & Rupr.) Maxim, although it is limited.

Fruits, Vegetables, and Herbs.
DOI: http://dx.doi.org/10.1016/B978-0-12-802972-5.00012-3

Six countries, China, Italy, New Zealand, Iran, Chile, and Greece, produce over 90% of the world's kiwifruit; 80% come from the northern hemisphere (Belrose, Inc., 2014; Ferguson, 2015). Total kiwifruit production is currently about 3.0 million metric tonnes, of which at least 70% or some 2 million tonnes are a single cultivar, *A. deliciosa* 'Hayward' ("green" kiwifruit). More than 90% of the kiwifruit in international trade are therefore fruit of 'Hayward.' The most commonly traded yellow-fleshed kiwifruit is *A. chinensis* 'Zesy002' (Gold3), sold as Zespri® SunGold Kiwifruit, which has now largely replaced the previous widely sold, yellow-fleshed kiwifruit, 'Hort16A' (sold as Zespri™ Gold Kiwifruit). This is because 'Hort16A' proved to be particularly susceptible to the disease, bacterial canker of kiwifruit, caused by *Pseudomonas syringae* pv. *actinidiae* (Psa).

In China, *Actinidia* species are generally referred to as *mihoutao*, a name used since the beginning of the Tang Dynasty (618–906 AD). According to Chinese pharmacopoeia, *mihoutao* were used to aid digestion, reduce irritability, relieve rheumatism, prevent kidney or urinary tract stones, and cure hemorrhoids, dyspepsia, and vomiting (Ferguson, 1990). They were also used for the treatment of many types of cancer, especially breast cancer and cancers of the digestive system (Motohashi et al., 2002). Some of the "anticancer" properties of kiwifruit (*A. chinensis*) recognized in traditional Chinese medicine may be attributable to their polysaccharide content (Chang, 2002). As populations age, there is increasing emphasis on maintenance of health and wellbeing, and more interest in developing functional foods based on traditional therapies. Kiwifruit have long been used in China for medicinal purposes and their potential for use in modern therapy and/or to promote health deserves detailed study.

Kiwifruit are often promoted for their high vitamin C (ascorbic acid) content, which probably contributes to the health benefits observed. *A. deliciosa* 'Hayward' typically contains 85 mg/100 g (fresh weight), and a single fruit can provide the recommended daily intake (RDI; Ferguson and Ferguson, 2003). Vitamin C levels vary amongst and within *Actinidia* species (Ferguson and Huang, 2007; Ferguson and Ferguson, 2003; Nishiyama et al., 2004b; Drummond, 2013; Huang et al., 2004; Ferguson and MacRae, 1992). The health benefits attributed to vitamin C include antioxidant, antiatherogenic, and anticarcinogenic activities, as well as immunomodulation (Vissers et al., 2013). However, kiwifruit also contain other vitamins and minerals that may contribute to possible health benefits, including folate, potassium and magnesium, dietary fiber and phytochemicals (Ferguson and Ferguson, 2003; Drummond, 2013). Phytochemicals are well recognized for their antioxidant and cell protection activity, and they are becoming increasingly recognized for immunomodulatory properties. However, the phytochemical composition of kiwifruit can vary greatly according to the particular species or genotype. Typically green-fleshed kiwifruit (*A. deliciosa*) contain chlorophylls *a* and *b*, and carotenoids such as β-carotene, lutein, violaxanthin, and 9'-*cis*-neoxanthin. Yellow-fleshed kiwifruits (eg, *A. chinensis* or *A. macrosperma*) also contain carotenoids, but little or no chlorophyll when ripe (McGhie, 2013), and red-fleshed genotypes (eg, *A. chinensis* 'Hongyang') contain anthocyanins (Montefiori et al., 2005). In addition, *A. deliciosa* 'Hayward' leaf tissue and juice prepared from the fruit have been shown to contain polyphenolics, specifically flavonols (McGhie, 2013; Webby, 1990; Dawes and Keene, 1999).

Most experimental studies give inadequate details of the species or cultivar of kiwifruit used, despite differences in the composition of their fruit having been noted (Ferguson and Huang, 2007; Huang et al., 2004; Nishiyama, 2007; Iwasawa et al., 2011; Park et al., 2011, 2014). Some authors do not even specify the plant part analyzed. Most studies, especially those from outside China, have probably used fruit of only *A. deliciosa* 'Hayward': such fruit are often referred to as "green" kiwifruit. Even so, the composition of 'Hayward' fruit could be affected by varying growing conditions, the maturity or ripeness of the fruit or different periods in coolstore (Park et al., 2014). Until recently, the most common "gold" kiwifruit available outside China were those of *A. chinensis* 'Hort16A.' Drummond (2013) presents comprehensive data on the nutrient composition of the edible flesh (ie, skin removed) of "ready-to-eat" 'Hayward' and 'Hort16A' kiwifruit (US Department of Agriculture, A. R. S., Nutrient Data Laboratory, 2015). Similar comprehensive data are not available for other *A. chinensis* or *A. deliciosa* cultivars or for other *Actinidia* species.

HEALTH BENEFITS FROM *ACTINIDIA* SPECIES

Consumers are becoming more interested in the health benefits of food, particularly fruits (Crawford and Mellentin, 2008). Studies using *in vitro* and animal models, and evidence from human epidemiological studies provide supporting information for developing marketing strategies. However, the most convincing evidence is ultimately that provided by clinical intervention trials, the type of evidence required to validate any health claims made about functional foods. The putative health benefits of kiwifruit will be summarized later, considering all levels of evidence available, but with greatest weight given to human intervention/clinical trials.

Cell protection and antimutagenic activity

Cells are continuously exposed to reactive oxygen species (ROS), produced during normal metabolism, and at higher concentrations as a result of infection, smoking, alcohol consumption, poor diet, and environmental pollution. The oxidative stress mediated by ROS can potentially cause oxidative damage to DNA, proteins, and lipids, contributing to inflammation and the development of a wide range of pathologies, including cancer (Kryston et al., 2011), cardiovascular disease (CVD), neurological disease, sensory impairment, and psychiatric disease (Brieger et al., 2012). High consumption of fruits and vegetables has been associated with a lower risk of death from diseases of the circulatory, respiratory, and digestive systems (Leenders et al., 2014). Similar associations between higher fruit and vegetable consumption and reduced risk have also been reported for CVD (Okuda et al., 2015), coronary heart disease (He et al., 2007), and stroke (He et al., 2006). As often suggested by the authors of these studies, the benefit of a high consumption of fruits and vegetables may be attributable to antioxidants within those foods reducing the effects of oxidative stress or inflammation.

Antioxidant capacity of fruits and vegetables can come from vitamin C, vitamin E, carotenoids, and phenolic compounds. In the past the antioxidant capacity of a given food or fruit, or their components, was measured using chemical assays, such as the Trolox™ equivalent antioxidant capacity (TEAC) assay, the ferric reducing antioxidant power (FRAP) assay, the DPPH (2,2'-diphenyl-1-picrylhydrazyl) free radical scavenging potential assay, the oxygen radical absorption capacity (ORAC) assay, and the total radical absorption potential (TRAP) assay. The performance of kiwifruit (presumably 'Hayward') in these assays is moderate compared with other types of fruit, ranking 5th highest out of 13 fruits on a fresh weight basis using the ORAC assay (Wang et al., 1996), and 10th out of 14 fruits using the TEAC assay (Chun et al., 2005). The various components of fruit are known to perform differently, depending on the discrete mechanism of the assay (Ozgen et al., 2006), but the antioxidant capacity of different kiwifruit cultivars correlates well with their total polyphenol content and vitamin C content (Lim et al., 2014; Du et al., 2009). These factors probably contribute to reports that fruit of other genotypes of kiwifruit have greater antioxidant capacity than 'Hayward,' eg, *A. eriantha* and *A. latifolia* (Du et al., 2009), and *A. eriantha* 'Bidan,' *A. chinensis* 'Haegeum,' and *A. chinensis* 'Haehyang' (Lim et al., 2014). However, the relevance of such chemical-based antioxidant assays to the activity of kiwifruit *in vivo* is limited, and results such as those described earlier may not necessarily be extrapolated to benefits for human health.

It is therefore important that the ability of extracts from kiwifruit to protect against oxidative stress has been demonstrated in cell-based bioassays. For example, juice concentrate from 'Hayward' extracts protected human, Jurkat T cells from cell death induced by hydrogen peroxide-mediated oxidative stress (Hunter et al., 2008), and a *n*-hexane extract from 'Hayward' reduced oxidative stress (DCF formation) and hydrogen peroxide-induced cytotoxicity in the neuronal rat cell line PC12 (Jin et al., 2014). Whilst more biologically relevant than a chemical-based antioxidant assay, such cell-based assays often do not account for digestion which may influence metabolism, uptake, and activity of compounds; hence *in vivo* evidence of biological activity from kiwifruit remains the strongest evidence available.

Indeed, *in vivo* evidence for an antioxidant benefit from kiwifruit is accumulating. A single consumption of kiwifruit juice and *A. deliciosa* 'Hayward' kiwifruit increased plasma antioxidant activity, tested using *ex vivo* chemical-based methods (Ko et al., 2005; Prior et al., 2007). A longer term intervention of consumption of one or two gold kiwifruit (*A. chinensis* 'Hort16A') per day for 4 weeks increased resistance of isolated lymphocytes toward hydrogen peroxide-induced DNA oxidation in an *ex vivo* challenge (Brevik et al., 2011). *In vivo* benefits have also been demonstrated with significant reductions in plasma lipid peroxidation following consumption of 2 'Hayward' kiwifruit daily for 4 or 8 weeks by hyperlipidemic subjects (Chang and Liu, 2009), and 4 gold kiwifruit ('Hort16A') daily for 4 weeks by healthy older adults (Hunter et al., 2012). Similarly, a reduction in endogenous DNA damage, demonstrated by a reduction in oxidized pyrimidines and purines from lymphocytes, was observed following consumption of gold kiwifruit (Brevik et al., 2011) and green kiwifruit (Collins, 2013). Although protection from ROS and oxidation by kiwifruit has been demonstrated, and is often reported in conjunction with higher concentrations of circulating antioxidant species, particularly vitamins C and E (eg, Hunter et al., 2012; Chang and Liu, 2009; Brevik et al., 2011), it should not be assumed that direct antioxidant activity is solely responsible for the protection from oxidative stress observed with kiwifruit consumption.

Phytochemicals can modulate processes involved in protection from oxidative stress and DNA damage, such as cell signaling, gene expression, and enzyme activity (Collins, 2013; Stevenson, 2012), with some examples evident with kiwifruit. The addition of three kiwifruit (species and cultivar not specified) per day to the usual diet of healthy male smokers resulted in significant upregulation of gene sets relating to DNA repair (such as nucleotide excision repair, mismatch repair, and double-stranded break repair), hypoxia and apoptosis, and immune response (Bohn et al., 2010). DNA repair has been used as a marker for susceptibility to mutagenicity (Collins and Galvão, 2007), and increased susceptibility to mutagenicity is positively correlated with incidence of cancer. However, the development of cancer is a complex process that may be stimulated by many genetic and/or environmental factors. Key intervention steps for chemoprevention have been identified based on (1) blocking carcinogen formation and absorption, (2) carcinogen activation, DNA damage, and mutagenesis, (3) detoxification of carcinogens, and (4) cell proliferation, promotion, and tumor formation (Trosko and Chang, 2001; Wattenberg, 1990).

Aside from directly protecting from, or mitigating DNA damage and mutagenesis, the constituents of kiwifruit may also assist with other key strategies for chemoprevention. Firstly, kiwifruit may contribute to the blocking of carcinogen formation and absorption. Dietary mutagens, including compounds in cooked meat, *N*-nitroso compounds, and fungal toxins, have been related to common cancers, such as colon, prostate, and breast cancers (Ferguson et al., 2004). Compounds present in kiwifruit may inhibit the production of dietary mutagens. For example, vitamins C and E, and plant polyphenols inhibited endogenous production of *N*-nitroso compounds from amino precursors (Bartsch et al., 1988). Indeed, ethanol extracts of kiwifruit prevented mutagenic activity *in vitro* of *N*-nitrosamines (Ikken et al., 1999). Furthermore, absorption of mutagens may be reduced or prevented by fecal bulking through reducing transit time and contact time of the mutagens in the gut (Ferguson et al., 2004). 'Hayward' kiwifruit contain relatively high amounts of lignin, which contribute to their insoluble dietary fiber content (Bunzel and Ralph, 2006). Lignin is hydrophobic and higher lignin content increases adsorption of heterocyclic aromatic amines, potential mutagenic compounds, and potential carcinogens following absorption and metabolism in the liver (Funk et al., 2007). The high lignin content of kiwifruit may therefore act as a dietary antimutagen. Finally, the prebiotic effect of dietary fiber of kiwifruit may modulate colonic bacteria populations. Such modulation may reduce production of mutagens following fermentation of dietary chemicals by gut bacteria (Ferguson et al., 2004). Specific evidence of this with kiwifruit is limited however.

Secondly, there is some evidence that kiwifruit may intervene in cell proliferation, promotion, and tumor formation. *In vitro* studies have demonstrated inhibition of proliferation of cancer cell lines. For example, ethanol extracts from *A. kolomikta*, *A. arguta*, and *A. chinensis* inhibited proliferation of a human hepatocellular carcinoma cell line (HepG2) and a human colorectal adenocarcinoma cell line (HT-29), with greatest efficacy demonstrated by *A. arguta* (Zuo et al., 2012). Similar results were demonstrated with methanol extracts of 'Hayward' kiwifruit and *A. eriantha* 'Bidan' using the human pulmonary carcinoma (Calu-6) and human gastric carcinoma (SNU-601) cell lines (Park et al., 2012). Whilst promising, such results should be viewed with caution because it has yet to be proven that active compounds from kiwifruit are absorbed during digestion in sufficient concentrations to exert an antiproliferative effect *in vivo*. Moreover, mechanisms other than cytotoxicity may also be at work. Gap junction intercellular communication (GJIC) is thought to regulate growth control, differentiation, and apoptosis, with most normal, contact-inhibited cells having functional GJIC (Trosko and Chang, 2001). Loss of GJIC occurs during the promotion/progression steps of the carcinogenic process, however, and results from an *in vitro* study suggest that kiwifruit may help preserve GJIC function. Extracts of both green and gold kiwifruit (presumably 'Hayward' and 'Hort16A') prevented hydrogen peroxide inhibition of GJIC in WB-F344 rat liver epithelial cells (Lee et al., 2010). Furthermore, phosphorylation of the proteins connexin 43 (Cx43) and extracellular signal-related protein kinase (ERK 1/2), known to be associated with impaired GJIC, was reduced by the kiwifruit extracts in the model described earlier. This activity was attributed to the quercetin content in the extracts because a similar effect was observed in cells treated with quercetin only (Lee et al., 2010), however, the quercetin concentration in each extract was not reported. Considering all the different constituents of kiwifruit and the activities reported in the studies described earlier, kiwifruit has the potential to protect from oxidative damage and mutagenesis via multiple pathways, when included as part of a healthy, balanced diet.

Gut health

The gastrointestinal tract is involved in the processing of food from when it is first eaten until it is digested, absorbed, or passed out as feces. Increasingly the roles of the gut microbiota are being recognized as we understand how it fulfils functions that have a direct impact on health. Traditionally kiwifruit have been used to aid digestion. There is now clear evidence that green kiwifruit ('Hayward') and the enzyme actinidin that it contains can provide enhanced upper-tract digestion, particularly gastric, of a variety of food proteins. *In vitro* digestion of proteins present in yoghurt, cheese, fish, and raw eggs in the presence of 'Hayward' kiwifruit compared to mammalian digestive enzymes was shown to result in a substantially greater digestion of intact protein, and different peptide patterns were produced (Kaur et al., 2010a,b). An *in vivo* study in pigs that included a positive control of added actinidin, and a negative control where the actinidin in 'Hayward' kiwifruit had been inactivated, showed conclusively that actinidin was responsible for the enhanced gastric hydrolysis of food proteins (Montoya et al., 2014).

Kiwifruit consumption may also influence absorption of food components. Minerals are essential nutrients and each is absorbed in the gut via unique and complex pathways. Kiwifruit, in comparison to other foods, naturally contains a high concentration of vitamin C, which increases the bioavailability of nonheme iron and can impact calcium absorption. Recent research in cells, animals, and humans has demonstrated that kiwifruit, particularly the cultivar 'Hort16A,' can increase the uptake and retention of the essential dietary minerals iron, calcium, phosphorus, and magnesium (Wolber et al., 2013).

Clinical studies in a range of adult populations consistently indicate that kiwifruit are a highly effective dietary option to promote laxation. Healthy elderly subjects fed 'Hayward' kiwifruit daily for 3 weeks, one fruit per 30 kg of body weight, reported an improvement in laxation parameters, such as frequency and ease of defecation, stool bulk, and stool softness (Rush et al., 2002). It was concluded that kiwifruit, eaten in these realistic quantities, could be useful in maintaining regularity in elderly people who otherwise have no major bowel problems. A subsequent trial indicated that 'Hayward' kiwifruit can relieve chronic constipation in both healthy individuals (Chan et al., 2007) and those with irritable bowel syndrome (Chang et al., 2010). More recently, kiwifruit-derived supplements at 2400 mg/day for 28 days were shown to increase stool frequency in healthy but not in functionally constipated individuals (Ansell et al., 2015). The supplements were powdered ingredients derived from either whole green ('Hayward') or gold (*A. chinensis* 'Zesy002') kiwifruit. This study demonstrated for the first time that gold kiwifruit-derived material, as well as green kiwifruit, was able to promote laxation in healthy individuals. The laxative effects of kiwifruit have been ascribed to their content of dietary fiber (Rush et al., 2002; Chan et al., 2007), which is approximately of 2–3% fresh weight (Fourie and Hansmann, 1992; Rupérez et al., 1995), and about 10% of the RDI (Ferguson and Ferguson, 2003). The cell walls of kiwifruit are unusual in that during ripening they swell considerably (Hallett et al., 1992), and this may reflect an exceptionally high water-holding capacity, important for fecal bulking and enhancement of laxation (Rush et al., 2002). Other kiwifruit components suggested as having laxative properties include the proteolytic enzyme actinidin, nondigestible oligosaccharides and polyphenols (Ansell et al., 2015). The strength of the clinical evidence in the literature has encouraged Zespri International Limited to notify Food Standards Australia New Zealand of a self-substantiated food–health relationship between *A. deliciosa* 'Hayward' and its contribution to normal bowel function (http://www.foodstandards.gov.au/industry/labelling/fhr/Pages/20140902-051315-ZespriInternationalLtd.aspx; accessed 20.07.15.). A self-substantiated food–health relationship is established by process of a systematic review, and is required when making a general level health claim in Australia and New Zealand.

Gut health and immune function are both strongly influenced by microbial colonization of the gastrointestinal tract. Gut microflora act as an effective barrier against opportunistic and pathogenic micro-organisms (Cummings et al., 2004), and stimulating proliferation of beneficial bacteria with prebiotic components in the diet (dietary fiber) could reduce colonization by harmful bacteria. Dietary fiber is the "… nondigestible food ingredient that beneficially affects the host by selectively stimulating the growth and/or activity of one or a limited number of bacteria in the colon" (Gibson and Roberfroid, 1995). Kiwifruit are a reasonable source of dietary fiber (Lund et al., 1983), mostly cellulose, pectin polysaccharides, and hemicelluloses such as glucuronoxylans and xyloglucans (Martín-Cabrejas et al., 1995). Kiwifruit polysaccharides have the potential to prevent adhesion of enteropathogens and enhance adhesion of probiotic bacteria to Caco-2 (human colon epithelial-derived) cells *in vitro* (Ying et al., 2007). A pectin from kiwifruit prepared by resolubilization with monopotassium phosphate was superior to inulin, a standard prebiotic, in enhancing the adhesion of *Lactobacillus rhamnosus* and decreasing the adhesion of *Salmonella typhimurium* to Caco-2 cells (Parkar et al., 2010). Similarly Parkar (unpublished data in Ansell et al., 2013) reported that a kiwifruit polyphenol extract could prevent the adhesion of *S. typhimurium* to Caco-2 cells. Aqueous solutions prepared from the edible flesh, and water extracts of 'Hayward' and 'Hort16A' also promoted the growth of lactic acid bacteria and reduced the growth of *Escherichia coli* using a fecal batch fermentation model (Molan et al., 2007). Using a similar model both 'Hayward' and 'Hort16A' kiwifruit were shown to increase *Bifidobacterium* spp. and the Bacteroides–Prevotella–Porphyromonas group. This was accompanied by an increase in microbial glycosidases, especially those with substrate specificities relating to the breakdown of kiwifruit oligosaccharides, and with increased generation of short chain fatty acids (SCFA). Kiwifruit fermenta supernatant was also shown to affect the *in vitro* proliferation of *Bifidobacterium longum* and its adhesion to Caco-2 intestinal epithelial cells (Parkar et al., 2012). Collectively, these data suggest that whole kiwifruit may modulate human gut microbial composition and metabolism to benefit the host.

Some of the proteins and polypeptides in kiwifruit may have specific biological effects and could have pharmacological benefits. One example is kissper, a small, cysteine-rich peptide, present in large amounts in ripe kiwifruit (*A. deliciosa*) (Ciardiello et al., 2008; Ciacci et al., 2014). When ingested, kissper might affect gastrointestinal physiology and, it is conjectured, might have potential for treatment of disorders such as cystic fibrosis, in which ion transport mechanisms are disturbed (Ciardiello et al.,

2008). Certainly, the efficiency of kissper at reducing oxidative stress and inflammatory responses in an *in vitro* gut cell (Caco-2) model and *ex vivo* model using biopsies from the colonic mucosa of subjects with Crohn's disease has been demonstrated. Taken together with evidence that kissper is resistant to enzymatic degradation during digestion (Ciacci et al., 2014), kissper appears a likely candidate for promoting gut integrity. Further research and clinical trials are required to determine if kissper is available in sufficient quantities in the gut and has a meaningful effect on gastrointestinal health *in vivo*.

Immune function and protection from infectious disease

Nutrient status is an important contributing factor to immune competence, and essential nutrients for efficient immune function include essential amino acids, linolenic acid, folic acid, vitamins A, B_6, B_{12}, C, and E, and the minerals zinc, copper, iron, and selenium (Calder and Kew, 2002). Kiwifruit (*A. deliciosa* and *A. chinensis*) provide a reasonable source of copper, vitamin E, and folate (*A. deliciosa* 'Hayward': 18%, 11%, and 10% U.S. RDI, respectively; *A. chinensis* 'Hort16A': 19%, 11%, and 8% U.S. RDI, respectively), and are an excellent source of vitamin C (Ferguson and Ferguson, 2003). In addition, kiwifruit also contain phytochemicals, in particular carotenoids, and some evidence suggests that higher carotenoid intake is associated with reduced incidence of infection (Cser et al., 2004; van der Horst-Graat et al., 2004).

Immune function can be broadly divided into innate immunity, defined as a nonspecific first line of defense, and adaptive immunity, a specific response that requires an element of memory. Markers of innate immunity that can be used for determining the effect of nutrition and functional foods on immune function include phagocytosis, oxidative burst, natural killer (NK) cell activity, and activation of $\gamma\delta$ cells; markers of adaptive immunity include lymphocyte proliferation and activation, cytokine production, and circulating immunoglobulins (Ig) (Albers et al., 2005). A first step by which kiwifruit may contribute to innate defenses is by direct antimicrobial action of the kiwifruit components which has been demonstrated *in vitro* (Cederlund et al., 2011; Lu et al., 2007; Basile et al., 1997), however, it is yet to be proven whether this antimicrobial activity can influence pathogenic bacterial infections *in vivo*. Direct mucosal antimicrobial activity is provided by the host in the form of antimicrobial peptides such as β-defensins. These small, highly cationic peptides are produced at high local concentrations and recognize negatively charged bacterial cell surface components, to which they bind and disrupt bacterial membranes

(O'Neil, 2003). Data suggest that kiwifruit indirectly stimulate human β-defensin-1 and 2 production by acting as a fermentation substrate to increase SCFA production, which in turn stimulates the production of antimicrobial peptides from colonic epithelial cells (Bentley-Hewitt et al., 2012). Recent *in vitro* studies have utilized rat blood cells to demonstrate that kiwifruit extracts may also modulate other innate immune cell function. A phenolic extract of kiwifruit (species and cultivar not defined) significantly increased the percentage of activated γδ T cells in blood across a wide age spectrum of rats (Skinner et al., 2013). This observation may have implications for maintaining innate immunity during aging, as the percentage of γδ T cells in blood declines with age (Colonna-Romano et al., 2002).

Most studies examining the influence of kiwifruit on immune function in the whole organism have used rodent models. For example, supplementation of the diet with up to 30% kiwifruit extract (plant part, species and cultivar not defined) stimulated phagocytosis in Kunming mice, and enhanced levels of the serum immunoglobulins IgA, IgG, and IgM (Ma et al., 2006). *A. macrosperma* has been used in Chinese medicine for treatment of cancer and stimulation of the immune system (Lu et al., 2007) but feeding an aqueous extract to mice did not affect tumor weight although lymphocyte proliferation, NK cytotoxic activity, and phagocytosis were significantly stimulated. Mice (BALB/c) were also used in studies which showed that aqueous and supercritical fluid extracts of 'Hort16A' and 'Hayward' fruit enhanced both innate and adaptive immunity (Shu et al., 2008). The extracts enhanced nonspecific NK cell activity and cytokine production (interferon γ; IFN-γ), and enhanced antigen-specific antibody production following vaccination. The effect of kiwifruit on an antigen-specific systemic antibody and gut-associated responses in mice has also been studied. Feeding a processed puree product prepared from gold kiwifruit ('Hort16A') enhanced a gut-associated adaptive immune response to a model protein, ovalbumin (OVA), in C57Bl/6 mice following oral immunization with OVA (Hunter et al., 2008). The puree stimulated antigen-specific antibody production (total Ig and IgG) and antigen-specific proliferation of mesenteric lymph node (MLN) cells. Carotenoids and possibly water-soluble polysaccharides were suggested to be implicated in modulation of the adaptive immune response.

Adaptive immune responses can be broadly classified as resulting from one of two pathways; T helper (Th) 1 and Th2 responses which produce their particular characteristic cytokines and antibody subtypes for dealing with different types of infectious organisms. Both pathways were affected by consumption of the gold kiwifruit puree, when investigated using the

C57Bl/6 murine model described earlier. Mice fed the puree produced higher levels of IgG1, which is effective at fixing complement and dealing with bacterial and viral infections, and interleukin (IL) 5, indicating a predominantly Th2-type response (Skinner et al., 2007). However, the mice also produced higher levels of IgG2c and IgG2b antibodies, typical of a Th1-type response, suggesting a general stimulation of the humoral response.

Imbalance of immune pathways toward a predominant Th2-type response has been implicated in the onset of some allergic responses and hyperresponsiveness. Extracts of dried fruit of *A. arguta* have shown promise as antiallergenic agents. In an OVA-sensitized mouse model that promotes a Th2-type response, feeding with the kiwifruit extracts was shown to decrease significantly the Th2 and increase Th1 cytokines and antibodies (Park et al., 2005). Consumption of the extracts downregulated the GATA-binding protein 3 (GATA-3) and induced T-box transcription factor (T-bet), transcription factors that control the differentiation of Th1 and Th2 cells. The potential of *A. arguta* fruit extracts as orally active immune modulators for the therapy of allergic diseases was further tested using a mouse model for atopic dermatitis, a chronic inflammatory skin disease (Park et al., 2007). The extracts reduced the severity of the dermatitis induced in NC/Nga mice. There was an associated decrease in plasma IgE, IgG1, and IL-4 levels, and an increase in IgG2a and IL-12.

Bronchial asthma is a chronic inflammatory disease in which there is relative overproduction of Th2 cytokines relative to Th1 cytokines, and one of the causes is accumulation of eosinophils in airways, resulting in symptoms like wheezing, coughing, and shortness of breath (Lee et al., 2006). Induced bronchial inflammation in mice was reduced by feeding with extracts of *A. polygama* fruit, which appeared to have both anti-inflammatory and antiasthmatic activities. Accumulation of eosinophils into airways and the levels of IL-4, IL-5, IL-13, and IgE in bronchoalveolar lavage fluid were reduced (Lee et al., 2006). Although the active compound in *A. polygama* was not identified, a human study indicates that intake of fruits rich in vitamin C (citrus fruit and kiwifruit) reduced wheezing, and even eating the fruits as infrequently as once a week was found to alleviate symptoms (Forastiere et al., 2000). Fruit of *A. polygama* can contain about the same concentration of vitamin C as 'Hayward' fruit (Ferguson and MacRae, 1992).

Traditionally, *A. polygama* fruit have been used to treat rheumatic diseases and inflammation (Kim et al., 2003). Extracts of *A. polygama* fruit were shown to inhibit acute inflammation and reduce edema formation in the carrageenan-induced hind paw edema model in rats (Kim et al., 2003), a model considered to predict reliably the efficacy of orally active anti-inflammatory agents. *In vitro* assays indicated that the anti-inflammatory activity was due to reduced expression of inducible nitric oxide synthase (*i*NOS) and cyclooxygenase 2 (COX-2) (Kim et al., 2003). The active agent was identified as α-linolenic acid (Ren and Chung, 2007), which acts by downregulating enzymes such as *i*NOS and COX-2 and expression of the inflammatory cytokine tumor necrosis factor-α (TNF-α) through blocking of the nuclear factor NF-κB. NF-κB is involved in the regulation of transcription of many genes involved in inflammation and its inhibition offers promising therapeutic possibilities for treatment of rheumatoid arthritis and inflammatory bowel disease (IBD), including Crohn's disease. Interestingly, both water and ethyl acetate extracts of kiwifruit ('Hayward' and 'Hort16A') exhibited anti-inflammatory activity in a model of IBD using IL-10 gene deficient mice (Edmunds et al., 2011). Inhibition of TNF-α production was also achieved by the same aqueous extracts ('Hayward' or 'Hort16A') in human monocyte cultured cells (THP-1 cells) or peripheral whole blood cells, stimulated with lipopolysaccharide or IL-1β (Farr et al., 2007). Recent results related to maintenance of gut epithelial cell integrity have demonstrated that fermentable products from green and gold kiwifruit can protect Caco-2 cell integrity from a proinflammatory insult (Skinner et al., 2013). These encouraging results suggest that kiwifruit consumption may play a potential role in preventing barrier damage such as that associated with IBD. Overall, these results demonstrate the potential anti-inflammatory properties of kiwifruit in general.

There have been few human intervention trials that have attempted to provide evidence that kiwifruit consumption can positively modulate the immune system. In an attempt to provide evidence, a novel technique "scored human immunological vigor" (SIV) was used to determine the effect of kiwifruit consumption on the immune system in individuals who were feeling fatigued on a daily basis. SIV was derived from numbers of T lymphocytes in blood and various markers of their activity (numbers of $CD8^+$ $CD28^+$ T cells; the ratio of $CD4^+$ $CD8^+$ T cells; numbers of naïve T cells; the ratio of naïve to memory T cells in the blood and T lymphocyte age). Consumption of three gold kiwifruit, banana, or a vitamin C supplement that contained the same amount of vitamin C as the kiwifruit per day for 4 weeks was compared. Consumption of kiwifruit resulted in an increase in the numbers of naïve T cells, the numbers of $CD8^+$ T cells and their activation state ($CD8^+$ $CD28^+$) compared to baseline values and there was a significant reduction in the age of T lymphocytes. There was also a low (4.3%) nonsignificant rise in SIV associated with kiwifruit consumption. None of these changes were associated with banana or vitamin C consumption. In addition subjects who consumed kiwifruit reported significantly less fatigue, better skin condition, improved bowel motions, and less eye fatigue (Skinner et al., 2013). These results suggested that consumption of three gold kiwifruit per day delivering 390 mg/day of vitamin C together with other compounds that modulate the function of the immune system (ie, carotenoids, polyphenols, and polysaccharides) could modulate markers of immune function, which might result in increased immunological vigor and decrease in T cell age. Supplementation with a similar dose of vitamin C alone had no effect, suggesting that vitamin C consumed from gold kiwifruit was more beneficial than vitamin C taken as a supplement.

Segments of the population that may have a weakened or suppressed immune system include pregnant women, athletes, students before exams, people with chronic health conditions, the young and the aged, and they are particularly susceptible to upper respiratory tract infections. Recent evidence suggests that fruit, vegetable (Li and Werler, 2010; Roll et al., 2011), and tea consumption (Rowe et al., 2007) can reduce the symptoms and incidence of colds and flu. Two randomized crossover studies demonstrated that consumption of gold kiwifruit ('Hort16A') reduced symptoms of colds and flu and their severity in two "at risk" populations, older adults aged 65 years or over (Hunter et al., 2012) and preschool children aged 2–5 years (Skinner, 2012). In the study of older adults, 32 participants consumed two fresh and two freeze-dried kiwifruit or two freeze-dried bananas per day for 4 weeks. When participants recorded symptoms of cold and flu there were two symptoms, sore throat and head congestion, which people had for significantly fewer days when they ate kiwifruit compared with banana. Consumption of gold kiwifruit compared with banana led to significantly higher concentrations of plasma vitamin C, α-tocopherol and lutein/zeaxanthin, which may have contributed to the reduced duration and severity of those symptoms (Hunter et al., 2012). In the study with 66 preschool children, the overall incidence of a cold or flu-like illness was considerably reduced when children ate two servings of kiwifruit compared with banana (5 days per week for 4 weeks). The odds ratio of having a cold or flu-like illness was 0.55 when kiwifruit was consumed compared with banana, which means that the children had almost a 50% reduction in the chance of having a cold or flu when they ate kiwifruit. When individual symptoms were analyzed, there were significant improvements in a number of symptoms. Children had a better appetite, did not feel so unwell, had more energy, cried less and suffered less from headaches and sore throats (Skinner, 2012). The reduction in these last two symptoms is in agreement with the reduced head congestion and sore throat symptoms observed in the study with the older adults (Hunter et al., 2012). In summary, individuals and segments of the population that have a weakened immune system owing to stress, age, or health status may benefit from kiwifruit consumption.

Cardiovascular disease

Modification of the diet by increased consumption of fruit and vegetables has been associated with reduced risk of CVD (Miura et al., 2004; Lauretani et al., 2008). The result is decreased mortality from CVD and also reduced risk of ischemic stroke (Miura et al., 2004; Shirosaki et al., 2008). This has been ascribed to phytochemicals in fruit and vegetables such as carotenoids, flavonoids, polyphenols, and other antioxidants (Shirosaki et al., 2008; Deters et al., 2005; Emsaillzadeh and Azadbakht, 2008). The antioxidant capacity of kiwifruit (Hunter et al., 2011) suggests that they could contribute to reduced risk of CVD. Kiwifruit might also help protect against arteriosclerosis, a complex disorder involving cholesterol oxidation, intracellular accumulation of oxidized cholesterol, raised blood pressure and platelet aggregation.

Crude ethanolic and aqueous extracts of kiwifruit (probably 'Hayward') have been shown to have antioxidant, antihypertensive, and to a lesser degree hypocholesterolemic and fibrinolytic activity using *in vitro* assays (Jung et al., 2005). Confirmation of the antioxidant activity of kiwifruit suggests that consumption of kiwifruit could reduce oxidation of cholesterol, thereby lowering the formation of atherosclerotic lesions. Antihypertensive activity was assessed by inhibition of angiotensin I-converting enzyme, ACE (Jung et al., 2005), which is important in regulation of blood pressure. There is increasing interest in the possibility of reducing hypertension through ACE inhibitors in food. Hypocholesterolemic activity was assayed by inhibition of 3-hydroxy-3-methyl-glutaryl coenzyme A (HMG-CoA), a key enzyme in the biosynthesis of cholesterol. Kiwifruit extracts were only weak inhibitors (Jung et al., 2005). The extracts also mildly stimulated fibrinolytic activity. Fibrinolysis is the process by which fibrin in blood clots is dissolved, and increased fibrinolytic activity is associated with a reduced risk of thromboembolic and cardiovascular diseases.

In vivo tests with mice and clinical trials with participants diagnosed with moderate dyslipidemia could indicate that kiwifruit have potential as cardiovascular protectants. A fruit extract prepared from hawthorn (*Crataegus pinnatifida*) and kiwifruit resulted in a significant reduction in blood triglycerides and low-density lipoprotein cholesterol (Xu et al., 2009; Sun et al., 2012). How much of this effect can be attributed to kiwifruit is unknown however; much of it may well have been due to the hawthorn, a Chinese medicine widely used for cardiac disorders.

The effects of kiwifruit consumption on hypertension and dyslipidemia have also been tested in other human trials. Karlsen et al. (2013) found that consumption of green kiwifruit resulted in a small but significant reduction in diastolic and systolic blood pressure in male smokers, the effect being strongest in those with hypertension. However, Gammon et al. (Gammon et al., 2013, 2014) concluded that there were no beneficial effects on blood pressure of nonhypertensive subjects consuming two kiwifruit a day against the background of a healthy diet. On the other hand, in subjects that were hypercholesterolemic kiwifruit consumption did have a favorable effect on plasma high-density lipoprotein cholesterol (HDL-C) concentrations and the total cholesterol (TC):HDL-C ratio (Gammon et al., 2013). These results support the earlier findings that kiwifruit consumption increased HDL-C and decreased the TC:HDL-C ratio (Chang and Liu, 2009) and decreased the plasma triglyceride concentrations (Brevik et al., 2011; Duttaroy and Jørgensen, 2004). This response to kiwifruit consumption appeared to be related to the genetic makeup of the subjects (Gammon et al., 2014).

Adhesion and aggregation of platelets at injury sites in atherosclerotic vessel walls is very important in the pathogenesis of CVD (Duttaroy, 2007). Drugs such as aspirin are commonly used to inhibit platelet aggregation, and treatment with aspirin reduces heart attacks, strokes, and death. However, aspirin has only relatively weak antiplatelet activity and, moreover, can cause serious side effects in some patients. *In vitro* data suggest that natural products, including fruit, may also inhibit platelets by a different mechanism with tomatoes and kiwifruit having particularly high inhibitory activity (Duttaroy, 2007). This has been confirmed in human trials where the consumption of two or three kiwifruit per day by healthy volunteers inhibited platelet aggregation (Duttaroy and Jørgensen, 2004). Somewhat equivocal results were obtained in a trial with consumption of one or two gold kiwifruit ('Hort16A') (Brevik et al., 2011; Stonehouse et al., 2013).

These results indicate that kiwifruit have potential as cardiovascular protectants through various mechanisms and although some effects observed were relatively minor, cumulatively they may represent a significant reduction in overall risk (Duttaroy and Jørgensen, 2004). However, it is important to acknowledge the limitations of *in vitro* studies, and the *in vivo* effects of kiwifruit consumption depend on the absorption and metabolism of bioactives in the fruit. Diet–gene interactions might also influence the outcomes. It is also unwise to extrapolate results obtained with one kiwifruit variety to others.

Other health benefits from kiwifruit

In addition to the "mainstream" health targets commonly used to define the benefits from functional foods and fruits, a small number of studies demonstrate more novel bioactive effects of kiwifruit.

Sleep

Many adults have difficulty in falling asleep or staying asleep, and their disturbed sleep can impair daytime functioning. Chronic insomnia may also lead to an increased risk of depression and overuse of hypnotic medications. Treatments that improve sleep quality but avoid the use of prescription medicines could therefore be of considerable benefit. Many insomniacs prefer "natural" sleep aids, foods, or extracts of medicinal plants, because it is considered that they have fewer adverse effects and do not require prescriptions. Consumption of 'Hayward' kiwifruit in the evening has been shown to improve sleep onset, duration, and efficiency in adults with self-reported sleep disturbances (Lin et al., 2011). The authors recommended that further research into the sleep-promoting properties of kiwifruit be undertaken. The mechanisms behind these effects have yet to be clarified (Peuhkuri et al., 2012). Possible constituents of kiwifruit that might improve sleep quality include the high concentrations of antioxidants such as vitamin C, serotonin, and folate. Experiments with mice indicate that flavonoids in the skin of both green ('Hayward') and gold ('Hort16A') kiwifruit have sleep-inducing qualities (Yang et al., 2013), but as kiwifruit skins are not normally consumed, these benefits, if effective in humans, would depend on kiwifruit processing.

Wound healing and skin

Evidence is emerging that demonstrates efficacy of kiwifruit as a wound healing and dermatological agent. Debridement, the process of removing dead tissue from wounds, is an important part of wound healing and may be achieved via surgical, mechanical, autolytic, biological, or enzymatic means. Application of kiwifruit flesh slices to burns has been shown to improve the healing process. Using a rat model, average time of debridement of necrotic tissue from full-thickness burns was significantly shorter when the wound was covered with kiwifruit flesh slices, compared with wounds where no treatment agent or fibrinolysin treatment was applied (Kooshiar et al., 2012). As well as demonstrating a significant reduction in the surface area of deep second-degree burns, and a significantly shorter time to healing completely in wounds treated with kiwifruit, Mohajeri et al. (2010) also reported considerable antibacterial activity from the kiwifruit treatment. Among the rats treated with kiwifruit, no positive cultures for *Pseudomonas*, *Streptococci*, or *Staphylococcus* were detected, compared with their presence in two to four rats treated with a Vaseline® control and one to two rats treated with sulfadiazine cream ($n = 20$ per treatment). Neither study reported the type of kiwifruit used, but it was probably 'Hayward,' given that the presence of proteolytic enzymes in kiwifruit was implicated in the improved wound healing by both groups of authors. Suggestions that kiwifruit dressings, in this case of *A. deliciosa*, would be helpful in other wounds involving necrotic tissue, such as pressure sores and diabetic wounds, were also made, and some evidence to support this has since been reported (Mohajeri et al., 2014).

Other dermatological activities from kiwifruit have also been demonstrated, although only using *in vitro* models. Polysaccharide extracts from *A. chinensis* stimulated proliferation of primary human keratinocyte, and fibroblast cells *in vitro*, and also promoted collagen synthesis within stable dermal equivalents (Deters et al., 2005). In addition, an extract from the skin of *A. chinensis* 'Hort16A' inhibited the formation of advanced glycoxidation endproducts (AGEs) *in vitro* (Lee et al., 2011). In the skin, AGEs are formed when blood sugar reacts with protein such as collagen, leading to a degradation of collagen and, therefore, aging. Taken together, these studies suggest kiwifruit have potential as dermatological agents, but *in vivo* evidence to support this is lacking.

Diabetes

The glycemic index (GI) is used to indicate the extent to which a food raises blood sugar levels after eating, with a high GI value indicating rapid digestion and absorption, and hence a large fluctuation in blood sugar levels. Low GI foods produce gradual rises in blood sugar and insulin levels, and have been shown to benefit people with diabetes (The University of Sydney, 2011). In a detailed examination of the carbohydrate availability and glycemic impact of kiwifruit, Monro (2013) reported a discrepancy between the calculated GI value and the measured GI value of kiwifruit, with the measured GI value being lower than that calculated. Any factors that reduce the rate at which carbohydrate is absorbed will reduce the glycemic response. Using an *in vitro* model of digestion, peristalsis and diffusion, Monro (2013) demonstrated that the digestion-resistant residue of kiwifruit, provided by the cell wall component, swells to four times its original volume during digestion and, once settled, reduces mixing and the rate of glucose diffusion by approximately 40%. The conclusion is that kiwifruit may be considered to have a low glycemic impact, and hence, be suitable for diabetics.

In addition to kiwifruit simply being a suitable food for diabetics, *in vitro* studies suggest that kiwifruit may contain bioactive compounds that influence processes involved in diabetes. Adipocyte dysfunction is associated with the development of insulin resistance and diabetes; adipocytes ordinarily express and secrete adipocytokines such as adiponectin, which increases insulin sensitivity and inhibits inflammatory processes (Abe et al., 2010; Díez and Iglesias, 2003). A methanol fraction from an unripe kiwifruit extract (*A. deliciosa* 'Kouryoku') promoted differentiation of a preadipocyte cell line (3T3-L1), also enhancing the mRNA expression levels of peroxisome proliferator-activated receptor γ (PPARγ), which regulates adiponectin gene transcription, and hence enhanced expression levels of adiponectin mRNA and protein (Abe et al., 2010). Furthermore, this kiwifruit extract reduced mRNA expression and secretion of proinflammatory adipocytokines, interleukin 6 (IL-6), and monocyte chemoattractive protein-1 (MCP-1), which are induced by insulin resistance. Using a skeletal muscle cell model, Kim et al. (2013) also demonstrated activity reducing insulin resistance by a kiwifruit extract. A methanol extract from *A. chinensis* 'Halla Gold' significantly reduced phosphorylation of Akt (also known as protein kinase B) and glycogen synthase kinase-3, and significantly increased phosphorylation of glycogen synthase in L6 rat skeletal muscle cells under a condition of insulin resistance induced by exposure to chronic insulin. In this model, glucose consumption and glucose transporter 4 translocation to the plasma membrane were also inhibited by the 'Halla Gold' extract. In each instance, these changes tended to restore conditions to those observed in cells treated with a single dose of insulin, which simulated responses that typically occur in a noninsulin-resistant situation. Taken together, these studies suggest that kiwifruit may have potential in reducing insulin resistance and hence, eventual onset of type-2 diabetes. Again, there is no evidence of such potential *in vivo* with kiwifruit or a kiwifruit-derived product, and the potential benefit of kiwifruit at this time should not be overstated.

Kiwifruit allergies and other detrimental health effects

As kiwifruit consumption has become more common around the world, so too has the incidence of kiwifruit allergy. Allergic responses to kiwifruit range from localized oral allergy syndrome to life threatening anaphylaxis (Lucas et al., 2003; Bublin, 2013) and are often associated with allergic responses to birch (*Betula*) and grass pollen as well as with responses to natural rubber latex. Several clinical subgroups have been identified (Alemán et al., 2004), and while the allergenicity of kiwifruit is not in doubt, it is currently ill defined and poorly understood (Lucas et al., 2007; Lucas and Atkinson, 2008). Eleven allergens from *A. deliciosa* 'Hayward' have been identified and three from *A. chinensis* 'Hort16A' (Bublin, 2013) but whether these identifications are justified has been challenged (Lucas and Atkinson, 2008). Three of the allergens identified, actinidin, thaumatin-like protein, and kiwellin, are proteins often present in kiwifruit in large amounts and their identification as allergens may simply reflect this abundance, rather than their allergenicity (Lucas and Atkinson, 2008). Actinidin content and protease activity, thaumatin-like protein content and kiwellin content vary in different *Actinidia* species or genotypes (Maddumage et al., 2013). For example, fruit of some *A. arguta* cultivars contain more actinidin than *A. deliciosa* 'Hayward,' whereas actinidin and protease activity were not detectable or barely detectable in two *A. rufa* selections (Nishiyama et al., 2004a) and some *A. chinensis* cultivars, including 'Hort16A' (Bublin et al., 2004). Further work on kiwifruit allergens is required as future commercial kiwifruit cultivars should preferably be less allergenic than the cultivars now available.

Kiwifruit contain small amounts of oxalate, and this is commonly associated with the "catch" in the throat sometimes experienced when fresh kiwifruit and especially processed kiwifruit products are eaten (Perera et al., 1990; Walker and Prescott, 2003). This irritant effect could result from a synergism between calcium oxalate and the protease, actinidin, in the fruit (Konno et al., 2014). Oxalate is present in fruit of cultivars of *A. deliciosa* (eg, 'Hayward') as insoluble, fine needle-like, calcium oxalate raphide crystals (Perera et al., 1990), but in other *Actinidia* species the crystal shape varies (Watanabe and Takahashi, 1998). Estimation of oxalate content is difficult (McGhie, 2013) and the total concentrations in kiwifruit are low: fruit of *A. chinensis* contain 18–45 mg/100 g fresh weight (Drummond, 2013), similar to levels in mature fruit of *A. deliciosa* and *A. eriantha* (Rassam and Laing, 2005). High dietary intake of oxalate may be a major risk factor for calcium oxalate kidney stone formation (Siener et al., 2006), and oxalate consumption also has an antinutritional effect, reducing the bioavailability of Ca^{2+}, Mg^{2+}, and Fe^{2+} (Massey, 2003). Normal dietary intake of oxalate is estimated to be 50–200 mg/day (Siener et al., 2006), and other foods, such as spinach, have considerably higher levels of total oxalate (1959 mg/100 g fresh weight) (Siener et al., 2006) than kiwifruit. Although kiwifruit contain oxalate, the amount is most likely not of concern to healthy individuals who maintain a well-balanced diet; the effect of oxalate raphides on kiwifruit palatability is probably more significant.

Some of the phytochemicals in kiwifruit may also have harmful physiological activities. For example, aqueous ethanol extracts of kiwifruit (probably 'Hayward') decreased sperm quality in rats. As a consequence, men with infertility or reproductive problems have been advised to abstain from eating kiwifruit (Panjeh-Shahin et al., 2005). It is ironic that some advertising campaigns have previously promoted kiwifruit for their libido enhancement.

CONCLUSION

Dietitians along with other health professionals have the responsibility of providing consumers with scientifically supported knowledge to help them make informed dietary decisions. The scientific information supporting the unique health benefits of kiwifruit is growing rapidly. Evidence from *in vitro* cell studies and animal models of health and disease indicates health benefits of kiwifruit in a number of target health areas. Such evidence must be validated by human intervention trials.

Two intervention trials have been described that provide evidence for improved oxidation status of the blood after consumption of kiwifruit, with subsequent studies reporting greater resistance to DNA oxidation from isolated cells following an *ex vivo* challenge, reduced endogenous DNA damage, and upregulation of genes associated with DNA repair. However, it is currently not clear how this influences the health of the individual. Oxidative stress may play a role in the pathogenesis of CVD, the leading cause of death in developed countries. Protection from DNA damage may also help prevent mutagenesis and cancer. However, there is no evidence to support the use of antioxidant supplements to prevent mortality in healthy subjects or patients with various diseases (Bjelakovic et al., 2012). It remains to be proven whether the antioxidant activity provided as a result of regular consumption of kiwifruit improves health outcomes in the long term for aging, but otherwise healthy subjects.

One intervention trial provided evidence for decreased platelet aggregation after consumption of green kiwifruit (Duttaroy and Jørgensen, 2004), and others indicated an improvement in blood pressure, particularly in hypertensive subjects (Karlsen et al., 2013), and improvement in HDL-C, reduction in the TC:HDL-D ratio (Chang and Liu, 2009; Gammon et al., 2013), and reduction in plasma triglyceride concentrations (Brevik et al., 2011; Duttaroy and Jørgensen, 2004). Collectively, regular kiwifruit consumption could result in an alteration in the natural course of atherosclerosis and reduce the risk of coronary arteriole disease, myocardial infarction, and stroke.

The strongest evidence for a health benefit of kiwifruit is in the area of intestinal wellbeing. Intestinal wellbeing is an ill-defined state often equated with an absence of symptoms. Bowel habit is a useful overall biomarker of gut function, particularly colonic function. Kiwifruit have been shown in intervention trials to contribute to gastrointestinal wellbeing by their positive effects on laxation in targeted groups of subjects: the elderly (Rush et al., 2002), those suffering from constipation (Chan et al., 2007), and those suffering from irritable bowel syndrome with constipation (Chang et al., 2010).

Building on the many *in vitro* and animal studies demonstrating that kiwifruit modulates numerous aspects of immune function, the benefit of regular kiwifruit consumption to immune function and recovery from colds and flu in humans, particularly those who may have weakened immune systems, is being realized. Human intervention studies suggest that regular consumption of 2–4 gold kiwifruit per day may reduce the feeling of fatigue (Skinner et al., 2013; Skinner, 2012) and reduce the length of time that symptoms of sore throat, head ache, and congestion are present when people are suffering from cold or flu-like symptoms (Hunter et al., 2012; Skinner, 2012). There is some evidence that these benefits extend beyond simply the vitamin C content of the fruit (Skinner et al., 2013).

A diet rich in fruits and vegetables offers health and wellness benefits that go beyond basic nutrition (Leenders et al., 2014; Okuda et al., 2015; He et al., 2006, 2007). Consumption of green kiwifruit ('Hayward') contributes by having positive effects on cardiovascular and gut health. As supporting evidence accumulates for other cultivars, it can be used to justify progression to human intervention trials. Validation of health claims that might be made about kiwifruit in the future may be based on consumption of the whole fruit, when the fruit is palatable, or processed functional products, when the fruit is not palatable (eg, *A. polygama*). As the potential benefit of kiwifruit consumption continues to be researched, in the future we can look forward to further ways that kiwifruit will contribute to our health.

REFERENCES

Abe, D., Saito, T., Kubo, Y., Nakamura, Y., Sekiya, K., 2010. A fraction of unripe kiwi fruit extract regulates adipocyte differentiation and function in 3T3-L1 cells. Biofactors 36, 52–59.

Albers, R., Antoine, J.-M., Bourdet-Sicard, R., Calder, P.C., Gleeson, M., Lesourd, B., et al., 2005. Markers to measure immunomodulation in human nutrition intervention studies. Br. J. Nutr. 94, 452–481.

Alemán, A., Sastre, J., Quirce, S., de las Heras, M., Carnés, J., Fernández-Caldas, E., et al., 2004. Allergy to kiwi: a double-blind, placebo-controlled food challenge study in patients from a birch-free area. J. Allergy Clin. Immunol. 113, 543–550.

Ansell, J., Butts, C.A., Paturi, G., Eady, S.L., Wallace, A.J., Hedderley, D., et al., 2015. Kiwifruit-derived supplements increase stool frequency in healthy adults: a randomized, double-blind, placebo-controlled study. Nutr. Res. 35, 401–408.

Ansell, J., Parkar, S., Paturi, G., Rosendale, D., Blatchford, P., 2013. Modification of the colonic microbiota. Adv. Food. Nutr. Res. 68, 205–217.

Bartsch, H., Ohshima, H., Pignatelli, B., 1988. Inhibitors of endogenous nitrosation mechanisms and implications in human cancer prevention. Mutat. Res-Fund. Mol. M. 202, 307–324.

Basile, A., Vuotto, M.L., Violante, U., Sorbo, S., Martone, G., Castaldo-Cobianchi, R., 1997. Antibacterial activity in *Actinidia chinensis*, *Feijoa sellowiana* and *Aberia caffra*. Int. J. Antimicrob. Agents. 8, 199–203.

Belrose, Inc., 2014. World Kiwifruit Review 2014. Belrose, Inc., Pullman.

Bentley-Hewitt, K.L., Blatchford, P.A., Parkar, S.G., Ansell, J., Pernthaner, A., 2012. Digested and fermented green kiwifruit increases human β-defensin 1 and 2 production *in vitro*. Plant Food Hum. Nutr. 67, 208–214.

Bjelakovic, G., Nikolova, D., Gluud Lise, L., Simonetti, R.G., Gluud, C., 2012. Antioxidant supplements for prevention of mortality in healthy participants and patients with various diseases. Cochrane Database Syst. Rev. 3, 1–288.

Bohn, S.K., Myhrstad, M.C., Thoresen, M., Holden, M., Karlsen, A., Tunheim, S.H., et al., 2010. Blood cell gene expression associated with cellular stress defense is modulated by antioxidant-rich food in a randomised controlled clinical trial of male smokers. BMC Med. 8, 54.

Brevik, A., Gaivão, I., Medin, T., Jørgenesen, A., Piasek, A., Elilasson, J., et al., 2011. Supplementation of a western diet with golden kiwifruits (*Actinidia chinensis* var. 'Hort 16A'): effects on biomarkers of oxidation damage and antioxidant protection. Nutr. J. 10, 54.

Brieger, K., Schiavone, S., Miller Jr., F.J., Krause, K.-H., 2012. Reactive oxygen species: from health to disease. Swiss. Med. Wkly. 142, w13659.

Bublin, M., 2013. Kiwifruit allergies. Adv. Food. Nutr. Res. 68, 321–340.

Bublin, M., Mari, A., Ebner, C., Knulst, A., Scheiner, O., Hoffmann-Sommergruber, K., et al., 2004. IgE sensitization profiles toward green and gold kiwifruits differ among patients allergic to kiwifruit from 3 European countries. J. Allergy Clin. Immunol. 114, 1169–1175.

Bunzel, M., Ralph, J., 2006. NMR characterization of lignins isolated from fruit and vegetable insoluble dietary fiber. J. Agric. Food. Chem. 54, 8352–8361.

Calder, P.C., Kew, S., 2002. The immune system: a target for functional foods? Br. J. Nutr. 88 (Suppl. 2), S165–S176.

Cederlund, A., Gudmundsson, G.H., Agerberth, B., 2011. Antimicrobial peptides important in innate immunity. FEBS J. 278, 3942–3951.

Chan, A.O.O., Leung, G., Tong, T., Wong, N.Y.H., 2007. Increasing dietary fiber intake in terms of kiwifruit improves constipation in chinese patients. World J. Gastroenterol. 13, 4771–4775.

Chang, C.-C., Lin, Y.-T., Lu, Y.-T., Liu, Y.-S., Liu, J.-F., 2010. Kiwifruit improves bowel function in patients with irritable bowel syndrome with constipation. Asia. Pac. J. Clin. Nutr. 19, 451–457.

Chang, R., 2002. Bioactive polysaccharides from traditional chinese medicine herbs as anticancer adjuvants. J. Altern. Complement. Med. 8, 559–565.

Chang, W.-H., Liu, J.-F., 2009. Effects of kiwifruit consumption on serum lipid profiles and antioxidative status in hyperlipidemic subjects. Int. J. Food. Sci. Nutr. 60, 709–716.

Chun, O.K., Kim, D.-O., Smith, N., Schroeder, D., Han, J.T., Lee, C.Y., 2005. Daily consumption of phenolics and total antioxidant capacity from fruit and vegetables in the American diet. J. Sci. Food. Agric. 85, 1715–1724.

Ciacci, C., Russo, I., Bucci, C., Iovino, P., Pellegrini, L., Giangrieco, I., et al., 2014. The kiwi fruit peptide kissper displays anti-inflammatory and anti-oxidant effects in *in-vitro* and *ex-vivo* human intestinal models. Clin. Exp. Immunol. 175, 476–484.

Ciardiello, M.A., Meleleo, D., Saviano, G., Crescenzo, R., Carratore, V., Camardella, L., et al., 2008. Kissper, a kiwi fruit peptide with channel-like activity: structural and functional features. J. Pept. Sci. 14, 742–754.

Collins, A.R., 2013. Kiwifruit as a modulator of DNA damage and DNA repair. Adv. Food. Nutr. Res. 68, 283–299.

Collins, A.R., Gaivão, I., 2007. DNA base excision repair as a biomarker in molecular epidemiology studies. Mol. Aspects Med. 28, 307–322.

Colonna-Romano, G., Potestio, M., Aquino, A., Candore, G., Lio, D., Caruso, C., 2002. Gamma/delta T lymphocytes are affected in the elderly. Exp. Gerontol. 37, 205–211.

Crawford, K., Mellentin, J., 2008. Successful Superfruit Strategy: How to Build a Superfruit Business. Woodhead Publishing, Cambridge.

Cser, M.A., Majchrzak, D., Rust, P., Sziklai-László, I., Kovács, I., Bocskai, E., et al., 2004. Serum carotenoid and retinol levels during childhood infections. Ann. Nutr. Metab. 48, 156–162.

Cummings, J.H., Antoine, J.-M., Azpiroz, F., Bourdet-Sicard, R., Brandtzaeg, P., Calder, P.C., et al., 2004. PASSCLAIM—Gut health and immunity. Eur. J. Nutr. 43 (Suppl. 2), II/118–II/173.

Dawes, H.M., Keene, J.B., 1999. Phenolic composition of kiwifruit juice. J. Agric. Food. Chem. 47, 2398–2403.

Deters, A.M., Schröder, K.R., Hensel, A., 2005. Kiwi fruit (*Actinidia chinensis* L.) polysaccharides exert stimulating effects on cell proliferation via enhanced growth factor receptors, energy production, and collagen synthesis of human keratinocytes, fibroblasts, and skin equivalents. J. Cell. Physiol. 202, 717–722.

Díez, J.J., Iglesias, P., 2003. The role of the novel adipocyte-derived hormone adiponectin in human disease. Eur. J. Endocrinol. 148, 293–300.

Drummond, L., 2013. The composition and nutritional value of kiwifruit. Adv. Food. Nutr. Res. 68, 33–57.

Du, G., Li, M., Ma, F., Liang, D., 2009. Antioxidant capacity and the relationship with polyphenol and vitamin C in *Actinidia* fruits. Food. Chem. 113, 557–562.

Duttaroy, A.K., 2007. Kiwifruits and cardiovascular health. Acta. Hortic. 753, 819–824.

Duttaroy, A.K., Jørgensen, A., 2004. Effects of kiwi fruit consumption on platelet aggregation and plasma lipids in healthy human volunteers. Platelets 15, 287–292.

Edmunds, S.J., Roy, N.C., Love, D.R., Laing, W.A., 2011. Kiwifruit extracts inhibit cytokine production by lipopolysaccharide-activated macrophages, and intestinal epithelial cells isolated from IL10 gene deficient mice. Cell. Immunol. 270, 70–79.

Emsaillzadeh, A., Azadbakht, L., 2008. Dietary flavonoid intake and cardiovascular mortality. Br. J. Nutr. 100, 695–697.

Farr, J.M., Hurst, S.M., Skinner, M.A., 2007. Anti-inflammatory effects of kiwifruit. Proc. Nutr. Soc. N. Z. 32, 20–25.

Ferguson, A.R., 1990. The kiwifruit in China. In: Warrington, I.J., Weston, G.C. (Eds.), Kiwifruit: Science and Management Ray Richards Publisher & New Zealand Society for Horticultural Science, Auckland, pp. 155–164.

Ferguson, A.R., 2015. Kiwifruit in the world – 2014 Acta. Hortic. 1096, 33–46.

Ferguson, A.R., Ferguson, L.R., 2003. Are kiwifruit really good for you? Acta. Hortic. 610, 131–138.

Ferguson, A.R., Huang, H., 2007. Genetic resources of kiwifruit: domestication and breeding. Hortic. Rev. 33, 1–121.

Ferguson, A.R., MacRae, E.A., 1992. Vitamin C in *Actinidia*. Acta. Hortic. 297, 481–487.

Ferguson, L.R., Philpott, M., Karunasinghe, N., 2004. Dietary cancer and prevention using antimutagens. Toxicology 198, 147–159.

Forastiere, F., Pistelli, R., Sestini, P., Fortes, C., Renzoni, E., Rusconi, F., et al., 2000. Consumption of fresh fruit rich in vitamin C and wheezing symptoms in children. Thorax 55, 283–288.

Fourie, P.C., Hansmann, C.F., 1992. Fruit composition of four South African-grown kiwifruit cultivars. N. Z. J. Crop Hortic. Sci. 20, 449–452.

Funk, C., Braune, A., Grabber, J.H., Steinhart, H., Bunzel, M., 2007. Model studies of lignified fiber fermentation by human fecal microbiota and its impact on heterocyclic aromatic amine adsorption. Mutat. Res-Fund. Mol. M. 624, 41–48.

Gammon, C.S., Kruger, R., Brown, S.J., Conlon, C.A., von Hurst, P.R., Stonehouse, W., 2014. Daily kiwifruit consumption did not improve blood pressure and markers of cardiovascular function in men with hypercholesterolemia. Nutr. Res. 34, 235–240.

Gammon, C.S., Kruger, R., Minihane, A.M., Conlon, C.A., von Hurst, P.R., Stonehouse, W., 2013. Kiwifruit consumption favourably affects plasma lipids in a randomised controlled trial in hypercholesterolaemic men. Br. J. Nutr. 109, 2208–2218.

Gammon, C.S., Minihane, A.M., Kruger, R., Conlon, C.A., von Hurst, P.R., Jones, B., et al., 2014. *TaqIB* polymorphism in the cholesteryl ester transfer protein (*CETP*) gene influences lipid responses to the consumption of kiwifruit in hypercholesterolaemic men. Br. J. Nutr. 111, 1077–1084.

Gibson, G.R., Roberfroid, M.B., 1995. Dietary modulation of the human colonic microbiota: introducing the concept of prebiotics. J. Nutr. 125, 1401–1412.

Hallett, I.C., MacRae, E.A., Wegrzyn, T.F., 1992. Changes in kiwifruit cell wall ultrastructure and cell packing during postharvest ripening. Int. J. Plant. Sci. 153, 49–60.

He, F.J., Nowson, C.A., MacGregor, G.A., 2006. Fruit and vegetable consumption and stroke: meta-analysis of cohort studies. Lancet 367, 320–326.

He, F.J., Nowson, C.A., Lucas, M., MacGregor, G.A., 2007. Increased consumption of fruit and vegetables is related to a reduced risk of coronary heart disease: meta-analysis of cohort studies. J. Hum. Hypertens. 21, 717–728.

Huang, H., Wang, Y., Zhang, Z., Jiang, Z., Wang, S., 2004. *Actinidia* germplasm resources and kiwifruit industry in China. HortScience 39, 1165–1172.

Hunter, D.C., Denis, M., Parlane, N.A., Buddle, B.M., Stevenson, L.M., Skinner, M.A., 2008. Feeding ZESPRI™ GOLD kiwifruit puree to mice enhances serum immunoglobulins specific for ovalbumin and stimulates ovalbumin-specific mesenteric lymph node cell proliferation in response to orally administered ovalbumin. Nutr. Res. 28, 251–257.

Hunter, D.C., Greenwood, J., Zhang, J., Skinner, M.A., 2011. Antioxidant and "natural protective" properties of kiwifruit. Curr. Top. Med. Chem. 11, 1811–1820.

Hunter, D.C., Skinner, M.A., Wolber, F.M., Booth, C.L., Loh, J.M.S., Wohlers, M., et al., 2012. Consumption of gold kiwifruit reduces severity and duration of selected upper respiratory tract infection symptoms and increases plasma vitamin C concentration in healthy older adults. Br. J. Nutr. 108, 1235–1245.

Hunter, D.C., Zhang, J., Stevenson, L.M., Skinner, M.A., 2008. Fruit-based functional foods. II: The process for identifying potential ingredients. Int. J. Food Sci. Tech. 43, 2123–2129.

Ikken, Y., Morales, P., Martínez, A., Marin, M.L., Haza, A.I., Cambero, M.I., 1999. Antimutagenic effect of fruit and vegetable ethanolic extracts against *N*-nitrosamines evaluated by the Ames test. J. Agric. Food. Chem. 47, 3257–3264.

Iwasawa, H., Morita, E., Yui, S., Yamazaki, M., 2011. Anti-oxidant effects of kiwifruit *in vitro* and *in vivo*. Biol. Pharm. Bull. 34, 128–134.

Jin, D.E., Kim, H.J., Ji Hee, J., Yu Na, J., Kwon, O.-J., Choi, S.-G., et al., 2014. Nutritional components of Zespri green kiwi fruit (*Actinidia delicosa*) and neuronal cell protective effects of the *n*-hexane fraction. Korean J. Food Sci. Technol. 46, 369–374.

Jung, K.-A., Song, T.-C., Han, D.-S., Kim, I.-H., Kim, Y.-E., Lee, C.-H., 2005. Cardiovascular protective properties of kiwifruit extracts *in vitro*. Biol. Pharm. Bull. 28, 1782–1785.

Karlsen, A., Svendsen, M., Seljeflot, I., Laake, P., Duttaroy, A.K., Drevon, C.A., et al., 2013. Kiwifruit decreases blood pressure and whole-blood platelet aggregation in male smokers. J. Hum. Hypertens. 27, 126–130.

Kaur, L., Rutherfurd, S.M., Moughan, P.J., Drummond, L., Boland, M.J., 2010a. Actinidin enhances gastric protein digestion as assessed using an *in vitro* gastric digestion model. J. Agric. Food. Chem. 58, 5068–5073.

Kaur, L., Rutherfurd, S.M., Moughan, P.J., Drummond, L., Boland, M.J., 2010b. Actinidin enhances protein digestion in the small intestine as assessed using an *in vitro* digestion model. J. Agric. Food. Chem. 58, 5074–5080.

Kim, J.H., Kim, J.W., Kim, S.C., Lee, Y.J., 2013. Kiwifruit (*Actinidia chinensis*) extract annuls chronic insulininduced insulin resistance in L6 skeletal muscle cells. Food. Sci. Biotechnol. 22, 1091–1096.

Kim, Y.K., Kang, H.J., Lee, K.T., Choi, J.G., Chung, S.H., 2003. Anti-inflammation activity of *Actinidia polygama*. Arch. Pharm. Res. 26, 1061–1066.

Ko, S.-H., Choi, S.-W., Ye, S.-K., Cho, B.-L., Kim, H.-S., Chung, M.-H., 2005. Comparison of the antioxidant activities of nine different fruits in human plasma. J. Med. Food. 8, 41–46.

Konno, K., Inoue, T.A., Nakamura, M., 2014. Synergistic defensive function of raphides and protease through the needle effect. PLoS One 9, e91341.

Kooshiar, H., Abbaspour, H., Al Shariati, S.M.M., Rakhshandeh, H., Rad, A.K., Esmaily, H., et al., 2012. Topical effectiveness of kiwifruit versus fibrinolysin ointment on removal of necrotic tissue of full-thickness burns in male rats. Dermatol. Ther. 25, 621–625.

Kryston, T.B., Georgiev, A.B., Pissis, P., Georgakilas, A.G., 2011. Role of oxidative stress and DNA damage in human carcinogenesis. Mutat. Res-Fund. Mol. M. 711, 193–201.

Lauretani, F., Semba, R.D., Dayhoff-Brannigan, M., Corsi, A.M., Di Iorio, A., Buiatti, E., et al., 2008. Low total plasma carotenoids are independent predictors of mortality among older persons. The InCHIANTI study. Eur. J. Nutr. 47, 335–340.

Lee, D.E., Shin, B.J., Hur, H.J., Kim, J.H., Kim, J., Kang, N.J., et al., 2010. Quercetin, the active phenolic component in kiwifruit, prevents hydrogen peroxide-induced inhibition of gap-junction intercellular communication. Br. J. Nutr. 104, 164–170.

Lee, Y., Hong, C.-O., Nam, M.-H., Kim, J.-H., Ma, Y., Kim, Y.-B., et al., 2011. Antioxidant and glycation inhibitory activities of gold kiwifruit, *Actinidia chinensis*. J. Korean Soc. Appl. Bi 54, 460–467.

Lee, Y.-C., Kim, S.-H., Seo, Y.-B., Roh, S.-S., Lee, J.-C., 2006. Inhibitory effects of *Actinidia polygama* extract and cyclosporine A on OVA-induced eosinophilia and bronchial hyperresponsiveness in a murine model of asthma. Int. Immunopharmacol. 6, 703–713.

Leenders, M., Boshuizen, H.C., Ferrari, P., Siersema, P.D., Overvad, K., Tjønneland, A., et al., 2014. Fruit and vegetable intake and cause-specific mortality in the EPIC study. Eur. J. Epidemiol. 29, 639–652.

Li, J.-Q., Li, X.-W., Soejarto, D.D., 2007. Actinidiaceae. in flora of china. hippocastanaceae through theaceae. In: Wu, Z.-Y., Raven, P.H., Hong, D.-Y. (Eds.), Science Press, Beijing, pp. 334–360. Missouri Botanic Gardens Press, St Louis.

Li, L., Werler, M.M., 2010. Fruit and vegetable intake and risk of upper respiratory tract infection in pregnant women. Public. Health. Nutr. 13, 276–282.

Lim, Y.J., Oh, C.-S., Park, Y.-D., Kim, D.-O., Kim, U.-J., Cho, Y.-S., et al., 2014. Physiological components of kiwifruits with *in vitro* antioxidant and acetylcholinesterase inhibitory activities. Food. Sci. Biotechnol. 23, 943–949.

Lin, H.-H., Tsai, P.-S., Fang, S.-C., Liu, J.-F., 2011. Effect of kiwifruit consumption on sleep quality in adults with sleep problems. Asia. Pac. J. Clin. Nutr. 20, 169–174.

Lu, Y., Fan, J., Zhao, Y.-P., Chen, S.-Y., Zheng, X.-D., Yin, Y.-M., et al., 2007. Immunomodulatory activity of aqueous extract of *Actinidia macrosperma*. Asia. Pac. J. Clin. Nutr. 16 (Suppl. 1), 261–265.

Lu, Y., Zhao, Y.P., Wang, Z.C., Chen, S.Y., Fu, C.X., 2007. Composition and antimicrobial activity of the essential oil of *Actinidia macrosperma* from china. Nat. Prod. Res. 21, 227–233.

Lucas, J.S.A., Atkinson, R.G., 2008. What is a food allergen? Clin. Exp. Allergy 38, 1095–1099.

Lucas, J.S.A., Lewis, S.A., Hourihane, J.O.B., 2003. Kiwi fruit allergy: a review. Pediatr. Allergy Immunol. 14, 420–428.

Lucas, J.S.A., Nieuwenhuizen, N.J., Atkinson, R.G., MacRae, E.A., Cochrane, S.A., Warner, J.O., et al., 2007. Kiwifruit allergy: actinidin is not a major allergen in the United Kingdom. Clin. Exp. Allergy 37, 1340–1348.

Lund, E.D., Smoot, J.M., Hall, N.T., 1983. Dietary fiber content of eleven tropical fruits and vegetables. J. Agric. Food. Chem. 31, 1013–1016.

Ma, A.-G., Han, X.-X., Zhang, Y., Gao, Y.-H., Lan, J., 2006. Effect of kiwifruit extract supplementation on levels of serum immunoglobulins and phagocytosis activity in mice (abstract only). FASEB J. 20, A1057.

Maddumage, R., Nieuwenhuizen, N.J., Bulley, S.M., Cooney, J.M., Green, S.A., Atkinson, R.G., 2013. Diversity and relative levels of actinidin, kiwellin, and thaumatin-like allergens in 15 varieties of kiwifruit (*Actinidia*). J. Agric. Food. Chem. 61, 728–739.

Martín-Cabrejas, M.A., Esteban, R.M., López-Andreu, F.J., Waldron, K., Selvendran, R.R., 1995. Dietary fiber content of pear and kiwi pomaces. J. Agric. Food. Chem. 43, 662–666.

Massey, L.K., 2003. Dietary influences on urinary oxalate and risk of kidney stones. Front. Biosci. 8, s584–s594.

McGhie, T.K., 2013. Secondary metabolite components of kiwifruit. Adv. Food. Nutr. Res. 68, 101–124.

Miura, K., Greenland, P., Stamler, J., Liu, K., Daviglus, M.L., Nakagawa, H., 2004. Relation of vegetable, fruit, and meat intake to 7-year blood pressure change in middle-aged men: The Chicago Western Electric study. Am. J. Epidemiol. 159, 572–580.

Mohajeri, G., Masoudpour, H., Heidarpour, M., Khademi, E.F., Ghafghazi, S., Adibi, S., et al., 2010. The effect of dressing with fresh kiwifruit on burn wound healing. Surgery 148, 963–968.

Mohajeri, G., Safaee, M., Sanei, M.H., 2014. Effects of topical Kiwifruit on healing of neuropathic diabetic foot ulcer. J. Res. Med. Sci. 19, 520–524.

Molan, A.L., Kruger, M.C., De, S., Drummond, L.N., 2007. The ability of kiwifruit to positively modulate key markers of gastrointestinal function. Proc. Nutr. Soc. N. Z. 32, 66–71.

Monro, J.A., 2013. Kiwifruit, carbohydrate availability, and the glycemic response. Adv. Food. Nutr. Res. 68, 258–271.

Montefiori, M., McGhie, T.K., Costa, G., Ferguson, A.R., 2005. Pigments in the fruit of red-fleshed kiwifruit (*Actinidia chinensis* and *Actinidia deliciosa*). J. Agric. Food. Chem. 53, 9526–9530.

Montoya, C.A., Rutherfurd, S.M., Olson, T.D., Purba, A.S., Drummond, L.N., Boland, M.J., et al., 2014. Actinidin from kiwifruit (*Actinidia deliciosa* cv. Hayward) increases the digestion and rate of gastric emptying of meat proteins in the growing pig. Br. J. Nutr. 111, 957–967.

Motohashi, N., Shirataki, Y., Kawase, M., Tani, S., Sakagami, H., Satoh, K., et al., 2002. Cancer prevention and therapy with kiwifruit in chinese folklore medicine: a study of kiwifruit extracts. J. Ethnopharmacol. 81, 357–364.

Nishiyama, I., 2007. Fruits of the *Actinidia* genus. Adv. Food. Nutr. Res. 52, 293–324.

Nishiyama, I., Fukuda, T., Oota, T., 2004a. Varietal differences in actinidin concentration and protease activity in the fruit juice of *Actinidia arguta* and *Actinidia rufa*. J. Jpn. Soc. Hortic. Sci. 73, 157–162.

Nishiyama, I., Yamashita, Y., Yamanaka, M., Shimohash, A., Fukuda, T., Oota, T., 2004b. Varietal difference in vitamin C content in the fruit of kiwifruit and other *Actinidia* species. J. Agric. Food. Chem. 52, 5472–5475.

Okuda, N., Miura, K., Okayama, A., Okamura, T., Abbott, R.D., Nishi, N., et al., 2015. Fruit and vegetable intake and mortality from cardiovascular disease in Japan: a 24-year follow-up of the NIPPON DATA80 Study. Eur. J. Clin. Nutr. 69, 482–488.

O'Neil, D.A., 2003. Regulation of expression of β-defensins: endogenous enteric peptide antibiotics. Mol. Immunol. 40, 445–450.

Ozgen, M., Reese, R.N., Tulio Jr., A.Z., Scheerens, J.C., Miller, A.R., 2006. Modified 2,2-azino-bis-3-ethylbenzothiazoline-6-sulfonic acid (ABTS) method to measure antioxidant capacity of selected small fruits and comparison to ferric reducing antioxidant power (FRAP) and 2,2'-diphenyl-1-picrylhydrazyl (DPPH) methods. J. Agric. Food. Chem. 54, 1151–1157.

Panjeh-Shahin, M.-R., Dehghani, F., Talaei-Khozani, T., Panahi, Z., 2005. The effects of hydroalcoholic extract of *Actinidia chinensis* on sperm count and motility, and on the blood levels of estradiol and testosterone in male rats. Arch. Iran. Med. 8, 211–216.

Park, E.-J., Kim, B.C., Eo, H.K., Park, K.C., Kim, Y.R., Lee, H.J., et al., 2005. Control of IgE and selective T_H1 and T_H2 cytokines by PG102 isolated from *Actinidia arguta.* J. Allergy Clin. Immunol. 116, 1151–1157.

Park, E.-J., Park, K.C., Eo, H.K., Seo, J.Y., Son, M.W., Kim, K.H., et al., 2007. Suppression of spontaneous dermatitis in NC/Nga murine model by PG102 isolated from *Actinidia arguta.* J. Invest. Dermatol. 127, 1154–1160.

Park, Y.S., Ham, K.-S., Kang, S.G., Park, Y.K., Namiesnik, J., Leontowicz, H., et al., 2012. Organic and conventional kiwifruit, myths versus reality: antioxidant, antiproliferative, and health effects. J. Agric. Food. Chem. 60, 6984–6993.

Park, Y.-S., Leontowicz, H., Leontowicz, M., Namiesnik, J., Suhaj, M., Cvikrová, M., et al., 2011. Comparison of the contents of bioactive compounds and the level of antioxidant activity in different kiwifruit cultivars. J. Food Compos. Anal. 24, 963–970.

Park, Y.-S., Namiesnik, J., Vearasilp, K., Leontowicz, H., Leontowicz, M., Barasch, D., et al., 2014. Bioactive compounds and the antioxidant capacity in new kiwifruit cultivars. Food. Chem. 165, 354–361.

Parkar, S.G., Redgate, E.L., Wibisono, R., Luo, X., Koh, E.T.H., Schröder, R., 2010. Gut health benefits of kiwifruit pectins: comparison with commercial functional polysaccharides. J. Funct. Foods 2, 210–218.

Parkar, S.G., Rosendale, D., Paturi, G., Herath, T.D., Stoklosinski, H., Phipps, J.E., et al., 2012. *In vitro* utilization of gold and green kiwifruit oligosaccharides by human gut microbial populations. Plant Food Hum. Nutr. 67, 200–207.

Perera, C.O., Hallett, I.C., Nguyen, T.T., Charles, J.C., 1990. Calcium oxalate crystals: the irritant factor in kiwifruit. J. Food. Sci. 55, 1066–1069.

Peuhkuri, K., Sihvola, N., Korpela, R., 2012. Diet promotes sleep duration and quality. Nutr. Res. 32, 309–319.

Prior, R.L., Gu, L., Wu, X., Jacob, R.A., Sotoudeh, G., Kader, A.A., et al., 2007. Plasma antioxidant capacity changes following a meal as a measure of the ability of a food to alter *in vivo* antioxidant status. J. Am. Coll. Nutr. 26, 170–181.

Rassam, M., Laing, W.A., 2005. Variation in ascorbic acid and oxalate levels in the fruit of *Actinidia chinensis* tissues and genotypes. J. Agric. Food. Chem. 53, 2322–2326.

Ren, J., Chung, S.H., 2007. Anti-inflammatory effect of α-linolenic acid and its mode of action through the inhibition of nitric oxide production and inducible nitric oxide synthase gene expression via NF-κB and mitogen activated protein kinase pathways. J. Agric. Food. Chem. 55, 5073–5080.

Roll, S., Nocon, M., Willich, S.N., 2011. Reduction of common cold symptoms by encapsulated juice powder concentrate of fruits and vegetables: a randomised, double-blind, placebo-controlled trial. Br. J. Nutr. 105, 118–122.

Rowe, C.A., Nantz, M.P., Bukowski, J.F., Percival, S.S., 2007. Specific formulation of *Camellia sinensis* prevents cold and flu symptoms and enhances γδ T cell function: a randomized, double-blind, placebo-controlled study. J. Am. Coll. Nutr. 26, 445–452.

Rupérez, P., Bartolomé, A.P., Fernández-Serrano, M.I., 1995. Dietary fibre in Spanish kiwifruit. Eur. J. Clin. Nutr. 49 (Suppl. 3), S274–S276.

Rush, E.C., Patel, M., Plank, L.D., Ferguson, L.R., 2002. Kiwifruit promotes laxation in the elderly. Asia. Pac. J. Clin. Nutr. 11, 164–168.

Shirosaki, M., Koyama, T., Yazawa, K., 2008. Anti-hyperglycemic activity of kiwifruit leaf (*Actinidia deliciosa*) in mice. Biosci. Biotechnol. Biochem. 72, 1099–1102.

Shu, Q., De Silva, U.M., Chen, S., Peng, W.-D., Ahmed, M., Lu, G.-J., et al., 2008. Kiwifruit extract enhances markers of innate and acquired immunity in a murine model. Food. Agric. Immunol. 19, 149–161.

Siener, R., Hönow, R., Seidler, A., Voss, S., Hesse, A., 2006. Oxalate contents of species of the polygonaceae, amaranthaceae and chenopodiaceae families. Food. Chem. 98, 220–224.

Skinner, M.A., 2012. Wellness foods based on the health benefits of fruit: gold kiwifruit for immune support and reducing symptoms of colds and influenza. J. Food Drug Anal. 20 (Suppl. 1), 261–264.

Skinner, M.A., Bentley-Hewitt, K., Rosendale, D., Naoko, S., Pernthaner, A., 2013. Effects of kiwifruit on innate and adaptive immunity and symptoms of upper respiratory tract infections. Adv. Food. Nutr. Res. 68, 301–320.

Skinner, M.A., Hunter, D.C., Denis, M., Parlane, N., Zhang, J., Stevenson, L.M., et al., 2007. Health benefits of ZESPRI™ GOLD Kiwifruit: effects on muscle performance, muscle fatigue and immune responses (abstract). Asia. Pac. J. Clin. Nutr. 16, S31.

Stevenson, D.E., 2012. New antioxidant mechanisms and functional foods (Part 1). Agro Food Ind. Hi Tech 23, 32–33.

Stonehouse, W., Gammon, C.S., Beck, K.L., Conlon, C.A., von Hurst, P.R., Kruger, R., 2013. Kiwifruit: our daily prescription for health. Can. J. Physiol. Pharmacol. 91, 442–447.

Sun, S., Xu, H., Ngeh, L., 2012. The evaluation of Chinese therapeutic food for the treatment of moderate dyslipidemia. Evid Based Complement Alternat. Med. 2012, 508683.

The University of Sydney, 2011. <glycemicindex.com> (accessed 13.07.15.).

Trosko, J.E., Chang, C.-C., 2001. Mechanism of up-regulated gap junctional intercellular communication during chemoprevention and chemotherapy of cancer. Mutat. Res-Fund. Mol. M. 480–481, 219–229.

US Department of Agriculture, A. R. S., Nutritent Data Laboratory, 2015 USDA National Nutrient Database for Standard Reference, *Release 27* (revised). Version Current: May 2015.

van der Horst-Graat, J.M., Kok, F.J., Schouten, E.G., 2004. Plasma carotenoid concentrations in relation to acute respiratory infections in elderly people. Br. J. Nutr. 92, 113–118.

Vissers, M.C.M., Carr, A.C., Pullar, J.M., Bozonet, S.M., 2013. The bioavailability of vitamin C from kiwifruit. Adv. Food. Nutr. Res. 68, 125–147.

Walker, S., Prescott, J., 2003. Psychophysical properties of mechanical oral irritation. J. Sens. Stud. 18, 325–345.

Wang, H., Cao, G.-H., Prior, R.L., 1996. Total antioxidant capacity of fruits. J. Agric. Food. Chem. 44, 701–705.

Watanabe, K., Takahashi, B., 1998. Determination of soluble and insoluble oxalate contents in kiwifruit (*Actinidia deliciosa*) and related species. J. Jpn. Soc. Hortic. Sci. 67, 299–305.

Wattenberg, L.W., 1990. Inhibition of carcinogenesis by naturally occurring and synthetic compounds. In: Kuroda, Y., Shankel, D.M., Waters, M.D. (Eds.), Antimutagenesis and anticarcinogenesis, mechanisms II Plenum Press, New York, pp. 155–166.

Webby, R.F., 1990. Flavonoid complement of cultivars of *Actinidia deliciosa* var. *deliciosa*, kiwifruit. N. Z. J. Crop Hortic. Sci. 18, 1–4.

Wolber, F.M., Beck, K.L., Conlon, C.A., Kruger, M.C., 2013. Kiwifruit and mineral nutrition. Adv. Food. Nutr. Res. 68, 233–256.

Xu, H., Xu, H.-E., Ryan, D., 2009. A study of the comparative effects of hawthorn fruit compound and simvastatin on lowering blood lipid levels. Am. J. Chin. Med. 37, 903–908.

Yang, H., Lee, Y.-C., Han, K.-S., Singh, H., Yoon, M., Park, J.-H., et al., 2013. Green and gold kiwifruit peel ethanol extracts potentiate pentobarbital-induced sleep in mice via a GABAergic mechanism. Food. Chem. 136, 160–163.

Ying, D.Y., Parkar, S., Luo, X.X., Seelye, R., Sharpe, J.C., Barker, D., et al., 2007. Microencapsulation of probiotics using kiwifruit polysaccharide and alginate chitosan. Acta. Hortic. 753, 801–808.

Zuo, L.-L., Wang, Z.-Y., Fan, Z.-L., Tian, S.-Q., Liu, J.-R., 2012. Evaluation of antioxidant and antiproliferative properties of three *Actinidia* (*Actinidia kolomikta*, *Actinidia arguta*, *Actinidia chinensis*) extracts *in vitro*. Int. J. Mol. Sci. 13, 5506–5518.

Chapter 13

Cocoa—past medicinal uses, current scientific evidence, and advertised health benefits

Dan Ju and Gertraud Maskarinec
University of Hawaii Cancer Center, Honolulu, HI, United States

CHAPTER OUTLINE

INTRODUCTION

Cocoa beans are the seeds contained in the pods harvested from *Theobroma cacao*, also known as the cacao or cocoa tree (Afoakwa, 2014). Cocoa differs from apples, oranges, berries, and other commonly consumed fruits in at least two important ways. Cocoa beans need to be fermented, dried, and processed to obtain an edible product (International Cocoa Organization, 2013) and they contain substantial amounts of energy from fat (>40%) and carbohydrates (>30%) in addition to bioactive

Fruits, Vegetables, and Herbs.
DOI: http://dx.doi.org/10.1016/B978-0-12-802972-5.00013-5

substances (Torres-Moreno et al., 2015). Both the geographical origin and the processing of beans influence the nutrient profile and fatty acid composition. In one comparative analysis, cocoa beans from Ecuador had a higher total fat content (435 g vs 419 g per 1 kg) and higher proportions of unsaturated fatty acids than samples from Ghana (Torres-Moreno et al., 2015). A comparison of specimens from nine different locations also showed considerable variation in the molecular species of triglycerides (Bertazzo et al., 2013). Once processed into confectionary, the nutritional profile of different products depends primarily on the proportion of cocoa solids as compared to sugar and milk (Table 13.1). The content of calories, total fat, and all types of fatty acids decreases from unsweetened to milk chocolate, whereas the carbohydrate concentration increases as cocoa solids are replaced with milk and sugar (U.S. Department of Agriculture, Agricultural Research Service, 2015).

In addition to theobromine and caffeine, products prepared from cocoa beans contain catechin and epicatechin, readily water soluble flavonoids classified as flavan-3-ols (Aron and Kennedy, 2008; Dreosti, 2000), which are polyphenolic compounds with antioxidative properties (Scalbert and Williamson, 2000). Flavan-3-ols are also found in substantial amount in grapes, wine, tea, apples, cranberries, and many other plant foods (Aron and Kennedy, 2008; Gu et al., 2004), but cocoa is unique because it also contains polymeric condensation products of catechins (dimers to decamers) formed during fermentation (Hammerstone et al., 2000), which constitute up to 60% of the total polyphenol content in cocoa (Rusconi and Conti, 2010). The content of catechins and procyanidins is high for cocoa powder and unsweetened chocolate (Table 10.1) but low for milk chocolate and cocoa powder processed with alkali (Neveu et al., 2010). The intake of flavan-3-ols varies considerably across populations, with high levels in some European countries (Gu et al., 2004; Perez-Jimenez et al., 2011; Zamora-Ros et al., 2013; Landberg et al., 2011). Within the European Prospective Investigation into Cancer and Nutrition (EPIC), the mean intake of chocolate was reported as 6–7 g/day with the highest intake of 10 and 12 g for British women and men and the lowest intake in Greece and Italy (Wirfalt et al., 2002). Plasma levels of catechins increase after intake of cocoa products by approximately 200 nmol/L after the intake of 100 mg catechins (Manach et al., 2005). In one trial, plasma levels of epicatechin rose by 133±27, 258±29, and 355±49 nmol/L in individuals who consumed 27, 53, and 80 g of chocolate containing 5.3 mg total procyanidins per 1 g, respectively (Wang et al., 2000). A 12-fold increase in plasma epicatechin from 22 to 257 nmol/L ($P < 0.01$) was seen after 2 h when volunteers consumed 80 g of semisweet chocolate (Rein et al., 2000).

Table 13.1 Nutrient Content of Cocoa and Chocolate Products According to USDA Database (U.S. Department of Agriculture, Agricultural Research Service, 2015)

Nutrient (Per 100 g)	Milk Chocolate	Dark Chocolate (45–59% Cacao Solids)	Dark Chocolate (70–85% Cacao Solids)	Baking Chocolate, Unsweetened	Cocoa, Dry Powder, Unsweetened	Cocoa, Dry Powder, Unsweetened, Processed with Alkali
Energy (kcal)	535	546	598	642	228	220
Protein (g)	7.7	4.9	7.8	14.3	19.6	18.1
Total lipid (fat) (g)	29.7	31.3	42.6	52.3	13.7	13.1
Carbohydrate (g)	59.4	61.2	45.9	28.4	57.9	58.3
Sugars, total (g)	51.5	47.9	24.0	0.91	1.75	1.76
Lipids (g)						
Fatty acids, total saturated (g)	18.5	18.5	24.5	32.3	8.1	7.76
Fatty acids, monounsaturated (g)	7.2	9.5	12.8	16.1	4.6	4.4
Fatty acids, polyunsaturated (g)	1.4	1.1	1.3	1.6	0.4	0.4
Cholesterol (mg)	23	8	3	2	0	0
Caffeine (mg)	20	43	80	80	230	78
Theobromine (mg)	205	493	802	1297	2057	2634
Flavan-3-ols (mg)						
(+) Catechin	4.2			64.3	64.8	36.7
(−) Epicatechin	10.9			141.8	196.4	56.6
Proanthocyanidins (mg)						
Monomers	23.5			199	317	
Dimers	23.1			207	184	
Trimers	14.6			131	160	
4–6mers	40.7			333	525	
7–10mers	17.6			216	189	
Polymers (>10mers)	32.8			551		

Throughout its history, cocoa and chocolate have been valued for medicinal purposes, some times probably more so than for their nutritional properties (Bruinsma and Taren, 1999; Keen, 2001). In Mesoamerican cultures, cocoa was primarily consumed as a beverage, often mixed with maize and/or spices (Coe and Coe, 2007). After colonialists encountered cocoa in the New World and enjoyed its flavor, they introduced the beverage to countries across Europe, where its popularity increased rapidly and many new recipes were developed. However, due to the high content of cocoa butter from solids, the drinks had a high fat content, a gritty texture, and an oily surface. Only in 1828, a process to separate the cocoa butter from the cocoa solids was developed in the Netherlands (Snyder et al., 2009). The production of solid bars and chocolate as a confectionary started toward the end of the century and developed into a flourishing industry in the 20th century (Coe and Coe, 2007).

Ancient populations in Central America and later the Spanish and other Europeans identified a variety of conditions, for which the healing properties of cocoa products would alleviate symptoms (Dillinger et al., 2000). With the rising interest in the role of bioactive food components in human health, the possible protective effects of cocoa products and flavan-3-ols have been investigated in many experimental and population-based studies (Aron and Kennedy, 2008; Cooper et al., 2008; Hooper et al., 2012; Ried et al., 2012; Corti et al., 2009). As a result of the emerging scientific evidence, manufacturers of cocoa products started to promote dark chocolates and cocoa supplements based on these potential health benefits. The current review compares medicinal uses of cocoa products in Central American and European history, current scientific evidence for disease prevention, and contemporary health-related statements offered as advertisement for modern cocoa products.

HISTORIC USES OF COCOA PRODUCTS

Several reviews by historians and anthropologists have provided insight into medicinal uses of cocoa products (Dillinger et al., 2000; Lippi, 2009, 2013a,b, 2015). In old manuscripts, early accounts of indigenous Mexica/Aztec views were compiled by Spanish priests who collected information when they arrived in Mexico (Grivetti, 2009). One example is the Badianus Manuscript (dated to 1552) consisting of detailed paintings of medicinal plants and a text describing Mexican diseases, nutritional problems, and healing techniques. Later, the Florentine Codex (dated to 1577) recorded different types and dosages of beverages consumed by the Mexican populations and advised against excessive drinking of cocoa prepared from unroasted beans but recommended the beverage as an invigorating and refreshing beverage if used in moderation (Lippi, 2015). The chocolate beverages were consumed to treat stomach and intestinal complaints, infections, childhood diarrhea, fever, cough, and skin eruptions, conditions that must have been very common at the time. Several texts presented the benefits of cocoa for very specific conditions, whereas others made recommendations for a wide range of medicinal complaints. Basically all organ systems were mentioned at one time or another (Dillinger et al., 2000). Once Europeans discovered and started to enjoy cocoa, accounts of medicinal benefits of chocolate drinks also described a wide range of conditions that were prevalent at the time: kidney disease, fever, liver disease, stomach problems, dysentery, consumption, chest ailments, weakness, and skin conditions (Dillinger et al., 2000). Both in precolonial times and in Europe, spices and substances believed to cure diseases were often added to the cocoa beverages or cocoa was used to improve the flavor of other medicinal plants.

An overarching theme over time was the attribution of nourishment and energy (Dillinger et al., 2000). In some accounts, cocoa products were regarded as a food that could solely sustain a person or even prolong life. Terms such as fortifying, refreshing, and invigorating emphasized the restorative and nutritious nature of the beverages. The British Medical Journal (1870) endorsed Cadbury Cocoa Essence with this notice: "The excess of fatty matter which makes cocoa indigestible to many stomachs is removed.... Cocoa treated thus will, we expect, prove to be one of most nutritious, digestible and restorative of drinks." In the early 20th century (Coe and Coe, 2007), advertisements for Cadbury products claimed that "Cocoa makes strong men stronger. The most refreshing nutritious and sustaining of all cocoas," while Hershey's Milk Chocolate was marketed as "A meal in itself." Energy provision was also an important consideration between 1940 and 1945, when Hershey produced over 3 billion chocolate bars for soldiers throughout the world (Hershey Community Archives, 2015). The US military had charged the company to develop a product that "was able to withstand high temperatures, high in food energy value, and tasting just a little better than a boiled potato." This resulted in the Ration D and later the Tropical bars with improved flavor (Lippi, 2015).

As summarized by a detailed historical review of medicinal uses for cocoa, three consistent therapeutic purposes in the prescription of cocoa products emerged over the centuries (Dillinger et al., 2000): promote weight gain and restore a person from exhaustion or depression; balance the nervous system, that is, stimulate or calm as needed; and improve digestion.

CURRENT SCIENTIFIC EVIDENCE

Given the rapidly increasing published research related to the beneficial effects of cocoa products, the current text needed to be selective in choosing sources. Whenever available, meta-analyses and reviews were selected. Among the wide range of conditions investigated during recent years, cardiovascular disease is certainly the most common disorder (Cooper et al., 2008; Hooper et al., 2012; Erdman et al., 2008). In addition to outlining research on cardiovascular disease and its risk factors, short summaries for antioxidant and anti-inflammatory effects, cancer, neurocognitive function, and intestinal health will also be presented.

Cardiovascular disease

In 1944, a report about Kuna Indians in Panama described an extraordinarily high cocoa consumption and low blood pressure in this population. The daily intake of flavan-3-ols was estimated at approximately 900mg (Kean, 1944). Since then, the health status of the Kuna Indians has been examined repeatedly (McCullough et al., 2006). The lower mortality rates for cancer and other chronic diseases among Kuna Indians living in the San Blas islands, where intake of cocoa-containing beverages was high as compared to the Kuna Indians in mainland Panama who did not consume cocoa drinks, were attributed to the high flavan-3-ol intake (Bayard et al., 2007).

Additional investigations have explored the association of cocoa and chocolate intake with risk and mortality for heart disease and stroke (Zhang et al., 2013). In a cohort of 470 elderly men, participants consuming >2.5g of cocoa per day reduced their 15-year cardiovascular mortality by half ($P = 0.004$) as compared to those consuming <0.5g per day (Buijsse et al., 2006). Similarly, deaths due to stroke and myocardial infarction were significantly lower for German adults consuming 7.5g versus 1.5g chocolate per day (Buijsse et al., 2010). In a meta-analysis of 10 observational studies reporting on cardiovascular outcomes (Zhang et al., 2013), a summary risk estimate of 0.75 (95% CI: 0.62, 0.91) was obtained for the highest versus the lowest chocolate intake category.

Several biologic mechanisms explaining how cocoa products may benefit the heart and blood vessels have been proposed (Keen, 2001; Cooper et al., 2008; Erdman et al., 2008). Foremost, it has been hypothesized that cocoa intake maintains a low cardiovascular risk profile due to the activation of nitric oxide synthesis sustained by flavan-3-ols (Grassi et al., 2013). In turn, nitric oxide may be responsible for vasodilation and lower blood pressure (Ried et al., 2012; Hollenberg et al., 2009), antioxidant protection (Prior and Gu, 2005; Gu et al., 2006), anti-inflammatory action (di Giuseppe et al., 2008), reduction in endothelial dysfunction (Engler et al., 2004), improvements in glucose metabolism (Grassi et al., 2015), and inhibition of lipoprotein oxidation (Mursu et al., 2004). We will review four major mechanisms of action that have been investigated widely while realizing that many other pathways may be involved: endothelial function, blood pressure, insulin resistance, and antioxidant/anti-inflammatory effects (Hooper et al., 2012; Corti et al., 2009).

The endothelium in blood vessels plays an important role in disease risk (Grassi et al., 2013). When the bioavailability of nitric oxide is reduced, endothelial dysfunction is a first step in the development of atherosclerosis and future cardiovascular events. Cocoa flavonoids may positively modulate these mechanisms and, thereby, protect against cardiovascular disease (Grassi et al., 2013). Flow-mediated dilation, a measure of endothelial function, was improved significantly in intervention with acute or chronic chocolate intake (Hooper et al., 2012; Corti et al., 2009). In a large meta-analysis, the mean difference in flow-mediated dilation in 11 short-term interventions was 3.19 (95% CI: 2.04, 4.33) while it was 1.34 (95% CI: 1.00, 1.68) in the trials that lasted several weeks (Hooper et al., 2012).

Blood pressure has been the subject of many investigations. Results from an observational study in Dutch men showed that those in the highest tertile of cocoa intake had a significantly lower mean systolic blood pressure (−3.7 mmHg; $P = 0.03$) and diastolic blood pressure (−2.1 mmHg; $P = 0.03$) than those in the lowest tertile (Buijsse et al., 2006). Similarly, blood pressure was significantly lower for German adults consuming 7.5 g versus 1.5 g chocolate per day (Buijsse et al., 2010). A random effects meta-analysis with 15 trial arms of 13 studies revealed a significant blood pressure-reducing effect of cocoa-chocolate compared with controls of -3.2 ± 1.9 mmHg for systolic ($P = 0.001$) and -2.0 ± 1.3 mmHg ($P = 0.003$) for diastolic blood pressure (Ried et al., 2010). However, this beneficial effect was restricted to individuals with hypertension and prehypertension. When 20 interventions with 856 participants were combined, the hypothesis that chocolate and cocoa products lowered blood pressure was supported; the respective mean differences in systolic and diastolic blood pressure were −2.8 mmHg ($P = 0.005$) and −2.2 mmHg ($P = 0.0006$) although this finding was restricted to 2-week trials as opposed to trials of longer duration (Ried et al., 2012). The effects on blood pressure were more pronounced on diastolic than systolic blood pressure and doses of >50 mg catechins had a greater effect than lower amounts (Hooper et al., 2012). However, in some clinical trials, significant decreases in blood pressure were observed with amounts as low as 6.3 g of dark chocolate (30 mg flavan-3-ols) per day (Taubert et al., 2007).

Insulin resistance is a well-known risk factor for cardiovascular disease and insulin sensitivity is dependent at least in part on insulin-mediated nitric oxide release (Grassi et al., 2013). Thus, flavan-3-ols may counteract insulin resistance by increasing the nitric oxide bioavailability and decreasing the formation of reactive oxygen species. Benefits on glucose tolerance and insulin resistance were described repeatedly (Hooper et al., 2012; Mastroiacovo et al., 2015; Almoosawi et al., 2012). A meta-analysis reported an improvement in glucose metabolism as assessed by a lowered homeostatic model assessment insulin resistance index (HOMA-IR: –0.67; 95% CI: –0.98, –0.36) due to significant reductions in fasting serum insulin by 22.7 IU/mL although the interventions had no effect on fasting glucose (Hooper et al., 2012). In a recent randomized trial, glucose and insulin levels as well as insulin resistance decreased significantly in the high (993 mg/day) and intermediate (520 mg/day) flavan-3-ol groups as compared to the low (48 mg/day) group after 8 weeks (Mastroiacovo et al., 2015). In a single-blind randomized placebo-controlled cross-over study, 20 g of dark chocolate with 500 mg polyphenols improved glucose regulation as indicated by the reduction in fasting glucose and HOMA-IR without affecting insulin levels (Almoosawi et al., 2012).

Antioxidant/antiinflammatory effects

As reviewed previously, the antioxidant action of flavan-3-ols has been investigated in many clinical trials using various biomarkers (Maskarinec, 2009). Despite the short duration of several trials, some favorable changes in biomarkers assessing antioxidant status were reported. Of the 11 studies that assessed antioxidant capacity, four studies showed an increase in antioxidant capacity (Wang et al., 2000; Rein et al., 2000; Wan et al., 2001; Serafini et al., 2003) but seven did not (Engler et al., 2004; Mursu et al., 2004; Mathur et al., 2002; Murphy et al., 2003; Wiswedel et al., 2004; Fraga et al., 2005; Heiss et al., 2007). Malondialdehyde, a marker for oxidative stress, decreased in two studies (Wiswedel et al., 2004; Fraga et al., 2005) but not in another one (Heiss et al., 2007). A role of flavan-3-ols appears likely because significant increases in plasma antioxidant activity were only described in volunteers who consumed 100 g dark chocolate, whereas no change was seen after the intake of 100 g milk chocolate (Serafini et al., 2003). Fewer changes in inflammatory markers have been reported. Observational data from an Italian cohort reported that concentrations of serum C-reactive protein (CRP), a well-established inflammatory marker, were significantly lower in dark chocolate consumers with a mean intake of 5.7 g/day than in nonconsumers even after adjustment for lifestyle factors and other nutrients (di Giuseppe et al., 2008). However, a meta-analysis of cardiovascular risk factors did not show a significant effect on CRP (Hooper et al., 2008).

Cancer

A limited number of observational epidemiologic studies offer weak support for a reduction in mortality and little information related to cancer incidence (Maskarinec, 2009) although cocoa and chocolate products may lower oxidative stress and chronic inflammation (di Giuseppe et al., 2008), which are considered risk factors for cancer (Coussens and Werb, 2002). Catechin and procyanidin intake from all sources, not specifically cocoa products, was associated with lower cancer risk, in particular lung and colorectal cancer in several population-based studies (Arts and Hollman, 2005; Theodoratou et al., 2007; Rossi et al., 2010a). In a report from Italy, procyanidins with a higher degree of polymerization were associated with a lower colorectal cancer risk, especially for rectal cancer, suggesting a local effect (Rossi et al., 2010a). In the same population, stomach cancer risk was also lower with higher intake of procyanidins (Rossi et al., 2010b). On the other hand, null reports (Rouillier et al., 2005; Thompson et al., 2010) and higher risks for colorectal (Boutron-Ruault et al., 1999) and pancreatic cancer (Chan et al., 2009) have been reported in relation to chocolate products. From a mechanistic point of view, the flavan-3-ols contained in cocoa products may be able to reduce cancer risk, but the concentrations of flavan-3-ols are low in most products and the evidence from epidemiologic studies is limited and contradictory.

Neurocognitive function

A review of published evidence found that a large proportion of these reports described significant beneficial associations between cocoa products and different aspects of cognitive functioning (Crews et al., 2013). In a more recent double-blinded trial conducted in 90 elderly individuals without clinical evidence of cognitive dysfunction, the participants were randomly assigned to consume daily drinks with high, intermediate, and low flavan-3-ol content for 8 weeks. Although the overall changes in cognitive function scores did not differ across groups, specific aspects of cognitive function improved more in the high flavan-3-ol group. The authors concluded that regular flavan-3-ol consumption can reduce some measures of age-related cognitive dysfunction, possibly through an improvement in insulin sensitivity (Mastroiacovo et al., 2015).

Intestinal health

As the importance of gut microbiota in health has emerged (Sekirov et al., 2010), a promising effect of procyanidins on the composition of gut microbiota appears possible (Tzounis et al., 2011; Etxeberria et al., 2013). Because procyanidins do not appear to be degraded in the stomach, they may interact directly with gut microbiota (Keen, 2001; Tzounis et al., 2011; Rios et al., 2002). For example, gut microbiota in rats were modified by the administration of procyanidins, demonstrating the possibility that these compounds alter the composition of microbiota (Smith and Mackie, 2004). In a study with healthy volunteers, a change in gut microbiota composition was observed in addition to an increase in plasma catechin levels and a decrease in CRP during the high-cocoa flavan-3-ol period (Tzounis et al., 2011). The bifidobacterial and lactobacilli populations increased, while the clostridia counts decreased. These observations are important in the context of recent evidence that different bifidobacteria and other gut microbiota may play a role in the development of gastrointestinal cancers (Lampe, 2008; Roberfroid et al., 2010). This process may be mediated by the renewal of gut epithelial cells or by altering cancer risk in other tissues through pathways such as nutrient harvesting, metabolism of xenobiotics, and the immune system (Turnbaugh et al., 2007).

ADVERTISED HEALTH BENEFITS

Currently, no authorized health claims for cocoa products or flavan-3-ols have been approved by the US Food and Drug Administration, but the European Union in 2013 permitted a claim, which is restricted to the use by Barry Callebaut in Belgium for 5 years (Official Journal of the European Union, 2013; EFSA Panel on Dietetic Products, Nutrition and Allergies (NDA), 2012). It states that "Cocoa flavanols help maintain the elasticity of blood vessels, which contributes to normal blood flow." The following conditions are attached to the claim: "Information shall be given to the consumer that the beneficial effect is obtained with a daily intake of 200 mg of cocoa flavan-3-ols. The claim can be used only for cocoa beverages (with cocoa powder) or for dark chocolate which provide at least a daily intake of 200 mg of cocoa flavan-3-ols with a degree of polymerization 1–10." Based on an unsystematic Internet search, we show sample statements from 15 companies (Table 13.2) that declare potential health benefits for cocoa and chocolate products (Barry Callebaut, 2015; Ludwig Weinrich GmbH & Co.KG, 2015; Mars Incorporated, 2015; MXI Corporation, 2013; Nestle, 2015; Reserveage Organics, 2015; Righteously Raw, 2015; Sweetriot, 2015; Taza Chocolate, 2015; JAK Native, 2015;

Table 13.2 Examples of Advertised Health Benefits for Cocoa and Chocolate Products

Health Benefit	Statement	Ref.
Cardiovascular disease	Theobromine dilates the cardiovascular system making the hearts job easier	Pure Natural Miracles (2015)
	Contains Theobromine which enhances blood flow to vital organs and provides a natural energy boost	JAK Native (2015)
	Helps protect the cardiovascular system, brain and other body systems	MXI Corporation (2013)
	Truly, as valentine's day suggests, chocolate could be considered good for our hearts	Sweetriot (2015)
	The unique combination of natural ingredients in this cocoa powder extract supports cardiovascular health, arterial health, healthy blood flow and digestive health, as well as support for the immune system and healthy energy levels	New Vitality (2015)
	Protect the heart and blood vessels	MXI Corporation (2013)
	Catechins may help to protect against heart disease and cancer	Ludwig Weinrich GmbH & Co.KG (2015)
	Supports heart and cognitive health and energy	Reserveage Organics (2015)
	Clinical studies suggest that cocoa, when combined with plant flavanols, can help support already normal healthy blood pressure levels	Reserveage Organics (2015)
	Studies have indicated that chocolate may relax vascular tissue and blood vessel walls, also aiding in general cardiovascular health	Taza Chocolate (2015)
	It provides an abundant source of iron and magnesium, which support healthy heart function	Righteously Raw (2015)
	Fortunately, the cocoa flavanols found in this supplement are scientifically proven to help support healthy circulation and healthy aging by helping your arteries keep their flexibility at any age	Mars Incorporated (2015)
	Cocoa flavanols help support cardiovascular health by maintaining the elasticity of blood vessels, helping support a normal blood flow	Barry Callebaut (2015)
	Given the official EU approved health claim, we can safely state that chocolate and cacao powder with cacao flavanols help maintain healthy blood circulation and can play a supporting role in the cardiovascular system	ChocoNature (2014)
	Kuna-Inspired. An indigenous people of coastal Panama, they followed a daily, sacred practice of drinking several cups of raw cacao sweetened with plantains. A major university's 20-year research study of the Kuna found they were able to maintain already normal blood pressure levels and enjoy good cardiovascular health longer	Reserveage Organics (2015)

(*Continued*)

Table 13.2 Examples of Advertised Health Benefits for Cocoa and Chocolate Products (Continued)

Health Benefit	Statement	Ref.
Antioxidant/ antiinflammatory effects	Flavonoids help body's cells resist damage by free radicals	MXI Corporation (2013)
	Nutritionally supports the body's protection against oxidative stress and free radicals	Reserveage Organics (2015)
	Superior antioxidant profile/ORAC score (75,456/serving)	MXI Corporation (2013)
	Catechins effectively catch free radicals and prevent deposits in the blood vessel walls, regulate the blood pressure, and stimulate the immune system	Ludwig Weinrich GmbH & Co.KG (2015)
	Cacao is one of the leading antioxidant rich substances on the planet known today	Righteously Raw (2015)
	Dark chocolate is a great source of antioxidants	Nestle (2015)
	Are rich in antioxidants and polyphenols	True Healthy Products LLC (2014)
	You're getting 4000 mg of concentrated cocoa that offers a powerhouse of antioxidant protection against free radical damage	New Vitality (2015)
	Contains antioxidants that protect our bodies from damage caused by free radicals. These unstable oxygen molecules are thought to be responsible for aging and some diseases	JAK Native (2015)
	Chocolate contains a high level of antioxidants in the form of flavanols	Taza Chocolate (2015)
	It is amazing to note the abundance of antioxidants present in chocolate in comparison to other well-known antioxidant rich foods	Sweetriot (2015)
	Contains more active flavanols than standard chocolate on the market. Helps to maintain healthy cells by neutralizing free radicals	ChocoNature (2014)
	The cocoa flavanols are natural and powerful antioxidants and help to strengthen your body's own natural defense against free radicals before they can cause any harm	Pure Natural Miracles (2015)
	Boost immune function and decrease inflammation	Reserveage Organics (2015)
	Minimize inflammation throughout the body	MXI Corporation (2013)
Cancer	Catechins may help to protect against heart disease and cancer	Ludwig Weinrich GmbH & Co.KG (2015)
	Antioxidants have the power to reduce the risks of cancer and heart disease	Sweetriot (2015)
	When you lower the number of free radicals in your cells, your risk of cancers and chronic diseases are lowered as well	Righteously Raw (2015)
	Phytochemicals reduce the risk of certain cancers	Reserveage Organics (2015)
Neurocognitive function	Supports healthy blood flow, helps maintain and enhance concentration and memory	Reserveage Organics (2015)
	Healthy circulation important for cognitive health	Mars Incorporated (2015)
	Increases mental alertness and focus	True Healthy Products LLC (2014)
	Cacao and chocolate supports memory and concentration	ChocoNature (2014)

(*Continued*)

Table 13.2 Examples of Advertised Health Benefits for Cocoa and Chocolate Products (Continued)

Health Benefit	Statement	Ref.
Emotional health	Cocoa boosts mood—Numerous studies show a positive correlation between mood and chocolate	The Healthy Chocolate Co, Inc. (2012)
	Promotes essential brain chemicals that improve mood	MXI Corporation (2013)
	Milk chocolate delights the senses and may help improve your mood	Nestle (2015)
	Endorphins make us happy. These so called "hormones of happiness" are released when eating chocolate	Ludwig Weinrich GmbH & Co.KG (2015)
	This "bliss chemical" is also found in the properties of chocolate, which could explain why we consider chocolate to be a natural mood enhancer	Sweetriot (2015)
	Lowers PMS irritability	True Healthy Products LLC (2014)
	Serotonin helps us build up our stress defense shield	Pure Natural Miracles (2015)
Skin health	Cocoa polyphenols protect the skin from UV radiation. These polyphenols likely minimize inflammation in skin tissue	MXI Corporation (2013)
	Cacao and chocolate keeps the skin soft and supple	ChocoNature (2014)
	Healthy circulation important for skin health	Mars Incorporated (2015)
Other effects	Protect and repair the liver	MXI Corporation (2013)
	Helps maintain already normal cholesterol levels	Reserveage Organics (2015)
	Modify blood sugar levels	MXI Corporation (2013)

ChocoNature, 2014; Pure Natural Miracles, 2015; New Vitality, 2015; True Healthy Products LLC, 2014; The Healthy Chocolate Co, Inc., 2012). This list is not considered all-inclusive. Whereas many large chocolate manufacturers do not refer to health on their websites, several companies market cocoa powders, drinks, capsules, and chocolate bars by stating potential health benefits.

Although food labels are available for all products, only three companies (Barry Callebaut, 2015; Mars Incorporated, 2015; Reserveage Organics, 2015) provide flavan-3-ol content and one (MXI Corporation, 2013) lists flavonoid content for their products. Several companies have a particular focus on cocoa and health while others may briefly mention a variety of potential health benefits. A majority of the websites market chocolate, especially dark chocolate, in the form of bars or nuggets. Serving sizes vary considerably across products, from 8 to 42 g, and one can expect to consume anywhere from 39 to 220 calories per serving. With the exception of one milk chocolate bar, most of these chocolates are advertised as healthy with low amounts of sugar (0–9 g per serving). Interestingly, some chocolate bars and most cocoa powders were classified as supplements by the manufacturers. Capsule supplements by two different companies revealed marked differences in nutritional labeling (Mars Incorporated, 2015; Reserveage Organics, 2015). One company presents specific amounts for catechins and epicatechins while another only lists flavan-3-ols.

The number of possible beneficial effects varies greatly across websites from a few specific statements to a long list of benefits. These statements were classified into groups similar to the scientific evidence discussed above (Table 13.2). Some websites list citations from the scientific publications that support health benefits of dark chocolate, but others lack clear references to support proclaimed benefits. A large proportion of statements refer to basic biologic functions, such as preventing free radical damage because ingredients of cocoa will capture the free radicals, protecting against oxidative stress, and improving inflammation. Many also refer to specific organ systems, such as cardiovascular disease, blood vessels, and neurocognitive function. However, general statements that the product is good for overall health and fitness are quite common. Very few statements address skin health and digestion.

CONCLUSIONS

The history of cocoa across centuries shows a range of uses for therapeutic, nutritional, and recreational purposes (Keen, 2001; Dillinger et al., 2000; Lippi, 2013, 2015). Looking at the attributed health effects over time, it appears that populations in different locations and during various eras made an effort to identify beneficial effects for the most common health problems in their environment. Infectious diseases and fevers were a predominant concern in earlier times, whereas the provision of energy was important in the 19th century when malnutrition and debilitating disease, such as tuberculosis, were highly prevalent as a result of the industrial revolution and poor working conditions. After developing from a beverage with more medicinal applications to a confectionary with high sugar content, cocoa products became associated with obesity, dental problems, unhealthy lifestyle, and other negative health effects. Only recently have the scientific evidence for potential beneficial effects of flavan-3-ols and the availability of dark chocolate products improved the perception of cocoa. As a historian stated recently, the appreciation of cocoa as the food of the gods, the name given to the plant *T. cacao* by Linnaeus, may be returning (Lippi, 2015).

The comparison of the three historic uses of cocoa (Dillinger et al., 2000) to the current scientific evidence indicates some continuity as well as changes in direction. The first theme of weight gain and restoration of health appears to have evolved into a wider concern of the prevention of chronic diseases, in particular cardiovascular disease. In the present time with obesity as a major health concern, risk factors for chronic diseases have become a major health issue for many populations. The second theme, that is, balancing the nervous system, has remained quite constant as can be seen by the research and statements related to neurocognitive function and emotional well-being. The third use, for digestion, appears to have receded; there is limited research in that area and few advertisements refer to stomach or intestines despite some interesting hypotheses related to procyanidins and gut microbiota (Tzounis et al., 2011; Etxeberria et al., 2013).

From a casual survey of companies online, a great variation in the scientific grounding of proclaimed health benefits among and even within websites becomes evident. By and large the statements used for advertisement reflect the ongoing scientific research although they convey more certainty than is justified based on the current literature. As a disease, cancer is mentioned repeatedly although the scientific evidence is insufficient and weaker than the research supporting preventive effects against cardiovascular disease. It may be challenging for the average consumer to evaluate if health effects are supported by substantial scientific evidence. It appears debatable whether quoting scientific articles in this instance is better practice than not. Customers may look at the original article, but the average consumer likely will not do so. The appearance of being scientifically proven can be deceptive if the evidence is cherry-picked or taken out of context. Furthermore, often the different statements are listed in such a fashion that one would assume equal weight of evidence behind each benefit. In addition, the nutritional advertising of bioactive compounds may prove confusing to consumers, especially considering the challenge of distinguishing technical terms such as flavan-3-ols and flavonoids.

Despite the large volume of published research papers, our knowledge about the health effects of cocoa products remains incomplete due to many methodological issues. The concentrations of flavan-3-ols need to be taken into account when assessing any health effects, but flavan-3-ol content varies widely in cocoa and chocolate products given its dependence on fermentation and processing of the cocoa beans (McShea et al., 2008). In population-based studies, the intake of cocoa products tends to be low and dietary assessment of flavan-3-ol intake is limited due to the lack of information about the type of cocoa and chocolate products collected by food frequency questionnaires. Other issues include the lack of knowledge about plasma concentrations of flavan-3-ols achieved in many investigations (Grassi et al., 2013). Also, substances in cocoa other than flavan-3-ols may be important and have been neglected. As shown for vascular endothelial function (Costello et al., 2014), outcomes are not always assessed in a standardized fashion. Despite obvious advantages and strengths, intervention studies are frequently limited by their short duration (Cooper et al., 2008), the failure to reflect normal patterns of consumption of cocoa products, and the difficulties in controlling food intake in humans.

Cocoa products deserve further investigation for a number of reasons. Although flavan-3-ols are present in green tea and a variety of fruits and vegetables, the high concentration of procyanidins is a unique property of cocoa products (Perez-Jimenez et al., 2010). Procyanidins may have distinct health effects, which have been primarily investigated in experimental systems so far, for example, local antioxidant activity in the gastrointestinal tract, regulation of signal transduction pathways, suppression of oncogenes, induction of apoptosis, modulation of enzyme activity related to detoxification, stimulation of the immune system, angiogenesis, and regulation of hormone metabolism (Aron and Kennedy, 2008; Prior and Gu, 2005; Gu et al., 2006). To capture the overall health effects, future nutritional trials need to assess a larger number of biomarkers that may be relevant for disease risk, whereas epidemiologic studies require valid dietary assessment methods to examine the association of cocoa products with cancer risk in larger populations and to distinguish possible protective effects of cocoa products from those due to other polyphenolic compounds. Long-term epidemiological investigations assessing intake of flavan-3-ols accurately are necessary to understand health effects throughout a lifetime of consumption. Given the increasing availability of dark chocolates with relatively low sugar content and high concentrations of flavan-3-ols, consuming cocoa and chocolate may contribute to the prevention of chronic conditions when consumed in moderation, in addition to provide pleasure as experienced by so many populations throughout history.

REFERENCES

Afoakwa, E., 2014. Cocoa Production and Processing Technology. CRC Press, Boca Raton, FL.

Almoosawi, S., Tsang, C., Ostertag, L.M., Fyfe, L., Al-Dujaili, E.A., 2012. Differential effect of polyphenol-rich dark chocolate on biomarkers of glucose metabolism and cardiovascular risk factors in healthy, overweight and obese subjects: a randomized clinical trial. Food Funct. 3, 1035–1043.

Aron, P.M., Kennedy, J.A., 2008. Flavan-3-ols: nature, occurrence and biological activity. Mol. Nutr. Food Res. 52, 79–104.

Arts, I.C., Hollman, P.C., 2005. Polyphenols and disease risk in epidemiologic studies. Am. J. Clin. Nutr. 81, 317S–325S.

Barry Callebaut, 2015. FAQ. <http://www.acticoa.com/faq> (accessed 17.07.15.).

Bayard, V., Chamorro, F., Motta, J., Hollenberg, N.K., 2007. Does flavanol intake influence mortality from nitric oxide-dependent processes? Ischemic heart disease, stroke, diabetes mellitus, and cancer in Panama. Int. J. Med. Sci. 4, 53–58.

Bertazzo, A., Comai, S., Mangiarini, F., Chen, S., 2013. Composition of cocoa beans. In: Watson, R., Preedy, V., Zibadi, S. (Eds.), Chocolate in Health and Nutrition Springer Humana Press, New York, pp. 105–118.

Boutron-Ruault, M.C., Senesse, P., Faivre, J., Chatelain, N., Belghiti, C., Meance, S., 1999. Foods as risk factors for colorectal cancer: a case-control study in Burgundy (France). Eur. J. Cancer Prev. 8, 229–235.

British Medical Journal, 1870. Cadbury's cocoa essence. <https://play.google.com/books/reader?id=9DFHAAAAYAAJ&printsec=frontcover&output=reader&hl=en&pg=GBS.PA48-IA1:49> (accessed 23.07.15.).

Bruinsma, K., Taren, D.L., 1999. Chocolate: food or drug? J. Am. Diet. Assoc. 99, 1249–1256.

Buijsse, B., Feskens, E.J., Kok, F.J., Kromhout, D., 2006. Cocoa intake, blood pressure, and cardiovascular mortality: the Zutphen Elderly Study. Arch. Intern. Med. 166, 411–417.

Buijsse, B., Weikert, C., Drogan, D., Bergmann, M., Boeing, H., 2010. Chocolate consumption in relation to blood pressure and risk of cardiovascular disease in German adults. Eur. Heart J. 31, 1616–1623.

Chan, J.M., Wang, F., Holly, E.A., 2009. Sweets, sweetened beverages, and risk of pancreatic cancer in a large population-based case-control study. Cancer Causes Control 20, 835–846.

ChocoNature, 2014. EU approved health claim. <https://choconature.com/preserving-health-benefits-taste/> (accessed 29.07.15.).

Coe, S., Coe, M., 2007. The True History of Chocolate. Thames & Hudson Ltd, London.

Cooper, K.A., Donovan, J.L., Waterhouse, A.L., Williamson, G., 2008. Cocoa and health: a decade of research. Br. J. Nutr. 99, 1–11.

Corti, R., Flammer, A.J., Hollenberg, N.K., Luscher, T.F., 2009. Cocoa and cardiovascular health. Circulation 119, 1433–1441.

Costello, R.B., Lentino, C.V., Saldanha, L., Engler, M.M., Engler, M.B., Srinivas, P., et al., 2014. A select review reporting the quality of studies measuring endothelial dysfunction in randomised diet intervention trials. Br. J. Nutr., 1–11.

Coussens, L.M., Werb, Z., 2002. Inflammation and cancer. Nature 420, 860–867.

Crews Jr., W.D., Harrison, D., Gregory, K., Kim, B., Darling, A., 2013. The Effects of cocoa- and chocolate-related products on neurocognitive functioning. In: Watson, R., Preedy, V., Zibadi, S. (Eds.), Chocolate in Health and Nutrition Springer Humana Press, New York, pp. 369–379.

di Giuseppe, R., Di, C.A., Centritto, F., Zito, F., De, C.A., Costanzo, S., et al., 2008. Regular consumption of dark chocolate is associated with low serum concentrations of C-reactive protein in a healthy italian population. J. Nutr. 138, 1939–1945.

Dillinger, T.L., Barriga, P., Escarcega, S., Jimenez, M., Salazar, L.D., Grivetti, L.E., 2000. Food of the gods: cure for humanity? A cultural history of the medicinal and ritual use of chocolate. J. Nutr. 130, 2057S–2072S.

Dreosti, I.E., 2000. Antioxidant polyphenols in tea, cocoa, and wine. Nutrition 16, 692–694.

EFSA Panel on Dietetic Products, Nutrition and Allergies (NDA), 2012. Scientific opinion on the substantiation of a health claim related to cocoa flavanols and maintenance of normal endothelium-dependent vasodilation pursuant to Article 13(5) of Regulation(EC) No 1924/2006. EFSA J. 10, 2809.

Engler, M.B., Engler, M.M., Chen, C.Y., Malloy, M.J., Browne, A., Chiu, E.Y., et al., 2004. Flavonoid-rich dark chocolate improves endothelial function and increases plasma epicatechin concentrations in healthy adults. J. Am. Coll. Nutr. 23, 197–204.

Erdman Jr., J.W., Carson, L., Kwik-Uribe, C., Evans, E.M., Allen, R.R., 2008. Effects of cocoa flavanols on risk factors for cardiovascular disease. Asia Pac. J. Clin. Nutr. 17 (Suppl. 1), 284–287.

Etxeberria, U., Fernandez-Quintela, A., Milagro, F.I., Aguirre, L., Martinez, J.A., Portillo, M.P., 2013. Impact of polyphenols and polyphenol-rich dietary sources on gut microbiota composition. J. Agric. Food Chem. 61, 9517–9533.

Fraga, C.G., ctis-Goretta, L., Ottaviani, J.I., Carrasquedo, F., Lotito, S.B., Lazarus, S., et al., 2005. Regular consumption of a flavanol-rich chocolate can improve oxidant stress in young soccer players. Clin. Dev. Immunol. 12, 11–17.

Grassi, D., Desideri, G., Ferri, C., 2013. Protective effects of dark chocolate on endothelial function and diabetes. Curr. Opin. Clin. Nutr. Metab. Care 16, 662–668.

Grassi, D., Desideri, G., Mai, F., Martella, L., De, F.M., Soddu, D., et al., 2015. Cocoa, glucose tolerance and insulin signalling: the cardiometabolic protection. J. Agric. Food Chem.

Grivetti, L.E., 2009. Medicinal chocolate in New Spain, Western Europe, and North America. In: Grivetti, L.E., Shapiro, H.-Y. (Eds.), Chocolate-History, Culture, and Heritage John Wiley & Sons, Hoboken, NJ, pp. 67–88.

Gu, L., House, S.E., Wu, X., Ou, B., Prior, R.L., 2006. Procyanidin and catechin contents and antioxidant capacity of cocoa and chocolate products. J. Agric. Food Chem. 54, 4057–4061.

Gu, L., Kelm, M.A., Hammerstone, J.F., Beecher, G., Holden, J., Haytowitz, D., et al., 2004. Concentrations of proanthocyanidins in common foods and estimations of normal consumption. J. Nutr. 134, 613–617.

Hammerstone, J.F., Lazarus, S.A., Schmitz, H.H., 2000. Procyanidin content and variation in some commonly consumed foods. J. Nutr. 130, 2086S–2092S.

Heiss, C., Finis, D., Kleinbongard, P., Hoffmann, A., Rassaf, T., Kelm, M., et al., 2007. Sustained increase in flow-mediated dilation after daily intake of high-flavanol cocoa drink over 1 week. J. Cardiovasc. Pharmacol. 49, 74–80.

Hershey Community Archives, 2015. Ration D Bars. <http://www.hersheyarchives.org/essay/details.aspx?EssayId=26> (accessed 03.07.15.).

Hollenberg, N.K., Fisher, N.D., McCullough, M.L., 2009. Flavanols, the Kuna, cocoa consumption, and nitric oxide. J. Am. Soc. Hypertens. 3, 105–112.

Hooper, L., Kay, C., Abdelhamid, A., Kroon, P.A., Cohn, J.S., Rimm, E.B., et al., 2012. Effects of chocolate, cocoa, and flavan-3-ols on cardiovascular health: a systematic review and meta-analysis of randomized trials. Am. J. Clin. Nutr. 95, 740–751.

Hooper, L., Kroon, P.A., Rimm, E.B., Cohn, J.S., Harvey, I., Le Cornu, K.A., et al., 2008. Flavonoids, flavonoid-rich foods, and cardiovascular risk: a meta-analysis of randomized controlled trials. Am. J. Clin. Nutr. 88, 38–50.

International Cocoa Organization, 2013. Harvesting and post-harvesting processing. <http://www.icco.org/about-cocoa/harvesting-and-post-harvest.html> (accessed 23.07.15.).

JAK Native, 2015. Benefits. <http://mayesa.com/our-product/> (accessed 29.07.15.).

Kean, B.H., 1944. The blood pressure of the Cuna Indians. Am. J. Top. Med. 24, 341–343.

Keen, C.L., 2001. Chocolate: food as medicine/medicine as food. J. Am. Coll. Nutr. 20, 436S–439S.

Lampe, J.W., 2008. The Human Microbiome Project: getting to the guts of the matter in cancer epidemiology. Cancer Epidemiol. Biomarkers Prev 17, 2523–2524.

Landberg, R., Sun, Q., Rimm, E.B., Cassidy, A., Scalbert, A., Mantzoros, C.S., et al., 2011. Selected dietary flavonoids are associated with markers of inflammation and endothelial dysfunction in U.S. women. J. Nutr. 141, 618–625.

Lippi, D., 2009. Chocolate and medicine: dangerous liaisons? Nutrition 25, 1100–1103.

Lippi, D., 2013a. Chocolate in history: food, medicine, medi-food. Nutrients 5, 1573–1584.

Lippi, D., 2013b. History of the medical use of chocolate. In: Watson, R., Preedy, V., Zibadi, S. (Eds.), Chocolate in Health and Nutrition Springer Humana Press, New York, pp. 11–21.

Lippi, D., 2015. Sin and pleasure: the history of chocolate in medicine. J. Agric. Food Chem.

Ludwig Weinrich GmbH & Co.KG, 2015. Enjoy life with chocolate. <http://www.vivani-chocolate.de/Gesundheit_e.html> (accessed 17.07.15.).

Manach, C., Williamson, G., Morand, C., Scalbert, A., Remesy, C., 2005. Bioavailability and bioefficacy of polyphenols in humans. I. Review of 97 bioavailability studies. Am. J. Clin. Nutr. 81, 230S–242S.

Mars Incorporated, 2015. What it does. <http://www.cocoavia.com/why-it-works/what-does-it-do> (accessed 17.07.15.).

Maskarinec, G., 2009. Cancer protective properties of cocoa: a review of the epidemiologic evidence. Nutr. Cancer 61, 573–579.

Mastroiacovo, D., Kwik-Uribe, C., Grassi, D., Necozione, S., Raffaele, A., Pistacchio, L., et al., 2015. Cocoa flavanol consumption improves cognitive function, blood pressure control, and metabolic profile in elderly subjects: the Cocoa, Cognition, and Aging (CoCoA) Study—a randomized controlled trial. Am. J. Clin. Nutr. 101, 538–548.

Mathur, S., Devaraj, S., Grundy, S.M., Jialal, I., 2002. Cocoa products decrease low density lipoprotein oxidative susceptibility but do not affect biomarkers of inflammation in humans. J. Nutr. 132, 3663–3667.

McCullough, M.L., Chevaux, K., Jackson, L., Preston, M., Martinez, G., Schmitz, H.H., et al., 2006. Hypertension, the Kuna, and the epidemiology of flavanols. J. Cardiovasc. Pharmacol. 47 (Suppl. 2), S103–S109.

McShea, A., Ramiro-Puig, E., Munro, S.B., Casadesus, G., Castell, M., Smith, M.A., 2008. Clinical benefit and preservation of flavonols in dark chocolate manufacturing. Nutr. Rev. 66, 630–641.

Murphy, K.J., Chronopoulos, A.K., Singh, I., Francis, M.A., Moriarty, H., Pike, M.J., et al., 2003. Dietary flavanols and procyanidin oligomers from cocoa (*Theobroma cacao*) inhibit platelet function. Am. J. Clin. Nutr. 77, 1466–1473.

Mursu, J., Voutilainen, S., Nurmi, T., Rissanen, T.H., Virtanen, J.K., Kaikkonen, J., et al., 2004. Dark chocolate consumption increases HDL cholesterol concentration and chocolate fatty acids may inhibit lipid peroxidation in healthy humans. Free Radic. Biol. Med. 37, 1351–1359.

MXI Corporation, 2013. Cacao: nature's supreme antioxidant source. <http://xocai.xocaistore.com/index.php/cacao/> (accessed 02.07.15.).

Nestle, 2015. Enjoyment and intrinsic goodness. <http://www.nestle.com/brands/chocolateconfectionery/chocolateandconfectionerynhw> (accessed 17.07.15.).

Neveu, V., Perez-Jimenez, J., Vos, F., Crespy, V., du Chaffaut, L., Mennen, L., et al., 2010. Phenol-Explorer: an online comprehensive database on polyphenol contents in foods. Database (Oxford) 2010, bap024.

New Vitality, 2015. Coco complete—cocoa tea. <http://www.newvitality.com/coco-complete/p/d84ebb11393118d/> (accessed 29.07.15.).

Official Journal of the European Union, 2013. Commission Regulation (EU) No 851/2013. <http://eur-lex.europa.eu/LexUriServ/LexUriServ.do?uri=OJ:L:2013:235:0003:0007:EN:PDF> (accessed 21.07.15.).

Perez-Jimenez, J., Fezeu, L., Touvier, M., Arnault, N., Manach, C., Hercberg, S., et al., 2011. Dietary intake of 337 polyphenols in French adults. Am. J. Clin. Nutr. 93, 1220–1228.

Perez-Jimenez, J., Neveu, V., Vos, F., Scalbert, A., 2010. Identification of the 100 richest dietary sources of polyphenols: an application of the Phenol-Explorer database. Eur. J. Clin. Nutr. 64 (Suppl. 3), S112–S120.

Prior, R.L., Gu, L., 2005. Occurrence and biological significance of proanthocyanidins in the American diet. Phytochemistry 66, 2264–2280.

Pure Natural Miracles, 2015. Raw organic cacao powder. <http://www.purenaturalmiracles.com/product/raw-organic-cacao-powder/> (accessed 29.07.15.).

Rein, D., Lotito, S., Holt, R.R., Keen, C.L., Schmitz, H.H., Fraga, C.G., 2000. Epicatechin in human plasma: in vivo determination and effect of chocolate consumption on plasma oxidation status. J. Nutr. 130, 2109S–2114S.

Reserveage Organics, 2015. Cocoa science capsules. <http://cocoawell.com/products/cocoawell-capsules/cocoa-science-capsules/> (accessed 17.07.15.).

Ried, K., Sullivan, T.R., Fakler, P., Frank, O.R., Stocks, N.P., 2010. Does chocolate reduce blood pressure? A meta-analysis. BMC Med. 8, 39.

Ried, K., Sullivan, T.R., Fakler, P., Frank, O.R., Stocks, N.P., 2012. Effect of cocoa on blood pressure. Cochrane Database Syst. Rev. 8, CD008893.

Righteously Raw, 2015. Organic raw cacao. <https://righteouslyrawchocolate.com/product/pure-dark-box-6-bars/> (accessed 17.07.15).

Rios, L.Y., Bennett, R.N., Lazarus, S.A., Remesy, C., Scalbert, A., Williamson, G., 2002. Cocoa procyanidins are stable during gastric transit in humans. Am. J. Clin. Nutr. 76, 1106–1110.

Roberfroid, M., Gibson, G.R., Hoyles, L., McCartney, A.L., Rastall, R., Rowland, I., et al., 2010. Prebiotic effects: metabolic and health benefits. Br. J. Nutr. 104 (Suppl. 2), S1–63.

Rossi, M., Negri, E., Parpinel, M., Lagiou, P., Bosetti, C., Talamini, R., et al., 2010a. Proanthocyanidins and the risk of colorectal cancer in Italy. Cancer Causes Control 21, 243–250.

Rossi, M., Rosato, V., Bosetti, C., Lagiou, P., Parpinel, M., Bertuccio, P., et al., 2010b. Flavonoids, proanthocyanidins, and the risk of stomach cancer. Cancer Causes Control 21, 1597–1604.

Rouillier, P., Senesse, P., Cottet, V., Valleau, A., Faivre, J., Boutron-Ruault, M.C., 2005. Dietary patterns and the adenomacarcinoma sequence of colorectal cancer. Eur. J. Nutr. 44, 311–318.

Rusconi, M., Conti, A., 2010. *Theobroma cacao* L., the food of the gods: a scientific approach beyond myths and claims. Pharmacol. Res. 61, 5–13.

Scalbert, A., Williamson, G., 2000. Dietary intake and bioavailability of polyphenols. J. Nutr. 130, 2073S–2085S.

Sekirov, I., Russell, S.L., Antunes, L.C., Finlay, B.B., 2010. Gut microbiota in health and disease. Physiol. Rev. 90, 859–904.

Serafini, M., Bugianesi, R., Maiani, G., Valtuena, S., De, S.S., Crozier, A., 2003. Plasma antioxidants from chocolate. Nature 424, 1013.

Smith, A.H., Mackie, R.I., 2004. Effect of condensed tannins on bacterial diversity and metabolic activity in the rat gastrointestinal tract. Appl. Environ. Microbiol. 70, 1104–1115.

Snyder, R., Olsen, B., Brindle, L., 2009. From stone metates to steel mills. In: Grivetti, L.E., Shapiro, H.-Y. (Eds.), Chocolate-History, Culture, and Heritage John Wiley & Sons, Hoboken, NJ, pp. 611–623.

Sweetriot, 2015. Health by chocolate. <http://sweetriot.com/riot/cacao-fun/health-by-chocolate/> (accessed 17.07.15.).

Taubert, D., Roesen, R., Lehmann, C., Jung, N., Schomig, E., 2007. Effects of low habitual cocoa intake on blood pressure and bioactive nitric oxide: a randomized controlled trial. JAMA 298, 49–60.

Taza Chocolate, 2015. Healthy dark chocolate. <http://www.tazachocolate.com/Process/Healthy_Dark_Chocolate> (accessed 17.07.15.).

The Healthy Chocolate Co, Inc., 2012. The Healthy Chococolate Co, Inc. company overview. <https://4noguilt.com/company> (accessed 29.07.95).

Theodoratou, E., Kyle, J., Cetnarskyj, R., Farrington, S.M., Tenesa, A., Barnetson, R., et al., 2007. Dietary flavonoids and the risk of colorectal cancer. Cancer Epidemiol. Biomarkers Prev. 16, 684–693.

Thompson, C.A., Habermann, T.M., Wang, A.H., Vierkant, R.A., Folsom, A.R., Ross, J.A., et al., 2010. Antioxidant intake from fruits, vegetables and other sources and risk of non-Hodgkin's lymphoma: the Iowa Women's Health Study. Int. J. Cancer 126, 992–1003.

Torres-Moreno, M., Torrescasana, E., Salas-Salvado, J., Blanch, C., 2015. Nutritional composition and fatty acids profile in cocoa beans and chocolates with different geographical origin and processing conditions. Food Chem. 166, 125–132.

True Healthy Products LLC, 2014. True healthy dark chocolate. <http://www.truehealthyproducts.com/products/dietary/true-healthy-dark-chocolate> (accessed 29.07.15.).

Turnbaugh, P.J., Ley, R.E., Hamady, M., Fraser-Liggett, C.M., Knight, R., Gordon, J.I., 2007. The human microbiome project. Nature 449, 804–810.

Tzounis, X., Rodriguez-Mateos, A., Vulevic, J., Gibson, G.R., Kwik-Uribe, C., Spencer, J.P., 2011. Prebiotic evaluation of cocoa-derived flavanols in healthy humans by using a randomized, controlled, double-blind, crossover intervention study. Am. J. Clin. Nutr. 93, 62–72.

U.S. Department of Agriculture, Agricultural Research Service, 2015. USDA National Nutrient Database for Standard Reference, Release 27 <http://www.ars.usda.gov/Services/docs.htm?docid=8964> (accessed 22.07.15.).

Wan, Y., Vinson, J.A., Etherton, T.D., Proch, J., Lazarus, S.A., Kris-Etherton, P.M., 2001. Effects of cocoa powder and dark chocolate on LDL oxidative susceptibility and prostaglandin concentrations in humans. Am. J. Clin. Nutr. 74, 596–602.

Wang, J.F., Schramm, D.D., Holt, R.R., Ensunsa, J.L., Fraga, C.G., Schmitz, H.H., et al., 2000. A dose-response effect from chocolate consumption on plasma epicatechin and oxidative damage. J. Nutr. 130, 2115S–2119S.

Wirfalt, E., McTaggart, A., Pala, V., Gullberg, B., Frasca, G., Panico, S., et al., 2002. Food sources of carbohydrates in a European cohort of adults. Public Health Nutr. 5, 1197–1215.

Wiswedel, I., Hirsch, D., Kropf, S., Gruening, M., Pfister, E., Schewe, T., et al., 2004. Flavanol-rich cocoa drink lowers plasma F(2)-isoprostane concentrations in humans. Free Radic. Biol. Med. 37, 411–421.

Zamora-Ros, R., Rothwell, J.A., Scalbert, A., Knaze, V., Romieu, I., Slimani, N., et al., 2013. Dietary intakes and food sources of phenolic acids in the European Prospective Investigation into Cancer and Nutrition (EPIC) study. Br. J. Nutr. 110, 1500–1511.

Zhang, Z., Xu, G., Liu, X., 2013. Chocolate intake reduces risk of cardiovascular disease: evidence from 10 observational studies. Int. J. Cardiol. 168, 5448–5450.

Chapter 14

Pomegranate juice and extract

Gene Bruno
Huntington College of Health Sciences, Knoxville, TN, United States

CHAPTER OUTLINE

INTRODUCTION

For thousands of years, pomegranate fruit (*Punica granatum*) has been used as a food and traditional medicine (Still, 2006). One of the earliest fruits to be domesticated, it originated in the Middle East and now can be found as a crop in the Far East, India, the Mediterranean, and the Americas where it is consumed fresh and in processed form as juice, wines, flavors, and extracts (Mertens-Talcott et al., 2006). Furthermore, pomegranate's use as a medicine is ancient. According to Jimenez del Rio et al. (2006), its phytotherapeutic history originated from the folk medicine of cultures in the Caucasus and Mediterranean basin. In fact, Pomegranate's medicinal use was discussed in the *Ebers Papyrus* from Egypt (c. 1500 BCE), one of the oldest medical texts (Jayaprakasha and Negi, 2006).

Fruits, Vegetables, and Herbs.
DOI: http://dx.doi.org/10.1016/B978-0-12-802972-5.00014-7

This chapter will address the chemistry, pharmacology, and human clinical research associated with pomegranate juice and extract.

PLANT PARTS AND CHEMISTRY

The skin (a.k.a. rind, husk, or pericarp) of the pomegranate fruit is tough and leathery. Membranous walls, known as carpels, compartmentalize the interior of the fruit, along with white spongy pith. The resulting compartments (a.k.a. locules) contain 600–800 sacs called arils. One seed and juicy pulp is contained in each aril. In total, the arils consist of approximately 80% juice pulp and 20% seeds (Tous and Ferguson, 1996; El-Nemr et al., 1990).

The parts of pomegranate which have been used medicinally include the fruit, fruit juice, seed, seed oil, bark, rind, root, stem, leaf, and flower (Schubert et al., 1999; Huang et al., 2005). These plant parts provide the following chemical constituents:

Plant Part	Chemical Constituents
Seeds and seed oil	Polyphenols and fatty acids, including punicic acid, palmitic acid, stearic acid, oleic acid, and linoleic acid (Schubert et al., 1999; Wang et al., 2004); estrone and other nonsteroidal estrogenic substances (Moneam et al., 1988)
Bark, leaf, and fruit husk	Ellagitannins and gallotannins (Gil et al., 2000)
Bark of the root and stem	Piperidine alkaloids: pelletierine, pseudopelletierine, isopelletierine, and methyl isopelletierine (Tripathi and Singh, 2000; Vidal et al., 2003)
Juice	0.2–1.0% polyphenols. These polyphenols primarily include anthocyanidins such as delphinidin, cyanidin, pelargonidin, and hydrolyzable tannins including punicalin, pedunculagin, punicalagin, gallagic, and ellagic acids (Esmaillzadeh et al., 2004; Malik et al., 2005; Miguel et al., 2004). The juice also contains citric acid, ascorbic acid, oxalic acid, and tartaric acid (Gil et al., 2000; Miguel et al., 2004)

PHARMACOLOGY/MECHANISM OF ACTION

Antioxidant The polyphenols in pomegranate have antioxidant activity (Schubert et al., 1999; Noda et al., 2002). In fact, pomegranate juice contains more polyphenols than red wine, blueberry, cranberry, green tea, or orange juice (Aviram, 2002), and its antioxidant activity can be as much as three times higher than red wine or green tea (Gil et al., 2000). In human clinical research, pomegranate ellagitannin-enriched polyphenol extract significantly reduced the production of thiobarbituric acid reactive substances (TBARS)[1] in plasma (Heber et al., 2007). Furthermore, human (Rosenblat et al., 2006) and animal (Kaplan et al., 2001) researches suggest that pomegranate juice may slow the progression of atherosclerosis, in association with reduced lipid peroxidation of low-density lipoproteins (LDL). In addition, *in vitro* research has shown that several seed constituents have antioxidant activity (Wang et al., 2004).

Nitric oxide Research demonstrates that pomegranate extract activates the nitric oxide synthetase pathway (Vilahur et al., 2015), and pomegranate juice can increase nitric oxide synthetase activity in the blood vessel endothelium (Esmaillzadeh et al., 2004). Nitric oxide synthetase increases the availability of nitric oxide, an antioxidant and vasodilator.

Anticholesterolemic Pomegranate juice has reduced total and LDL cholesterol in diabetic subjects, possibly due to its polyphenol constituents which may decrease cholesterol synthesis in the liver (Al-Jarallah et al., 2013). Pomegranate extract reduced aortic sinus and coronary artery atherosclerosis in mice (de Nigris et al., 2005).

Antihypertensive Pomegranate juice has reduced the activity of angiotensin converting enzyme (ACE) by about 36%, and reduced blood pressure (BP) in patients with hypertension (Aviram and Dornfeld, 2001). Similar results have been seen in animal research as well (Mohan et al., 2010).

Antiviral *In vitro* testing suggests pomegranate juice might have inhibitory activity against infection by HIV-1 BaL (Neurath et al., 2005), targeting the viral envelope to prevent cellular viral entry (Neurath et al., 2004). *In vitro* testing also found that pomegranate polyphenol extract (PPE) suppresses replication of influenza A virus as well as inhibiting viral RNA replication. In this instance, punicalagin was demonstrated to be the effective, anti-influenza component of PPE (Haidari et al., 2009).

Antibacterial Pomegranate fruit extract was shown to have good activity against *Staphylococcus aureus in vitro* (Holetz et al., 2002) (and subsequent enterotoxin production; Braga et al., 2005), as well as against 35 hospital isolates of methicillin-resistant *S. aureus* (MRSA) (Voravuthikunchai and Kitpipit, 2005).

Anticandidal Anticandidal activity was detected *in vitro* with pomegranate fruit extract (Holetz et al., 2002), and a pomegranate gel was shown to have efficacy as a topical antifungal agent for the treatment of candidosis associated with denture stomatitis (Vasconcelos et al., 2003).

---

[1] TBARS are formed as a byproduct of lipid peroxidation.

Anticancer Various pomegranate materials have demonstrated anticancer activity. Aggressive prostate cancer cell growth was inhibited *in vitro* and apoptosis induced with pomegranate fruit extract, and tumor growth was likewise inhibited while prostate-specific antigen (PSA) levels were reduced in animals implanted with prostate cancer cells (Malik et al., 2005; Albrecht et al., 2004). Fermented pomegranate juice polyphenols and pomegranate extracts were shown to have activity against malignant breast cancer cells (Kim et al., 2002; Jeune et al., 2005), and pomegranate seed oil demonstrated activity against skin cancer cells (Hora et al., 2003). Pomegranate juice was found to have greater *in vitro* effectiveness against oral, colon, and prostate cancer cells than individual pomegranate constituents (Seeram et al., 2005).

HUMAN CLINICAL RESEARCH

A fairly significant body of human research has been conducted on pomegranate juice and extract. This includes research on various aspects of cardiovascular health, prostate cancer, exercise, dental health, and ultraviolet ray (UV)-induced skin pigmentation. In this chapter, the research discussed in regard to these disease states will be limited to human research.

Cardiovascular health

Modulating risk and progression of atherosclerosis/coronary heart disease

Various clinical approaches exist for modulating the risk as well as the progression of atherosclerosis/coronary heart disease (CHD). Among these include reduction of oxidative stress, improvement in antioxidant status, reduction in intima-media thickness (IMT), protection against lipid peroxidation, improvement in myocardial perfusion, and reducing the atherogenicity of human monocyte-derived macrophages (HMDM). Pomegranate juice and extract may play a role in this modulation process, as discussed later. While modulation of serum lipids and BP also play major roles in reducing risk and disease progression, this will be addressed separately in a subsequent section.

In a 3-month open trial, Rosenblat et al. (2006) assessed the effects of pomegranate juice (50 mL/day) on serum glucose, cholesterol, and triglyceride levels, and on measures of oxidative stress in serum and macrophages of 10 type-2 diabetic patients; 10 healthy subjects served as controls. Results showed that pomegranate juice consumption did not affect serum glucose, cholesterol, and triglyceride levels, but it did significantly:

- Reduce serum lipid peroxide and thiobarbituric acid reactive substance (TBARS) levels by 56% and 28%, respectively

- Increase serum sulfhydryl groups[2] and paraoxonase 1 (PON1)[3] activity by 12% and 24%, respectively
- Reduce cellular peroxides by 71%
- Increase glutathione levels by 141% in HMDM
- Decrease the extent of oxidized LDL (Ox-LDL) cellular uptake by 39%.

Researchers concluded that pomegranate juice consumption by diabetic patients resulted in an antioxidant effect on serum and macrophages, which may help attenuate atherosclerosis development without worsening diabetic parameters.

The effects of 50 mL/day of pomegranate juice consumption by atherosclerotic patients with carotid artery stenosis (CAS) on the progression of carotid lesions and changes in oxidative stress and BP were also investigated in a controlled study by Aviram et al. (2004), with 10 patients supplemented for 1 year and 5 patients continuing for up to 3 years, while 9 patients served as the control group. Blood samples were collected before treatment and during pomegranate juice consumption. Results after 1 year showed that pomegranate juice consumption resulted in:

- A significant reduction in IMT up to 30%, while IMT increased by 9% in the control group ($P < 0.01$)
- An increase in serum PON 1 activity by 83% ($P < 0.01$) and a further 10% increase after 3 years
- A significant decrease in serum LDL basal oxidative state and LDL susceptibility to copper ion-induced oxidation by 90% and 59%, respectively ($P < 0.01$)
- A decrease in serum levels of antibodies against oxidized LDL by 19% ($P < 0.01$)
- A significant reduction in serum lipid peroxidation by 59% and a further 16% reduction after 3 years
- An increase in serum total antioxidant status (TAS) was increased by 130%
- A reduction in systolic BP by 12% ($P < 0.05$), with no significant change in the control group.

No further changes occurred in association with 3 years of pomegranate juice consumption. The researchers concluded that the antioxidant characteristics

---

[2] Sulfhydryl groups are part of the structure of certain antioxidants such as the amino acid cysteine.

[3] Due to its ability to remove harmful oxidized lipids, PON1 protects against the development of atherosclerosis.

of pomegranate juice polyphenols likely resulted in the decrease in carotid IMT and systolic BP in patients with CAS.

Conversely, Davidson et al. (2009) reported the results of another randomized, double-blind, parallel trial using 240 mL/day of pomegranate juice, showing no significant effect on overall anterior and posterior carotid intima-media thickness (CIMT) progression rate in subjects at moderate risk for CHD, but may have slowed CIMT progression in subjects with increased oxidative stress and disturbances in the triglyceride-rich lipoprotein/HDL (high-density lipoprotein) axis.

Aviram et al. (2000) tested the effects of pomegranate juice consumption on lipoprotein oxidation, aggregation and retention, macrophage atherogenicity, platelet aggregation and atherosclerosis *ex vivo* in two human studies. In the first study, 13 healthy, nonsmoking men (20–35 years) were supplemented with 50 mL/day of pomegranate juice (1.5 mmol total polyphenols) for 2 weeks. In the second study, performed for $\leq$ 10 weeks, 3 subjects were supplemented with increasing doses of 20–80 mL/day of pomegranate juice (0.54–2.16 mmol total polyphenols). The results were that pomegranate juice consumption decreased LDL susceptibility to aggregation and retention, while increasing the activity of serum paraoxonase[4] by 20%.

A 3-month, randomized, placebo-controlled, double-blind study by Sumner et al. (2005) investigated the effects of 240 mL/day of pomegranate juice on myocardial perfusion in 45 patients who had ischemic CHD and myocardial ischemia. The summed difference score was calculated by subtracting the summed score at rest from the summed stress score, and this was used to assess the amount of inducible ischemia. Although the experimental and control groups had similar levels of stress-induced ischemia (SDS) at baseline, the extent of SDS decreased in the pomegranate group but increased in the control group ($P < 0.05$) after 3 months. The average improvement in myocardial perfusion was about 17% with pomegranate juice compared with an 18% worsening of myocardial perfusion in patients treated with placebo.

A 2-month, double-blind, placebo-controlled, randomized, prospective pilot study was conducted by Hamoud et al. (2014) to examine the effect of pomegranate extract on cholesterol and oxidative stress in serum and in HMDM[5] in simvastatin-treated patients. Subjects received simvastatin

[4] An HDL-associated esterase that can protect against lipid peroxidation.

[5] HMDM are involved in creating the progressive plaque lesions of atherosclerosis.

(20 mg/day) and a placebo pill ($n = 11$), or simvastatin and pomegranate extract (1 g/day, $n = 12$). After 2 months, simvastatin + placebo significantly decreased HMDM cholesterol biosynthesis rate by 33%, and simvastatin + pomegranate extract decreased it by 44%. HMDM reactive oxygen species (ROS) levels decreased by 18% in the simvastatin + placebo group, while it decreased up to 30% in the simvastatin + pomegranate extract group. Also, macrophage triglycerides significantly decreased by 48% versus baseline levels with simvastatin + pomegranate extract, but not with simvastatin + placebo therapy. Researchers concluded that adding pomegranate extract to simvastatin therapy in hypercholesterolemic could reduce the risk for atherosclerosis.

Modulation of serum lipids

Esmaillzadeh et al. (2006) conducted an 8-week open pilot study to examine the effects of concentrated pomegranate juice on the lipid profiles of 22 type-2 diabetic patients with hyperlipidemia who were free of any other chronic diseases. Food recall and food records were completed and anthropometric and biochemical assessments were taken, and the patients consumed 40 g concentrated pomegranate juice daily. Results demonstrated that consumption of concentrated pomegranate juice significantly reduced total cholesterol ($P < 0.006$), low-density lipoprotein cholesterol (LDL-C) ($P < 0.006$), LDL-C/high-density lipoprotein cholesterol (HDL-C) ($P < 0.001$), and total cholesterol/HDL-C ($P < 0.001$), but there were no significant changes in serum triacylglycerol and HDL-C concentrations. Researchers concluded that concentrated pomegranate juice consumption could modify heart disease risk factors in hyperlipidemic patients.

Similarly, Esmaillzadeh et al. (2004) conducted an earlier open study with 22 type-2 diabetic patients with hyperlipidemia, to examine the effect of consuming 40 g/day of concentrated pomegranate juice on lipid profiles. During the initial 8-week period, a baseline for normal dietary intake was established using 24-hour food recall and food records. Consumption of concentrated pomegranate juice commenced during the following 8-week period. Anthropometric and blood indices evaluated at baseline and upon conclusion of the study. Results demonstrated that concentrated pomegranate juice consumption significantly reduced total cholesterol ($P < 0.006$), LDL-C ($P < 0.006$), LDL-C/HDL-C ($P < 0.0001$), and total cholesterol/HDL-C ($P < 0.001$), but had no significant effect on concentrations of serum triglycerides and HDL-C. Researchers concluded that concentrated pomegranate juice consumption may modify heart disease risk factors in hyperlipidemic patients.

Blood pressure modulation

To examine the effect of consuming 50 mL/day of pomegranate juice (providing 1.5 mmol of total polyphenols per day) by hypertensive patients on BP and on serum ACE activity, Aviram and Dornfeld (2001) conducted a 2-week open trial. Results showed a 36% decrease in serum ACE activity and a 5% reduction in systolic BP. In an accompanying in–vitro study, pomegranate juice demonstrated a similar dose-dependent, 31% inhibitory effect of pomegranate juice on serum ACE activity.

Since high-fat meals are known to initiate a transitory increase in BP, Mathew et al. (2012) conducted a randomized, controlled cross-over trial in 19 young, healthy men to examine the effects of pomegranate extract in a test drink consumed 15 min before (ET-PRE) or during a high-fat meal (ET-DUR) compared to placebo on postprandial triglyceride levels, vascular function and BP. Results showed that, compared to the placebo group, there was a lesser increase in systolic BP in the ET-PRE and ET-DUR groups ($P = 0.041$), with other parameters unaffected.

To determine the effects of 200 mL/day pomegranate juice (sugar or additives free) consumption compared to a control on BP in 61 type-2 diabetic patients, Sohrab et al. (2008) conducted a 6-week, randomized clinical trial study. Results demonstrated that the pomegranate juice consumption group experienced a significant decrease in mean systolic BP and diastolic BP compared with baseline ($P < 0.001$ and $P < 0.05$, respectively), and compared to the control group ($P < 0.02$ and $P < 0.03$, respectively). Researchers concluded that pomegranate juice consumption may be recommended for hypertension prevention in these patients.

Wright and Pipkin (2008) examined the effects of antioxidants in pomegranate juice and kiwifruit (KW) on the renin–angiotensin system (RAS) and BP in a randomized, placebo-controlled study with 45 student volunteers (aged 20.7 ± 1.2) assigned the control group (no supplementation) or the KW (2 fruits per day) or pomegranate juice (166 mL/day) groups. Results were that, in the control and KW groups, there was no significant change in DBP. In the pomegranate juice group, however, there was a significant ($P = 0.037$) reduction of −6.0 mmHg in DBP. No significant changes in SBP were seen in any group. Plasma ACE and plasma antioxidant concentrations did not change significantly overall.

A randomized double-blind placebo-controlled trial was conducted by Carpenter et al. (2010) to examine the effect of 2 weeks of supplementation with either pomegranate juice (300 mL/day) or placebo on BP in 46 healthy students (mean age 20.4 ± 1.1). While results found that pomegranate juice had no significant effect on SBP in the overall student sample, the reduction in SBP in students with systolic pre-hypertension was significantly greater in those supplemented with pomegranate juice (−9.1 vs − 2.2 mmHg; $P = 0.039$). No effect was found on diastolic BP.

Modulation of endothelial function

Hashemi et al. (2010) conducted a 1-month, randomized, controlled clinical trial with 30 metabolic syndrome (MetS) adolescents (age: 12–15 years) to determine the acute and long-term effects of consuming grape (18 mL/kg/day) and pomegranate (240 mL/day) juices on endothelium function by assessing basal brachial artery dimension and flow-mediated dilation (FMD). Endothelial-dependent dilation was also measured after receiving nitroglycerin spray before juice consumption, as well as 4 hours and 30 days after regular daily consumption. Results showed that FMD at 90 seconds and after nitroglycerin significantly improved at 4 hours and at 1 month in both juice groups (not significant between group differences).

In a similar 1-month, randomized, controlled clinical trial, Kelishadi et al. (2011) examined the short- and long-term effects of consumption of grape and pomegranate juices (same quantity as in previous study) on markers of endothelial function and inflammation in adolescents with MetS. Assessment methods included measurements of inflammatory factors and FMD at baseline, 4 hours after first juice consumption and after 1 month of juice consumption. Results showed significant short- and long-term improvement in FMD in both groups. Hs-CRP had a nonsignificant decrease. Regarding inflammatory markers, there was a significant decrease in sE selectin and interleulkin-6 after 4 hours in the pomegranate juice group and after 1 month in both groups. Likewise, there was a significant decrease in sICAM-1 after 4 hours and after 1 month in pomegranate juice group. Furthermore, the decline in inflammation was associated with improvement in FMD.

Prostate cancer

A phase II, Simon two-stage clinical trial was conducted by Pantuck et al. (2006) to determine the effects of consuming 8 oz/day of pomegranate juice (Pom Wonderful, 570 mg total polyphenol gallic acid equivalents) on PSA progression in men with a rising PSA following primary therapy. Results demonstrated a significant increase in mean PSA doubling time from a mean of 15 months (baseline) to 54 months (posttreatment, $P < 0.001$). Furthermore, treatment was well tolerated and there were no serious adverse events reported. In addition, pre- and post-treatment *in vitro* assays of patient serum on the growth of LNCaP showed a 12% decrease in cell proliferation ($P = 0.0048$) and a 17% increase in apoptosis ($P = 0.0004$), as well as a 23% increase in nitric oxide ($P = 0.0085$) with significant reductions in oxidative state and sensitivity to oxidation of serum lipids ($P < 0.02$). The researchers suggested that the significant results warrant further testing in a placebo-controlled study.

Subsequently, Stenner-Liewen et al. (2013) conducted a phase IIb, double-blinded, randomized placebo-controlled trial in 98 patients with histologically confirmed prostate cancer who consumed 500 mL/day of pomegranate juice (equivalent to 1147 mg polyphenol gallic acid) or placebo beverage for a 4-week period. In the second open phase of the study, all subjects received 250 mL/day of pomegranate juice (equivalent to 573 mg polyphenol gallic acid) daily for another 4 weeks. No differences were detected between the two groups with regard to PSA kinetics and pain scores.

One major difference between these two studies was the source of the pomegranate juice. While both provided similar amounts of polyphenol gallic acid equivalents, these are not the only active phytochemical constituents of pomegranate juice. In the Pantuck et al. (2006) study, Pom Wonderful was the source of the pomegranate juice, providing flavonoids which constituted 40% (anthocyanins, catechins, and phenols) of total polyphenols. Conversely, in the Stenner-Liewen et al. (2013) study Biotta AG of Switzerland provided the pomegranate juice which contained pear purée, white tea, agave concentrate and aronia berry juice and 27.5% pomegranate extract (not pomegranate juice); but other phytochemical constituents of the pomegranate juice were not identified in the study. It appears that the pomegranate juice used in the two studies was not phytochemically equivalent, and therefore the latter study cannot reasonably be said to have been an accurate follow-up to the Pom Wonderful study.

In addition to pomegranate juice, pomegranate extract has also been used in human prostate cancer-related research. To assess the effect of pomegranate extract on prostate oxidative stress, Freedland et al. (2013) conducted a placebo-controlled trial with 70 men who were randomized to two daily tablets of pomegranate extract (POMx, 2 g/day) or placebo for up to 4 weeks before radical prostatectomy. Results showed that POMx was associated with a nonstatistically significant 16% lower benign tissue 8-hydroxy-2'-deoxyguanosine (an oxidative stress biomarker), and POMx was well tolerated. Researchers indicated that future larger longer studies are needed to more definitively test whether POMx reduces prostate oxidative stress.

To assess the biological activity of two doses of pomegranate extract (POMx) on PSA doubling time (PSADT) in men with recurrent prostate cancer (n = 104, median age 74.5 years) with a rising PSA and without metastases, Paller et al. (2013) conducted a randomized, multi-center, double-blind phase II, dose-exploring trial. Subjects received 1 or 3 g of POMx, stratified by baseline PSADT and Gleason score, for up to 18 months. Results demonstrated a significant lengthening of median PSADT ($P < 0.001$). In the low-dose group, PSADT lengthened from 11.9 to 18.8 months, and in the high-dose group PSADT lengthened from 12.2 to 17.5 months, with no significant difference between dose groups ($P = 0.554$). Furthermore, 43% of patients had PSADT increases greater than 100% of baseline, and declining PSA levels were observed in 13 patients. Primarily due to a rising PSA, 42% of patients discontinued treatment before meeting the protocol-definition of PSA progression (or 18 months). Treatment was associated with ≥ 6 months increases in PSADT in both treatment arms without adverse effects.

Musculoskeletal/joint health

Balbir-Gurman et al. (2011) investigated rheumatoid arthritis (RA) disease activity in relation to serum oxidative status in 6 RA patients consuming pomegranate extract (POMx, 10 mL/day) during a 12-week, pilot open-labeled study. Results showed that pomegranate extract significantly ($P <$ 0.02) reduced the composite Disease Activity Index (DAS28) by 17%. This could be predominantly related to a significant ($P < 0.005$) 62% reduction in the tender joint count. In addition, there was a significant ($P < 0.02$) reduction in serum oxidative status as well as a moderate but significant ($P < 0.02$) increase in serum HDL-associated PON1 activity. Researchers concluded that supplementation may be useful in attenuating clinical symptoms in RA.

Exercise

To determine if pomegranate juice consumption would improve recovery of skeletal muscle strength after eccentric exercise in subjects who routinely performed resistance training, Trombold et al. (2011) conducted a randomized, cross-over, placebo-controlled study with resistance trained men (n = 17). Subjects performed 3 sets of 20 unilateral eccentric elbow flexion and 6 sets of 10 unilateral eccentric knee extension exercises to produce delayed onset muscle soreness. Compared to placebo, results showed that elbow flexion strength was significantly higher during the 2- to 168-hour period postexercise with pomegranate juice ($P = 0.031$), and elbow flexor muscle soreness was significantly reduced ($P = 0.006$), as well as at 48 and 72 hours postexercise ($P = 0.003$ and $P = 0.038$, respectively).

There was no significant improvement with isometric strength and muscle soreness in the knee extensors compared to placebo.

To determine the effect of supplementation with Wonderful variety pomegranate extract (POMx, 500 mL twice daily at 12-hour intervals) compared to placebo on recovery of skeletal muscle strength after eccentric exercise, Trombold et al. (2010) conducted a double-blind, randomized, placebo-controlled cross-over study with recreationally active males during a period of 9 days, subjects performed two sets of 20 maximal eccentric elbow flexion exercises with one arm to produce delayed onset muscle soreness. Measures of maximal isometric elbow flexion strength and muscle soreness, as well as serum markers of inflammation and muscle damage were taken at baseline and 2, 24, 48, 72, and 96 hours after exercise. Results showed that, after exercise, strength was significantly higher in POMx compared to placebo at 48 hours (85.4% ± 2.5% and 78.3% ± 2.6%, $P = 0.01$) and 72 hours (88.9% ± 2.0% and 84.0% ± 2.0%, $P = 0.009$). There were no significant changes in serum markers of inflammation and muscle damage.

In an 8-day study, Machin et al. (2014) set out to determine if there is a dose response effect of pomegranate juice concentrate supplementation after eccentric exercise isometric strength recovery in 45 nonresistance trained, recreationally active men assigned to once-daily pomegranate juice (650 mg gallic acid equivalents), twice-daily pomegranate juice (1300 mg gallic acid equivalents), or placebo. Throughout the postexercise time period, isometric knee extensor and elbow flexor strength were similar between once-daily and twice-daily pomegranate juice supplementation groups. Isometric strength, however, was significantly higher in pomegranate juice groups than placebo. Researchers concluded that once-daily pomegranate juice supplementation is not different from twice-daily supplementation in regards to strength recovery after eccentric exercise.

Dental health

In a placebo-controlled study, DiSilvestro et al. (2009) compared the effects of 4 weeks of thrice daily mouth rinsing with the pomegranate extract (PomElla) dissolved in water or placebo on young adults ($n = 32$). Results showed changes in salivary measures relevant to oral health, including gingivitis:

- Reduced total protein (may correlate with plaque forming bacteria readings)
- Reduced activities of aspartate aminotransferase (may indicate cell injury)

- Reduced alpha-glucosidase activity (sucrose degrading enzyme)
- Increased activities of the antioxidant enzyme ceruloplasmin (may give better protection against oral oxidant stress)
- Increased radical scavenging capacity (increase was significant by nonparametric statistical analysis).

The placebo had no effect on these measures.

To examine the effect of the pomegranate extract on dental plaque microorganisms, Menezes et al. (2006) conducted a study with 60 healthy patients (age: 9–25 years) using fixed orthodontic appliances. Subjects were randomized into three groups: (1) distilled water (control), (2) chlorhexidine (standard) mouthwash, and (3) pomegranate mouthwash. Before and after a 1-min mouthrinse with 15 mL, dental plaque material was collected from each subject. Results showed that pomegranate extract effectively decreased dental plaque microorganisms (CFU/mL) by 84%, and similar values were observed with chlorhexidine at 79% inhibition. Comparatively the control group only experienced an 11% inhibition of CFU/mL. In addition, pomegranate extract demonstrated antibacterial activity against selected microorganisms.

Similarly, Bhadbhade et al. (2011) evaluated the effect of a pomegranate-containing mouthrinse on plaque on 30 periodontally healthy volunteers in a randomized, placebo-controlled trial. Subjects were randomized into three mouthrinse groups: (1) pomegranate, (2) chlorhexidine, or (3) distilled water (placebo), used twice daily in all cases. Plaque Index (PI) was assessed at days 0 and 5, and pomegranate extract was tested *in vitro* against *Aggregatibacter actinomycetemcomitans*, *Porphyromonas gingivalis*, and *Prevotella intermedia*. Results showed no statistically significant difference between chlorhexidine and pomegranate rinse groups with respect to PI, but both were significantly superior to placebo ($P < 0.05$). In addition, pomegranate extract inhibited all three strains of periodontopathogens at various concentrations.

To evaluate the effect of a gel containing pomegranate extract of *P. granatum* as an antifungal agent against candidosis associated with denture stomatitis, Vasconcelos et al. (2003) conducted a positive control study with 60 denture stomatitis patients randomized to two groups: (1) miconazole (Daktarin® gel oral) and (2) pomegranate gel, both of which were used three times daily for 15 days. Results showed a satisfactory and regular response in 27 subjects using miconazole and in 21 subjects using pomegranate gel. Likewise, negativity of yeasts was observed in 25 subjects using miconazole and in 23 subjects using pomegranate gel. Researchers concluded that pomegranate extract may be used as a topical antifungal agent for the treatment of candidosis associated with denture stomatitis.

UV-induced skin pigmentation

To examine the protective and ameliorative effects of ellagic acid-rich pomegranate extract on pigmentation in the skin after UV irradiation, Kasai et al. (2006) conducted a 4-week, double-blind, placebo-controlled trial using 39 female subjects (age range: 20–40s) randomized to three groups: high dose (200 mg/day ellagic acid), low dose (100 mg/day ellagic acid), and control (0 mg/day ellagic acid: placebo). A 1.5 MED (minimum erythema dose) of UV irradiation was administered to each subject on an inside region of the right upper arm, based on the MED value measured on the previous day, and measurements of luminance (L), melanin and erythema values were taken at 0 week and after 1, 2, 3 and 4 weeks. Additionally, subjects responded to questionnaires regarding skin condition before at the termination of the pomegranate extract intake. Results were as follows:

- Compared to control group, luminance values were inhibited by 1.35% and 1.73% in the low- and high dose groups, respectively.
- In subjects with a slight sunburn, stratified analysis revealed a decrease of luminance values compared with the control group at 1, 2 ($P < 0.01$, respectively), and 4 weeks ($P < 0.05$) in the low dose group, and at 2 and 3 weeks ($P < 0.05$) in the high dose group.
- Ameliorating tendencies in test groups in "brightness of the face" and "stains and freckles."

Researchers suggested that oral ingestion of ellagic acid-rich pomegranate extract has an inhibitory effect on a slight pigmentation in the human skin caused by UV irradiation.

DISCUSSION

The pomegranate materials used in the aforementioned studies vary in type and potency. Table 14.1 delineates those specific materials by study.

A significant body of human research was conducted using the Wonderful variety of pomegranate juice (ie, POM Wonderful®) as well as POMx™ pomegranate extract, although nonproprietary pomegranate juices and extracts were also studied. Since pomegranate materials differ with regard to their respective profiles of active phytochemicals, it makes sense to consider the specific materials studied when determining an appropriate material to utilize for a specific application.

Table 14.1 Types of Pomegranate Materials Used in Clinical Studies and Daily Doses

Study	Pomegranate Material Used	Daily Dose
Rosenblat et al. (2006)	Pomegranate juice—Wonderful variety[a]	50 mL
Aviram et al. (2004)	Pomegranate juice—Wonderful variety	50 mL
Davidson et al. (2009)	Pomegranate juice—Wonderful variety	240 mL
Aviram et al. (2000)	Pomegranate juice—Wonderful variety	50 mL
Sumner et al. (2005)	Pomegranate juice—POM Wonderful®	240 mL
Hamoud et al. (2014)	Pomegranate extract—POMx™	1 g
Esmaillzadeh et al. (2006)	Concentrated pomegranate juice	40 g
Esmaillzadeh et al. (2004)	Concentrated pomegranate juice	40 g
Aviram and Dornfeld (2001)	Pomegranate juice (providing 1.5 mmol of total polyphenols/50 mL)	50 mL
Mathew et al. (2012)	Pomegranate extract—POMx™ in test drink	652–948 mg pomegranate polyphenols (expressed as gallic acid equivalents)/237 mL
Sohrab et al. (2008)	Sugar/additive-free pomegranate juice	200 mL
Wright & Pipkin (2008)	Pomegranate juice—POM Wonderful®	166 mL
Carpenter et al. (2010)	Pomegranate juice—POM Wonderful®	300 mL
Hashemi et al. (2010)	Pomegranate juice—Home-made without added sweetener	240 mL
Kelishadi et al. (2011)		240 mL
Pantuck et al. (2006)	Pomegranate juice—POM Wonderful®	8 oz (237 mL)
Stenner-Liewen et al. (2013)		500 mL 250 mL

(Continued)

Table 14.1 Types of Pomegranate Materials Used in Clinical Studies and Daily Doses (Continued)

Study	Pomegranate Material Used	Daily Dose
Freedland et al. (2013)	Pomegranate extract—POMx™	2 g
Paller et al. (2013)	Pomegranate extract—POMx™	1 or 3 g
Balbir-Gurman et al. (2011)	Pomegranate extract—POMx™	10 mL
Trombold et al. (2011)	Pomegranate juice	650 mg gallic acid equivalents
Trombold et al. (2010)	Pomegranate extract—POMx™	1000 mL
Machin et al. (2014)	Concentrated pomegranate juice	650–1300 mg gallic acid equivalents
DiSilvestro et al. (2009)	PomElla® extract mouthwash	Thrice daily rinse
Menezes et al. (2006)	Pomegranate extract	15 mL
Bhadbhade et al. (2011)	Pomegranate mouthwash	Thrice daily rinse
Vasconcelos et al. (2003)	Pomegranate gel	Thrice daily application
Kasai et al. (2006)	Pomegranate extract	2 tablets providing 100–200 mg ellagic acid

[a]Providing 1979 mg/L of tannins (1561 mg/L punicalagin and 417 mg/L hydrolysable tannins), 384 mg/L of anthocyanins (delphinidin 3,5-diglucoside, cyanidin 3,5-diglucoside, delphinidin-3-glucoside, cyanidin 3-glucoside, and pelargonidine 3-glucoside), and 121 mg/L of ellagic acids derivatives.

REFERENCES

Albrecht, M., Jiang, W., Kumi-Diaka, J., Lansky, E.P., Gommersall, L.M., Patel, A., et al., 2004. Pomegranate extracts potently suppress proliferation, xenograft growth, and invasion of human prostate cancer cells. J. Med. Food 7, 274–283.

Al-Jarallah, A., Igdoura, F., Zhang, Y., Tenedero, C.B., White, E.J., MacDonald, M.E., et al., 2013. The effect of pomegranate extract on coronary artery atherosclerosis in SR-BI/APOE double knockout mice. Atherosclerosis 228, 80–89.

Aviram, M., 2002. Polyphenolic flavonoids content and anti-oxidant activities of various juices: a comparative study. In: Proceedings of the 11th Biennial Meeting of the Society for Free Radical Research International, pp. 1–9.

Aviram, M., Dornfeld, L., 2001. Pomegranate juice consumption inhibits serum angiotensin converting enzyme activity and reduces systolic blood pressure. Atherosclerosis 158, 195–198.

Aviram, M., Dornfeld, L., Rosenblat, M., Volkova, N., Kaplan, M., Coleman, R., et al., 2000. Pomegranate juice consumption reduces oxidative stress, atherogenic modifications to LDL, and platelet aggregation: studies in humans and in atherosclerotic apolipoprotein E-deficient mice. Am. J. Clin. Nutr. 71, 1062–1076.

Aviram, M., Rosenblat, M., Gaitini, D., Nitecki, S., Hoffman, A., Dornfeld, L., et al., 2004. Pomegranate juice consumption for 3 years by patients with carotid artery stenosis reduces common carotid intima-media thickness, blood pressure and LDL oxidation. Clin. Nutr. 23, 423–433.

Balbir-Gurman, A., Fuhrman, B., Braun-Moscovici, Y., Markovits, D., Aviram, M., 2011. Consumption of pomegranate decreases serum oxidative stress and reduces disease activity in patients with active rheumatoid arthritis: a pilot study. Isr. Med. Assoc. J. 13, 474–479.

Bhadbhade, S.J., Acharya, A.B., Rodrigues, S.V., Thakur, S.L., 2011. The antiplaque efficacy of pomegranate mouthrinse. Quintessence Int. 42, 29–36.

Braga, L.C., Shupp, J.W., Cummings, C., Jett, M., Takahashi, J.A., Carmo, L.S., et al., 2005. Pomegranate extract inhibits *Staphylococcus aureus* growth and subsequent enterotoxin production. J. Ethnopharmacol. 96, 335–339.

Carpenter, L.A., Conway, C.J., Pipkin, F.B., 2010. Pomegranates (*Punica granatum*) and their effect on blood pressure: a randomised double-blind placebo-controlled trial. Proc. Nutr. Soc. 69, 95.

Davidson, M.H., Maki, K.C., Dicklin, M.R., Feinstein, S.B., Witchger, M., Bell, M., et al., 2009. Effects of consumption of pomegranate juice on carotid intima-media thickness in men and women at moderate risk for coronary heart disease. Am. J. Cardiol. 104, 936–942.

de Nigris, F., Williams-Ignarro, S., Lerman, L.O., Botti, C., Mansueto, G., D'Armiento, F.P., et al., 2005. Beneficial effects of pomegranate juice on oxidation-sensitive genes and endothelial nitric oxide synthase activity at sites of perturbed shear stress. Proc. Natl. Acad. Sci. USA 102, 4896–4901.

DiSilvestro, R.A., DiSilvestro, D.J., DiSilvestro, D.J., 2009. Pomegranate extract mouth rinsing effects on saliva measures relevant to gingivitis risk. Phytother. Res. 23, 1123–1127.

El-Nemr, S.E., Ismail, I.A., Ragab, M., 1990. Chemical composition of juice and seeds of pomegranate fruit. Nahrung 34, 601–606.

Esmaillzadeh, A., Tahbaz, F., Gaieni, I., Alavi-Majd, H., Azadbakht, L., 2004. Concentrated pomegranate juice improves lipid profiles in diabetic patients with hyperlipidemia. J. Med. Food 7, 305–308.

Esmaillzadeh, A., Tahbaz, F., Gaieni, I., Alavi-Majd, H., Azadbakht, L., 2006. Cholesterol-lowering effect of concentrated pomegranate juice consumption in type II diabetic patients with hyperlipidemia. Int. J. Vitam Nutr. Res. 76, 147–151.

Esmaillzadeh, A., Tahbaz, F., Gaieni, I., Azadbakht, L., 2004. Concentrated pomegranate juice improves lipid profiles in diabetic patients with hyperlipidemia. J. Med. Food 7, 305–308.

Freedland, S.J., Carducci, M., Kroeger, N., Partin, A., Rao, J.Y., Jin, Y., et al., 2013. A double-blind, randomized, neoadjuvant study of the tissue effects of POMx pills in men with prostate cancer before radical prostatectomy. Cancer Prev. Res. (Phila) 6, 1120–1127.

Gil, M.I., Tomas-Barberan, F.A., Hess-Pierce, B., Holcroft, D.M., Kader, A.A., 2000. Antioxidant activity of pomegranate juice and its relationship with phenolic composition and processing. J. Agric. Food Chem. 48, 4581–4589.

Haidari, M., Ali, M., Ward Casscells 3rd, S., Madjid, M., 2009. Pomegranate (*Punica granatum*) purified polyphenol extract inhibits influenza virus and has a synergistic effect with oseltamivir. Phytomedicine 16, 1127–1136.

Hamoud, S., Hayek, T., Volkova, N., Attias, J., Moscoviz, D., Rosenblat, M., et al., 2014. Pomegranate extract (POMx) decreases the atherogenicity of serum and of human monocyte-derived macrophages (HMDM) in simvastatin-treated hypercholesterolemic patients: a double-blinded, placebo-controlled, randomized, prospective pilot study. Atherosclerosis 232, 204–210.

Hashemi, M., Kelishadi, R., Hashemipour, M., Zakerameli, A., Khavarian, N., Ghatrehsamani, S., et al., 2010. Acute and long-term effects of grape and pomegranate juice consumption on vascular reactivity in paediatric metabolic syndrome. Cardiol. Young 20, 73–77.

Heber, D., Seeram, N.P., Wyatt, H., Henning, S.M., Zhang, Y., Ogden, L.G., et al., 2007. Safety and antioxidant activity of pomegranate ellagitannin-enriched polyphenol dietary supplement in overweight individuals with increased waist size. J. Agric. Food Chem. 55, 10050–10054.

Holetz, F.B., Pessini, G.L., Sanches, N.R., Cortez, D.A., Nakamura, C.V., Filho, B.P., 2002. Screening of some plants used in the Brazilian folk medicine for the treatment of infectious diseases. Mem. Inst. Oswaldo Cruz. 97, 1027–1031.

Hora, J.J., Maydew, E.R., Lansky, E.P., Dwivedi, C., 2003. Chemopreventive effects of pomegranate seed oil on skin tumor development in CD1 mice. J. Med. Food 6, 157–161.

Huang, T.H., Yang, Q., Harada, M., Li, G.Q., Yamahara, J., Roufogalis, B.D., et al., 2005. Pomegranate flower extract diminishes cardiac fibrosis in Zucker diabetic fatty rats: modulation of cardiac endothelin-1 and nuclear factor-kappaB pathways. J. Cardiovasc. Pharmacol. 46, 856–862.

Jayaprakasha, G.K., Negi, P.S., Jena, B.S., 2006. Antimicrobial activities of pomegranate. In: Seeram, N., Schulman, R., Heber, D. (Eds.), Pomegranates: Ancient Roots to Modern Medicine CRC Press, Boca Raton, pp. 167–183.

Jeune, M.A., Kumi-Diaka, J., Brown, J., 2005. Anticancer activities of pomegranate extracts and genistein in human breast cancer cells. J. Med. Food 8, 469–475.

Jimenez del Rio, M., Ramazanov, A., Sikorski, S., Ramozanov, Z., Chkhikvishvili, I., 2006. A new method of standartization of health-promoting pomegranate fruit (*Punica granatum*) extract. Georgian Med. News 11, 70–76.

Kaplan, M., Hayek, T., Raz, A., Coleman, R., Dornfeld, L., Vaya, J., et al., 2001. Pomegranate juice supplementation to atherosclerotic mice reduces macrophage lipid peroxidation, cellular cholesterol accumulation and development of atherosclerosis. J. Nutr. 131, 2082–2089.

Kasai, K., Yoshimura, M., Koga, T., Arii, M., Kawasaki, S., 2006. Effects of oral administration of ellagic acid-rich pomegranate extract on ultraviolet-induced pigmentation in the human skin. J. Nutr. Sci. Vitaminol. (Tokyo) 52, 383–388.

Kelishadi, R., Gidding, S.S., Hashemi, M., Hashemipour, M., Zakerameli, A., Poursafa, P., 2011. Acute and long term effects of grape and pomegranate juice consumption on endothelial dysfunction in pediatric metabolic syndrome. J. Res. Med. Sci. 16, 245–253.

Kim, N.D., Mehta, R., Yu, W., Neeman, I., Livney, T., Amichay, A., et al., 2002. Chemopreventive and adjuvant therapeutic potential of pomegranate (*Punica granatum*) for human breast cancer. Breast Cancer Res. Treat. 71, 203–217.

Machin, D.R., Christmas, K.M., Chou, T.-H., Hill, S.C., Van Pelt, D.W., Trombold, J.R., et al., 2014. Effects of differing dosages of pomegranate juice supplementation after eccentric exercise. Physiol. J. 2014, 1–7.

Malik, A., Afaq, F., Sarfaraz, S., Adhami, V.M., Syed, D.N., Mukhtar, H., 2005. Pomegranate fruit juice for chemoprevention and chemotherapy of prostate cancer. Proc. Natl. Acad. Sci. USA 102, 14813–14818.

Mathew, A.S., Capel-Williams, G.M., Berry, S.E., Hall, W.L., 2012. Acute effects of pomegranate extract on postprandial lipaemia, vascular function and blood pressure. Plant Foods Hum. Nutr. 67, 351–357.

Menezes, S.M., Cordeiro, L.N., Viana, G.S., 2006. *Punica granatum* (pomegranate) extract is active against dental plaque. J. Herb Pharmacother. 6, 79–92.

Mertens-Talcott, S.U., Jilma-Stohlawetz, P., Rios, J., Hingorani, L., Derendorf, H., 2006. Absorption, metabolism, and antioxidant effects of pomegranate (*Punica granatum* L.) polyphenols after ingestion of a standardized extract in healthy human volunteers. J. Agric. Food Chem. 54, 8956–8961.

Miguel, G., Dandlen, S., Antunes, D., Neves, A., Martins, D., 2004. The effect of two methods of pomegranate (*Punica granatum* L.) juice extraction on quality during storage at 4°C. J. Biomed. Biotechnol. 2004 (5), 332–337.

Mohan, M., Waghulde, H., Kasture, S., 2010. Effect of pomegranate juice on angiotensin II-induced hypertension in diabetic Wistar rats. Phytother. Res. 24, S196–S203.

Moneam, N.M., el Sharaky, A.S., Badreldin, M.M., 1988. Oestrogen content of pomegranate seeds. J. Chromatogr. 438, 438–442.

Neurath, A.R., Strick, N., Li, Y.Y., Debnath, A.K., 2004. *Punica granatum* (Pomegranate) juice provides an HIV-1 entry inhibitor and candidate topical microbicide. BMC Infect. Dis. 4, 41.

Neurath, A.R., Strick, N., Li, Y.Y., Debnath, A.K., 2005. *Punica granatum* (pomegranate) juice provides an HIV-1 entry inhibitor and candidate topical microbicide. Ann. N. Y. Acad. Sci. 1056, 311–327.

Noda, Y., Kaneyuki, T., Mori, A., Packer, L., 2002. Antioxidant activities of pomegranate fruit extract and its anthocyanidins: delphinidin, cyanidin, and pelargonidin. J. Agric. Food Chem. 50, 166–171.

Paller, C.J., Ye, X., Wozniak, P.J., Gillespie, B.K., Sieber, P.R., Greengold, R.H., et al., 2013. A randomized phase II study of pomegranate extract for men with rising PSA following initial therapy for localized prostate cancer. Prostate Cancer Prostatic Dis. 16, 50–55.

Pantuck, A.J., Leppert, J.T., Zomorodian, N., Aronson, W., Hong, J., Barnard, R.J., et al., 2006. Phase II study of pomegranate juice for men with rising prostate-specific antigen following surgery or radiation for prostate cancer. Clin. Cancer. Res. 12, 4018–4026.

Rosenblat, M., Hayek, T., Aviram, M., 2006. Anti-oxidative effects of pomegranate juice (PJ) consumption by diabetic patients on serum and on macrophages. Atherosclerosis 187, 363–371.

Schubert, S.Y., Lansky, E.P., Neeman, I., 1999. Antioxidant and eicosanoid enzyme inhibition properties of pomegranate seed oil and fermented juice flavonoids. J. Ethnopharmacol. 66, 11–17.

Seeram, N.P., Adams, L.S., Henning, S.M., Niu, Y., Zhang, Y., Nair, M.G., et al., 2005. *In vitro* antiproliferative, apoptotic and antioxidant activities of punicalagin, ellagic acid and a total pomegranate tannin extract are enhanced in combination with other polyphenols as found in pomegranate juice. J. Nutr. Biochem. 16, 360–367.

Sohrab, G., Sotoodeh, G., Siasi, F., Neiestani, T., Rahimi, A., Chamari, M., 2008. Effect of pomegranate juice consumption on blood pressure in type 2 diabetic patients. IJEM 9 (399–405), 470.

Stenner-Liewen, F., Liewen, H., Cathomas, R., Renner, C., Petrausch, U., Sulser, T., et al., 2013. Daily pomegranate intake has no impact on PSA levels in patients with advanced prostate cancer—results of a phase IIb randomized controlled trial. J. Cancer 4, 597–605.

Still, D.W., 2006. Pomegranates: a botanical perspective. In: Seeram, N., Schulman, R., Heber, D. (Eds.), Pomegranates: Ancient Roots to Modern Medicine CRC Press, Boca Raton, pp. 199–209.

Sumner, M.D., Elliott-Eller, M., Weidner, G., Daubenmier, J.J., Chew, M.H., Marlin, R., et al., 2005. Effects of pomegranate juice consumption on myocardial perfusion in patients with coronary heart disease. Am. J. Cardiol. 96, 810–814.

Tous, J., Ferguson, L., 1996. Mediterranean fruits. In: Janick, J. (Ed.), Progress in New Crops ASHS Press, Arlington, VA, pp. 416–430.

Tripathi, S.M., Singh, D.K., 2000. Molluscicidal activity of *Punica granatum* bark and *Canna indica* root. Braz. J. Med. Biol. Res. 33, 1351–1355.

Trombold, J.R., Barnes, J.N., Critchley, L., Coyle, E.F., 2010. Ellagitannin consumption improves strength recovery 2–3 d after eccentric exercise. Med. Sci. Sports Exerc. 42, 493–498.

Trombold, J.R., Reinfeld, A.S., Casler, J.R., Coyle, E.F., 2011. The effect of pomegranate juice supplementation on strength and soreness after eccentric exercise. J. Strength Cond. Res. 25, 1782–1788.

Vasconcelos, L.C., Sampaio, M.C., Sampaio, F.C., Higino, J.S., 2003. Use of *Punica granatum* as an antifungal agent against candidosis associated with denture stomatitis. Mycoses 46, 192–196.

Vidal, A., Fallarero, A., Peña, B.R., Medina, M.E., Gra, B., Rivera, F., et al., 2003. Studies on the toxicity of *Punica granatum* L. (Punicaceae) whole fruit extracts. J. Ethnopharmacol. 89, 295–300.

Vilahur, G., Padró, T., Casaní, L., Mendieta, G., López, J.A., Streitenberger, S., et al., 2015. Polyphenol-enriched diet prevents coronary endothelial dysfunction by activating the Akt/eNOS pathway *Rev. Esp. Cardiol.* (*Engl Ed*), 68216–225

Voravuthikunchai, S.P., Kitpipit, L., 2005. Activity of medicinal plant extracts against hospital isolates of methicillin-resistant *Staphylococcus aureus*. Clin. Microbiol. Infect. 11, 510–512.

Wang, R.F., Xie, W.D., Zhang, Z., Xing, D.M., Ding, Y., Wang, W., et al., 2004. Bioactive compounds from the seeds of *Punica granatum* (pomegranate). J. Nat. Prod. 67, 2096–2098.

Wright, H., Pipkin, F.B., 2008. Pomegranates (*Punica granatum*), kiwifruit (*Actinidia deliciosa*) and blood pressure: a pilot study. Proc. Nutr. Soc. 67, 1.

Chapter 15

Berries and blood pressure

Greg Arnold
Complete Chiropractic Healthcare, Hauppauge, NY, United States

CHAPTER OUTLINE

INTRODUCTION

Blood pressure is the pressure exerted by blood against arterial walls as blood circulates through the body. Blood pressure is regulated by a number of body systems such as nerve and hormone signals from the heart, blood vessels, brain, kidneys, and digestive organs (Piper, 2014). Blood pressure is expressed in a two-number format and measured in millimeters of mercury (mmHg). The top number, called systolic blood pressure, is the highest pressure exerted against blood vessel walls when the heart contracts (called systole) while the bottom number, called diastolic blood pressure, is the lowest pressure exerted against blood vessel walls when the heart relaxes between contractions (called diastole). The average blood pressure is currently regarded as 120/80 mmHg, between 120/80 and 140/90 mmHg

Fruits, Vegetables, and Herbs.
DOI: http://dx.doi.org/10.1016/B978-0-12-802972-5.00015-9

as "prehypertension" and >140/90 mmHg and above as high blood pressure, or "hypertension" (Piper, 2014).

HIGH BLOOD PRESSURE: A HIDDEN EPIDEMIC

The latest statistics from the Centers for Disease Control state that nearly one in three US adults (29% = ~70 million) have high blood pressure (Nwankwo et al., 2013). Even more alarming is that barely more than half (52%) of those with high blood pressure have it under control and one in five US adults with high blood pressure still do not know they suffer from the condition (Mozzafarian et al., 2015). High blood pressure costs the nation $46 billion each year in the form of doctor's visits, medications for high blood pressure, and missed days of work (Mozzafarian et al., 2015).

The danger of having high blood pressure lies in the fact that it is the largest contributing risk factor to death from all-causes as well as cardiovascular disease (Yang et al., 2012). In 2010, high blood pressure was listed as a primary or contributing cause of death for more than 362,000 Americans (Go et al., 2014). In addition, poor control of high blood pressure has been identified as the third ranked factor for disability-adjusted life years (Ezzati et al., 2002).

THE ONSET OF HIGH BLOOD PRESSURE

A foundation of the onset of high blood pressure lies in the progressive decline of normal blood vessel function (Kimura et al., 1999). The entire structure of blood vessels makes it the body's largest organ, with its total area equal to six tennis courts and its total length would be 100,000 km, equal to two and half times around the earth (Higashi et al., 2009).

There are three primary contributors to a decline in blood vessel function: cell damage (oxidative stress), aging cells (called "senescence"), and inflammation (Wei, 1992; Folkow and Svanborg, 1993; Butt et al., 2010). Regarding oxidative stress, its increase in the body inactivates nitric oxide, a potent vasodilator (Touyz, 2004) which has been shown in both animal and human studies of hypertension (Cai and Harrison, 2000). Regarding free radical production, NADPH oxidase, a major source of free radicals in blood vessel walls, is activated in rats with high blood pressure (Hegde et al., 1998). Therefore, enhanced production of reactive oxygen species and an attenuated antioxidant system may contribute to endothelial dysfunction in patients with hypertension.

BERRIES FOR HIGH BLOOD PRESSURE

Because of their low calories, high content of antioxidants called polyphenols as well as fiber, minerals, and vitamins, berry fruits have been subject to significant research on their potential to maintain health. Strawberries, blueberries, and cranberries contain abundant levels of anthocyanins and ellagitannins in their skin and flesh, flavonoids which give berries their bright colors (Basu et al., 2010a). We will now examine the research examining individual berry consumption as well as combinations of berries on blood pressure.

BLUEBERRIES: BEST FOR BLOOD PRESSURE

Research by Rodriguez-Mateos et al. (2013) and Rodriguez-Mateos (2014) suggests that the antioxidants in blueberries may have a positive effect on blood pressure by increasing the effectiveness of nitric oxide through the inhibition of an enzyme called NAPDH-oxidase. This increased effectiveness in nitric oxide is thought to improve blood vessel function and possibly lower blood pressure, though "further work is needed to confirm whether this is indeed the case" (Rodriguez-Mateos, 2014).

Research examining blueberry consumption on blood pressure suggests two groups of patients, those with metabolic syndrome and those with prehypertension, may benefit most from blueberry consumption. Metabolic syndrome is estimated to be 39% (Grundy et al., 2004) and is an important risk factor for the development of both coronary artery disease (Malik et al., 2004) and type-2 diabetes mellitus (Laaksonen et al., 2002).

A study by Basu et al. (2010a) looked at 48 subjects (4 males, 44 females) between the ages of 47 and 53 with metabolic syndrome (body mass index between 35.5 and 41.1 kg/m^2) consumed 50 g of freeze-dried blueberries [equal to 350 g (2.3 cups) of fresh blueberries] in 960 mL of water with vanilla extract or Splenda based on the preference of the participants. They consumed 480 mL of the beverage in the morning and then 480 mL 6–8 h later. The composition of the beverage was as follows (Table 15.1).

The control group consumed 960 mL water to match the fluid intake of the blueberry group.

After 8 weeks, those in the blueberry group saw a 6% decrease (7.8 mmHg) in systolic blood pressure compared to 1.5% decrease (2.0 mmHg) in the control group ($P < 0.05$). For diastolic blood pressure, the blueberry group saw a 4% decrease (2.5 mmHg) compared to a 1.2% decrease (0.7 mmHg) in the control group ($P < 0.05$).

The researchers concluded that "our study is the first to our knowledge to report that blueberries have antihypertensive effects in people with metabolic syndrome" and that "because hypertension is an independent and significant CVD risk factor (Wright et al., 2005) and can be mitigated by

Table 15.1 Blueberry Beverage Composition

Composition of Beverage	Unit
Calories	174
Protein (g)	1.7
Carbohydrates (g)	42.3
Total sugars (g)	30
Fiber (g)	9.3
Vitamin C (mg)	86
Calcium (mg)	15
Iron (mg)	0.5
Potassium (mg)	204
Sodium (mg)	8
Phenols (mg)	1624
Anthocyanins (mg)	742

Table 15.2 Blueberry Beverage Composition

Composition of Beverage	Unit
Calories	87
Protein (g)	0.59
Carbohydrates (g)	20.57
Fiber (g)	4.73
Vitamin C (mg)	2.27
Calcium (mg)	7.5
Potassium (mg)	103.18
Phenols (mg)	844.58
Anthocyanins (mg)	469.48

dietary practices (Levitan et al., 2009), blueberry supplementation may be a potential therapeutic dietary measure and needs further confirmation in larger controlled studies."

Regarding blueberries and prehypertension, a study by Johnson (2015) examined the effect of 22 g of freeze-dried blueberry powder or 22 g of a control powder for 8 weeks in 48 postmenopausal women between the ages of 53 and 63 with prehypertension (average blood pressure 138/80 mmHg), with the blueberry powder containing the following (Table 15.2).

After 8 weeks, those in the blueberry powder group noted a 5.1% decrease (7 mmHg) in systolic blood pressure compared to a 0.7% increase

(1 mmHg) in the control group ($P < 0.05$). For diastolic blood pressure, the blueberry group had a 6.25% decrease (5 mmHg) compared to a 2.5% increase (2 mmHg) in the control group ($P < 0.01$). These results led the researchers to conclude that "This suggests that regular consumption of blueberries over the long term could potentially delay the progression of hypertension and reduce cardiovascular risk in postmenopausal women."

While blueberry supplementation for those with metabolic syndrome and prehypertension has proven beneficial, research in chronic smokers and obese insulin-resistant individuals has proven less "fruitful." McAnulty et al. (2005) supplied 10 male smokers (smoking one pack per day for 1 year, average blood pressure 130/81 mmHg) with 250 g of blueberries or placebo (10 subjects, average blood pressure 128/81 mmHg) per day for 3 weeks. While no differences were seen regarding either systolic ($P = 0.740$) or diastolic blood pressure ($P = 0.680$) compared to the placebo group, a note should be made for the short duration of the study (3 weeks) as a possible explanation for a lack of blood-pressure benefit compared to the 8 weeks conducted in the Basu and Johnson studies.

Regarding insulin-resistant obese subjects, Stull et al. (2010) supplemented 15 obese (body mass index between 32 and 45 kg/m^2, average blood pressure 117/73 mmHg), nondiabetic, and insulin-resistant subjects a smoothie containing 22.5 g blueberry powder or a placebo smoothie of equal nutritional value without the blueberry powder (17 subjects, average blood pressure 123/76 mmHg) two times daily for 6 weeks. The blueberry powder was made from a 50/50 mixture of two varieties of highbush blueberries, Tifblue (*Vaccinium ashei*) and Rubel (*Vaccinium corymbosum*), which were freeze-dried, milled, and contained 1462 mg of total phenolics and 668 mg of anthocyanins, equal to the amount of antioxidants found in two cups of fresh whole blueberries.

The composition of each smoothie (consumed two times daily) was as follows (Table 15.3).

After 6 weeks, while insulin sensitivity improved significantly in the blueberry group versus the placebo group [22.2% vs 4.9% improved sensitivity ($P = 0.02$), no significant differences were noted between the two groups ($P > 0.05$)].

Finally, regarding healthy subjects (Rodriguez-Mateos, 2013), 21 men consumed a blueberry beverage containing up to 1791 mg of polyphenols (10 men) or a placebo drink that was matched for calories and sugar (10 men, no specific data on the smoothie drink provided). Each subject consumed their drink and then had their blood pressure and a measure of

Table 15.3 Beverage Compositions

Composition of Beverage	Blueberry Smoothie	Placebo Smoothie
Calories	239	234
Protein (g)	11.9	11.1
Carbohydrates (g)	48.5	48.6
Fiber (g)	4.2	4.3
Fat (g)	0.08	0.08
Dannon Light & Fit yogurt (g)	245	245
Skim milk (g)	105	105
Freez-dried blueberry powder	22.5	0
Imitation vanilla flavor (g)	5	0
Splenda (g)	1	0
Benefiber	0	5
Sugar (g)	0	12
Red food color (g)	0	1.5
Blue food color (g)	0	0.7

blood vessel relaxation (called "flow-mediated dilatation") 6h later. While those in the blueberry group saw a 1.2% increase in flow-mediated dilatation compared to no change in the placebo group ($P < 0.05$), no significant changes were seen with blood pressure between the two groups ($P > 0.05$). Although the researchers admit the very short time frame of the study "limited the biological significance of the finding and did not predict the benefits of longer-term consumption on endothelial function," they did admit that "our data provide the first evidence that circulating small phenolic metabolites derived from blueberry polyphenols may be partly responsible for acute improvements in endothelial function in healthy individuals."

Grapes

The research examining grapes and blood pressure has shown a mostly beneficial effect. In a 2004 study by Park et al. (2004), 40 hypertensive men were given either 5.5mL of Concord grape juice per kilogram of bodyweight (21 men, average blood pressure 145.5/93.9mmHg) or a calorie-matched placebo drink (19 men, average blood pressure 147.5/94mmHg) every day for 8 weeks. Those in the grape juice group saw a 5% decrease in their systolic pressure (145.5–138.3mmHg) compared to a 2.4% decrease in the placebo group (147.5–144mmHg, $P = 0.005$) while diastolic blood pressure decreased by 6.7% in the grape juice group (93.9–87.7 mmHg) compared to a 3.5% decrease (94–90.8 mmHg, $P = 0.001$).

The researchers cited animal studies showing the flavonoids in purple grape juice and red wine increase the production of nitric oxide "which cause relaxation of the adjacent vascular smooth muscle cells in animal model" (Fitzpatrick et al., 1993) by inhibiting the effect of angiotensin-converting enzyme (Keider et al., 1994). The researchers concluded that "consuming Concord grape juice, which is high in polyphenolic compounds, may favorably affect BP in hypertensive individuals."

A 2010 study by Dohadwala et al. (2010) produced mixed results in 64 prehypertensive subjects (44 men, 20 women) between the ages of 31 and 55 given either 7 mL/kg of bodyweight of Concord grape juice or a placebo for 8 weeks, with each 8-oz serving of grape juice containing 160 calories, 39 g natural sugar (52% fructose and 48% glucose), and 472.8 mg total polyphenols. This resulted in a 150-lb subject consuming 490 mL/day (16 oz) and providing 965 mg of polyphenols.

While the researchers noted no significant differences between groups in 24-h ambulatory blood pressure [when your blood pressure is being measured as you move around, living your normal daily life ("24-hour ambulatory blood pressure monitoring (ABPM)")] for either systolic ($P = 0.67$) or diastolic ($P = 0.90$) blood pressure, there was a 20.5% increase in the systolic blood pressure dip at night (6.8–8.2 mmHg dip) compared to a 23.3% decrease in the placebo group (9.9–7.6 mmHg, $P = 0.005$) as well as a 15.1% increase in the diastolic blood pressure dip at night (9.9–11.4 mmHg) compared to a 14.7% decrease in the placebo group (13–11.1 mmHg, $P = 0.03$).

The value in this improved nocturnal dip researched by Ohkubo (2002) showing each 5% decrease in the decline in nocturnal systolic/diastolic blood pressure increased the risk of death from a cardiovascular even by 20%. In healthy subjects, blood pressure drops by at least 10% when sleeping at night (Sayk et al., 2007). Conditions like obstructive sleep apnea syndrome (Veerman et al., 1995) increase activity of the sympathetic nervous system that produces consistent arterial constriction and prevent a healthy drop in nocturnal blood pressure (Peppard et al., 2000), thereby affecting the morning increase in blood pressure (Dodt et al., 1997) and resulting in the early morning as the most common time of day for cardiovascular events for those with blood-pressure problems (Kario et al., 2003).

Regarding grape seed extract, those with either prehypertension or metabolic syndrome benefit most from berry supplementation. In a 2009

Table 15.4 Effect of Supplementation on Blood Pressure

	Systolic BP	Diastolic BP
150 mg GSE/day	8.3% decrease (134–123 mmHg)	7.3% decrease (83–77 mmHg)
300 mg GSE/day	8.7% decrease (127–116 mmHg)	9% decrease (78–71 mmHg)
Placebo	1.7% decrease (123–121 mmHg)	5.5% decrease (74–70 mmHg)
P-value	0.003	0.007

study by Sivaprakasapillai et al. (2009), 27 subjects (11 men, 16 women) between the ages of 43 and 51 with metabolic syndrome were given either grape seed extract [150 mg (nine subjects) or 300 (nine subjects)] of grape seed extract or placebo (nine subjects) per day for 4 weeks. After 4 weeks, the following was observed (Table 15.4).

For subjects with prehypertension, a 2013 study by Ras et al. (2013) supplemented 70 prehypertensive subjects (32 men, 38 women) between the ages of 53 and 71 with either 300 mg of grape seed extract (35 subjects) or placebo (35 subjects) per day for 8 weeks. After 8 weeks, those in the grape seed extract group saw a 4.1% decrease in systolic blood pressure (135.8–130.3 mmHg) compared a 2.4% decrease in the placebo group (135.7–132.5 mmHg, $P < 0.01$) while the diastolic blood pressure decreased by 3.5% in the grape seed extract group (81.9–79.1 mmHg) compared to a 1.4% decrease in the placebo group (81.1–80 mmHg, $P < 0.01$).

When looking at the effect of grape seed extract on blood pressure in healthy subjects, the results have shown a lack of effectiveness. In a 2007 study by van Mierlo et al. (2010), 35 healthy males between the ages of 22 and 40 receiving 500 mg of grape solids (containing 800 mg total polyphenols) or placebo for 2 weeks followed by a 1-week washout period followed by a switch to the other supplement for two more weeks. Although no differences were noted between supplementation and the grape solids for systolic ($P = 0.70$) or diastolic blood pressure ($P = 0.44$), neither did they see a difference in flow-mediated dilatation between the two groups ($P = 0.94$) and the researchers did acknowledge 2 weeks of supplementation to be a limitation to the study, though "we expected to show benefits of polyphenols within 2 weeks, because previous studies investigated acute and several weeks' effects on flow-mediated vasodilatation with positive outcomes (Karatzi et al., 2007; Papamichael et al., 2004)."

Strawberries

While blueberry and grape supplementation benefited blood pressure most in prehypertensives and metabolic syndrome, strawberry ingestion does not seem to bestow the same blood-pressure benefits. In a 2010 study by Basu et al. (2010c), 27 subjects (2 men, 25 women) between the ages of 44 and 50 with metabolic syndrome consumed either four cups (50 g) of freeze-dried strawberries (equivalent to three cups of fresh strawberries) or placebo per day for 8 weeks. While significant decreases were found for total cholesterol (10.4%, $P < 0.05$) and LDL cholesterol (11.5%, $P < 0.05$) compared to changes in the placebo group, no significant benefits were seen for blood pressure between the two groups ($P > 0.05$).

In an another study by Basu (2009), 16 females between the ages of 42 and 60 with metabolic syndrome were given either 25 g of freeze-dried strawberries blended into a drink or placebo per day for 4 weeks. As in the previous study by Basu, those in the strawberry group saw significant decreases in total cholesterol (5.1% decrease, $P < 0.05$) and LDL cholesterol (6.25% decrease, $P < 0.05$) but no significant differences in either systolic or diastolic blood pressure between groups ($P > 0.05$).

Finally, in a 2012 study by Zunino et al. (2012), 20 healthy subjects (7 men, 13 women) between the ages of 20 and 50 and a body mass index between 30 and 40 kg/m^2 received either a strawberry powder equivalent to four servings of frozen strawberries or a placebo for 3 weeks. As in the previous two studies, significant benefits were found for total cholesterol levels (4% decrease, $P < 0.05$) but no benefits to blood pressure ($P > 0.05$). For the researches, "the alterations in lipid subfractions that were observed may represent a beneficial reduction in risk factors for cardiovascular disease, stroke, and the metabolic syndrome/diabetes in our obese volunteers, suggesting a role for strawberries as a dietary means to decrease obesity-related disease."

Cranberries

Cranberry juice is a rich source of polyphenolic compounds, particularly anthocyanins (Milbury et al., 2010; Vinson et al., 2001). And while research on cranberries has uncovered several blood-vessel benefits with supplementation, those benefits did not extend to blood pressure. In a 2011 study by Basu (Veerman et al., 1995), 32 women between the ages of 44 and 60 with metabolic syndrome (average body mass index of 40 kg/m^2) were given either 480 mL (two cups) of cranberry juice per day (16 women) or placebo (16 women) for 8 weeks. The two cups of 27% cranberry juice provided 80 calories, 11.4 g of natural sugars, and

458 mg of total phenolics. After 8 weeks, those in the cranberry juice saw a 50% decrease in levels of cell damage (malondialdehyde, 3.4–1.7 μM) compared to a 6.7% increase in the placebo group (3.0–3.2, $P < 0.05$) but no significant differences between the two groups for blood pressure ($P > 0.05$).

Regarding cranberry's effect on those with heart disease, a 2011 study by Dohadwala et al. (2011) examined 15 subjects (13 men, 2 women) between the ages of 54 and 70 with heart disease (53% with hypertension, 67% with a history of smoking, 33% with type-2 diabetes) who were given either a double-strength cranberry supplement (54% juice with 80 calories, 20 g natural sugar, 1770 mg total polyphenols, 188 mg anthocyanins) or placebo for 4 weeks. And while those in the cranberry group saw a 12.9% increase in flow-mediation dilatation (7.7–8.7%) compared to no change in the placebo group ($P = 0.003$), no significant differences were seen for either systolic ($P = 0.274$) or diastolic ($P = 0.503$) blood pressure.

An important cardiovascular benefit noted in the cranberry juice group in addition to improved flow-mediated dilatation was a 6.1% decrease in a measure of blood-vessel health called carotid-femoral pulse wave velocity (8.3–7.8 m/s) compared to a 5% increase in the placebo group (8.0–8.4 m/s, $P = 0.003$). Research is starting to identify carotid-femoral pulse wave velocity as "an important measure of vascular function that relates to cardiovascular disease risk." It predicted cardiovascular events in the Framingham Heart Study after adjustment for other cardiovascular disease risk factors and was a stronger predictor than other measures of arterial stiffness, including the augmentation index and central pulse pressure (Mitchell et al., 2010).

For type-2 diabetics, a randomized, double-blind, placebo-controlled study by Lee et al. (2008) studied 30 subjects (16 men, 14 women), with an average age of 65 with type-2 diabetes and supplemented their diets with either 1500 mg of cranberry extract (15 subjects) or placebo (15 subjects) for 12 weeks. As in previous research, significant decreases were seen for total cholesterol (7.5% decrease) and LDL cholesterol (12.2% decrease) compared to the placebo group (5.8% increase in total cholesterol and 6.7% increase in LDL cholesterol, $P < 0.01$) with no significant benefits were seen for either systolic ($P = 1.000$) or diastolic ($P = 0.441$) blood pressure.

Black currants

Very little research has been done with black currants and blood pressure, with a 2011 study by Jin et al. (2011) on 20 healthy subjects (9 men, average blood pressure 121/72 mmHg; 11 women, average blood pressure

110/68 mmHg) between the ages of 32 and 57 with an average blood pressure of showed no benefit from a single ingestion of 250 mL of 20% black currant juice compared to a placebo ($P > 0.05$).

BEYOND HYPERTENSION: BERRIES FOR ORTHOSTATIC HYPOTENSION

While this chapter has focused on the ability of berries to attain a healthier blood pressure by lowering it out of a prehypertensive or hypertensive range, research has also showed berry intake can help to maintain a healthier blood pressure by raising it, specifically in a condition called orthostatic hypotension.

Defined as "a fall in systolic blood pressure by at least 20 mmHg or in diastolic blood pressure by at least 10 mmHg after 3 min of standing upright or on a tilt table" (Masaki et al., 1998), orthostatic hypotension is estimated to be present in as little as 4% but as much as 33% of the elderly (Masuo et al., 1993). The cause of orthostatic hypotension is a compromise of the mechanisms that prevent from pooling in the lower extremities when one goes from a supine (lying down) to a standing position when nearly 1 L of blood shifts downward to the legs. In a normal functioning nervous system, pressure receptors in the heart, lungs, and a blood vessel called the aorta instantly induce a constriction of blood vessels within seconds that causes blood to be sent up from the legs to the brain and rest of the upper body (Lamarre-Cliché and Cusson, 2001).

The effect of orthostatic hypotension on risk of death is significant. Research by Masaki et al. (1998) each orthostatic drop in systolic blood pressure by 10 mmHg increases the risk of death in men by 18%, a risk that has been found in other populations as well (Raiha et al., 1995). In addition, data from the ARIC study showed orthostatic hypotension to be a predictor of stroke and coronary heart disease (Eigenbrodt et al., 2000).

Crataegus berries with D-camphor

In a 2002 study by Belz et al. (2002), 24 men and women with orthostatic hypotension underwent a tilt-table test, receiving either a extract of 97.5 g of fluid extract of crataegus berries 2 with 2.5 g of natural D-camphor or a placebo after 1, 3, and 5 min of being on the tilt table (Tables 15.5 and 15.6).

When suggesting how the camphor and crataegus berries produced these changes in blood pressure, the researches pointed to research suggesting "neuronal mechanisms, eg, via partial activation of the sympatho-adrenergic system" (Belz et al., 2000; Gabard and Trunzler, 1983) and concluded that

Table 15.5 Systolic Blood Pressure Readings

	Crataegus/ D-Camphor	Placebo	*P*-Value
Initial systolic BP (mmHg)	110.1	111.2	
1 min after tilt-table exposure	102.6 (6.9% drop)	97.5 (12.4% drop)	<0.02
3 min	100.5 (8.8% drop)	96.6 (13.2% drop)	<0.02
5 min	99.7 (9.5% drop)	96.1 (13.6% drop)	<0.02

Table 15.6 Diastolic Blood Pressure Readings

	Crataegus/ D-Camphor	Placebo	*P*-Value
Initial systolic BP (mmHg)	69	69.2	
1 min after tilt-table exposure	73.4 (6.3% increase)	70.1 (1.3% increase)	<0.02
3 min	72.6 (5.2% increase)	69.1 (0.1% drop)	<0.02
5 min	71.5 (3.6% increase)	68 (1.2% drop)	<0.02

D-camphor and crataegus berries "may be administered as a rationally reasoned phytopharmaceutical agent with proven effectiveness in acute indications such as hypotensive circulatory dysregulation or orthostatic circulatory dysregulation with fall in blood pressure."

CONCLUSIONS

As a whole, research on the heart-healthy benefits to berry consumption is beneficial for those with prehypertension, hypertension, type-2 diabetes, with blood pressure improvements were seen mostly for subjects with metabolic syndrome. As well as helping decrease blood pressure into healthy ranges, berry intake may also increase blood pressure into healthy ranges for those suffering from orthostatic hypotension.

Health benefits of berry consumption in healthy subjects are yet to demonstrate an improvement in healthy subjects but long-term studies should be conducted to discover a possible protective effect against the onset of chronic disease.

REFERENCES

"24-hour ambulatory blood pressure monitoring (ABPM)" posted on <http://www.bloodpressureuk.org/BloodPressureandyou/Medicaltests/24-hourtest>.

Basu, A., 2009. Freeze-dried strawberry powder improves lipid profile and lipid peroxidation in women with metabolic syndrome: baseline and post intervention effects. Nutr. J. 8, 43. http://dx.doi.org/10.1186/1475-2891-8-43.

Basu, A., Du, M., Leyva, M.J., Sanchez, K., Betts, N.M., Wu, M., et al., 2010a. Blueberries decrease cardiovascular risk factors in obese men and women with metabolic syndrome. J. Nutr. 140, 1582–1587. <http://jn.nutrition.org/content/140/9/1582.long> (accessed 1.05.15.).

Basu, A., Fu, D.X., Wilkinson, M., Simmons, B., Wu, M., Betts, N.M., et al., 2010b. Strawberries decrease atherosclerotic markers in subjects with metabolic syndrome. Nutr. Res. (NY) 30, 462–469.

Basu, A., Rhone, M., Lyons, T.J., 2010c. Berries: emerging impact on cardiovascular health. Nutr. Rev. 68 (3), 168–177. http://dx.doi.org/10.1111/j.1753-4887.2010.00273.x.

Belz, G.G., Breithaupt-Grögler, K., Butzer, R., Herrmann, V., Malerczyk, C., Mang, C., et al., 2000. In: Phyto-pharmaka, V.I., Rietbrock, N. (Eds.), Klinische Pharmakologie von D-Campher Steinkopff Verlag, Darmstadt, pp. 21–28.

Belz, G.G., Butzer, R., Gaus, W., Loew, D., 2002. Camphorcrataegus berry extract combination dose-dependently reduces tilt induced fall in blood pressure in orthostatic hypotension. Phytomedicine 9, 581–588.

Butt, H.Z., Atturu, G., London, N.J., Sayers, R.D., Bown, M.J., 2010. Telomere length dynamics in vascular disease: a review. Eur. J. Vasc. Endovasc. Surg. 40, 17–26.

Cai, H., Harrison, D.G., 2000. Endothelial dysfunction in cardiovascular diseases: the role of oxidant stress. Circ. Res. 87, 840–844.

Dodt, C., Breckling, U., Derad, I., Fehm, H.L., Born, J., 1997. Plasma epinephrine and norepinephrine concentrations of healthy humans associated with nighttime sleep and morning arousal. Hypertension 30, 71–76.

Dohadwala, M.M., Hamburg, N.M., Holbrook, M., Kim, B.H., Duess, M.-A., Levit, A., 2010. Effect of grape juice on ambulatory blood pressure in pre-hypertension and stage 1 hypertension. Am. J. Clin. Nutr. 92, 1052–1059.

Dohadwala, M.M., Holbrook, M., Hamburg, N.M., Shenouda, S.M., Chung, W.B., Titas, M., et al., 2011. Effects of cranberry juice consumption on vascular function in patients with coronary artery disease. Am. J. Clin. Nutr. 93, 934–940.

Eigenbrodt, M.L., Rose, K.M., Couper, D.J., Arnett, D.K., Smith, R., Jones, D., 2000. Orthostatic hypotension as a risk factor for stroke. The atherosclerosis risk in communities (ARIC) study, 1987–1996. Stroke 31, 2307–2313.

Ezzati, M., Lopez, A.D., Rodgers, A., Vander Hoorn, S., Murray, C.J., 2002. Comparative risk assessment collaborating group. Selected major risk factors and global regional burden of disease. Lancet 360, 1347–1360.

Fitzpatrick, D.F., Hirschfield, S.L., Coffey, R.G., 1993. Endothelium-dependent vasorelaxing activity of wine and other grape products. Am. J. Physiol. 265, H774–H778.

Folkow, B., Svanborg, A., 1993. Physiology of cardiovascular aging. Physiol. Rev. 73, 725–764.

Gabard, B., Trunzler, G., 1983. Zur Pharmakologie von Crataegus. In: Rietbrock, N., Schnieders, B., Schuster, J. (Eds.), Wandlungen in der Therapie der Herzinsuffizienz Friedr. Vieweg & Sohn, Braunschweig, pp. 43–53.

Go, A.S., Mozaffarian, D., Roger, V.L., et al., 2014. Heart disease and stroke statistics—2014 update: a report from the American Heart Association. Circulation 129 (3), e28–292. PMID: 24352519.

Grundy, S.M., Brewer Jr, H.B., Cleeman, J.I., et al., 2004. Definition of metabolic syndrome: report of the National Heart, Lung, and Blood Institute/American Heart Association conference on scientific issues related to definition. Circulation 109, 433–438.

Hegde, L.G., Srivastava, P., Kumari, R., Dikshit, M., 1998. Alterations in the vasoreactivity of hypertensive rat aortic rings: role of nitric oxide and superoxide radicals. Clin. Exp. Hypertens. 20, 885–901.

Higashi, Y., Noma, K., Yoshizumi, M., Kihara, Y., 2009. Oxidative stress and endothelial function in cardiovascular diseases. Circ. J. 73, 411–418.

Jin, Y., Alimbetov, D., George, T., Gordon, M.H., Lovegrove, J.A., 2011. A randomised trial to investigate the effects of acute consumption of a blackcurrant juice drink on markers of vascular reactivity and bioavailability of anthocyanins in human subjects. Eur. J. Clin. Nutr. 65, 849–856.

Johnson, S.A., 2015. Daily blueberry consumption improves blood pressure and arterial stiffness in postmenopausal women with pre- and stage 1-hypertension: a randomized, double-blind, placebo-controlled clinical trial. J. Acad. Nutr. Diet. Mar. 115 (3), 369–377. http://dx.doi.org/10.1016/j.jand.2014.11.001. Epub 2015 Jan 8.

Karatzi, K., Papamichael, C., Karatzis, E., Papaioannou, T.G., Voidonikola, P.T., Lekakis, J., et al., 2007. Acute smoking induces endothelial dysfunction in healthy smokers. Is this reversible by red wine's antioxidant constituents? J. Am. Coll. Nutr. 26, 10–15.

Kario, K., Pickering, T.G., Umeda, Y., Hoshide, S., Hoshide, Y., Morinari, M., et al., 2003. Morning surge in blood pressure as a predictor of silent and clinical cerebrovascular disease in elderly hypertensives. Circulation 107, 1401–1406.

Keider, S., Kaplan, M., Shapira, H., Brook, J.G., Aviram, M., 1994. Low density lipoprotein isolated from patients with essential hypertension exhibits increased propensity for oxidation and enhanced uptake by macrophages: a possible role for angiotensin II. Atherosclerosis 107, 71–84.

Kimura, Y., Matsumoto, M., Den, Y.B., Iwai, K., Munehira, J., Hattori, H., et al., 1999. Impaired endothelial function in hypertensive elderly patients evaluated by high resolution ultrasonography. Can. J. Cardiol. 15, 563–568.

Laaksonen, D.E., Lakka, H.M., Niskanen, L.K., et al., 2002. Metabolic syndrome and development of diabetes mellitus: application and validation of recently suggested definitions of the metabolic syndrome in a prospective cohort study. Am. J. Epidemiol. 156, 1070–1077.

Lamarre-Cliché, M., Cusson, C., 2001. The fainting patient: value of the head-upright tilt-table test in adult patients with orthostatic intolerance. CMAJ 164, 372–376.

Lee, I.T., Chan, Y.C., Lin, C.W., Lee, W.J., Sheu, W.H., 2008. Effect of cranberry extracts on lipid profiles in subjects with type 2 diabetes. Diabetic Med. 25, 1473–1477.

Levitan, E.B., Wolk, A., Mittleman, M.A., 2009. Relation of consistency with the dietary approaches to stop hypertension diet and incidence of heart failure in men aged 45 to 79 years. Am. J. Cardiol. 104, 1416–1420.

Malik, S., Wong, N.D., Franklin, S.S., et al., 2004. Impact of the metabolic syndrome on mortality from coronary heart disease, cardiovascular disease, and all causes in United States adults. Circulation 110, 1245–1250.

Masaki, K.H., Schatz, I.J., Burchfield, C.M., Sharp, D.S., Chiu, D., Foley, D., et al., 1998. Orthostatic hypotension predicts mortality in elderly men: the Honolulu. Heart Program. Circulation 98, 2290–2295.

Masuo, K., Mikami, H., Ogihara, T., 1993. The frequency of orthostatic hypotension in elderly patients with essential hypertension, isolated systolic hypertension and borderline hypertension. J. Hypertens. 11 (Suppl. 5), 306–307.

McAnulty, S.R., McAnulty, L.S., Morrow, J.D., Khardouni, D., Shooter, L., Monk, J., et al., 2005. Effect of daily fruit ingestion on angiotensin converting enzyme activity, blood pressure, and oxidative stress in chronic smokers. Free Radic. Res. 39, 1241–1248.

Milbury, P.E., Vita, J.A., Blumberg, J.B., 2010. Anthocyanins are bioavailable in humans following an acute dose of cranberry juice. J. Nutr. 140, 1099–1104.

Mitchell, G.F., Hwang, S.J., Vasan, R.S., et al., 2010. Arterial stiffness and cardiovascular events: the Framingham Heart Study. Circulation 121 (4), 505–511.

Mozzafarian, D., Benjamin, E.J., Go, A.S., et al., 2015. Heart disease and stroke statistics-2015 update: a report from the American Heart Association. Circulation, e29–322.

Nwankwo, T., Yoon, S.S., Burt, V., Gu, Q., 2013. Hypertension among adults in the US: National Health and Nutrition Examination Survey, 2011–2012. NCHS Data Brief, No. 133. National Center for Health Statistics, Centers for Disease Control and Prevention, US Dept of Health and Human Services, Hyattsville, MD.

Ohkubo, T., 2002. Prognostic significance of the nocturnal decline in blood pressure in individuals with and without high 24-h blood pressure: the Ohasama study. J. Hypertens. 20 (11), 2183–2189.

Papamichael, C., Karatzis, E., Karatzi, K., Aznaouridis, K., Papaioannou, T., Protogerou, A., et al., 2004. Red wine's antioxidants counteract acute endothelial dysfunction caused by cigarette smoking in healthy nonsmokers. Am. Heart J. 147, E5.

Park, Y.K., Kim, J.S., Kang, M.H., 2004. Concord grape juice supplementation reduces blood pressure in Korean hypertensive men: double-blind, placebo controlled intervention trial. Biofactors 22, 145–147.

Peppard, P.E., Young, T., Palta, M., Skatrud, J., 2000. Prospective study of the association between sleep-disordered breathing and hypertension. N. Eng. J. Med. 342, 1378–1384.

Piper, M.A., 2014. Screening for high blood pressure in adults: a systematic evidence review for the U.S. Preventive Services Task Force [Internet]. Rockville (MD): Agency for Healthcare Research and Quality (US); Dec. Report No.: 13-05194-EF-1. U.S. Preventive Services Task Force Evidence Syntheses, formerly Systematicb Evidence Reviews.

Raiha, I., Luutonen, S., Piha, J., Seppanen, A., Toikka, T., Sourander, I., 1995. Prevalence, predisposing factors, and prognostic importance of postural hypotension. Arch. Intern. Med. 155, 930–935.

Ras, R.T., Zock, P.L., Zebregs, Y.E., Johnston, N.R., Webb, D.J., Draijer, R., 2013. Effect of polyphenol-rich grape seed extract on ambulatory blood pressure in subjects with pre- and stage I hypertension. Br. J. Nutr. 110, 2234–2241.

Rodriguez-Mateos, A., 2013. Intake and time dependence of blueberry flavonoid-induced improvements in vascular function: a randomized, controlled, double-blind, crossover intervention study with mechanistic insights into biological activity. Am. J. Clin. Nutr. 98 (5), 1179–1191. http://dx.doi.org/10.3945/ajcn.113.066639. Epub 2013 Sep 4.

Rodriguez-Mateos, A., 2014. Berry (poly)phenols and cardiovascular health. J. Agric. Food Chem. 62 (18), 3842–3851. http://dx.doi.org/10.1021/jf403757g. Epub 2013 Oct 7.

Rodriguez-Mateos, A., Rendeiro, C., Bergillos-Meca, T., Tabatabaee, S., George, T., Heiss, C., et al., 2013. Intake and time dependence of blueberry flavonoid-induced improvements in vascular function: a randomized, controlled, double-blind, crossover intervention study with mechanistic insights into biological activity. Am. J. Clin. Nutr. http://dx.doi.org/10.3945/ajcn.113.066639.

Sayk, F., Becker, C., Teckentrup, C., Fehm, H.-L., Struck, J., Wellhoener, J.P., et al., 2007. To dip or not to dip: on the physiology of blood pressure decrease during nocturnal sleep in healthy humans. Hypertension 49, 1070–1076.

Sivaprakasapillai, B., Edirisinghe, I., Randolph, J., Steinberg, F., Kappagoda, T., 2009. Effect of grape seed extract on blood pressure in subjects with the metabolic syndrome. Metabolism 58, 1743–1746.

Stull, A.J., Cash, K.C., Johnson, W.D., Champagne, C.M., Cefalu, W.T., 2010. Bioactives in blueberries improve insulin sensitivity in obese, insulin-resistant men and women. J. Nutr. 140, 1764–1768.

Touyz, R.M., 2004. Reactive oxygen species, vascular oxidative stress, and redox signaling in hypertension: what is the clinical significance? Hypertension 44, 248–252.

van Mierlo, L.A.J., Zock, P.L., van der Knaap, H.C.M., Draijer, R., 2010. Grape polyphenols do not affect vascular function in healthymen. J. Nutr. 140, 1769–1773.

Veerman, D.P., Imholz, B.P., Wieling, W., Wesseling, K.H., van Montfrans, G.A., 1995. Circadian profile of systemic hemodynamics. Hypertension 26, 55–59.

Vinson, J.A., Su, X., Zubik, L., Bose, P., 2001. Phenol antioxidant quantity and quality in foods: fruits. J. Agric. Food Chem. 49, 5315–5321.

Wei, J.Y., 1992. Age and the cardiovascular system. N. Engl. J. Med. 327, 1735–1739.

Wright Jr, J.T., Dunn, J.K., Cutler, J.A., Davis, B.R., Cushman, W.C., Ford, C.E., et al., 2005. Outcomes in hypertensive black and nonblack patients treated with chlorthalidone, amlodipine, and lisinopril. JAMA 293, 1595–1608.

Yang, Q., Cogswell, M.E., Flanders, W.D., et al., 2012. Trends in cardiovascular health metrics and associations with all-cause and CVD mortality among US adults. JAMA 307 (12), 1273–1283. PMID: 22427615.

Zunino, S.J., Parelman, M.A., Freytag, T.L., Stephensen, C.B., Kelley, D.S., Mackey, B.E., et al., 2012. Effects of dietary strawberry powder on blood lipids and inflammatory markers in obese human subjects. Br. J. Nutr. 108, 900–909.

Section 3

Vegetables in Health and Diseases

Chapter 16

Poi history, uses, and role in health

Amy C. Brown[1], Salam A. Ibrahim[2] and Danfeng Song[3]
[1]*University of Hawaii at Manoa, Honolulu, HI, United States*
[2]*North Carolina Agricultural and Technical State University, Greensboro, NC, United States*
[3]*AUI Fine Foods, Gaithersburg, MD, United States*

CHAPTER OUTLINE

INTRODUCTION

Historical Review of Taro

Taro (*Colocasia esculenta* L.) has been cultivated for thousands of years. Originating in Asia, taro is now found in tropical and subtropical regions where it was historically a major dietary staple on the islands of the Pacific, especially Hawaii, New Zealand, and west to Indonesia. Taro became especially important to the Hawaiians who called it kalo, associated it with their gods and the original ancestor of the Hawaiian people, and even used it for medicinal purposes (Brown and Valiere, 2004b). The taro plant is particularly connected to the culture of the indigenous Hawaiian people, the Kanaka Maoli. They believed that taro had the greatest life force of all foods. *Poi* is a Hawaiian word for the primary Polynesian staple food made from the corm of the taro plant (Fig. 16.1).

Fruits, Vegetables, and Herbs.
DOI: http://dx.doi.org/10.1016/B978-0-12-802972-5.00016-0

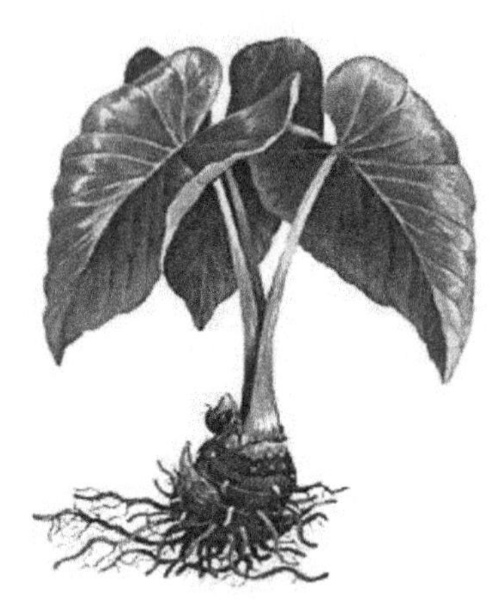

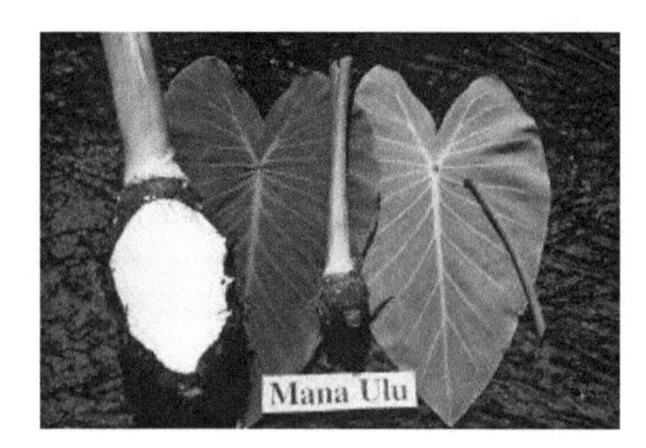

FIGURE 16.1 The taro (*Colocasia esculenta* L.) plant yields a starchy taro corm. *Courtesy of www.ndsu.edu and www.ctahr.hawaii.edu.*

Taro and *poi* became symbols and means of survival for the Hawaiian people. Ritual consumption of *poi* is an integral part of a ceremony of life that brings people together and supports a relationship of `ohana (family) and of appreciation of the `aumakua (ancestors).

Poi Preparation

In the traditional native Hawaiian diet, *poi* is made by first steaming taro corms which are then peeled, mashed, and mixed with a small amount of water to form a smooth paste (Fig. 16.2). Raw taro corms are generally not edible due to their high oxalate content that can cause intense burning sensations in the mouth and throat, but heating reduces oxalate levels and increases palatability. *Poi* produced from cooked corms is thick and starchy. When fresh, *poi* tastes rather bland, but if allowed to cool for 2 to 3 days it begins to ferment and develops a sour taste. This souring occurs due to the yeast and lactic acid bacteria naturally found on the plant's corm surface (Huang et al., 1994). During the "souring" process, acid production changes the pH from 6.3 to 4.5 within 24 hours and reaches its lowest pH on the fourth or fifth day of fermentation. At this point, *poi* is usually discarded. In recent years, however, innovations in *poi* production have resulted in methods that allow *poi* to stay fresh longer and have a sweeter taste. This has produced a new group of products similar to yogurt that generally require refrigeration (Huang et al., 2002).

Like yogurt, bacteria are responsible for the transformation of *poi* into an edible food. As early as 1933, Allen and Allen were able to identify the

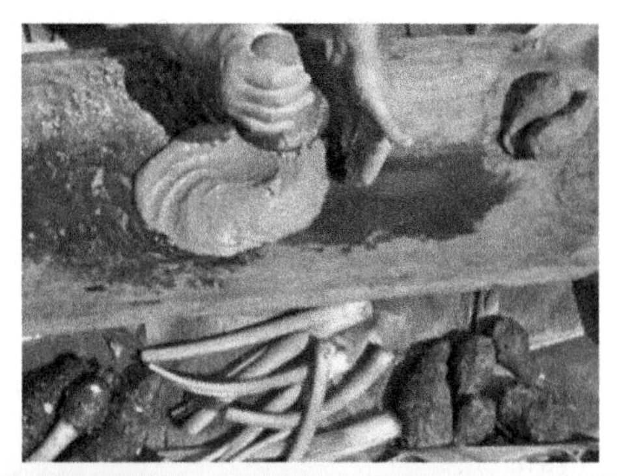

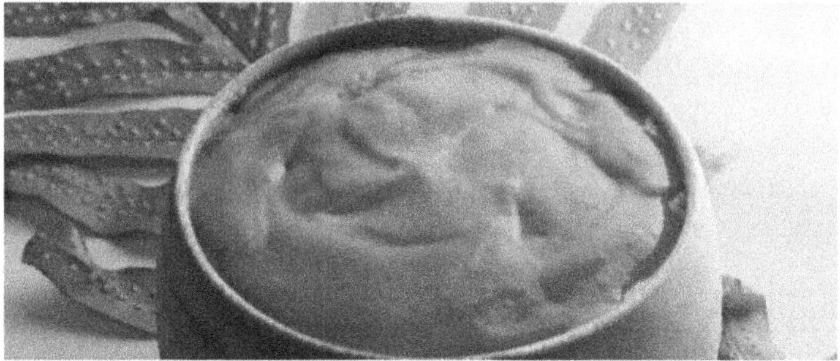

■ **FIGURE 16.2** *Poi* is made by cooking, peeling, and mashing the corms. *Courtesy of Uncle John Lind of the Kipahula Ohana, and photographer Scott Crawford; and Tomas del Amo.*

presence of three *Lactobacillus* species and two *Streptococcus* (recently renamed *Lactococcus*) bacteria, which included the *L. lactis* species, in *poi* (Allen and Allen, 1933). Bilger and Young (1935) later identified the actions of lactic acid, acetic acid, formic acid, alcohol, and acetaldehyde as being the primary agents for why *poi* "sours" (Bilger and Young, 1935). Huang et al. later identified the predominant species in sour *poi* as *L. lactis* (approximately 6.00 log CFU/g) and the major acids as lactic and acetic acids (Huang et al., 1994).

MEDICAL USE REVIEW

In the first part of the 20th century, researchers believed that, due to its easy digestibility, *poi* might have beneficial health effects for certain gastrointestinal conditions such as diarrhea and as an infant food. Studies conducted in the mid-1960s suggested that due to its high caloric content of easily digestible starch, *poi* might also be useful for the treatment of allergies and failure-to-thrive in infants (United States Department of Agriculture). The nutrient composition of *poi* primarily includes carbohydrates (65 g/cup or 27 g/100 g), potassium (439 mg/cup or 183 mg/100 g), fiber (1 g/cup or 0.4 g/100 g), and a few other nutrients. Very few foods have the high carbohydrate content of *poi* which delivers 269 calories per cup (112 calories/100 g), an amount that exceeds the 220 calories found in 8 ounces of Ensure. *Poi*'s easy digestibility is due to its extremely small starch granules and hypoallergenic nature because of its very low protein content of only 1 g/cup (0.38 g/100 g). The high concentrations of alkaline-forming elements such as Na, K, Ca, Mg and low concentrations of acid-forming elements such as S, P, Cl make *poi* an alkaline food product (Derstine and Rada, 1952). In addition, the microorganisms that make up *poi* have probiotic properties. According to the World Health Organization, these microorganisms are described as "live organisms which when administered in adequate amounts confer a health benefit to the host." Consequently, due to poi's probiotic capability, some researchers speculate that *poi* might also be useful for other digestive disorders such as gastroenteritis, irritable bowel syndrome, ulcerative colitis, and reducing the risk of colon cancer (Song et al., 2012).

Digestive disorders

Poi is easily digested, and this may have a beneficial impact on certain health conditions involving the gastrointestinal tract. However, research on digestive tract issues has been extremely limited to include two studies on food allergies of which one addresses failure-to-thrive and one is an *in vitro* study on the antiproliferative action of *poi* on colorectal cells (Table 16.1) (Brown et al., 2005a). These studies were preceded by food science research evaluating the digestibility of *poi* in the laboratory. MacCaughey recognized how easily *poi* was digested which he attributed to the small size of the taro starch granule (MacCaughey, 1917). Langworthy and Deuel (1922) confirmed this finding and further established that the raw starches of rice and taro root were notably more digestible as the result of the smaller size of the starch granules. Taro starches have irregular, polygonal shapes and very small granular sizes. The average diameter of taro starches ranges from 2.60 to 3.76 μm (Jane et al., 1992). This small size makes *poi* an excellent food for patients with digestive disorders. Further evidence of the high digestibility of *poi* has been demonstrated in human studies which have reported of undigested starch in the feces, even when large quantities of *poi* were consumed (Langworthy and Deuel, 1922). Derstine and Rada also reported that the easy digestibility of *poi* and the high absorbability of its minerals, such as calcium and phosphorus, appear to be related to its rapid fermentation process (Derstine and Rada, 1952).

Table 16.1 Studies Utilizing *Poi* for Health Conditions

Medical Conditions	Refs	Study Objective	Subject Type	Subject #	Study Length	Treatment	Results
Food Allergies	Derstine and Rada (1952)	Not a study, but observations of *poi* being used as a food source	Human	NA	NA	None	Use of *poi* in Hawaii hospitals during WWII
	Glaser et al., (1967)	Compare *poi* versus rice as food source for ill infants	Human	100	6 months	Fed *poi* or rice instead of cereal	Equal thriving between *poi* and rice-fed groups
	Roth et al. (1967)	Compared *poi* versus cereal for allergic reactions	Human	132	NA	Fed *poi*/rice instead of cereal	Only 7% of both groups had allergic reactions
Failure-to-thrive	Glaser et al. (1967)	Case studies of *poi* as cereal substitute for infants	Human	12	11–45 days	Fed *poi* and formula	All gained enough weight to be discharged
Probiotic	Brown et al., (2005b)	Cross-over clinical feeding study	Human	18 (19–64 years)	14 weeks 2 week washout 4 week treatment or control (twice)	Fed 1- to 2-day-old poi (390 g or 1.5 cups per day)	No significant difference in microbial fecal culture analysis
Cancer	Brown et al. (2005a)	Antiproliferation effect of *poi*	*In vitro* colon cancer cells (rat YYT)	NA	NA	*Poi* extract (water soluble)	Antiproliferative and lymphocyte stimulation effects
	Kai et al. (2011)	Inhibition of adult T-cell leukemia cells	*In vitro* adult T-cell leukemia cells (Su9T01)	NA	NA	*Poi* extract	Inhibited adult T-cell leukemia cells

(*Continued*)

Table 16.1 Studies Utilizing *Poi* for Health Conditions (Continued)

Medical Conditions	Refs	Study Objective	Subject Type	Subject #	Study Length	Treatment	Results
	Okabe et al. (1996)	Inhibition of bacterial mutations	*In vitro Salmonella typhimurium* exposed to carcinogen	NA	NA	*Poi* extract (water soluble)	Highest inhibition compared to yam and jinenjo
	Botting et al. (1999)	Inhibition of bacterial mutations	*In vitro Salmonella typhimurium* exposed to carcinogen	NA	NA	Taro leaf extract	Protected bacteria from mutagenicity
	Nakamura et al. (1998)	Inhibition of bacterial mutations	*In vitro E. coli* exposed to UV	NA	NA	*Poi* extract (water soluble)	Protected bacteria from UV mutagenicity
	Kundu et al. (2012)	Inhibition of metastasis from implanted mammary gland tumors	Mice plus *in vitro*	14 control 10 treatment	NA	*Poi* extract (water soluble)	Antimutagenic and antimetastatic activities against breast cancer
	Ferguson et al. (2012)	Effect of 10% *poi* diet on inhibiting tumors	Rats	10 per group	1 year	10% taro diet	Increased risk of skin tumors

This article was reprinted in part from Nutr Clin Care 7, 69–74, 2004, with permission from Wiley.

Infant allergies

Because of its very low protein content, *poi* is hypoallergenic. Alverez in 1939 was the first to suggest that *poi* be used as a substitute food for people allergic to certain foods (Alverez, 1939). During World War II, *poi* was used as a substitute starch for people allergic to cereal or grain (Derstine and Rada, 1952). Feingold was one of the first to suggest that *poi* be considered as a substitute for soy milk in infants allergic to both soy and cow's milk (Feingold, 1942). Physicians in Hawaii were some of the first to research *poi* as a substitute for infant food allergies. In a 1961 paper by Dr. Jerome Glaser, he noted the common use of *poi* for infants showing allergic reactions and those with gastrointestinal disorders and theorized that infants suspected of being allergic to cereal grains could eat *poi* as a substitute. Glaser conducted a 6-month study of 100 infants, in which 50 infants were fed *poi* compared with 50 babies fed rice, which was the conventional food allergy therapy at the time, and found that both groups of infants thrived equally well (Glaser et al., 1967).

Roth et al. (1967) confirmed Glaser's findings after they tested 132 potentially allergic infants. Of the infants fed cow's milk substitutes ($n = 132$), about 7% of the rice-fed infants (4/55) and *poi*-fed infants (5/73) showed signs of allergy. Roth concluded that *poi* was well tolerated by the babies and had potential as a food alternative for infants with a family history of cereal allergy.

Failure-to-thrive

Weight gain is often the desired outcome for pediatric patients with failure-to-thrive. The lack of gluten in *poi* makes it an ideal substitute for cereals in patients with celiac disease or nonceliac gluten sensitivity (Glaser et al., 1967). Since the mid-1960s, a few studies have been conducted on the use of *poi* and failure-to-thrive. Glaser et al. reported two case studies in which *poi* proved to be helpful to failure-to-thrive infants due to allergies. One infant boy had severe multiple food intolerances and was diagnosed with failure-to-thrive. At the age of 9 months, he was started on *poi* as the main dietary carbohydrate, and by the age of 19 months, he was at the lower limit of weight for his height. By age 4 years and 3 months (the last observation of the boy), he had achieved a normal weight and height for his age, appeared healthy, and was regularly consuming large amounts of *poi* (Glaser et al., 1967).

The other case study involved an infant girl experiencing severe gastrointestinal problems attributed to cow's milk allergy (Glaser et al., 1967). The premature female infant weighed 1500 g at birth was placed on various formulas but only gained 100 g in 54 days, so her risk of failing to thrive became acute. She was then given *poi*, quickly responded positively, and was able to be discharged from the hospital after achieving and maintaining a healthy weight (2250–2500 g). However, because these studies were dated further research is warranted for the use of *poi* as a hypoallergenic food source for infants and children with food allergies and/or failure-to-thrive. *Poi* is not a complete food nutritionally for infants who are not breast fed, and these infants should always receive an American Academy of Pediatric approved formula for the first year of life to avoid potentially serious nutrient deficiencies.

Probiotic effects

Poi can be used as a probiotic in medical nutrition therapy (Brown and Valiere, 2004a,b). The predominant bacteria in *poi* are *L. lactis* (95%) and *Lactobacilli* (5%) (Huang et al., 1994), both of which are lactic acid-producing bacteria. *Poi* contains significantly more of these bacteria per gram than yogurt. Brown et al. (2005b) were the first to investigate the effect of *poi* consumption on gastrointestinal tract bacterial concentration was a cross-over clinical study involving 18 subjects (a *poi* group of 10 and a control group of 8). This study found no significant differences in total bacterial counts following a fresh *poi* diet versus following a control diet, nor were significant differences found in counts of specific bacterial species. However, measuring colonic bacteria is an evolving field, and researchers expect that a "sour *poi*" might have a greater effect than fresh *poi* as a potential probiotic. More studies are needed to confirm *poi*'s probiotic function.

Cancer inhibiting properties

Like many plants, *poi* contains a unique collection of compounds that can impact chemoprotection and anticancer activity. Taro corms have been reported to contain anthocyanins, cyanidin 3-glucoside, pelargonidin 3-glucoside, and cyanidin 3-rhamnoside. These substances have antioxidant and anti-inflammatory properties which may protect the intestine from carcinogens (Cambie and Ferguson, 2003). Taro has also been suggested to have anticancer potential based on findings that taro extracts have significant antioxidative effects against xanthine oxidase, one of the major enzymes responsible for oxidative stress through superoxide O_2^- generation (Kim et al., 2002).

Another study revealed that the taro plant's edible fiber could adsorb mutagens (Ferguson et al., 1992). As a result, the fiber content might also contribute to anticancer effects against colon cancers including colorectal cancer (Baena and Salinas, 2015) which continues to be a leading cause of morbidity and mortality in the Western World (DeSantis et al., 2014). Hawaiians consume more *poi* than most other groups in Hawaii and tend to have a lower incidence of colorectal cancer. In addition to the epidemiological data linking *poi* and low colon cancer incidence, *poi* has several properties including fiber content, novel phytochemical contents, pH influences, and possible probiotic chemoprotection that may play a significant role in decreasing the risk of carcinogenesis. Colon cancer prevention has long been associated with plant rich diets, especially diets supplemented with probiotics. Brown was the first to discover that *poi* extract can have two distinct inhibitory *in vitro* effects toward colon cancer cells (Brown et al., 2005a). *Poi* can directly inhibit the proliferation of mammalian colon cancer cells by (1) inducing their apoptosis and (2) stimulating the immune system by activating lymphocytes which have previously been shown to kill numerous types of colon cancer cells, both in humans and in rodents.

Additional support for *poi*'s *in vitro* anticancer activity was reported by researchers who found that an extract from the edible portion of taro showed markedly greater inhibitory effects than the phytoestrogen control of genistein on adult T-cell leukemia cells (Su9T01) (Kai et al., 2011). This may be promising because adult T-cell leukemia cancer is often resistant to conventional chemotherapy. Other *in vitro* research suggests that *poi* may be useful in controlling laboratory-induced carcinogenity in bacteria. Okabe et al. investigated the antimutagenicity effects of different preparation bases on the Trp-P2-induced mutagenicity to *Salmonella typhimurium* (Okabe et al., 1996). Water extracts, EtOH extracts, and gummy materials were prepared from four root crops: Chinese yam (*Dioscorea opposita* Thumb.), jinenjo (*D. japonica* Thunb.), taro (*C. esculenta* (L.) Schott), and processed freeze-dried *poi*. The gummy processed taro showed the highest inhibition of mutagenicity among the plant specimens used (Okabe et al., 1996). Another bacteria-based study revealed that an extract from taro leaves, not *poi*, protected carcinogen exposed *S. typhimurium* against mutagenicity (Botting et al., 1999). *E. coli* bacteria exposed to UV radiation were less likely to mutate when exposed to the water-soluble extraction of taro. Taro showed the most robust effects of all the vegetable samples tested and surpassed the antimutagenic ability of eggplant and melon (Nakamura et al., 1998).

Kundu et al. demonstrated for the first time in a mouse model that a water-soluble extract from uncooked taro corms had potent antimetastatic activity against metastatic breast cancer (Kundu et al., 2012). However, in another animal study, it was reported that rats fed a 10% taro diet and then exposed to a carcinogen developed higher rates of skin tumors (Ferguson et al., 2012).

Future research

Very limited research exists on utilizing *poi* for its potential health benefits making *poi* investigation a promising area in food science research. Studies from the mid-1960s first suggested that *poi* may have great potential for treating food allergies and failure-to-thrive in infants. *Poi*'s unique combination as a probiotic, high caloric content, hypoallergenic due to low protein content, and easy digestibility due to small starch granules suggest that new *poi*-containing products could be developed to assist with weight loss-related health conditions such as failure-to-thrive, cancer cachexia, AIDS, pancreatitis, cystic fibrosis, Crohn's disease, and ulcerative colitis. Its probiotic qualities could also be explored in treating antibiotic-associated diarrhea, traveler's diarrhea, gastroenteritis, irritable bowel syndrome, pouchitis, and digestive tract cancers.

Its role as a probiotic is enhanced by a high polysaccharide concentration and other substances that support the growth of *Lactobacillus* and *Bifidobacteria* (Song et al., 2012). There is a need to develop and evaluate the viability of new *poi* probiotic products. For example, a recent study found that fermented sweet potato contains several probiotic strains that produced functional ingredients with health benefits (Hayek et al., 2013). *Poi* also contains several functional ingredients that can be investigated for their effect on probiotics and human health.

Poi's initial anticancer properties, which were revealed in a few *in vitro* and animal studies, suggest the need for further research. *Poi*'s combination of antioxidant and anti-inflammatory compounds suggests that it may have cancer fighting properties, especially against colorectal cancer.

As a food supplement, *poi* is a probiotic that needs to be researched in terms of a complementary treatment for several health conditions, and also in health promotion and disease prevention by the possible risk reduction of certain cancers.

SUMMARY POINTS

- *Poi* can provide extra calories as a supplemental food for infants born with an allergy to dairy products as long as all of the infants' essential nutrient needs, including protein intake, are being met by commercial infant formulas approved by the American Academy of Pediatrics.
- Sour *poi* is a nondairy probiotic that warrants further research.
- *Poi*, as a functional food, has antiproliferative and antimetastatic properties that warrant further investigation.

REFERENCES

Allen, O.N., Allen, E.K., 1933. The manufacture of *poi* from taro in Hawaii: with special emphasis upon its fermentation. Hawaii Agric. Exp. Stn. Bull. No. 70.

Alverez, W.C., 1939. Problems of maintaining nutrition in the highly food-sensitive person. Am. J. Dig. Dis. 5, 801–803.

Baena, R., Salinas, P., 2015. Diet and colorectal cancer. Maturitas 80, 258–264.

Bilger, L.N., Young, H.Y., 1935. The chemical investigation of the fermentations occurring in the process of *poi* manufacture. J. Agric. Res. 51, 45–50.

Botting, K.J., Young, M.M., Pearson, A.E., Harris, P.J., Ferguson, L.R., 1999. Antimutagens in food plants eaten by Polynesians: micronutrients, phytochemicals and protection against bacterial mutagenicity of the heterocyclic amine 2-amino-3-methylimidazo[4,5-f]quinoline. Food Chem. Toxicol. 37, 95–103.

Brown, A.C., Valiere, A., 2004a. Probiotics and medical nutrition therapy. Nutr. Clin. Care 7, 56–68.

Brown, A.C., Valiere, A., 2004b. The medicinal uses of *poi*. Nutr. Clin. Care 7, 69–74.

Brown, A.C., Reitzenstein, J.E., Liu, J., Jadus, M.R., 2005a. The antiproliferative effect of diluted *poi* (*Colocasia esculenta*) on colonic adenocarcinoma cells *in vitro*. Phytother. Res. 19, 767–771.

Brown, A.C., Shovic, A., Ibrahim, S.A., Holck, P., Huang, A., 2005b. A non-dairy probiotics's (*poi*) influence on changing the gastrointestinal tract's microflora environment. Altern. Ther. Health Med. 11, 58–64.

Cambie, R.C., Ferguson, L.R., 2003. Potential functional foods in the traditional Maori diet. Mutat. Res. 523–524, 109–117.

Derstine, V., Rada, E., 1952. Some dietetic factors influencing die market for *poi* in Hawaii "Agricultural Economics", Bulletin No. 3, vol. 3. University of Hawaii Agricultural Experiment Station, Hawaii.1–43

DeSantis, C.E., Lin, C.C., Mariotto, A.B., Siegel, R.L., Stein, K.D., Kramer, J.L., et al., 2014. Cancer treatment and survivorship statistics, 2014. CA Cancer J. Clin. 64, 252–271.

Feingold, B.F., 1942. A vegetable milk substitute: taro. J. Allergy 13, 488.

Ferguson, L.R., Roberton, A.M., McKenzie, R.J., Watson, M.E., Harris, P.J., 1992. Adsorption of a hydrophobic mutagen to dietary fiber from taro (*Colocasia esculenta*), an important food plant of the South Pacific. Nutr. Cancer 17, 85–95.

Ferguson, L.R., Zhu, S., Han, D.Y., Harris, P.J., 2012. Inhibition or enhancement by 4 Pacific Island food plants against cancers induced by 2 amino-3-methylimidazo[4,5-f]quinoline in male Fischer 344 rats. Nutr. Cancer 64, 218–227.

Glaser, J., Lawrence, R.A., Harrison, A., Ball, M.R., 1967. *Poi*—its use as a food for normal, allergic and potentially allergic children. Ann. Allergy 25, 496–500.

Hayek, S.A., Shahbazi, A., Awaisheh, S.S., Shah, N.P., Ibrahim, S.A., 2013. Sweet potatoes as a basic component in developing a medium for the cultivation of *Lactobacilli*. Biosci. Biotechnol. Biochem. 77, 2248–2254.

Huang, A.S., Lam, S.Y., Nakayama, T.M., Lin, H., 1994. Microbiological and chemical changes in *poi* stored at 20°C. J. Agric. Food Chem. 42, 45–48.

Huang, A.S., Karthik, K., Liu, X.X., 2002. Textural and sensory properties of α-amylase treated *poi* stored at 4°C. J. Food Process. Pres 26, 1–10.

Jane, J., Shen, L., Kasemsuwan, T., 1992. Physical and chemical studies of taro starches and flours. Cereal Chem. 69, 528–535.

Kai, H., Akamatsu, E., Torii, E., Kodama, H., Yukizaki, C., Sakakibara, Y., et al., 2011. Inhibition of proliferation by agricultural plant extracts in seven human adult T-cell leukaemia (ATL)-related cell lines. J. Nat. Med. 65, 651–655.

Kim, H.W., Murakami, A., Nakamura, Y., Ohigashi, H., 2002. Screening of edible Japanese plants for suppressive effects on phorbol ester-induced syperoxide generation in differentiated HL-60 cells and AS52 cells. Cancer Lett. 176, 7–16.

Kundu, N., Campbell, P., Hampton, B., Lin, C.Y., Ma, X., Ambulos, N., et al., 2012. Antimetastatic activity isolated from *Colocasia esculenta* (taro). Anticancer Drugs 23, 200–211.

Langworthy, C.F., Deuel, H.J., 1922. Digestibility of raw rice, arrowroot, canna, cassava, taro, tree-fern, and potato starches. J. Biol. Chem. 52, 251–261.

MacCaughey, V., 1917. The Hawaiian taro as food. Hawaiian Forester Agric. 14, 265–268.

Nakamura, Y., Suganuma, E., Kuyama, N., Sato, K., Ohtsuki, K., 1998. Comparative bio-antimutagenicity of common vegetables and traditional vegetables in Kyoto. Biosci. Biotechnol. Biochem. 62, 1161–1165.

Okabe, Y., Shinmoto, H., Tsushida, T., Tokuda, S., 1996. Antimutagenicity of the extracts from four root crops on the Trp-p 2-induced mutagenicity to *Salmonella* typhimurium TA 98. J. Jpn. Soc. Food Sci. Technol. 43, 36–39.

Roth, A., Worth, R.M., Lichton, I.J., 1967. Use of *poi* in the prevention of allergic disease in potentially allergic infants. Ann. Allergy 25, 501–506.

Song, D., Ibrahim, S.A., Hayek, S., 2012. Recent applications of probiotics in food and agricultural science In: Rigobelo, E.C. (Ed.), Probiotics, vol. 10 InTech, Manhattan, NY, pp. 1–34. (Chapter 1).

United States Department of Agriculture. Agricultural Research Service. National Database for Standard Reference Release 27. Basic Report: 11349, Poi. <http://ndb.nal.usda.gov/ndb/foods/> (accessed 05.05.15.).

Chapter 17

Bioactive potential of two wild edible mushrooms of the Western Ghats of India

N.C. Karun, K.R. Sridhar, V.R. Niveditha and S.D. Ghate

Mangalore University, Mangalagangotri, Mangalore, Karnataka, India

CHAPTER OUTLINE

Fruits, Vegetables, and Herbs.
DOI: http://dx.doi.org/10.1016/B978-0-12-802972-5.00017-2

INTRODUCTION

In the interest of human health, exploration of natural products gained utmost importance than synthetic drugs. Although fungi are the diverse dominant group of life forms, a fraction of them are described (~7%) and a few species are explored for bioactive metabolites (De Silva et al., 2013). However, success of many fungal-derived secondary metabolites (eg, antibiotics, cholesterol-lowering agents, immunosuppressive drugs, and mycotoxins) projects their future potential. Mushrooms are believed to be an important natural source of remedial products for a variety of human ailments (Abraham, 2001; Aly et al., 2011; Wasser, 2011). Asian countries are historically depending on indigenous macrofungi for several centuries to treat many of human diseases (Aly et al., 2011; Ying et al., 1987; Xu et al., 2011). A variety of potential compounds possessing useful biological activities (eg, antibiotics, antiviral, cytotoxic, and pharmacological) were isolated from macrofungi (De Silva et al., 2013; Bao et al., 2001; Zhang et al., 2007; Jeong et al., 2011). Many edible mushrooms besides serving as potential nutritional value, they are known to serve as nutraceuticals through diet management in prevention of cardiovascular diseases, hypocholesterolemia, and atherosclerosis due to their high fiber and low fat content (De Silva et al., 2013). Western Ghats of India is endowed with a variety of macrofungi of nutritional, medicinal, and industrial importance (Mohanan, 2011; Farook et al., 2013; Thatoi and Singdevsachan, 2014). Although they are traditionally used for nutrition and medicinal purposes, a precise picture on their importance is yet to emerge. Besides nutritional attributes, wild edible mushrooms are potential source of bioactive compounds aids in combating human ailments. Therefore, the present study attempts to evaluate two wild edible mushrooms in the Western Ghats of India to link their bioactive components with functional attributes. As they are edible, dry flours of uncooked as well as cooked mushrooms are evaluated for their potent components and antioxidant potential.

MUSHROOMS AND PROCESSING

Auricularia auricula-judae (Bull.) Quél. (Auriculariaceae-Basidiomycotina) and *Termitomyces umkowaan* (Cooke & Massee) D.A. Reid (Lyophyllaceae-Basidiomycotina) were collected from Kadnur, Virajpet of the Western Ghats (12°13'N, 75°46'E; 891m asl) and from mixed forest of Mangalore University Campus, Mangalore, west coast (12°48'N, 74°55'E; 112.4m asl), respectively, during July–August 2013 (Fig. 17.1). *A. auricula-judae* was gregarious on decomposing standing dead and fallen logs, bark and twigs (eg, *Artocarpus heterophyllus*), while *T. umkowaan* was common in and around the termite mounds in mixed forests.

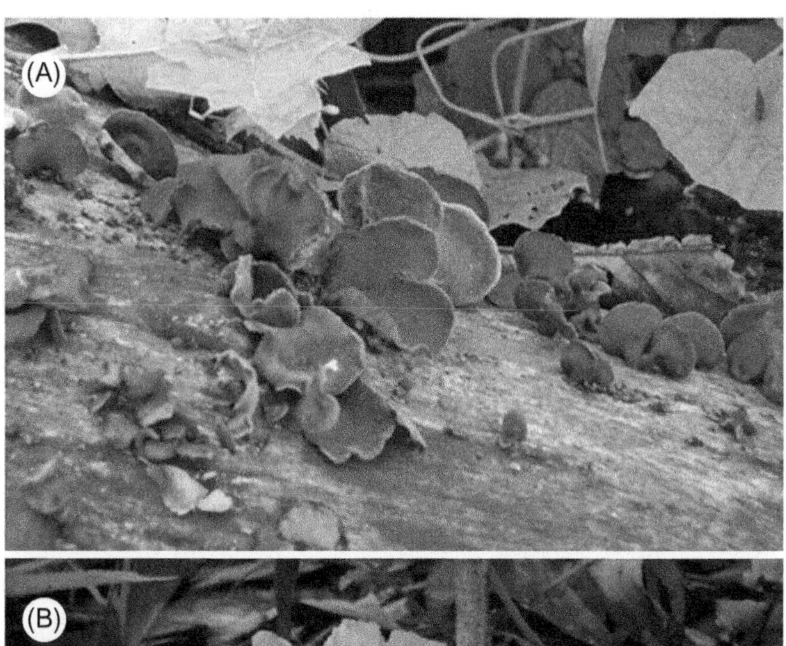

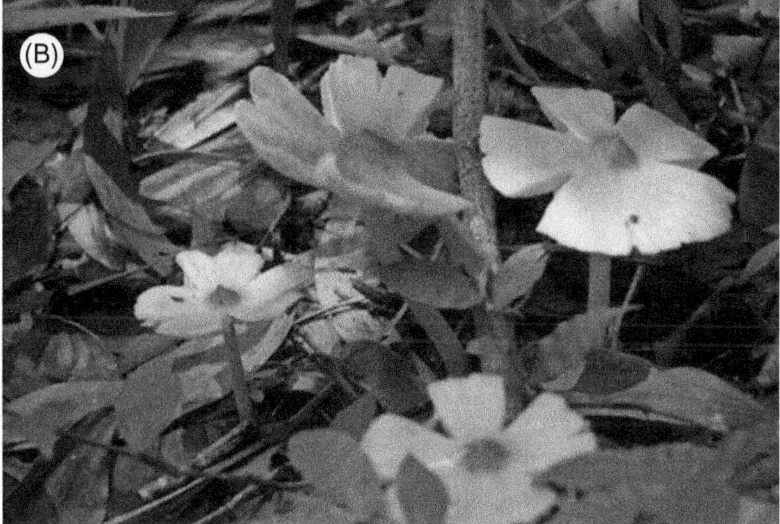

■ **FIGURE 17.1** Mushrooms assessed for bioactive potential: *Auricularia auricula* grown on a decaying log (A) and *Termitomyces umkowaan* grown in the vicinity of termite mound (B).

For assessment of bioactive potential, freshly collected mushroom samples ($n = 5$) were blotted and grouped into two portions in each replicate. One portion of each replicate was oven dried (50–55°C) and another portion was cooked using a household pressure cooker with limited water (6.5L, Deluxe stainless steel, TTK Prestige™; Prestige Ltd., Hyderabad, India) and oven dried on aluminum foil (50–55°C). Dried mushroom samples were milled (Wiley Mill, mesh #30) and refrigerated (4°C) in airtight containers.

BIOACTIVE PRINCIPLES

Total phenolics

Total phenolics of mushroom samples were determined based on the method outlined by Rosset et al. (1982). Mushroom flours of 50mg each were extracted in 5mL methanol (50%) in water bath (95±1°C) for 10min followed by centrifugation (1500rpm) and collection of supernatant. Methanol extraction was repeated once again for the flour pellet and pooled supernatant was made up to 10mL. Aliquots of 0.5mL extract was mixed with 0.5mL distilled water, mixed with 5mL Na_2CO_3 (in 0.1N NaOH) and incubated for 10min at laboratory temperature. Folin-Ciocalteu's reagent 0.5mL (diluted, 1:2 v/v with distilled water) was added and absorbance was read at 725nm (UV-VIS Spectrophotometer-118; Systronics, Ahmedabad, Gujarat, India) with tannic acid as standard. The results were expressed in mg of tannic acid equivalents per g of the sample (mgTAEs/g).

Tannins

To assess tannins in mushroom flours, vanillin–HCl method by Burns (1971) was used. Mushroom flour (1g) was extracted with methanol (50mL) at 28°C up to 24h, followed by centrifugation (1500rpm) and collection of supernatant. Aliquots of 1mL supernatant was treated with 5mL vanillin hydrochloride reagent (mixture of 4% vanillin in methanol and 8% concentrated HCl in methanol; ratio, 1:1). On incubation up to 20min, the developed color was read at 500nm and catechin (98% HPLC grade; Sigma Aldrich, USA) served as standard. The results were expressed in mg of catechin equivalents per g of the sample (mgCEs/g).

Flavonoids

Content of flavonoids in mushroom flours was evaluated by following the procedure by Chang et al. (2002). Mushroom flours were extracted in methanol at a concentration of 1mg/mL. Aliquots of 0.5mL methanolic extract was mixed with methanol (1.5mL), aluminum chloride (10%, 0.1mL), potassium acetate (1M, 0.1mL), and distilled water (2.8mL). Absorbance was measured at 415nm after incubation for 30min at laboratory temperature. Quercetin served as standard and the results were expressed in mg of quercetin equivalents per g of the sample (mgQEs/g).

Vitamin C

Content of vitamin C of mushroom flours was determined based on Roe (1954) with a slight modification. One gram of mushroom sample was extracted with trichloroacetic acid (TCA; 5%, 10 mL). Aliquots of 0.2 mL was made up to 1 mL with TCA (5%) and 2,4-dinitrophenylhydrazine (DNPH) (1 mL) was added. This reaction mixture was boiled up to 10 min, cooled to laboratory temperature, sulfuric acid was added (65%, 4 mL) and incubated up to 30 min at laboratory temperature followed by measurement of absorbance at 540 nm with ascorbic acid as standard. Vitamin C content was expressed as ascorbic acid equivalents in mg/g of mushroom flour (mg AAEs/g).

L-DOPA

L-DOPA (L-3,4-Dihydroxyphenylalanine) was determined according to the protocol by Fujii et al. (1991) (Fig. 17.2). Aliquots of mushroom powder was mixed with 1 mL distilled water followed by incubation up to 2 h at laboratory temperature. After centrifugation (1500 rpm), supernatant was concentrated using rotary evaporator to dryness. The extract was dissolved in distilled water, filtered (Ultrafilter; Toyo Roshi Kaisha Ltd., Japan) and kept for overnight to eliminate compounds of higher molecular weight. The low molecular weight fraction was further purified using a ODS mini

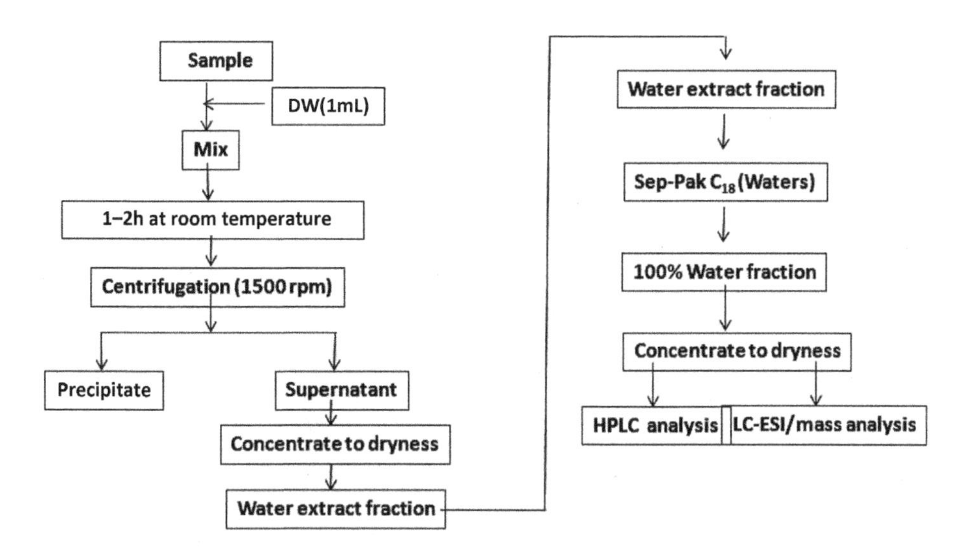

■ **FIGURE 17.2** Protocol employed for extraction of L-DOPA from *Auricularia auricula* and *Termitomyces umkowaan* using HPLC and LC-ESI/MS (DW, distilled water).

column (C18 Sep-Pak Cartridge; Waters) with 100% water. After concentrating the extract to dryness, L-DOPA was analyzed by HPLC and LC-ESI/MS.

Trypsin inhibition

To determine trypsin inhibition activity of mushroom flours, enzymatic assay proposed by Kakade et al. (1974) was employed. One gram of mushroom flour was extracted with NaOH (0.01 N, 50 mL), 1 mL of the extract was made up to 2 mL using distilled water. Two mL of trypsin solution (4 mg in 200 mL 0.001 M HCl) was added followed by incubation in a water bath (37°C) up to 10 min. To each tube, 5 mL of BAPNA [(40 mg N-a-Benzoyl-DL-Arginine p-nitroanilide hydrochloride in 1 mL dimethyl sulfoxide diluted to 100 mL with Tris-buffer at 37°C)] was added. On incubation up to 10 min, the reaction was terminated by adding 1 mL acetic acid (30%). After thorough mixing, it was filtered and absorbance was measured at 410 nm against reagent blank (1 mL, 30% acetic acid containing 2 mL each of trypsin and distilled water+5 mL BAPNA). One unit of trypsin inhibition (TIu/mg) is defined as release of 1 μM of p-nitroanilide per min by the enzyme.

Hemagglutination

The hemagglutinin activity of mushroom flours was evaluated according to the method by Occenã et al. (2007). Mushroom flour (500 mg) was suspended in NaCl (10 mL, 0.9%) followed by vigorous shaking, allowed to stand for 1 h and centrifuged (2000 g, 10 min) to obtain clear solution. It was filtered and the filtrate was used as crude agglutinin extract. The RBCs were separated from the whole human blood suspension (5 mL) (A, B, AB, and O groups) followed by centrifugation (2000 g, 10 min). The RBCs were diluted with cold saline (0.9%) (1:4), centrifuged (2000 g, 10 min), and the supernatant was eliminated. The RBC pellet was washed using saline until the supernatant became colorless. Four mL of washed erythrocytes was suspended in 100 mL phosphate buffer (0.0006 M, pH 8.4). One mL trypsin solution (2%) was added to 10 mL washed erythrocytes, mixed and incubated at 37°C up to 1 hour. The trypsinized erythrocytes were washed (four to five times in saline) to remove traces of trypsin. The packed cells (1.2–1.5 mL) were suspended in 100 mL saline.

Microtiter plates (8 rows of 12 wells) were used to assess hemagglutinin activity of mushroom flours. In the first well, the crude agglutinin extract was added and the well 12 served as control as it has no crude agglutinin extract. The saline (0.3 mL) was dispensed to well # 2–12. Serial dilution was followed from the well # 2–11. Trypsinized RBC (in saline 2%,

0.3 mL) was dispensed to well # 1–12. The contents were mixed and incubated at laboratory temperature up to 4 h. The pattern of hemagglutination in each well was noted and the hemagglutinating unit per gram (Hu/g) was determined by the following formula:

$$\mathrm{Hu/g} = (\mathrm{D_a} \times \mathrm{D_b} \times \mathrm{S})/\mathrm{V} \tag{17.1}$$

where D_a, dilution factor of extract in well # 1 is the crude agglutinin extract it remains as 1 if the original extract is not diluted; D_b, dilution factor of well containing 1 Hu is the well in which hemagglutination is first seen; S, mL original extract/g mushroom flour; V, volume of extract in well # 1.

ANTIOXIDANT ASSAY

Antioxidant capacity of test sample is influenced by various factors and demands at least two methods have to be adapted for assessment (Wong et al., 2006). Thus, in the present study four assay methods were employed to evaluate antioxidant properties of mushroom samples: (1) reduction of Mo(VI) to Mo(V) by antioxidant compounds (total antioxidant activity, TAA); (2) reduction of Fe(III) to Fe(II) ions (Fe^{2+} ion chelating capacity); (3) DPPH (diphenyl-1-picrylhydrazyl) radical absorption on exposure to radical scavengers (radical-scavenging activity); (4) conversion of Fe^{3+}/ferricyanide complex into the ferrous form (reducing power).

Methanol extract of mushroom flour was prepared by extracting 0.5 g flour in 30 mL methanol (shaken at 150 rpm for 48 h). After incubation, the extract was centrifuged and supernatant was collected in a preweighed Petri dish and allowed to dry at laboratory temperature. The weight of the extract was determined gravimetrically and dissolved in methanol to get the desired concentration (1 mg/mL) to perform antioxidant assays.

Total antioxidant activity

For TAA, extract (0.1 mL) was mixed with 1 mL reagent mixture (sulfuric acid, 0.6 M+ sodium phosphate, 28 mM+ ammonium molybdate, 4 mM) (Prieto et al., 1999). It was incubated at 95°C up to 90 min, cooled and absorbance of phosphomolybdenum complex was measured at 695 nm with methanol blank. The TAA was expressed as μM equivalent of ascorbic acid per g of the mushroom flour (mg AAEs/g).

Ferrous ion chelating capacity

Method outlined by Hsu et al. (2003) was employed to determine Fe^{2+} chelating capacity of mushroom samples. To 1 mL of extract, $FeCl_2$ (2 mM,

0.1 mL) and ferrozine (5 mM, 0.2 mL) were added followed by making up to 5 mL in methanol. After incubation up to 10 min at laboratory temperature absorbance of Fe^{2+}–ferrozine complex was determined at 562 nm. The sample devoid of extract served as control to calculate ferrous ion chelating capacity:

$$\text{Ferrous ion chelating capacity (\%)} = 1 - (A_{s562}/A_{c562}) \times 100 \quad (17.2)$$

where A_c, absorbance of the control; A_s, absorbance of sample.

DPPH free radical-scavenging activity

Free radical-scavenging activity of mushroom extracts was evaluated based on the method by Singh et al. (2002). Concentrations ranging from 200 to 1000 μg (0.2–1 mL) of test sample were made up to 1 mL in methanol, 4 mL DPPH (0.01 mM) was added and allowed to react at room temperature up to 20 min. Reagents devoid of extract served as control, the absorbance of mixture was measured at 517 nm and free radical-scavenging activity was calculated as

$$\text{Free radical-scavenging activity (\%)} = \left[(A_{c517} - A_{s517})/(A_{c517})\right] \times 100 \quad (17.3)$$

where A_c, absorbance of the control; A_s, is absorbance of sample.

Effective concentration (EC_{50}; concentration of sample required to scavenge 50% of DPPH radicals) (μg extract/mL) was obtained on plotting percent radical-scavenging activity against concentration of the extracts.

Reducing power

Reducing power of the extract was determined according to the method by Pulido et al. (2000) with minor modification. Concentrations ranging from 200 to 1000 μg (0.2–1 mL) of mushroom flour extracted in methanol were mixed with 2.5 mL phosphate buffer (0.2 M, pH 6.6) and 2.5 mL potassium ferricyanide (1%). After mixing the contents, it was incubated at 50°C up to 20 min, 2.5 mL of TCA (10%) was added, centrifuged (3000 rpm) up to 10 min and 2.5 mL supernatant was mixed with 2.5 mL distilled water. Ferric chloride (0.1%, 0.5 mL) was added to the mixture followed by measurement of absorbance at 700 nm. Increase in absorbance of the reaction mixture indicates increase in reducing power.

Data analysis

Difference in bioactive components between uncooked and cooked mushroom flours was assessed by *t*-test using Statistica version # 8.0 (StatSoft, 2008).

OBSERVATIONS AND DISCUSSION

As in foods of plant origin, extensive interest has been developed to investigate bioactive potential of wild and cultivated mushrooms. Therapeutic potential of many macrofungi growing in wild or in cultivation is still not clearly understood although they are consumed and used for medicinal purposes. Considerable studies have been performed especially in the East Asian countries to employ many macrofungi for therapeutic purposes as they are traditionally used (Kalač, 2009). Nutritional and health-promoting/disease resistance (or nutraceutical) power of macrofungi is more valuable than the synthetic antioxidants like butylated hydroxytoluene (BHT), butylated hydroxyanisole (BHA), and tertiary butyl hydroquinone (TBHQ). Synthetic antioxidants used widely in food industry have been reported to be carcinogenic and their use needs to be restricted (Botterweck et al., 2000).

Total phenolics of many macrofungi serve as major antioxidants as well as free radical scavengers. The quantity of total phenolics was substantially lower in *A. auricula* than in *T. umkowaan* without significant change on cooking (Fig. 17.3). In uncooked samples of *T. umkowaan*, total phenolics was high and decreased significantly to one-third on cooking. Total phenolics of *T. umkowaan* is higher than many termitomycetes (*T. badius*, *T. medius*, *T. radicatus*, and *T. striatus*) (21.4 vs 15–20.1 mg/g), comparable with *T. heimii* (21.3 mg/g) and lower than *T. mammiformis* and *T. microcarpus* (21.4 vs 22.5–37 mg/g) (Kumari, 2012). Interestingly, although high quantities of total phenolics were reported in *T. mammiformis* and *T. robustus* from Nigeria, their antioxidant potential was not considerably high (Unekwa et al., 2014).

Tannin content was higher in *T. umkowaan* than in *A. auricula* with significant decrease on cooking (Fig. 17.3). However, its content in mushrooms of the same genera was higher as reported by Abdullah et al. (2012) (*A. auricula*: 0.37 vs 6.2 mg/g; *T. umkowaan* vs *T. heimii*: 0.37 vs 11.3 mg/g). The tannin content reported in other termitomycetes in Nigeria was substantially high (*T. mammiformis* and *T. robustus*: 169.2 and 170.6 mg/g, respectively), but their antioxidant activity was not higher than other mushrooms (Unekwa et al., 2014).

Flavonoids consist of several biologically active compounds like flavones, isoflavones, flavonols, flavanols, and anthocyanins possessing antidiabetic, anti-inflammatory, hepatoprotective, antithrombotic, antiatherosclerotic, antineoplastic, and cardioprotective properties (Champ, 2002; Tapas et al., 2008). In spite of flavonoids are nutritionally important, their reports in mushrooms are sporadic (Barros et al., 2008; Gursoy et al., 2009). Flavonoids were higher in *A. auricula* than in *T. umkowaan*

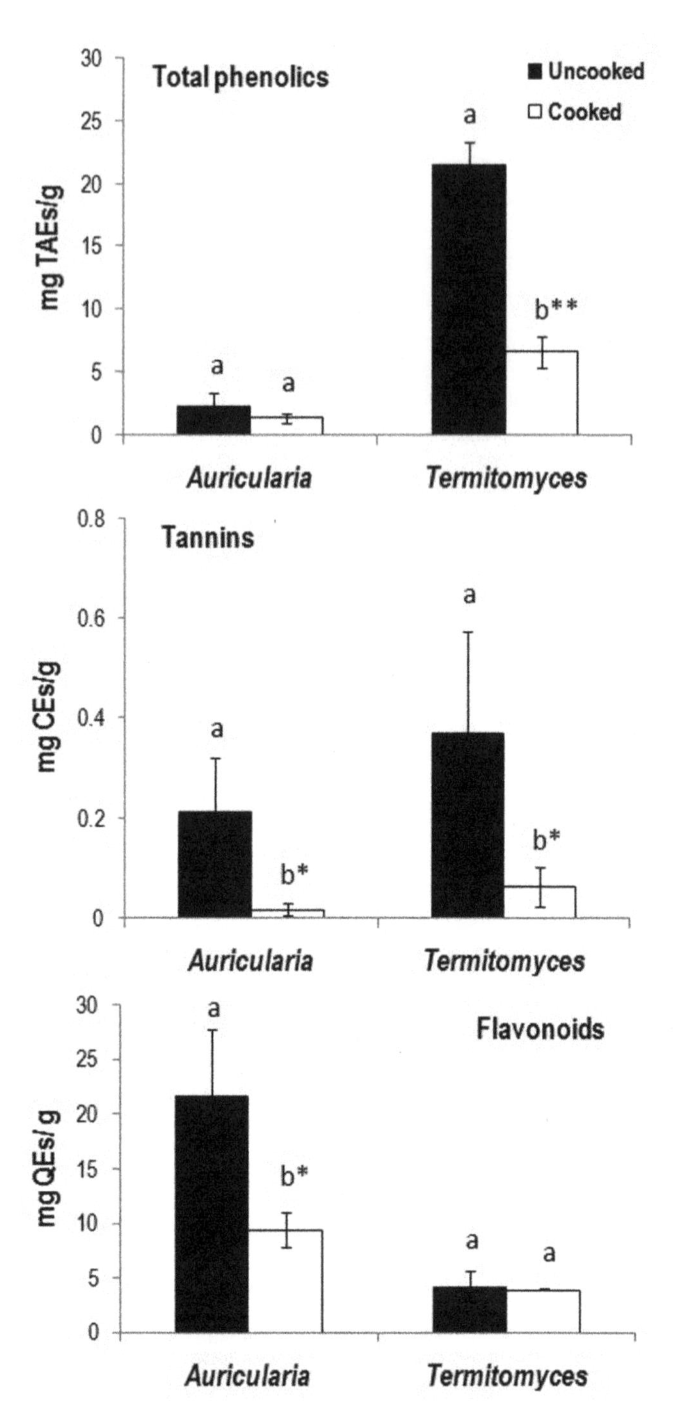

■ **FIGURE 17.3** Total phenolics (TAEs, tannic acid equivalents), tannins (CEs, catechin equivalents) and flavonoids (QEs, quercetin equivalents) in uncooked and cooked *Auricularia auricula* and *Termitomyces umkowaan* ($n = 5$, mean±SD) (different letters on the bars represent significant difference: *, $P < 0.05$; **, $P < 0.01$; t-test).

with significant decrease up to 50% on cooking, while cooking has no significant change in the latter (Fig. 17.3). The flavonoids in uncooked *A. auricula* of Nigeria is extremely low compared to the uncooked as well as cooked *A. auricula* in the present study (6.4 vs 9.4–21.6 mg/g) (Unekwa et al., 2014). Flavonoids of uncooked *T. umkowaan* is higher than other termitomycetes (*T. badius*, *T. heimii*, *T. medius*, *T. mammiformis*, *T. microcarpus*, *T. radicatus*, and *T. striatus*) (4–4.1 vs 1.4–2 mg/g) (Kumari, 2012). Flavonoids were as high as 23.9 and 25.7 mg/g in termitomycetes in Nigeria (*T. robustus* and *T. mammiformis*) (Unekwa et al., 2014).

Natural products rich in total phenolics have the capacity to decrease the incidence of atherosclerosis, cancer, and coronary heart diseases (Randhir et al., 2004; Alothman et al., 2009). In the present study, uncooked *T. umkowaan* consists of high quantities of total phenolics, tannins, and flavonoids, so also the flavonoids in uncooked *A. auricula*. Decrease in phenolics and tannins in these mushrooms on cooking can be attributed to leaching as well as formation of complexes with proteins on pressure cooking. The results on total phenolics clearly reveal such a change occurred only in *T. umkowaan* than in *A. auricula* possibly due to higher quantity of total proteins (18.9–21.5% vs 6.1–6.4%) (Karun, 2014). In uncooked *A. auricula*, total phenolics was low and its quantity did not significantly varied on cooking may be due to low protein content (6.1–6.4%) (Karun, 2014). Unlike total phenolics, cooking resulted in significant drastic decrease in tannins of both mushrooms.

Although vitamin C serves as a potent antioxidant, pro-oxidant, and radical scavenger, its loss takes place due to thermal treatment of foodstuffs (Podmore et al., 1998; Gregory, 1996). Vitamin C was higher in *A. auricula* than in *T. umkowaan* without significant change on cooking (Fig. 17.4). The vitamin C content in uncooked *T. umkowaan* was lower than other termitomycetes (*T. heimii*, *T. mammiformis*, *T. radicatus*, and *T. reticulatus*) (0.12 vs 0.24–1.45 mg/g). Interestingly, even though pressure cooking drastically reduced the vitamin C content in *T. umkowaan*, it was not significantly decreased in *A. auricula* as seen in total phenolics.

The L-DOPA is biologically inactive nonprotein amino acid useful in treatment of Parkinson's disease (Hornykiewicz, 2002). Its content was substantially higher in *T. umkowaan* compared to *A. auricula* and decreased substantially in both mushrooms on cooking (Fig. 17.4).

According to Acharya et al. (2004), *A. auricula* has very high potential of inhibition of lipid peroxidation as well as hydroxyl radical-scavenging ability. In *A. auricula* of Nigeria, the total phenolics, tannins, and flavonoids were high (116, 66.9, and 6.4 mg/g, respectively), but the

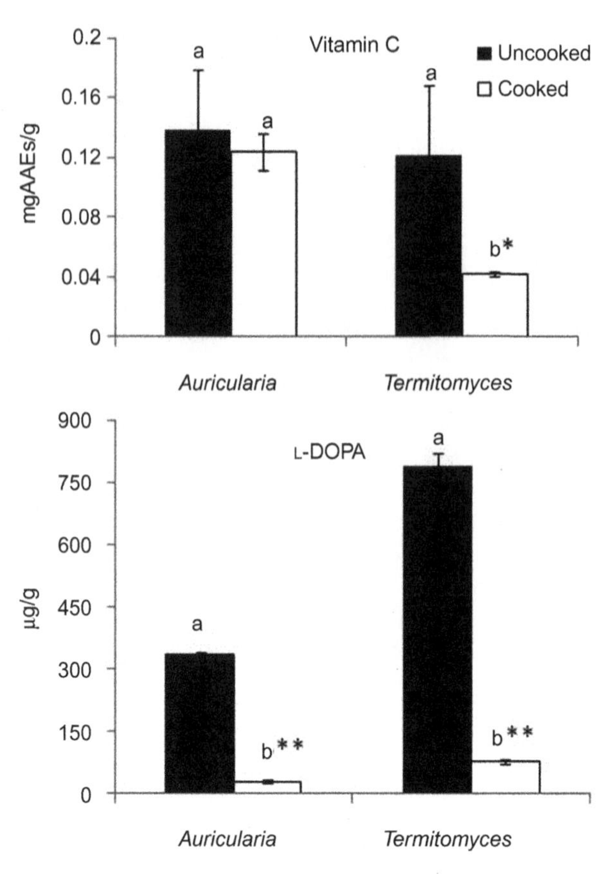

■ **FIGURE 17.4** Vitamin C (AAEs, ascorbic acid equivalents) and L-DOPA in uncooked and cooked *Auricularia auricula* and *Termitomyces umkowaan* ($n = 5$, mean$\pm$SD) (different letters on the bars represent significant difference: *, $P < 0.05$; **, $P < 0.001$; *t*-test).

antioxidant activity was not much elevated (Unekwa et al., 2014). Purified water-soluble polysaccharide obtained from *A. auricula* showed potent antioxidant activity *in vivo* in mice model and in turn serve as valuable agent for antiaging therapy (Zhang et al., 2011). Similarly, water-soluble β-D-glucan isolated from *A. auricula* serve as potent antitumor agent by inducing apoptosis against Sarcoma-180 solid tumor based on *in vitro* and *in vivo* antitumor assays (Ma et al., 2010). The mycelial methanol extract of *T. albuminosus* showed high antioxidant activity, reducing power, and radical-scavenging potential (Mau et al., 2004). Evaluation of 23 species of indigenous species of mushrooms (encompassing five species from the Western Ghat forests of Kerala, India) showed good nutraceutical properties (Puttaraju et al., 2006). In particular, *Termitomyces heimii* and *T. mammiformis* showed maximum antioxidant potential encompassing

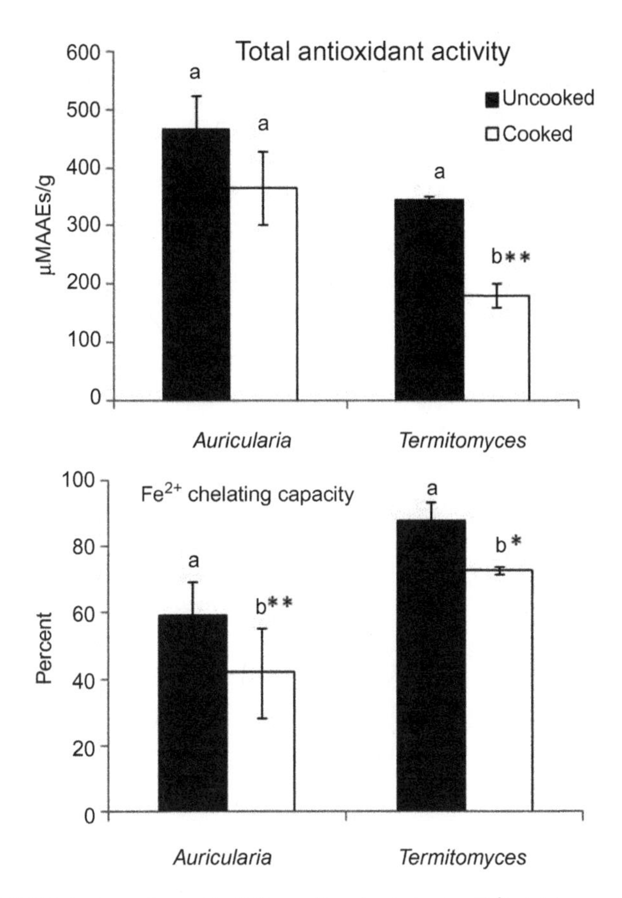

■ **FIGURE 17.5** Total antioxidant activity (AAEs, ascorbic acid equivalents) and Fe^{2+} chelating capacity (600 μg/mL) in uncooked and cooked *Auricularia auricula* and *Termitomyces umkowaan* ($n = 5$, mean±SD) (different letters on the bars represent significant difference: *, $P < 0.05$; **, $P < 0.01$; *t*-test).

high content of active principles like tannic, gallic, protocatacheuic, and gentisic acids.

The TAA was higher in *A. auricula* than in *T. umkowaan* without significant decrease on cooking, while it decreased significantly about 50% in cooked *T. umkowaan* (Fig. 17.5). It is likely the polysaccharides of *A. auricula* might be responsible for higher TAA in uncooked as well as cooked samples as reported by Zhang et al. (2011). Metal-ion chelating capacity becomes important because such ions cause lipid peroxidation leading to food deterioration and in turn causing arthritis and cancer (Gordon, 1990; Halliwell et al., 1995). In this study, ferric-ion chelating activity was higher in *T. umkowaan* than in *A. auricula* with significant decrease on cooking (Fig. 17.5). The DPPH radical-scavenging assay helps to evaluate the capacity of bioactive components in mushrooms to serve as radical scavengers especially the hydrogen donors. Radical-scavenging activity was higher in *A. auricula* than in *T. umkowaan* with significant decrease on cooking only in *A. auricula*. The reducing power was also higher in uncooked than in cooked mushrooms, which significantly decreased on cooking (Fig. 17.6). The reducing power of uncooked *A. auricula* was higher than the report by Abdullah et al. (2012) (1 mg/mL, absorbance at 700 nm: 0.207 vs 0.110) (Fig. 17.6).

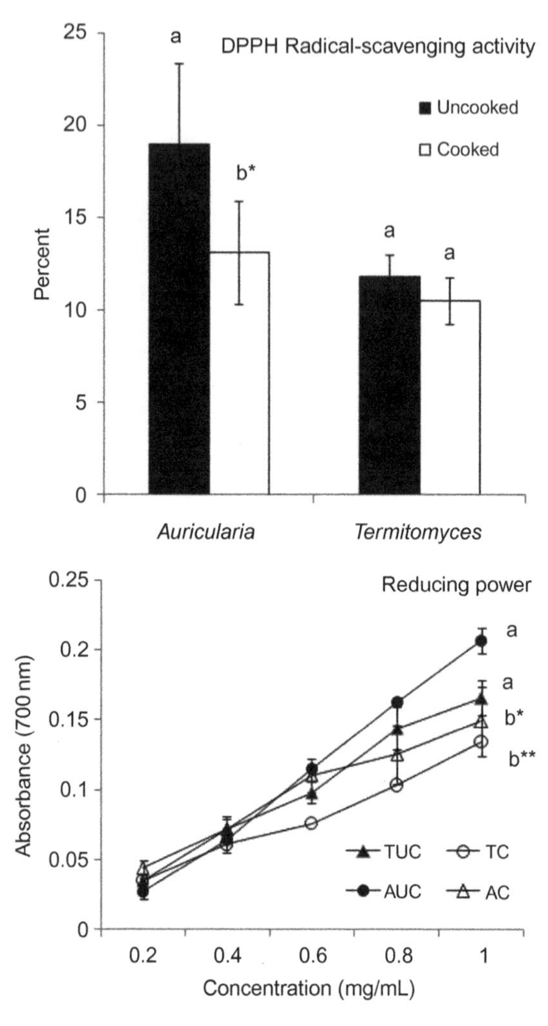

FIGURE 17.6 The DPPH radical-scavenging activity (1 mg/mL) and reducing power in uncooked and cooked *Auricularia auricula* and *Termitomyces umkowaan* ($n = 5$, mean±SD) (different letters on the bars or lines represent significant difference: *, $P < 0.05$; **, $P < 0.01$ (*t*-test).

In spite of low total phenolics and tannins, uncooked as well as cooked *A. auricula* showed higher TAA, DPPH radical-scavenging capacity and reducing power than *T. umkowaan*. It is likely the quantities of flavonoids, vitamin C, and L-DOPA in *A. auricula* could be responsible for such results. Similarly, high quantities of total phenolics, tannins, vitamin C, and L-DOPA especially in uncooked *T. umkowaan* might be responsible for good TAA as well as ferrous ion chelating capacity. Interestingly, total phenolics, tannins, flavonoids, vitamin C, and L-DOPA contents were lower in cooked than in uncooked *T. umkowaan*, but ferric-ion chelating capacity as well as the DPPH radical-scavenging activity were considerably high in cooked samples denotes the possibilities of involvement of other bioactive principles not affected by pressure cooking.

Uncooked and cooked samples of both mushrooms did not show trypsin inhibition activity (Table 17.1), which is nutritionally advantageous. In addition, the hemagglutination activity was substantially low (4–16 Hu/g) in both mushrooms (Table 17.1) qualify them as better source of nutrition than those mushrooms possessing high hemagglutination activity. There was no change in hemagglutination of blood group A+ve in uncooked and cooked mushrooms (16 Hu/g), so also in *A. auricula* and *T. umkowaan* against AB+ve and B+ve blood groups (8 Hu/g), respectively. Decrease in hemagglutination was seen between uncooked and cooked *A. auricula* against O+ve (8 vs 4 Hu/g), *T. umkowaan* against AB+ve (16 vs 8 Hu/g) and O+ve (16 vs 4 Hu/g) blood groups. However, *A. auricula* showed increased hemagglutination activity on cooking against B+ve blood group (8 vs 16 Hu/g).

Table 17.1 Trypsin Inhibition and Hemagglutinin Activity of Uncooked and Cooked Mushrooms (Based on Three Independent Observations)

	Auricularia auricula-judae		***Termitomyces umkowaan***	
	Uncooked	**Cooked**	**Uncooked**	**Cooked**
Trypsin Inhibition Activity				
	NP	NP	NP	NP
Hemagglutinin Activity (Hu/g)				
A+ve	16	16	16	16
B+ve	8	16	8	8
AB+ve	8	8	16	8
O+ve	8	4	16	4

NP, not present.

CONCLUSION

Now-a-days dyslipidemia is responsible for antioxidant stress and atherosclerosis, which can be combated using functional diet developed by blending polysaccharide derived from *A. auricula* with processed Hawthorn fruits (*Crataegus*) (4:1%) (Luo et al., 2009). It showed increased radical scavenging, inhibition of low density lipoprotein-cholesterol oxidation, lowered serum total cholesterol, and low atherogenic index. Besides, such functional formulations showed several additional pharmaceutical advantages (Luo et al., 2011). Microwave-assisted extraction of polysaccharides from *A. auricula* (showed no influence on their structure and molecular weight) possesses remarkable *in vitro* antioxidant activity and generally regarded as safe (GRAS) to use in food products based on toxicological evaluation (Zeng et al., 2012).

The products derived from uncooked *A. auricula* and *T. umkowaan* will be more beneficial than cooked ones. Besides, the nutritional qualities (eg, proximal features and minerals) will be reduced in pressure-cooked mushrooms (Karun, 2014). Other than medicinal uses, there are several innovative applications of wild mushrooms for health benefits especially in formulation of functional foods. For example, blending polysaccharide flour derived from *A. auricula* at 9% with bread did not alter the nutritional and sensory qualities, which resulted in marked increase in antioxidant property (DPPH radical scavenging) (Fan et al., 2007). Thus, alternate methods of cooking (eg, partial conventional/microwave cooking) should be applied to retain maximum quantity of bioactive compounds as well as nutritional qualities to derive maximum multifunctional nutraceutical benefits from these traditional wild mushrooms. Further, it is necessary to test the relevance of these mushrooms as antioxidant agents *in vivo* with appropriate markers. In addition to bioactive components evaluated in the present study, the antioxidant potential of *A. auricula* and *T. umkowaan* might have been influenced by other potential components like stilbenes, lignans, phytates, amino acids, peptides, vitamin E, carotinoids, specific fatty acids and specific minerals needs further precise investigation.

ABBREVIATIONS

AAEs ascorbic acid equivalents
asl above sea level
BAPNA N-a-Benzoyl-DL-Arginine p-nitroanilide hydrochloride
BHA butylated hydroxyanisole
BHT butylated hydroxytoluene
CEs catechin equivalents
DNPH dinitrophenylhydrazine

DPPH	dihydroxyphenylalanine
Fe	iron
$FeCl_2$	ferrous chloride
GRAS	generally regarded as safe
HCl	hydrochloric acid
HPLC	high performance liquid chromatography
Hu	hemagglutinating unit
LC-ESI/MS	liquid chromatography-electrospray ionization-tandem mass spectrometry
L-DOPA	L-dihydroxyphenylalanine
Mo	molybdenum
Na_2CO_3	sodium carbonate
NaCl	sodium chloride
NaOH	sodium hydroxide
ODS	octadecyl-bonded silica
QEs	quercetin equivalents
RBC	red blood corpuscles
TAA	total antioxidant activity
TAEs	tannic acid equivalents
TBHQ	tertiary butyl hydroquinone
TCA	trichloroacetic acid
TIu	trypsin inhibition units
UV-VIS	ultraviolet visible

ACKNOWLEDGMENTS

Authors are grateful to Mangalore University for permission to carry out this study in the Department of Biosciences. NCK acknowledges Mangalore University for partial fellowship under the Promotion of University Research and Scientific Excellence (PURSE), Department of Science Technology, New Delhi. KRS is grateful to University Grants Commission, New Delhi, for the award of UGC-BSR Faculty Fellowship. SDG acknowledges the award of an INSPIRE Fellowship by the Department of Science and Technology, New Delhi (Award # IF130237).

REFERENCES

Abdullah, N., Ismail, S.M., Aminudin, N., Shuib, A.S., Lau, B.F., 2012. Evaluation of selected culinary-medicinal mushrooms for antioxidant and ACE inhibitory activities. Evid. Based Complement Alternat. Med. Article ID # 464238, 1–12: http://dx.doi.org/10.1155/2012/464238.

Abraham, W.R., 2001. Bioactive sesquiterpenes produced by fungi: are they useful for humans as well? Curr. Med. Chem. 8, 583–606.

Acharya, K., Samul, K., Rai, M., Dutta, B.B., Acharya, R., 2004. Antioxidant and nitric oxide synthase activation properties of *Auricularia auricula*. Indian J. Exp. Biol. 42, 538–540.

Alothman, M., Bhat, R., Karim, A.A., 2009. Effects of radiation processing on phytochemicals and antioxidants in plant produce. Trends Food Sci. Technol. 20, 201–212.

Aly, A.H., Debbab, A., Proksch, P., 2011. Fifty years of drug discovery from fungi—review. Fungal Divers. 50, 3–19.

Bao, X., Duan, J., Fang, X., Fang, J., 2001. Chemical modifications of the (1→3)-α-D-glucan from spores of *Ganoderma lucidum* and investigation of their physicochemical properties and immunological activity. Carbohydr. Res. 336, 127–140.

Barros, L., Correia, D.M., Ferreira, I.C.F.R., Baptista, P., Santos-Buelga, C., 2008. Optimization of the determination of tocopherols in *Agaricus* sp. edible mushrooms by a normal phase liquid chromotographic method. Food. Chem. 110, 1046–1050.

Botterweck, A.A.M., Verhagen, H., Goldbohm, R.A., Kelinjans, J., Brandt, P.A.V.D., 2000. Intake of butylated hydroxyanisole and butylatedhydroxytoluene and stomach cancer risk: results from analyses in the Netherlands cohort study. Food Chem. Toxicol. 38, 599–605.

Burns, R., 1971. Methods for estimation of tannins in grain sorghum. Agron. J. 63, 511–512.

Champ, M.M., 2002. Non nutrient bioactive substances of pulses. Br. J. Nutr. 88, 307–319.

Chang, C., Yang, M., Wen, H., Chern, J., 2002. Estimation of total flavonoid content in propolis by two complementary colorimetric methods. J. Food Drug Anal. 10, 178–182.

De Silva, D.D., Rapior, S., Sudarman, E., Stadler, M., Xu, J., Alias, S.A., et al., 2013. Bioactive metabolites from macrofungi: ethnopharmacology, biological activities and chemistry. Fungal Divers. 62, 1–40.

Fan, L., Zhang, S., Yu, L., Ma, L., 2007. Evaluation of antioxidant property and quality of breads containing *Auricularia auricula* polysaccharide flour. Food. Chem. 101, 1158–1163.

Farook, V.A., Khan, S.S., Manimohan, P., 2013. A checklist of agarics (gilled mushrooms) of Kerala state, India. Mycosphere 4, 97–131.

Fujii, Y., Shibuya, T., Yasuda, T., 1991. L 3,4-dihydroxyphenylalanine as an allelochemical from *Mucuna pruriens* (L.) DC. var. *utilis*. Agric. Biol. Chem. 55, 617–618.

Gordon, M.H., 1990. The mechanism of antioxidant action *in vitro*. In: Hudson, B.J.F. (Ed.), "Food Antioxidants" Elsevier Applied Science, London, pp. 1–18.

Gregory, J.F., 1996. Vitamins. In: Fennema, O.R. (Ed.), "Food Chemistry", third ed. Dekker, New York, pp. 531–616.

Gursoy, N., Sarikurkcu, C., Cengiz, M., Solak, M.H., 2009. Antioxidant activities, metal contents, total phenolics and flavonoids of seven *Morchella* species. Food Chem. Toxicol. 47, 2381–2388.

Halliwell, B., Murcia, H.A., Chico, S., Aruoma, O.I., 1995. Free radicals and antioxidants in food an *in vivo*: what they do and how they work. CRC Crit. Rev. Food Sci. Nutr. 35, 7–20.

Hornykiewicz, O., 2002. L-DOPA: from a biologically inactive amino acid to a successful therapeutic agent. Amino. Acids. 23, 65–70.

Hsu, C.L., Chen, W., Weng, Y.M., Tseng, C.Y., 2003. Chemical composition, physical properties and antioxidant activities of yam flours as affected by different drying methods. Food. Chem. 83, 85–92.

Jeong, J.W., Jin, C.Y., Park, C., Hong, S.H., Kim, G.Y., Jeong, Y.K., et al., 2011. Induction of apoptosis by cordycepin via reactive oxygen species generation in human leukemia cells. Toxicol. In Vitro 25, 817–824.

Kakade, M.L., Rackis, J.J., McGhee, J.E., Puski, G., 1974. Determination of trypsin inhibitor activity of soy products, a collaborative analysis of an improved procedure. Cereal Chem. 51, 376–382.

Kalač, P., 2009. Chemical composition and nutritional value of European species of wild growing mushrooms: a review. Food. Chem. 113, 9–16.

Karun, N.C., 2014. Studies on Macrofungi and Aquatic Hyphomycets of the Western Ghats and West Coast of India. Mangalore University, Mangalore, India, PhD Thesis.

Kumari, B., 2012. Diversity, Sociobiology and Conservation of Lepiotoid and Termitophilous Mushrooms of North West India. Punjabi University, Patiala, India, PhD Thesis.

Luo, Y., Chen, G., Li, B., Ji, B., Guo, Y., Tian, F., 2009. Evaluation of antioxidative and hypolipidemic properties of a novel functional diet formulation of *Auricularia auricula* and Hawthorn. Innov. Food Sci. Emerg. Technol. 10, 215–221.

Luo, Y., Xiao, Z., Wang, Q., Li, B., Ji, B., 2011. Antioxidant activities and inhibitory effects of *Auricularia auricula* and its functional formula diet against vascular smooth muscle cell *in vitro*. Food Nutr. Sci. 2, 265–271.

Ma, Z., Wang, J., Zhang, L., Zhang, Y., Ding, K., 2010. Evaluation of water soluble β-D-glucan from *Auricularia auricula-judae* as potential anti-tumor agent. Carbohydr. Polym. 80, 877–983.

Mau, J.-L., Chang, C.-N., Huang, S.-J., Chen, C.-C., 2004. Antioxidant properties of methanolic extracts from *Grifola frondosa, Morchella esculenta* and *Termitomyces albuminosus* mycelia. Food. Chem. 87, 111–118.

Mohanan, C., 2011. "Macrofungi of Kerala" Handbook # 27. Kerala Forest Research Institute, Peechi, India.

Occenã, I.V., Majica, E.-R.E., Merca, F.E., 2007. Isolation of partial characterization of a lectin from the seeds of *Artocarpus camansi* Blanco. Asian J. Plant Sci. 6, 757–764.

Podmore, I.D., Griffiths, H.R., Herbert, K.E., Mistry, N., Mistry, P., Lunec, J., 1998. Vitamin C exhibits pro-oxidant properties. Nature 392, 559–560.

Prieto, P., Pineda, M., Aguilar, M., 1999. Spectrophotometric quantitation of antioxidant capacity through the formation of a phosphomolybdenum complex: specific application to the determination of vitamin E. Anal. Biochem. 269, 337–341.

Pulido, R., Bravo, L., Saura-Calixto, F., 2000. Antioxidant activity of dietary polyphenols as determined by a modified ferric reducing/antioxidant power assay. J. Agric. Food Chem. 48, 3396–3402.

Puttaraju, N.G., Venkateshaiah, S.U., Dharmesh, S.M., Urs, S.M., Somasundaram, R., 2006. Antioxidant activity of indigenous edible mushrooms. J. Agric. Food. Chem. 54, 9764–9772.

Randhir, R., Lin, Y.T., Shetty, K., 2004. Stimulation of phenolics, antioxidant and antimicrobial activities in dark germinated mung bean sprouts in response to peptide and phytochemical elicitors. Proc. Biochem. 39, 637–646.

Roe, J.H., 1954. Chemical determination of ascorbic, dehydroascorbic and diketogluconic acids In: Glick, D. (Ed.), "Methods of Biochemical Analysis", Vol. 1 InterScience Publishers, New York, pp. 115–139.

Rosset, J., Bärlocher, F., Oertli, J.J., 1982. Decomposition of conifer needles and deciduous leaves in two Black Forest and two Swiss Jura streams. Int. Rev. Gesamten Hydrobiol. 67, 695–711.

Singh, R.P., Murthy, C.K.N., Jayaprakasha, G.K., 2002. Studies on antioxidant activity of pomegranate (*Punica granatum*) peel and seed extracts using *in vitro* methods. J. Agric. Food. Chem. 50, 81–86.

StatSoft, 2008. "Statistica" Version # 8. StatSoft Inc., Oklahoma, USA.

Tapas, A.R., Sakarkar, D.M., Kakde, R.B., 2008. Flavonoids as nutraceuticals: a review. Trop. J. Pharm. Res. 7, 1089–1099.

Thatoi, H., Singdevsachan, S.K., 2014. Diversity, nutritional composition and medicinal potential of Indian mushrooms: a review. Afr. J. Biotechnol. 13, 523–545.

Unekwa, H.R., Audu, J.A., Makun, M.H., Chidi, E.E., 2014. Phytochemical screening and antioxidant activity of methonolic extract of selected wild edible mushrooms. Asian J. Trop. Dis. 4, S153–S157.

Wasser, S.P., 2011. Current findings, future trends, and unsolved problems in studies of medicinal mushrooms. Appl. Microbiol. Biotechnol. 89, 1323–1332.

Wong, S.P., Leong, L.P., Koh, J.H.W., 2006. Antioxidant activities of aqueous extracts of selected plants. Food. Chem. 99, 775–783.

Xu, X., Wu, Y., Chen, H., 2011. Comparative antioxidative characteristics of polysaccharide-enriched extracts from natural sclerotia and cultured mycelia in submerged fermentation of *Inonotus obliquus*. Food. Chem. 127, 74–79.

Ying, J., Mao, X., Ma, Q., Zong, Y., Wen, H., 1987. "Icones of medicinal fungi from china". Science Press, Beijing, Translated (X. Yuehan).

Zeng, W.-C., Zhang, Z., Gao, H., Jia, L.-R., Chen, W.-Y., 2012. Characterization of antioxidant polysaccharides from *Auricularia auricula* using microwave-assisted extraction. Carbohydr. Polym. 89, 694–700.

Zhang, H., Wang, Z.-Y., Zhang, Z., Wang, X., 2011. Purified *Auricularia auricula-judae* polysaccharide (AAP I-a) prevents oxidative stress in an ageing mouse model. Carbohydr. Polym. 84, 638–648.

Zhang, M., Cui, S.W., Cheung, P.C.K., Wang, Q., 2007. Anti-tumor polysaccharides from mushrooms: a review on their isolation, structural characteristics and antitumor activity. Trends Food Sci. Technol. 18, 4–19.

Section 4

Herbs in Health and Diseases

Chapter 18

Nutrient profile, bioactive components, and functional properties of okra (*Abelmoschus esculentus* (L.) Moench)

Sa'eed Halilu Bawa[1,2] and Neela Badrie[1]

[1]*The University of the West Indies, St. Augustine, Trinidad and Tobago, West Indies*

[2]*Warsaw University of Life Sciences, Warsaw, Poland*

CHAPTER OUTLINE

Fruits, Vegetables, and Herbs.
DOI: http://dx.doi.org/10.1016/B978-0-12-802972-5.00018-4

MANY NAMES

The okra plant, *Abelmoschus esculentus* (L.) Moench (syn, *Hibiscus esculentus* L.), is a flowering plant which belongs to the Malvaceae or mallow family having chromosome number ($2n$) = 130 (Ndunguru and Rajabu, 2004). It is an important vegetable crop widely grown in the tropical and subtropical regions of the world (Tindall, 1983). It is a perennial native plant from Africa which is now grown in many parts of the world (Lamont, 1999), such as Thailand, the Middle East, the Caribbean, and the Southern States of the United States. The term okra has been used in English by the late 18th century (Arapitsas, 2008). In its origin of Ethiopia, it is also called Kenkase (Berta), Andeha (Gumuz), and Bamia (Oromica/Amharic). The name okra was probably derived from one of Niger-Congo group of languages (the name for okra in the Twi language is nkuruma) (Benjawan et al., 2007). In Portugal and Angola, okra is known as "quiabo," Cuba as "quimbombo," Japan as "okura" (Kaur et al., 2013), and in Bosnia and most of West Asia, it is also known as "bamia" or "bamya." Table 18.1 shows the many names of okra in various languages.

Its scientific classification (Jain, 2012) is as follows:

Biological name: *Hibiscus esculentus*, *Abelmoschus esculentus*.

Scientific classification:

Kingdom: Plantae
Division: Magnoliophyta
Class: Magnoliopsida
(Unranked): Rosids
Order: Malvales
Genus: Abelmoschus
Species: *A. esculentus*
Binomial name: *Abelmoschus esculentus*

Table 18.1 Common and Vernacular Names of Okra

English	Portuguese	Spanish	Indian
bamia	gombô	ají turco	bindi
bandakai	gombó	algalia	bhendi
common okra	guibeiro	bombey	bhindi
gobbo	quigombô	candia	bhindiin
gombo	quigombó	candiá	
guino-gombo	quiabo	chaucha turca	
gumbo		chicombó	
lady's fingers		chimbombo	
ochro		gombo	
ocoro		guicombo	
ocro		guingambó	
okra		guino-gombo	
okro		lagarto	
okro		molondrón	
		naju	
		ñajú	
		ñangú	
		quiabo	
		quimbombó	
		quimgombó	
		quingombó	
		ruibarbo	

Ndunguru and Rajabu (2004), Jain (2012), Rattray (2001), Sahoo and Srivastava (2002), Mateus (2011), Sorapong (2012), Kermath et al. (2014).

AGRONOMY

For 2012, the world production of okra as fresh fruit vegetable was estimated to be at 9.5 million tonnes/year and for okra seeds at 65 tonnes/year (FAOSTAT, 2012). In 2006, the five highest okra producing countries were India, Nigeria, Sudan, Iraq, and Côte d'Ivoire (FAOSTAT, 2012). The okra fruits can be classified based on the shape, angular or circular (Mota et al., 2000). Depending on the cultivar, fruits of okra mature after 60–180 days of sowing (alternatively can also be counted 5–10 days after flowering of plant). Fruits are detached from the stacks by applying slight twist (Tindall, 1983). Irritating hairs are sometimes present on leaves, stems, and on the fruit surface.

Okra as a tropical to subtropical crop is sensitive to frost, low temperature, water logging, and drought conditions, and the cultivation practices have varied in different countries (Mota et al., 2000). The effect of presowing magnetic treatments (99 mT for 11 minutes exposure) on okra seeds showed a significant increase ($P < 0.05$) in the germination percentage, number of flowers per plant, leaf area (cm^2), plant height (cm) at maturity, number of fruits per plant pod mass per plant, and number of seeds per plant (Naz et al., 2012). Calisir et al. (2005) found that the physical properties of mature Turkish okra seeds increased as the moisture content levels increased (6.35%, 9.87%, and 15.22% dry basis). With the increase in the moisture content, the seed length, width, thickness, mass, and geometric diameter increased from 5.178 to 5.507 mm, 4.786 to 4.960 mm, 4.121 to 4.362 mm, 0.059 to 0.067 g, and 4.665 to 4.913 mm, respectively. A narrower intrarow plant spacing of 30 cm was found to significantly increase the plant height and produced weaker plants while a wider plant spacing of 90 cm significantly increased the plant weight, number of branches and leaves (Madisa et al., 2015).

Akanbi et al. (2010) suggested that inorganic fertilizers could improve okra crop yields and soil pH, total nutrient content, and nutrient availability, but their use is limited due to scarcity, high cost, nutrient imbalance and soil acidity. Farm yard manure has been applied at 25 tonnes/ha was found to be a suitable treatment for growth, yield, and economic returns for cultivation of okra under the agroclimatic condition of Allahabad, India (Amran et al., 2013). In a greenhouse experiment, the relative effect of organic and inorganic fertilizers on okra plant, the application of poultry droppings gave plants with the greatest plant height, leaf area, and fresh weight, while cow dung application gave the greatest dry weight (Uka et al., 2013). Organic fertilizers were better than the NPK mineral fertilizer. The treatment with poultry droppings was found to be the best, and the treatment with cow dung was better than the NPK treatment. Hence, the use of organic manure in the production of vegetables like okra should be encouraged (Uka et al., 2013). However, in another study, the growth of okra was not significantly affected by poultry manure but had a significant effect on the yield and yield components of okra (Ogundiran, 2013). It was found that liquid seaweed fertilizer extract, applied as a foliar spray to okra showed a significant increase per net plot in fruit field (20.47%), besides significant increase in length (31.77%), and diameter (18.26%) of fruit and number of fruits (37.47%) per net plot (Zodape et al., 2008). In Guyana, the combined application of organic fertilizers, vermicompost and vermiwash, and chemical fertilizers had greater influence on okra plant growth parameters compared with control, with as an average yield of okra of 64.27% during trial compared to the control (Ansari and Sukhraj, 2010).

Also, the fruits were found to have a greater percentage of fats and protein content when compared with those grown with chemical fertilizers by 23.86% and 19.86%, respectively.

The foliar application of gibberellic GA_3 (25 and 50 ppm) and $FeSO_4$ (0.5%) at 60 days after sowing indicated significantly higher fresh okra fruit yield over other treatments. This increase in okra yield was attributed to the increase in total number of flowers, fruits per plant, fruit length, seed number per fruit, seed weight, and harvest index (Surendra et al., 2006). Also, foliar applied glycine betaine and sugar beet extract improved the growth and yield of salt-stressed okra plants (Habib et al., 2012).

NUTRIENT PROFILE AND BIOACTIVE COMPONENTS OF OKRA AND THEIR HEALTH EFFECTS

As can be noticed in Table 18.2, okra contains many vital nutrients. These nutrients may confer a number of health advantages, including a decreased risk for the development of chronic noncommunicable diseases, such as obesity, hypertension, hypercholesterolemia, coronary heart diseases, and gastrointestinal (GI) disorders.

Table 18.2 Nutrient Content of Okra (100 g, raw)

Nutrient	Amount	%DV
Energy (kcal)	31	2
Total fat (g)	0.1 (0)	
Carbohydrate (g)	7	2
Fiber (g)	3.2	13
Protein (g)	2	4
Sugar (g)	1.2	
Calcium (mg)	81	8
Manganese (mg)	1	50
Magnesium (mg)	57	14
Potassium (mg)	303	9
Sodium (mg)	8	0
Vitamin C (mg)	21.1	35
Thiamin (mg)	0.2	13
Vitamin B6 (mg)	0.2	11
Folate (mcg)	88	22
Vitamin A (IU)	375	7
Vitamin K (mcg)	53	66
Vitamin E (α tocopherol) (mg)	0.4	2

USDA SR-21 Nutrient Database (2015).

Dietary fiber

Dietary fiber is one of the most important bioactive components present in vegetables, including okra. A 100-g serving of sliced, raw okra provides more than 3 g of dietary fiber. This amount supplies approximately 13% of the U.S. Department of Agriculture (USDA) recommended daily allowance of fiber for healthy adult men and women consuming a 2000-calorie diet.

Okra contains both soluble and insoluble fibers. Dietary fiber provides a multitude of health benefits and has been recommended by the Institute of Medicine (IOM) and the American Heart Association (AHA) as an essential component of a healthy diet (King et al., 2012). The USDA and other national health agencies as well as WHO recognize the health benefits of fiber and provide guidelines based on factors such as sex, age, and energy intake for daily fiber intake (Chucktan et al., 2012). Table 18.3 shows the recommended daily intake of dietary fiber for both genders and various age groups.

Fiber-rich diets and/or foods, such as okra, are usually characterized by lower energy density due to lower content of fat and added sugar. High-fiber foods provide bulk, are more satiating, and have been linked to lower body weights or decreased weight gain (ADA, 2008).

Howarth et al. (2001) estimated that increasing fiber intake by 14 g/day was associated with a 10% decrease in energy intake and a 2-kg weight loss over about a 4-month period. The observed changes in energy intake and body weight occurred without regard to the fiber's source as a naturally high-fiber food or a functional fiber supplement.

Table 18.3 Adequate Dietary Fiber Intake by Gender and Age

Sex	Age (years)	Fiber Intake (Total Fiber, g/day)
Women	19–30	25
	31–50	25
	51–70	21
	>70	21
Men	19–30	38
	31–50	38
	51–70	30
	>70	30

IOM (Institute of Medicine, 2005a).

There are multiple mechanisms, whereby fiber-rich foods, such as okra, exert and impact on satiation and satiety (Slavin and Green, 2007). Greater satiation may be a product of the increased time required to chew certain fiber-rich foods. Increased time chewing promotes saliva and gastric acid production, which requires energy and may increase gastric distention. Some soluble or viscous types of dietary fiber bind water, which also may increase distention. Stomach distension is believed to trigger afferent vagal signals of fullness, which likely contributes to satiation during meals and satiety in the postmeal period.

Furthermore, certain types of dietary fiber may slow gastric emptying and decrease the rate of glucose absorption in the small intestine. When glucose is released slowly, the insulin response may also be blunted. Slow, steady postprandial glucose and insulin responses are sometimes correlated with satiation and satiety.

In addition, as food moves through the upper and lower GI tract, various satiety-related hormones are released and signals are sent to the brain. Many of these gut hormones (ie, ghrelin, polypeptide YY, glucagon-like peptide) are thought to regulate satiety, food intake, and overall energy balance (Chaudhri and Salem, 2008).

Studies have found that okra, when provided as part of meal, possesses hypocholestorelemic properties. The Portfolio diet, designed to lower LDL (low-density lipoprotein), consisted of foods high in soluble or viscous fiber, soy protein, plant sterols, and nuts. These foods are known to reduce cholesterol. The study by Jenkins et al. (2003) compared a control diet composed of very low saturated fat, dairy and whole wheat cereal diet; the same diet plus lovastatin 20 mg; and the Portfolio diet. The four major components of the Portfolio diet contained a margarine enriched in plant sterol esters providing 1 g/1000-calorie diet, viscous fibers 10 g/1000-calorie diet from oats, barley and psyllium, okra, and eggplant were included. Soy protein was included in the form of soy burgers, soy dogs, and soy deli slices and 14 g of whole almonds/1000-calorie diet. The three diets were essentially equivalent in energy. Within 4 weeks of the study, weight was maintained in the three groups. The results showed a reduction in LDL in the Portfolio group and the statin group; the latter group had a slight edge, but was not statistically significant. More participants attained their National Cholesterol Education Program goal on the Portfolio diet than on statin group. High-density lipoprotein was not significantly affected.

The short-chained fatty acids (SFCAs), including acetate, propionate, butyrate, and valerate, which are released after the fermentation of soluble or viscous fiber can suppress cholesterol synthesis by the liver and may reduce serum levels of low-density lipoprotein cholesterol (LDL-C) and triglycerides (Anderson et al., 1991). Soluble or viscous fibers are also thought to exert their hypocholesterolemic action by increasing fecal sterol excretion and stimulating hepatic bile acid synthesis (Marlett, 2001; Trautwein et al., 1999). In a meta-analysis of 67 controlled trials, consumption of 2–10 g/day of fiber (ie, pectin, oat bran, guar gum, psyllium) reduced total cholesterol by 4% and LDL-C by 7% compared with placebo (Marlett, 2001). No significant effect was observed on serum high-density lipoprotein cholesterol (HDL-C) and triacylglycerol concentrations.

Butyrate, one of the SCFAs produced as a result of fermentation of soluble dietary fiber or prebiotics, has multiple beneficial effects on human health. At the intestinal level, butyrate plays a regulatory role on the transepithelial fluid transport, ameliorates mucosal inflammation and oxidative status, reinforces the epithelial defense barrier, and modulates visceral sensitivity and intestinal motility. In addition, a growing number of studies have stressed the role of butyrate in the prevention and inhibition of colorectal cancer (CRC). At the extraintestinal level, butyrate exerts potentially useful effects on many conditions, including hemoglobinopathies, genetic metabolic diseases, hypercholesterolemia, insulin resistance, and ischemic stroke. The mechanisms of action of butyrate are different; many of these are related to its potent regulatory effects on gene expression. These data suggest a wide spectrum of positive effects exerted by butyrate, with a high potential for a therapeutic use in human medicine (Sun and Chang, 2014).

Fiber-rich foods, including okra, can help reduce constipation by adding bulk to the stool. Bulky feces move through the gut faster, resulting in an increased stool weight and improved regularity. The increase in fecal bulk also "dilutes" the effect of toxic substances in the colon. Stool consistency, stool weight, and frequency of defecation are indicators of colonic function. Increased bulking and decreased transit time are considered as the most widely known beneficial effects of consuming fiber-rich diets and foods. Different kinds of dietary fiber can have different bulking capacities, depending on the underlying mechanism. The bulking effect of dietary fiber that is poorly fermented in the colon is associated with the mass of fiber itself and enhanced in some cases by water binding, which is maintained throughout the whole GI tract. Fermentable dietary fibers provide a bulking effect mainly due to increased bacterial mass. Dietary components that stimulate fermentation lead to an increase in bacterial mass and consequently fecal mass and, thus have a stool bulking effect. It is estimated that about 30 g of bacteria are produced for every 100 g of carbohydrate that is fermented.

Okra consumption and diabetes mellitus

Traditionally, okra has been used as an alternative treatment for diabetes in many countries including Thailand (Palanuvej et al., 2009). It is assumed that this effect of okra is due to the presence of large amount of soluble dietary fibers which retard glucose absorption from the GI tract. Similar to lowering cholesterol levels, soluble or viscous dietary fiber also decreases the absorption of glucose and can lower the glycemic impact of foods, thereby causing lower rise in blood glucose levels.

Unlike foods comprised of carbohydrates that are rapidly digested and absorbed in the small intestine, foods containing viscous dietary fiber, such as okra, are associated with a much slower rise in serum glucose that does not reach as high a maximum level. Similarly, the decline in serum glucose levels after reaching the peak is less rapid. Reduced postprandial blood glucose levels are considered one of the traditional beneficial physiological effects related to consumption of foods that are rich in viscous dietary fiber.

Palanuvej et al. (2009) showed that the ability of okra fruit to control glycemia is due to its ability to decrease the activity of α-glucosidase. The viscous characteristics of okra, due to its excellent water-holding and gel-forming capabilities, have been proposed as an important mechanistic factor to delay gastric emptying and delay absorption of glucose in GI tract. Many types of dietary fiber lower the glycemic impact of foods, because they substitute for high glycemic flours and sugars in food formulations. Thus, the possible interaction of the soluble dietary fiber fraction of okra with oral metformin is a matter of concern because this vegetable is being widely used by the people with diabetes mellitus as an adjunction to the treatment of this metabolic disorder.

Minerals in okra and their role in the prevention and management of noncommunicable diseases

Calcium, potassium, and magnesium are found in okra, providing about 8%, 9% and 14%, respectively, of the daily value (Table 18.2). Calcium is well known for its function in maintaining bone and teeth health, but is also critical to cell signaling, blood clotting, muscle contraction, and nerve function. Dietary potassium intake has been demonstrated to significantly lower blood pressure (BP) in a dose-responsive manner in both hypertensive and normotensive individuals in observational studies (Ascherio et al., 1992; Van Leer et al., 1995; He et al., 1991), clinical trials (Appel et al., 1997; Appel, 2010; Sacks et al., 2001; Sacks and Campos, 2010), and several meta-analyses (Whelton et al., 1997; Dickinson et al., 2006).

In hypertensive patients, the linear dose–response relationship is a 1.0-mmHg reduction in systolic BP and a 0.52-mmHg reduction in diastolic BP per 0.6 g per day increase in dietary potassium intake that is independent of baseline potassium deficiency (Appel, 2010). The average reduction in BP with 4.7 g (120 mmol) of dietary potassium per day is 8.0/4.1 mmHg, depending on race and on the relative intakes of other minerals such as sodium, magnesium, and calcium. If the dietary sodium chloride intake is high, there is a greater BP reduction with an increased intake of dietary potassium. Blacks have a greater decrease in BP than Caucasians with an equal potassium intake (Appel, 2010).

Potassium-induced reduction in BP significantly lowers the incidence of stroke, being a cerebrovascular accident (CVA), coronary heart disease, myocardial infarction, and other cardiovascular events. However, potassium also reduces the risk of CVA independent of BP reductions. Increasing consumption of potassium to 4.7 g/day predicts lower event rates for future cardiovascular disease (CVD), with estimated decreases of 8–15% in CVA and 6–11% in myocardial infarction (World Health Organization, 2012; Aburto et al., 2013).

Mechanisms by which potassium lowers BP

The metabolism of sodium and potassium plays a significant role in endothelium-dependent vasodilatation (Fujiwara et al., 2000). Sodium retention decreases the synthesis of nitric oxide, an arteriolar vasodilator elaborated by endothelial cells, and increases the plasma level of asymmetric dimethyl L-arginine, an endogenous inhibitor of nitric oxide production (Fujiwara et al., 2000). Sodium restriction induces the opposite effects.

A diet rich in potassium and increase in serum potassium (even within the physiologic range) cause endothelium-dependent vasodilatation by hyperpolarizing the endothelial cell through stimulation of the sodium pump and opening of potassium channels (Haddy et al., 2006; Amberg et al., 2003). Endothelial hyperpolarization is transmitted to the vascular smooth muscle cells, resulting in decreased cytosolic calcium, which in turn promotes vasodilatation. In contrast, experimental potassium depletion inhibits endothelium-dependent vasodilatation (Haddy et al., 2006).

In addition to increased vasodilatation, other proposed mechanisms by which potassium can influence BP include natriuresis, alterations in intracellular sodium and tonicity, modulation of baroreceptor sensitivity, reduced vasoconstrictive sensitivity to norepinephrine and angiotensin II, increased serum and urinary kallikrein, increased sodium/potassium ATPase activity and alteration in DNA synthesis and proliferation in vascular smooth muscle and sympathetic nervous system cells, improved insulin sensitivity, reduction in cardiac diastolic dysfunction, decrease in vascular neointimal formation, reduction in transforming growth factor (TGF)-β, and decrease in NADPH oxidase, oxidative stress, and inflammation (Ying et al., 2009; Ando et al., 2010).

As mentioned earlier, okra is a good source of magnesium with a 100-g serving providing 57 mg. Magnesium is an essential mineral critical for many metabolic functions in the body. Magnesium is primarily found in many unprocessed foods, such as whole grains, green leafy vegetables, including okra as well as legumes and nuts (Vaquero, 2002). The Recommended Dietary Allowances (RDA) for magnesium is 420 mg/day for adult men and 320 mg/day for women. Magnesium requirement increases during pregnancy and lactation (Table 18.4).

Suboptimal intake of dietary magnesium has long been observed in the general population of both developing and industrialized countries (Ford and Mokdad, 2003). Because magnesium content is low in diets high in meats and dairy products and tends to be lost substantially during the refining and processing of foods, the adoption of a "Western diet" characterized by low consumption of vegetables, including okra, but by high intakes of red meat, dairy products and other highly refined or prepared foods, is believed to contribute to the decline in magnesium intake during the 20th and 21st centuries.

Table 18.4 Magnesium Requirement Across Life Cycle, Age Groups, and Gender

		RDA	
Life stage	**Age (years)**	**Males (mg/day)**	**Females (mg/day)**
Children	1–3	80	80
Children	4–8	130	130
Children	9–13	240	240
Adolescent	14–18	410	380
Adult	19–30	400	310
Adult	31–50	420	320
Adult	>51	420	350
Pregnant	19–30	–	350
Pregnant	31–50	–	360
Lactating	19–30	–	310
Lactating	31–50	–	320

IOM (Institute of Medicine, 2005b).

Magnesium

Magnesium is a cofactor for hundreds of enzymes, particularly for those cellular reactions involved in the transfer, storage, and utilization of energy. Low intakes of magnesium as well as abnormalities in intracellular magnesium homeostasis have been linked to the increase in risk for the development of insulin resistance, type-2 diabetes mellitus, hypertension, and CVD (Shechter, 2010). The beneficial effects of magnesium intake may be explained by several mechanisms, including improvement of glucose and insulin homeostasis, lipid metabolism, vascular or myocardial contractility, endothelium-dependent vasodilation, antiarrhythmic effects, and anticoagulant or antiplatelet effects, which are partly present in Fig. 18.1 (Khan et al., 2010; Arnaud, 2008).

Okra, as a good source of magnesium, can be incorporated in the diet of patients with hypertension, since mineral has been shown to be very effective in reducing BP. One of the mechanisms by which magnesium lowers BP is by acting like a natural calcium channel blocker. Magnesium competes with sodium for binding sites on vascular smooth muscle cells, increases prostaglandin E1 (PGE1), binds to potassium in a cooperative manner, induces endothelial-dependent vasodilation, improves endothelial dysfunction in hypertensive and diabetic patients, decreases intracellular calcium and sodium, and reduces BP (Barbagallo et al., 2010). Magnesium is more effective in reducing BP when administered as multiple minerals

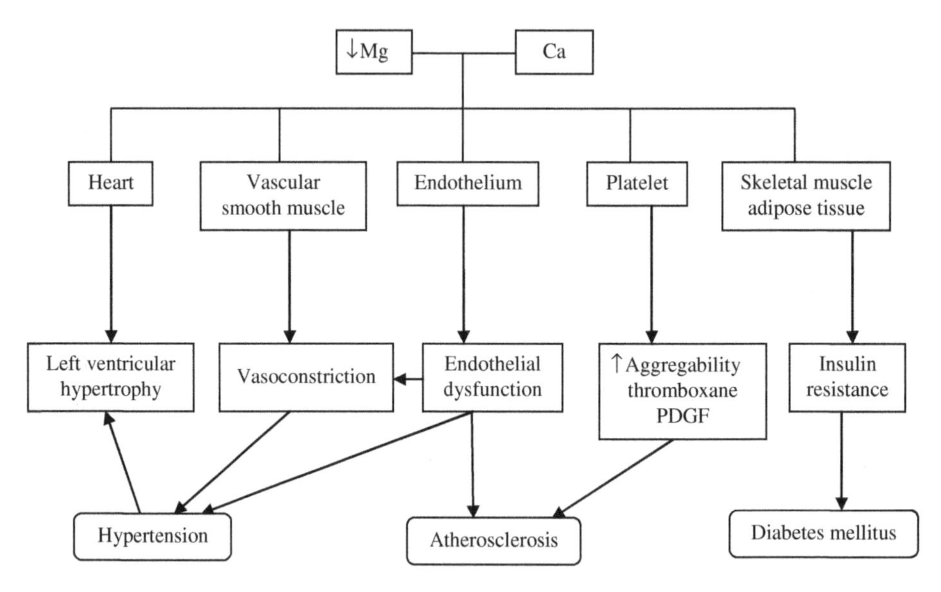

■ **FIGURE 18.1** Mechanisms, whereby deficiency of magnesium and excess calcium, may lead to hypertension, diabetes mellitus, and atherosclerosis.

in a natural form and as a combination with magnesium, potassium, and calcium than when given alone (Preuss, 1997).

Magnesium is also an essential cofactor for the delta-6-desaturase enzyme, which is the rate-limiting step for the conversion of linoleic acid (LA) to gamma-LA (GLA) (Das, 2006). GLA, in turn, elongates to form DGLA (dihomo-gamma-lineleic acid), the precursor for PGE1, is both a vasodilator and platelet inhibitor (Das, 2006). Low magnesium states lead to insufficient amounts of PGE1, causing vasoconstriction and increased BP (Das, 2006).

In addition to BP, magnesium regulates intracellular calcium, sodium, potassium, and pH as well as left ventricular mass, insulin sensitivity, and arterial compliance (Hatzistavri et al., 2001). Magnesium also suppresses circulating Na^+ K^+ ATPase inhibitory activity that reduces vascular tone (Haga, 1992).

Manganese

Okra pods or fruits are a very good source of manganese (Mn) with 100 g serving providing 1 mg, which constitutes 50% of the daily recommended intake of this mineral. Mn is an essential mineral. It is present in virtually all diets at low concentrations. The principal route of intake for Mn is through food consumption, but in occupational cohorts, inhalation exposure may also occur (Aschner and Aschner, 2005).

This trace mineral has a significant role as a cofactor for several critical enzymes. For example, Mn superoxide dismutase (MnSOD) is an antioxidant enzyme that is critical for the prevention and/or reduction of oxidative stress, facilitating the control of chronic diseases such as diabetes mellitus. Arginase is a Mn-dependent enzyme that regulates urea production in the liver and nitric oxide synthase in smooth muscle cells (Sarban et al., 2007). Other enzymes that require Mn as a cofactor or activator are involved in the metabolism of carbohydrates, amino acids, and cholesterol, the formation of bone and cartilage, and wound healing (Freeland-Graves et al., 2005). They include pyruvate carboxylase, transferases, hydrolases, kinases (Freeland-Graves et al., 2005), lyases, oxido-reductases, isomerases, ligases, glutamine synthetase, and phosphoenolpyruvate decarboxylase (Aschner and Aschner, 2005). Another Mn-dependent enzyme is the reverse transcriptase that some retroviruses use to multiply by transcription of the genetic material (Wilhelm et al., 2002). Finally, Mn assumes a significant role in digestion, development, reproduction, immune function, and regulation of cellular energy and blood glucose.

Though not frequently encountered, inadequate dietary intake and Mn deficiency lead to impaired growth, poor bone formation and skeletal defects, reduced fertility and birth defects, abnormal glucose tolerance, and altered lipid and carbohydrate metabolism (Keen et al., 1999).

Vitamin C

One cup of okra contains almost 35% of the recommended daily allowance of vitamin C, which plays significant functions in the human body, though its function at the cellular level is not very clear. Vitamin C is needed for collagen synthesis, the protein that serves so many connective functions in the body. The framework of bone, gums and binding materials in skin muscle or scar tissue is among the body's collagen-containing materials and structures. Production of certain hormones and of neurotransmitters and the metabolism of some amino acids and vitamins require vitamin C. This vitamin also helps the liver in the detoxification of toxic substances in the system and the blood in fighting infections. Ascorbic acid is important in the proper function of the immune system. As an antioxidant, it reacts with compounds like histamines and peroxides to reduce inflammatory symptoms. Its antioxidant property is associated with the reduction of cancer incidences (Arrigoni and De Tullio, 2002).

Claims for a positive link between vitamin C intake and health status are frequently made, but results from intervention studies are inconsistent. Low plasma levels have been reported in patients with diabetes (Afkhami-Ardekani and Shojaoddiny-Ardekani, 2007) and infections (Thurnham, 1994) and in smokers (Faruque, 1995), but the relative contribution of diet and stress to these situations is uncertain. Epidemiological studies indicate that diets with high vitamin C content, such as okra, have been associated with lower cancer risk, especially for cancers of the oral cavity, esophagus, stomach, colon, and lung. However, there appears to be no effect of consumption of vitamin C supplements on the development of colorectal adenoma and stomach cancer, and data on the effect of vitamin C supplementation on coronary heart disease and cataract development are conflicting (Li and Schellhorn, 2007). Currently there is no consistent evidence from population studies that heart disease, cancers, or cataract development are specifically associated with vitamin C status. This of course does not preclude the possibility that other components in vitamin C-rich fruits and vegetables, such as phytochemicals, provide health benefits, but it is not yet possible to isolate such effects from other factors such as lifestyle patterns of people who have a high vitamin C intake.

Folate

Okra pods or fruit contain a substantial amount of folate, with 100g serving providing 88mg, which is 22% of the daily value of this important vitamin. Folate in natural foods is in the form of polyglutamates (pteroylpolyglutamate), whereas folic acid is in monoglutamate (pteroylmonoglutamate) form. Polyglutamates have higher metabolic activity and are better retained by cells, while monoglutamates pass through cell walls more rapidly (Sanderson et al., 2003; Gregory, 1997). In humans, the metabolism of polyglutamates requires their deconjugation to monoglutamates within enterocytes, explaining their low bioavailability (~50%) compared to monoglutamates (~85%). The low bioavailability and, more importantly, the poor chemical stability of the natural folates have a profound influence on the development of nutrient recommendations. This is particularly true if some of the dietary intake is as the more stable and bioavailable synthetic form, folic acid. Fortification of foods such as breakfast cereals and flour can add significant amounts of folic acid to the diet (Selhub and Rosenberg, 2008).

Adequate folate intake is vital for cell division and homeostasis due to the essential role of folate coenzymes in nucleic acid synthesis, methionine regeneration, and in the shuttling, oxidation and reduction of one-carbon units required for normal metabolism and regulation (Chandra, 2010).

Inadequate folate intake or malabsorption, biochemical changes associated with low folate status may precipitate the onset of abnormalities in one-carbon metabolism. These abnormalities (eg, hyperhomocysteinemia or DNA hypomethylation) may result in deleterious consequences, including increased risk for certain types of chronic diseases, including anemia, neural tube defects (NTDs), CVD, neurological disorders, and CRC (Blom et al., 2006; Beaudin and Stover, 2009).

Low folate status has been linked with the development of several clinical disorders. From a nutritional point of view, deficiencies in iron, vitamins B_{12}, A, and folate can cause hematologic changes, which if untreated can lead to anemia. Clinically, severe folate deficiency yields a specific type of anemia, a megaloblastic anemia (Chandra, 2010). Megaloblasts are large, abnormal, nucleated cells that are precursors of erythrocytes; in a folate deficiency, they accumulate and are found in the bone marrow. These cells arise as a result of a failure of the red cell precursors to divide normally. The resulting anemia is not the only manifestation of diminished cell division. There are also decreased numbers of white cells and platelets. There is general impairment of cell division related to folate's role in nucleic acid synthesis, which is more apparent in tissues that turn over rapidly, such as the hematopoietic system and the cells lining the digestive tract.

There is now conclusive evidence that most NTDs can be prevented by the ingestion of adequate amount of folate or folic acid near the time of conception (Chen, 2008). It is now agreed that a supplement of 400 μg of folic acid taken near the time of conception will prevent most NTDs. The recommendation to prevent recurrence in women with a previous NTD birth remains 4.0 mg/day because of the high increase in risk in such cases and because that was the amount used in the most definitive trial (MRC Vitamin Study Research Group, 1991). Levels of red cell folate previously considered to be in the adequate or normal range are now associated with an increased risk of spina bifida and other NTDs. Red cell folate levels greater than 150 mg/L, which are completely adequate to prevent anemia, are nevertheless associated with increased risk of NTDs (Blom et al., 2006; Beaudin and Stover, 2009).

Folate deficiency can increase the risk for the development of CVD due to an elevation in the level of homocysteine, an amino acid arising from the metabolism of methionine. Plasma homocysteine concentration, if only moderately elevated, is an independent risk factor for CVD and stroke (Antoniades et al., 2009). Increased risk has been associated with values higher than 11 mmol/L, which is well within what is generally considered to be the normal range (5–15 mmol/L) of plasma homocysteine levels (Antoniades et al., 2009).

Evidence suggests a link between CRC and dietary folate intake and folate status (Koren, 2011). Studies have shown that women who take multivitamin supplements containing folic acid for prolonged periods have a significantly reduced risk of CRC (Wu et al., 2009). Currently, however, the scientific evidence is not sufficiently clear for recommending increased folate intake in populations at risk for CRC.

Proposed hypotheses regarding folate's role in carcinogenesis relate to DNA structure, stability, and transcriptional regulation; they include increased susceptibility of DNA to strand breakage, uracil misincorporation in DNA, and hypomethylation of DNA. Misincorporation of uracil into DNA with chronic folate deficiency is expected to stress the mechanism of DNA repair and thus result in subsequent increases in DNA strand breaks and chromosomal instability (Keum and Giovannucci, 2014).

Folate is essential for the formation of biogenic amines and pterins in the central nervous system. Folate deficiency produces a variety of neurologic symptoms, including neuropsychiatric disturbances and movement disorders. In healthy adults, cerebrospinal fluid (CSF) folate levels do not decline with age, but CSF folate levels have been found to be lower in patients with late-onset Alzheimer's disease (AD) than in age-matched control subjects (Serot et al., 2001).

Vitamin K

Okra can be considered to be a rich source of vitamin K, because 100 g serving of this vegetable supplies 53 µg of this essential vitamin, which is equivalent to almost 70% the daily recommended intake (Table 18.1).

Vitamin K is not a single compound, but a group name for a family of related structures that all share a methylated naphthoquinone ring system substituted with a variable aliphatic side chain (Shearer and Newman, 2008). In phylloquinone (vitamin K1), the side chain is composed of four isoprenoid residues, the last three of which are saturated. Menaquinones (vitamin K2) form a subfamily in which the length of the side chain may range from 1 to 13 isoprene residues, all of which are unsaturated.

Vitamin K1 is formed in plants and important sources in our diet are green leafy vegetables such as spinach, broccoli, Brussels sprouts, kale, collard greens, iceberg lettuce, and okra. It is located in the chloroplasts where it forms part of the electron transport system and about 90% of the total vitamin K in the western diet is formed by K1. Menaquinone forms of vitamin K are produced by bacteria in the lower bowel, where the forms appear in large amounts. However, their contribution to the maintenance of vitamin K status has been difficult to assess. Although the content is extremely variable, the human liver contains about 10 times as much vitamin K as a mixture of menaquinones than as phylloquinone.

Vitamin K functions as a coenzyme for biological reactions involved in blood coagulation and bone metabolism. It also plays an essential role in the conversion of certain residues in proteins into biologically active forms. These proteins include plasma prothrombin (coagulation factor II) and the plasma procoagulants, factors VII, IX, and X. Two structurally related vitamin K-dependent proteins have received recent attention as being proteins with possible roles in the prevention of chronic disease. They are osteocalcin, found in bone, and matrix Gla protein, originally found in bone, but now known to be more widely distributed.

It has been suggested that vitamin K may have roles in osteoporosis and vascular health (Gast et al., 2009; Shearer et al., 2012). However, this is difficult to establish on the basis of the studies performed thus far. Clinical intervention studies investigating the relationship between vitamin K and osteoporosis are currently being conducted mainly in North America and Europe. Whether vitamin K status within the range of normal intake plays a significant role in the development of atherosclerosis requires further investigation and should be verified in studies that employ rigorous experimental designs.

Vitamin B1

Thiamin (or thiamine) is one of the water-soluble B vitamins commonly known as vitamin B1. Thiamin is naturally present in some foods, added to some food products, and available as a dietary supplement. Okra can be considered as a good source of thiamine, because a 100 g serving of this vegetable provides 0.2 mg, which is 13% of recommended daily intake for this vitamin.

Thiamin pyrophosphate (TPP), the active form of thiamin, is involved in several enzyme functions associated with the metabolism of carbohydrates, branched chain amino acids, and fatty acids and, therefore, in the growth, development, and function of cells (Said, 2010).

Adequate intakes of vitamin B1 may reduce the risk for the development of cataract and diabetes complications as well as in the management of AD, congestive failure, and cancer. For example, a cross-sectional study carried out in Australian men and women aged 49 years found that those in the highest quintile of thiamin intake were 40% less likely to have nuclear cataracts than those in the lowest quintile (Cumming et al., 2000). In addition, a recent study in 408 US women found that higher dietary intakes of thiamin were inversely associated with 5-year change in lens opacification (Jacques et al., 2005).

Low plasma concentrations and high renal clearance of thiamin have been observed in diabetic patients compared to healthy subjects (Thornalley et al., 2007), suggesting that individuals with type-1 or type-2 diabetes mellitus are at increased risk for thiamin deficiency. Two thiamin transporters, thiamin transporter-1 (THTR-1) and THTR-2, are involved in thiamin uptake by enterocytes in the small intestine and re-uptake in the proximal tubules of the kidneys. A recent study suggested that hyperglycemia in diabetic patients could affect thiamin re-uptake by decreasing the expression of thiamin transporters in the kidneys (Larkin et al., 2012). Conversely, thiamin deficiency appears to impair the normal endocrine function of the pancreas and exacerbate hyperglycemia.

Some elderly people are at increased risk for developing subclinical thiamin deficiency secondary to poor dietary intake, reduced GI absorption, and multiple medical conditions (Ito et al., 2012). Since thiamin deficiency can result in a form of dementia called Wernicke–Korsakoff syndrome, its relationship to AD and other forms of dementia have been investigated. AD is characterized by a decline in cognitive function in elderly people, accompanied by pathologic features that include β-amyloid plaque deposition and tangles formed by phosphorylated Tau protein (Prvulovic and Hampel, 2011).

Thiamin deficiency has been linked to increased β-amyloid production in cultured neuronal cells and to plaque formation in animal models (Zhang et al., 2011). These pathological hallmarks of AD could be reversed by thiamin supplementation, suggesting that thiamin could be protective in AD.

Thiamin deficiency has been observed in some cancer patients with rapidly growing tumors. Research in cell culture and animal models indicates that rapidly dividing cancer cells have a high requirement for thiamin (Comin-Anduix et al., 2001). All rapidly dividing cells require nucleic acids at an increased rate, and some cancer cells appear to rely heavily on the TPP-dependent enzyme, transketolase, to provide the ribose-5-phosphate necessary for nucleic acid synthesis.

Vitamin B6

Okra is one of the best plant dietary sources of vitamin B6, since a 100 g serving of this vegetable provides 0.2 mg, which is 11% of recommended daily intake for this vitamin.

Vitamin B6 is a mixture of 6 inter-related forms: pyridoxine (or pyridoxol), pyridoxal, pyridoxamine and their 5′-phosphates. Interconversion is possible between all forms (Da Silva et al., 2012). The active form of the vitamin is pyridoxal phosphate (PLP), which plays a vital role in the function of over 100 enzymes that catalyze essential chemical reactions in the human body. The many biochemical reactions catalyzed by PLP-dependent enzymes are involved in essential biological processes, such as hemoglobin and amino acid biosynthesis, as well as fatty acid metabolism (Da Silva et al., 2012). Of note, PLP also functions as a coenzyme for glycogen phosphorylase, an enzyme that catalyzes the release of glucose from stored glycogen. Much of the PLP in the human body is found in muscle bound to glycogen phosphorylase. PLP is also a coenzyme for reactions that generate glucose from amino acids, a process known as gluconeogenesis (McCormick, 2006).

Adequate intakes of vitamin B6 has been reported to play an important role in the prevention of immune dysfunction, CVD, inflammation, dementias, depression, cancer, and kidney stones.

Several enzymatic reactions in the tryptophan–kynurenine pathway are dependent on vitamin B6 coenzyme, PLP. This pathway is known to be activated during proinflammatory immune responses and plays a critical role in immune tolerance of the fetus during pregnancy (Paul et al., 2013).

There is evidence to suggest that adequate vitamin B6 intake is important for optimal immune system function, especially in older individuals (Meydani et al., 1991). However, chronic inflammation that triggers tryptophan degradation and underlies many diseases (eg, CVD and cancers) may precipitate the loss of PLP and increase vitamin B6 requirements.

High levels of circulating homocysteine, which is derived from methionine metabolism, are associated with an increased risk of CVD. Randomized controlled trials have demonstrated that supplementation with B vitamins, including vitamin B6, could effectively reduce homocysteine levels. However, homocysteine lowering by B vitamins has failed to lower the risk of adverse cardiovascular outcomes in high-risk individuals (Gerhard and Duell, 1999). For details on vitamin B6 and homocysteine metabolism and their relation to CVD, see review by Gerhard and Duell (1999).

A few observational studies have linked cognitive decline and AD in the elderly with inadequate status of folate, vitamin B12, and vitamin B6 (Selhub et al., 2000). Yet, the relationship between B vitamins and cognitive health in aging is complicated by both the high prevalence of hyperhomocysteinemia and signs of systemic inflammation in elderly people (Pawelec et al., 2014). On the one hand, since inflammation may impair vitamin B6 metabolism, low serum PLP levels may well be caused by processes related to aging rather than by malnutrition. On the other hand, high serum homocysteine may possibly be a risk factor for cognitive decline in the elderly, although the matter remains under debate.

As earlier mentioned, chronic inflammation that underlies most cancers may enhance vitamin B6 degradation. In addition, the requirement of PLP in the methionine cycle, homocysteine catabolism, and thymidylate synthesis that lowers vitamin B6 status may contribute to the onset and/or progression of tumors. The systematic review of nine prospective studies found either inverse or positive associations between vitamin B6 intakes and CRC risk (Wu et al., 2013). Inconsistent evidence regarding the link between vitamin B6 intakes and breast cancer was also recently reported in a meta-analysis (Wu et al., 2013).

Effects of processing pretreatments on nutrients

Different pretreatments such as soaking, blanching, malting, and roasting have been applied to okra seeds and their effects on the mineral and functional properties of flour were investigated (Adelakun et al., 2010). Soaking reduced the content of minerals such as P, K, Ca, Mg, Na, Fe, Cu, Zn, and Mn. Blanching reduced level of all the earlier mentioned minerals except Mg. Malting reduced the amount of P, K, Mg, and Fe while it increased the content of Ca, Na, Zn, and Mn. Roasting increased the level of all the minerals except P and Mg. In another study, which investigated the effects of soaking and blanching on the yield, proximate composition and antioxidant activity of okra seed flour found increase yield which was time dependent (Adelakun et al., 2009). Slight but significant 2,2-diphenyl-1-picrylhydrazyl radical scavenging activity increased in soaked samples at 18th hour while blanching resulted in progressive decrease (Adelakun et al., 2009). The roasting of okra seed flour at 160ºC for up to 40 min caused an increase in antioxidant activity as determined by free radical scavenging using the DPPH assay (Adelakun et al., 2009).

The effects of blanching of okra (100°C for 3 minutes) and vacuum frying (frying the okra at 100°C for 20 minutes) on the quality of organic and conventionally grown okra (Arlai, 2009) were compared before and after processing. The blanching treatment increased the fiber and β-carotene content, while the carbohydrate, protein, fat, ash, pH, the total soluble solids as Brix, total sugar, and vitamin C levels decreased after processing (Arlai, 2009). The rate of vitamin C loss from the organic okra was less than in conventional okra, ie, 14.2 and 58.1 (% wet basis). While the rate of β-carotene increase in organic okra was higher than conventional okra, ie, 10.1 and 4.9 (% wet basis). The vacuum frying treatment reduced the physical and chemical quality of okra, but increased β-carotene content. In addition, the rate of protein, fiber, and vitamin C loss from the organic okra was lower than those in conventionally grown. In conclusion, the results show that the processing affects the chemical quality of organic okra less than conventionally grown okra.

The effects of slice thicknesses (5.0, 10.0, and 15.0 mm) had a significant effect ($P < 0.01$) on moisture, crude fiber, and ash contents but not on vitamin C content, viscosity, color, and microbial load of okra during solar drying (Adom et al., 1997). The study showed that a slice thickness of 10.0 mm and a drying time of 48 h were suitable for the solar drying of okra (Adom et al., 1997).

BIOACTIVE COMPONENTS—DISEASE PREVENTION AND MANAGEMENT

Flavonoids

Okra fruits have phenolic compounds with total flavonoids being between 18% and 22% of the total phenols contents for the analyzed samples

(Olivera et al., 2012). The total highest phenolics content was found in young okra leaves (0.99 mgTNE/1 g) and the total flavonoid was highest in mature leaves (0.79 mgQE/1 g) (Nwachukwu et al., 2014). For the total flavonoids, mature leaves showed a distinct highest flavonoids content mean percentage of 0.8 mgQE/0.1 g while mature fruit recorded a negligible mean value of 0.007 mgQE/0.1 g (Nwachukwu et al., 2014).

The total flavonoid in the red portion of the petal was 0.48% of fresh weight and in the white portion was 2.5% (Hedin et al., 1968). The two anthocyanins comprised 28.5% of the flavonoid content of the red flower but only a trace of the content of the white quercetin 4′-glucoside (Hedin et al., 1968). Flavonol glycosides and anthocyanins have been isolated from the flower petals of okra. These were quercetin 4′-glycoside, quercetin 7-glucoside, quercetin 5-glucoside, quercetin 3-diglucoside, quercetin 4′-diglucoside, quercetin 3-triglucoside, quercetin 5-rhamnoglucoside, gossypetin 8-glucoside, gossypetin 8-rhamnoglucoside, gossypetin 3-glucosido-8-rhamnoglucoside, cyanidin 4′-glucoside, and cyaniding 3-glucosido-4′ glucoside.

Okra seeds had 10 times higher concentration of flavonols and almost 15 times of higher concentration of catechins compared to skins (Arapitsas, 2008). The phenolic content as expressed as mg chlorogenic acid per equivalent per g of wet weight of okra seeds was 2.85 compared to the skin of 0.20.

Antiobesity, antidiabetic, and antihypertensive effects of quercetin

Obesity, defined as an excess of adipose tissue when body mass index is >30 kg/m^2, is due to an imbalance between energy intake and energy expenditure. Obesity is a major health problem in the industrialized world and it has reached epidemic proportions globally. The World Health Organization estimates that worldwide, obesity has more than doubled since 1980. In 2014, more than 1.9 billion adults, 18 years and older, were overweight. Of these, over 600 million were obese. 39% of adults aged 18 years and over were overweight in 2014, and 13% were obese. Overall, about 13% of the world's adult populations (11% of men and 15% of women) were obese in 2014. Most of the world's populations live in countries where overweight and obesity kill more people than underweight. 42 million children under the age of 5 were overweight or obese in 2013 (World Health Organization, 2015). Moreover, its prevalence is likely to increase as a result of changes in lifestyle, decreased physical activity, and socioeconomic development, among others.

In addition, obesity is a complex multifactorial and chronic disease that is considered to be a risk factor for the genesis or development of various diseases including hypertension, type-2 diabetes, coronary heart disease, cancer, respiratory complications, and osteoarthritis. Despite current intensive efforts to reduce obesity by diet, exercise, education, drug therapies, and surgery, an effective long-term solution to this problem has yet to be provided.

Scientists in various fields are constantly looking for new molecules that could be used as dietary functional ingredients in the prevention and management of overweight and obesity and studies with flavonoids, including quercetin, have shown promising results. As can be seen in Table 18.5, okra is a good source of quercetin.

Results of *in vitro* studies have demonstrated that apart from the indirect effects of quercetin in lipogenesis through the action of insulin, this flavonoid can also diminish or inhibit this metabolic pathway by acting directly on the expression of genes controlling this metabolic route. The results of studies by Ahn et al. (2008) revealed that quercetin decreased the expression of sterol regulatory element-binding proteins (SREBP)-1 and fatty acid synthase (FAS), and by increasing acetyl-CoA carboxylase (ACC) phosphorylation. This research group also showed that quercetin attenuated adipogenesis as a consequence of the decrease in the expression of CCAAT/enhancer binding protein α (C/EBPα) and peroxisome proliferator-activated receptor γ (PPARγ).

Quercetin has been shown to be a potent inhibitor of the stimulating effect of vanadate on lipoprotein lipase (LPL) activity. It is worth mentioning

Table 18.5 Quercetin Content of Selected Foods

Food	Quercetin Content (mg/100 g)
Capers	233
Onions	22
Okra	21
Cocoa powder	20
Cranberries	14
Lingonberries	7.4
Apples	4.57
Green tea	2.69
Black tea	1.99
Catsup	0.86

USDA Database for the Flavonoid Content of Selected Foods, Release 3.1 (2014).

that vanadate shows insulin-mimetic effects, such as increases in LPL and suppression of hormone-dependent lipolysis, in isolated rat adipocytes. Consequently, the inhibition of vanadate action leads to inhibition of LPL and thus to the incorporation of fatty acids which circulate as triacylglycerols in lipoproteins to adipocyte triacylglycerols (Motoyashiki et al., 1996).

Besides the effects on metabolic pathway involved in triacylglycerol accumulation, quercetin has been demonstrated to stimulate lipid mobilization. Studies by Kuppusamy and Das (1992) demonstrated that quercetin induced a dose- and time-dependent increase in lipolysis, which was synergic with epinephrine-induced lipolysis. Thus, it can be said that this flavonoid produces a competitive phosphodiesterase (PDE) inhibition. The competitive nature of the kinetics suggests that quercetin could compete with cAMP for the same binding sites in the adipocyte PDE, thus increasing the concentration of cAMP, being an activator of protein kinase A (PKA), which in turn activates the hormone sensitive lipase (HSL).

An increase in adipocyte apoptosis due to a down regulation of Poly(ADP-ribose) polymerases (PARPs) was demonstrated by Hsu and Yen (2006). PARPs are a set of protein that has several roles in cellular processes, most notably in DNA repair and programmed cell death, Bcl-2 proteins (apoptosis regulator proteins), Bax, and Bak proteins. The activation of caspase-3 and 9, as well as the inhibition of adenosine monophosphate-activated protein kinase (AMPK) pathway, also play a role in the induction of apoptosis (see Figs. 18.2 and 18.3 for mechanisms of actions of quercetin).

Steward et al. (2009) conducted an *in vivo* study in C57BL/6J mice fed a high-fat diet supplemented with quercetin (0.8%) for 3 and 8 weeks. Dietary supplementation with this quercetin produced a transient increase in energy expenditure, which diminished after 8 weeks. A decrease in circulating quercetin levels between 3 and 8 weeks indicated a metabolic adaptation. Furthermore, quercetin, at the concentrations provided, was effective in reducing circulating markers of inflammation, including IFN-γ, TNF-α, IL1, and IL4 after 8 weeks of treatment.

Kobori et al. (2011) performed *in vivo* studies, during which they fed C57/BL6J mice Western-style diet. They found that chronic dietary intake of quercetin reduced body weight gain, as well as visceral and liver fat accumulation, and improved systemic parameters related to metabolic syndrome (hyperglycemia, hyperinsulinemia, and dyslipidemia), probably by decreasing oxidative stress and increasing PPARα expression. In addition, quercetin suppressed the expression of PPARγ and CD36, as well as SREBP-1c and its target FAS in the liver. The reduction in PPARγ expression suggests a reduction in adipogenesis, because genes involved in this

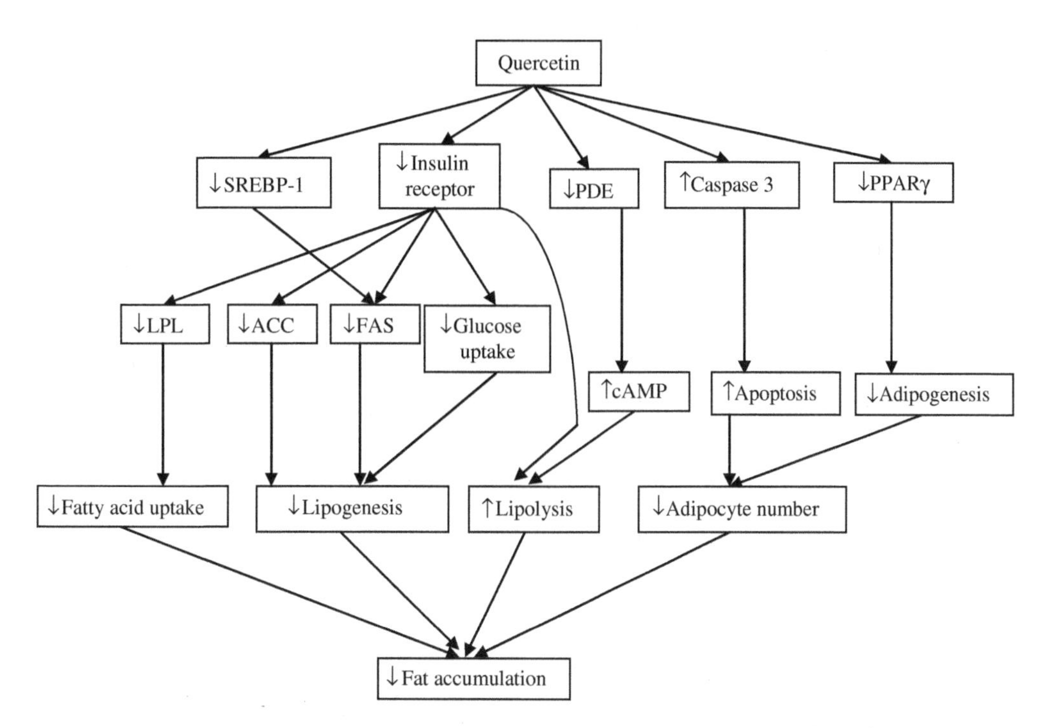

■ **FIGURE 18.2** Body-fat lowering effects of quercetin in adipose tissue with mechanisms of action. ↓ = decrease in process or activity; ↑ = increase in process or activity.

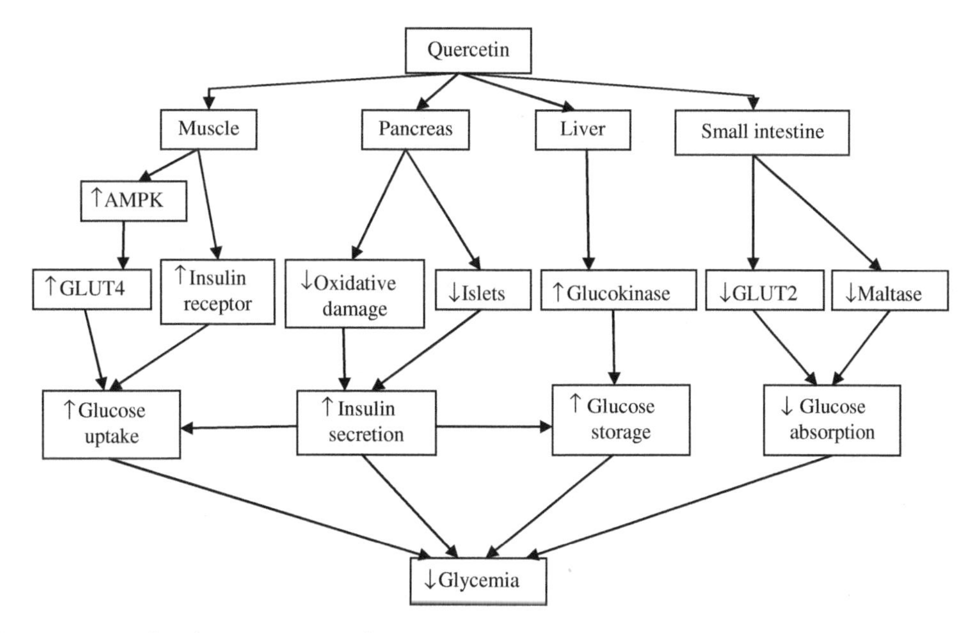

■ **FIGURE 18.3** Antidiabetic effects of quercetin: mechanisms of action. ↓ = decrease in process or activity; ↑ = increase in process or activity.

process are controlled by this transcriptional factor. However, the reduction in SREBP expression, as well as the gene of the lipogenic enzyme FAS, indicate a decrease in the *de novo* lipogenesis in liver. Consequently, a reduced amount of triacylglycerols in plasma, coming from liver and available for adipose tissue uptake, can be expected.

Not all studies have demonstrated favorable effects of quercetin on body weight and fat. For example, in an experiment carried out by Kim et al. (2011) in db/db mice treated with quercetin (100 mg/kg of body weight/day) for 7 weeks, this flavonoid led to a reduction in plasma glucose without changes in body weight. In another experiment performed in Wistar rats treated with 25 mg of quercetin/kg body weight/day and fed high-fat diet, body weight also remained unchanged (Wein et al., 2010).

Unfortunately, there is scarcity of data on the effects of quercetin on humans. The only published study carried out in humans revealed that nutritional status, namely: body weight, waist circumference, fat mass, and fat-free mass remained unchanged in participants with a body mass index between 25 and 35 kg/m^2, who consumed 150 mg/day of quercetin for 6 weeks (Egert et al., 2010).

Quercetin is a potent antioxidant agent that inhibits pro-oxidant enzymes and upregulates the expression of genes encoding enzymes involved in drug metabolism and antioxidant defense, such as γ-glutamylcysteine synthetase, the rate-limiting enzyme in glutathione synthesis. Reduced glutathione (rGSH) as an antioxidant is usually found in low concentrations in individuals with diabetes, which may be the result of the presence of high oxidative stress (Sekhar et al., 2011). rGSH influences the redox status of the cell, therefore affecting biochemical functions. The lack of rGSH or its decrease could lead to physiological imbalance and may predispose cells to oxidative damage and eventually diabetic complications.

Recently, Nájera et al. (2013) investigated the effect of daily administration of quercetin, in two different doses (15 vs 30 mg/kg), on the levels of rGSH and lipid peroxidation in rats, 2 weeks after induction of diabetes. Both doses of quercetin significantly increased blood rGSH levels and reduced lipid peroxidation in liver. Low quercetin doses increased superoxide dismutase activity (SOD) levels in liver and reduced lipid peroxidation in the heart. High quercetin doses induced recovery of rGSH levels in pancreas.

Several *in vivo* studies with the use of quercetin have been performed in animal models with diabetes. For example, Kim et al. (2011) found a reduction in serum glucose concentrations and blood glycated hemoglobin in C57BL/KsJdb-db mice fed with a diet supplemented with 0.08% quercetin for 7 weeks. The decline in serum glucose concentrations and blood glycated hemoglobin was attributed to the inhibition of small intestine maltase activity without changes in serum insulin levels. Mechanisms of the antidiabetic effects of quercetin are shown in Fig. 18.3.

Alpha-glucosidase and α-amylase inhibitors help retard postprandial blood glucose increase. Food compounds with such properties include tannins, anthocyanins, chlorogenic acid, and many other polyphenols, including quercetin present in okra (Boath et al., 2012). Recently, Rifaai et al. (2012) showed that quercetin exerted a protective effect against β-cell damage by its anti-inflammatory, antiapoptotic, antioxidant, and regenerative effects in rats with experimentally induced diabetes.

Wein et al. (2010), in a study carried out on male Wistar rats fed with a high-fat diet supplemented daily with 25 mg quercetin/kg body weight, showed an increase in adiponectin expression in white adipose tissue and its circulating concentration, despite an inhibition of PPARγ expression. The authors concluded that the effects of quercetin on adiponectin were PPARγ independent. Taking into account that adiponectin is an adipokine that facilitates insulin action, the authors proposed that the increase in adiponectin levels was involved in the improvement in insulin sensitivity induced by quercetin.

However, Stewart et al. (2008) induced insulin resistance in rats by feeding animals on a high-fat diet. They noticed that at the dose of 0.8% in the diet, quercetin exacerbated diet-induced insulin resistance at 3 weeks. After 8 weeks, insulin resistance in the quercetin supplemented group was not worse, when compared with animals fed on high fat alone. These results suggest that the inhibitory effect of insulin signaling at 3 weeks was further eliminated by an adaptive increase hepatic metabolism and/or excretion of the compound between 3 and 8 weeks. At the doses used, quercetin inhibited insulin-dependent activation of PI-3K.

Phytosterols

Okra is one of the best sources of phytosterols with 200 kcal serving providing 155 mg of these bioactive compounds (Table 18.6).

Phytosterols are plant compounds with similar chemical structure and biological functions as cholesterol (Piironen et al., 2000). Plant sterols contain an extra methyl, ethyl group or double bond. The most abundant plant sterols are sitosterol, campesterol, and stigmasterol (Ostlund, 2002). The daily dietary intake of plant sterol is 160–400 mg among different populations

Table 18.6 Phytosterol Content of Selected Foods

Food	Phytosterol Content (mg/200 kcal Serving)
Lettuce, green leaf, raw	507
Asparagus, raw	240
Beet greens, raw	191
Cucumber with peel, raw	187
Okra, raw	155
Cauliflower, raw	144
Lettuce, iceberg, raw	143
Pumpkin, raw	92
Sweet peppers, green	90
Cabbage, raw	88
Pimento, canned	78
Spinach, raw	78

www.nutritiondata.self.com

(Ostlund, 2002). However, in the earlier stages of human evolution, some 5–7 million years ago, plant sterol intake in Myocene diets would have been considerably higher, up to 1 g/day (Jenkins et al., 2005). Dietary sources of phytosterols include vegetable oils (especially unrefined oils), nuts, seeds, vegetables, and grains (Ostlund, 2002). Absorption efficiency for plant sterols in humans is considerably less than that of cholesterol. Percent absorption of the former is 25% versus 60% for the latter (Ostlund et al., 2002).

Studies have found that consuming a minimum dose of 0.8–1.0 g of free sterol and free sterol equivalents will reduce LDL cholesterol by 5% or more, and that this reduction in LDL cholesterol will correlate with an approximate 6–10% reduction in coronary heart disease risk at age 70 (Law et al., 1994). Phytosterols are also effective when combined with cholesterol-lowering medication; adding these bioactive compounds to statin medications can lower LDL more than doubling the statin dose (Talati et al., 2010).

Phytosterols work by reducing the amount of cholesterol that is absorbed in the small intestine. This includes cholesterol from dietary sources, as well as cholesterol from bile that would normally be reabsorbed and reused (Katan et al., 2003). The decrease in absorbed cholesterol upregulates LDL receptors, which in turn removes more LDL from circulation. It also causes an increase in endogenous production of cholesterol, although not enough to compensate for the increased blood clearance. The end result is lower LDL cholesterol (Katan et al., 2003).

In addition to their hypocholesterolemic and antiatherosclerotic effects, phytosterols have been shown in some *in vivo* and *in vitro* studies to exert other biological activities, such as (1) anticarcinogenic effects, protecting against colon, breast, and prostate cancers (Awad et al., 2008); (2) immunomodulatory and anti-inflammatory properties (Navarro et al., 2001); (3) antioxidant potential (Marineli et al., 2012); and (4) antidiabetogenic effects (Misawa et al., 2008).

Screening and extraction techniques for bioactive compounds

Several novel extraction techniques have been developed as an alternative to conventional extraction methods, offering advantages with respect to extraction time, solvent consumption, extraction yields, and reproducibility. An ethyl acetate–*n*-butanol gradient solvent system composed of *n*-hexane–ethyl acetate–*n*-butanol–water was successfully applied to the screening of antiproliferative compounds against cancer cells in okra (Ying et al., 2014). The multisteps of elution could separate the components with a large difference of polarity. The fractions collected from High-Speed Counter-Current Chromatography separation with the gradient solvent system were assayed for antiproliferative activity against cancer cells. The bioactive components identified: a major anticancer compound, 4-hydroxy phenethyl trans-ferulate, with middle activity, and a minor anticancer compound, carolignan, with strong activity.

Supercritical fluid extraction of okra seeds was carried out at a pilot scale using carbon dioxide as solvent, at temperatures of 40, 50, and 60°C and pressures of 150, 300, and 450 bar. The yields of supercritical fluid extraction and *n*-hexane Soxhlet extractions were similar. The fatty acid profiles of the extracts indicated a high unsaturated/saturated ratio (András et al., 2005). SFE with carbon dioxide was found to be a suitable technique for concentration of biologically active compounds (β-sitosterol, sitosterol esters, and tocopherols) from okra seeds. The overall yields of oil and sterols by SFE were very similar to those obtained using *n*-hexane as solvent, but the extraction temperature in the case of SFE is lower. The best process parameters were determined with the response surface method as $P = 450$ bar and $T = 60$°C, but, to avoid the possibility of thermal degradation of valuable components, it is recommended to use the intermediate temperature $T = 50$°C, because the yield decrease in this case is unimportant (András et al., 2005).

FUNCTIONAL PROPERTIES

Medicinal

Okra mucilage from the immature pods is suitable for industrial and medicinal applications (Akinyele and Temikotan, 2007). Industrially, okra mucilage is usually used for paper production and also has a confectionery use. Okra has medical application as a plasma replacement therapy (Savello et al., 1980; Markose and Peter, 1990). Carbohydrates are mainly present in the form of mucilage (Kumar et al., 2009) and in the young fruits consist of long chain molecules with a molecular weight of about 170,000 made up of sugar units and amino acids. The main components are galactose (25%), rhamnose (22%), galacturonic acid (27%), and amino acids (11%) (Kumar et al., 2009; Woolfe et al., 1977). The hot buffer soluble solid (HBSS) fraction was shown to be rich in galactose, rhamnose, and galacturonic acid in the ratio 1.3:1:1.3 (Sengkhamparn et al., 2009). The chelating agent soluble solids (CHSS) fraction contained much higher levels of methyl esterified galacturonic acid residues (63% galacturonic acid; DM = 48) in addition to minor amounts of rhamnose and galactose. The ratio of galactose to rhamnose to galacturonic acid was 1.3:1.0:1.3 and 4.5:1.0:1.2 for HBSS and CHSS, respectively (Sengkhamparn et al., 2009). These results indicated that the HBSS and CHSS fractions contain rhamnogalacturonan type I next to homogalacturonan, while the latter is more prevailing in CHSS (Sengkhamparn et al., 2009, 2010). The unusual slimy behavior of the nonsaponified samples may be related to the tendency of these pectins to associate, driven by hydrophobic interactions (Sengkhamparn et al., 2010).

The mucilage is highly soluble in water and has an intrinsic viscosity value of about 30% (Kumar et al., 2009) and has been employed as stabilizer and thickener of choice when high viscosity is desired especially in cosmetic, pharmaceutical, and food industries. Okra mucilage extract has been used to produce tablets (Kumar et al., 2009) and which could retard the release of water-soluble drug as pentoxifylline to decrease dosing frequency using novel retarding agent obtained from cheap available source (Hussein, 2015). Okra extract resulted in a sustained release tablet with acceptable retardation value. The addition of carboxy methyl cellulose (CMC) extended the disintegration time and lead pentoxifylline. Pentoxifylline is completely absorbed after oral administration but it undergoes first-pass metabolism results in a low bioavailability of 20% and short half-life of 0.4–0.8 h, so that, PTX formulation in sustained release tablets could solve the problem of low oral bioavailability (International Board for Plant Genetic Resources, 1990). These results show the emerging of a novel retardant for sustained release (Hussein, 2015). The use of mucoadhesive microspheres, using okra polysaccharide as a novel carrier for safe and effective delivery of rizatriptan benzoate into nasal cavity, was evaluated (Sharma et al., 2013). These microspheres were prepared by emulsification, followed by cross-linking using epichlorohydrin and were found to release 50% of drug within 15 min and rest of the drug was released within 60 min. The drug release was found to decrease with increasing concentration of polysaccharide (Sharma et al., 2013). The synthesis of gold nanoparticles (Au NPs) using okra seed aqueous extract and its antifungal activity was investigated (Jayaseelan et al., 2013). The antifungal activity of Au NPs was tested against *Puccinia graminis tritci*, *Aspergillus flavus*, *Aspergillus niger*, and *Candida albicans* using standard well diffusion method. The maximum zone of inhibition was observed in the Au NPs against *P. graminis* (17 mm) and *C. albicans* (18 mm). The results suggested that the synthesized Au NPs act as an effective antifungal agent. It is confirmed that Au NPs are capable of rendering high antifungal efficacy and hence have a great potential in the preparation of drugs used against fungal diseases (Jayaseelan et al., 2013). The methanol extract of okra showed that the dried fruit had inhibitory effects against Helicobacter strains with diameters zone of inhibition between 13 and 28 mm on 32 out of the 42 isolates tested (Taiye et al., 2013). The anti-*H. pylori* activities exhibited by okra suggested its use in the treatment of GI diseases associated with the *H. pylori* species.

The immature okra pods have been used in traditional medicine as a diuretic agent, the treatment of dental disease, and to reduce/prevent gastric irritations (Sengkhamparn et al., 2009; Ndjouenkeu et al., 1996).

The antitumor effects of a newly discovered lectin, isolated from okra, were investigated in human breast cancer (MCF7) and skin fibroblast (CCD-1059 sk) (Monte et al., 2014). The okra induced significant cell growth inhibition (63%) in MCF7 cells. The expression of pro-apoptotic caspase-3, caspase-9, and p21 genes was increased in MCF7 cells treated with AEL, compared to those treated with control. Thus okra in its native form promotes selective antitumor effects in human breast cancer cells and may represent a potential therapeutic to combat human breast cancer (Monte et al., 2014).

Food uses

The effects of adding okra extract on the physical properties of chickpeas (*Cicer arietinum* var. surutato) and Turkish dry beans (*Phaseolus vulgaris* var. pinto) starches (Alamri et al., 2013) were investigated. The okra extract was added at 5%, 10%, and 15% of the starch to develop dry or wet blends. The properties of the starches were changed by decreasing viscosity, setback, and pseudoplasticity, gel hardness, and increasing syneresis of gels.

Studies have indicated that okra mucilage may be used as a suspending agent at 4% w/v, depending on its suspending ability and the stability of the resulting suspension (Kumar et al., 2009). Okra seed coagulant was effective in the removal of turbidity of surface water (Raji et al., 2015). The turbidities of the water samples were removed effectively at an optimum dose of 300 mg/L of the seed extract with optimum pH of about 7.0 from 745 NTU to 11 NTU for one water sample and from 580 NTU to 5 NTU in another sample. The coagulant in samples with initial turbidity of not more than 580 NTU could be reduced to WHO limit of 5 NTU (Raji et al., 2015).

Pectin was extracted from okra pods by using response surface methodology (Chen et al., 2014). The optimal extraction conditions that maximized the pectin yield were at a pH of 3.9, an extraction time of 64 min, an extraction temperature of 60°C, and a liquid–solid ratio of 42:1. Under these processing conditions, the pectin yield was at 2.71%. In another study, extracts rich in pectin were isolated by aqueous extraction at pH 4.0 and 6.0 from okra pods (Alba et al., 2013). They were examined in terms of their composition and emulsion stabilizing capacity in model acidic emulsions (hexadecane-in-water at pH 3.0). The okra extracts were strong in emulsification in acidic environments (Alba et al., 2013).

The extract from okra seeds is an alternative source for edible oil. Okra seeds contain 40% oil contents which could be an alternative source of edible oil (Chauhan, 1972). The greenish yellow edible oil has a pleasant taste and odor, and is high in unsaturated fats such as oleic acid and linoleic acid (Chauhan, 1972) which is essential for human nutrition (Kumar et al., 2013). Okra seed oil is rich in palmitic, oleic, and linoleic acids. The reported composition of okra seed oil is approximately (g/kg): 255–297 linoleic acids, 415–419 oleic acids, and 288–297 saturated acids (Crossley and Hilditch, 1951; Chisholm and Hopkins, 1957). Using time-domain nuclear magnetic resonance, the oil content of okra seeds was found to range between 12.36% and 21.56%, with values of linoleic acid being 23.6–50.65% and palmitic acids of 10.3–36.35% (Jarret et al., 2011). Brazilian okra oil has significant amounts of protein (22.14%), lipids (14.01%), and high amounts of unsaturated lipids (66.32%), especially the oleic (20.38%) and linoleic acids (44.48%) (de Sousa Ferreira Soares et al., 2012). The Brazilian okra oil was found to be similar to industrially used consumable oils, such as soybean oil when considering both oleic and linoleic acids, which are essential for human health. The high degree of unsaturation in the oil favors its use for consumption or for use in the pharmaceutical and chemical industries (Jarret et al., 2011). Oil analysis through pressurized differential scanning calorimetry revealed an oxidation temperature of 175.2°C (Jarret et al., 2011).

Okra gum was found to be an acceptable fat replacer in chocolate bar cookies (Romanchik-Cerpovicz et al., 2002). The moisture contents of fresh okra gum (28.3±0.4%) cookies were higher than high-fat cookies (8.5±0.3%) and remained higher after 48 hours ($P < 0.001$). The sensory scores for color, smell, flavor, aftertaste, moistness, and overall acceptability for fresh cookies were acceptable, yet lower for flavor and after taste in fat-free cookies than high fat ($P < 0.01$).

Maize ogi was supplemented with 10% and 20% toasted and untoasted okra meals. Yields of ogi were 67.8% while yields of the toasted and untoasted okra seed meals were 35.1% and 39.9%, respectively. Supplementing ogi with okra meal increased protein, ash, oil, and fiber contents, but reduced ogi viscosity (Akingbala et al., 2003).

The mature okra seeds are eaten cooked and when dried and ground are used as a coffee substitute called *café de pobre* in some Spanish-speaking areas (Kermath et al., 2014).

OKRA FOOD DISHES

Okra is cultivated for its green nonfibrous fruits or pods containing round seeds. The edible, elongated seed pods are harvested when immature and eaten like a gelatinous vegetable (Medagam et al., 2012). The leaf buds and flowers are also edible (Doijode, 2001). The relative amount (g/100 g fresh okra pods) of different parts of the okra pods by fresh weight and dry weight, respectively, are the calyx of 14.6 and 1.4, pulp of 71.9 and 7.4, and seed of 9.1 and 1.3 (Sengkhamparn et al., 2009). The okra pulp yields about 5.8 g/100 g fresh okra of alcohol-insoluble solid representing cell wall materials (Sengkhamparn et al., 2009).

The immature fruit pods are consumed as vegetables and can be served raw, marinated in salads, dried, fried, boiled, and consumed in different forms (Ndunguru and Rajabu, 2004; Youssef, 2008; Akintoye et al., 2011). Often the young pods and leaves and fruit extract are added to different recipes like slimy soups and sauces, and stews to increase the consistency (Awodoyin and Olubode, 2009; Gemede et al., 2014; Roy et al., 2014). Fibrousness of the pods increases rapidly after harvest, rendering them inedible.

In Thailand, okra is usually boiled in water resulting in slimy soups and sauces, which are relished. The fruits are also served as soup thickeners. Okra seed can be dried and is a nutritious material that can be used to prepare vegetable curds, or roasted and ground to be used as coffee additive (Moekchantuk and Kumar, 2004).

Some regional dishes containing okra are: (1) "callaloo," a thick soup-like dish in Trinidad and Tobago; (2) "cou-cou" as the main ingredient in the cornmeal-based dish in some West Indian islands, like Trinidad and Tobago and West Indies; (3) "bamya" dried okra as a starter in Turkey; (4) "bhindi ghosht" and "sambar" chopped pieces are stir-fried with spices, pickled, salted, or added to gravy-based preparations in India and Pakistan; (5) "yong tau foo" a dish stuffed with processed fish paste (surimi) and boiled with vegetables; (6) "pinakbet," "dinengdeng," and "sinigang" on the Philippines; (7) "jambo" a soup which is primarily prepared from okra mucilage with fish and "funchi," a dish made out of cornmeal in Curacao; (8) "bamia" or "bamya," cooked whole young okra pods in Bosnia and most of West Asia; (9) "Frango com quiabo" (chicken with okra) in Brazil; (10) "gumbo" a stew in the Gulf Coast of the United States and South Carolina; and (11) "canh chua" in Vietnam.

CONCLUDING REMARKS

The immature fruit pods are consumed as vegetables and could be served raw, marinated in salads, dried, fried, boiled, and served in various regional food dishes. Often the young pods and leaves and fruit extract are added to different recipes like slimy soups and sauces, and stews to increase the consistency.

Okra is one of the low fat foods with unique nutrients and phytochemical profiles and is particularly rich in dietary fiber, potassium, magnesium, manganese, vitamin C, folate, B1, B6, and vitamin K as well as bioactive components, such as flavonoids, especially quercetin and phytosterols. In fact, okra is one of the richest dietary sources of quercetin and phytosterols (β-sitosterol, sitosterol esters). Okra seeds have been reported to contain 10 times higher concentration of flavonols and almost 15 times of higher concentration of catechins compared to the skins. However, further research should be focused to find out the mechanism of action of the bioactive components at the molecular level. Okra seeds contain 40% oil, which is high in oleic acid and linoleic acid and therefore could be an alternative source of edible oil. Some pretreatments of okra seeds have been shown to reduce some nutrients and increase others.

The daily incorporation of okra to a diet may help in improving its quality and subsequently reduce the risk for the development of chronic noncommunicable diseases, such as obesity, diabetes, atherosclerosis, hypertension, cancer, and neurological disorders as well as NTDs. Increasing evidence suggests that the health benefits of fruits, whole grains, and vegetables including okra as well as other plant foods are attributed to the synergy or interactions of bioactive compounds and other nutrients in whole foods. Therefore, consumers should obtain their nutrients, antioxidants, bioactive compounds, or phytochemicals from their balanced diet with a wide variety of fruits, vegetables, whole grains, and other plant foods for optimal nutrition, health, and well-being, not from dietary supplements. Most of the studies with promising results on the health benefits of okra consumption in relation to disease prevention and management, especially diabetes, were either performed *in vitro* or *in vivo* with the use of animal models. Most of the scientific studies are *in vitro* which do provide some evidence to support the potential beneficial effects of okra components in lowering the risk for various chronic diseases, although the mechanisms of action are limited to date. Therefore, further research on the health benefits of okra is warranted, especially in human subjects.

There are many uses of okra mucilage, including its application for paper production, confectionery as well as medical applications (production of tablets, plasma replacement therapy, and antifungal drugs). Among the functional food applications, okra pectin and gum are used as fat replacer in cookies, which helps in reducing their energy content.

REFERENCES

Aburto, N.J., Hanson, S., Gutierrez, H., Hooper, L., Elliott, P., Cappuccio Cephalon, F.P., 2013. Effect of increased potassium intake on cardiovascular risk factors and disease: systematic review and meta-analyses. BMJ 346, f1378. http://dx.doi.org/10.1136/bmj.f1378.

ADA, 2008. Position of the American Dietetic Association: health implications of dietary fiber. J. Am. Diet Assoc. 108, 1716–1731.

Adelakun, O.E., Ade-Omowaye, B.I.O., Adeyemi, I.A., Van de Venter, M., 2010. Functional properties and mineral contents of a Nigerian okra seed (*Abelmoschus esculentus* Moench) flour as influenced by pretreatments. J. Food Technol. 8, 39–45.

Adelakun, O.E., Oyelade, O.J., Ade-Omowaye, B.I.O., Adeyemi, I.A., Venter, M., Van de Koekemoer, T.C., 2009. Influence of pre-treatment on yield chemical and antioxidant properties of a Nigerian okra seed (*Abelmoschus esculentus* moench) flour. Food Chem. Toxicol. 47, 657–661.

Adom, K.K., Dzogbefia, V.P., Ellis, W.O., 1997. Combined effect of drying time and slice thickness on the solar drying of okra. J. Sci. Food Agric. 73, 315–320.

Afkhami-Ardekani, M., Shojaoddiny-Ardekani, A., 2007. Effect of vitamin C on blood glucose, serum lipids and serum insulin in type 2 diabetes patients. Indian J. Med. Res. 126, 471–474.

Ahn, J., Lee, H., Suna, K., Park, J., Ha, T., 2008. The anti-obesity effect of quercetin is mediated by the AMPK and MAPK signaling pathways. Biochem. Biophys. Res. 373, 545–549.

Akanbi, W.B., Togun, A.O., Adediran, J.A., Ilupeju, E.A.O., 2010. Growth, dry matter and fruityields components of okra under organic and inorganic sources of nutrients. Am. Eur. J. Sustain. Agric. 4, 1–13.

Akingbala, J.O., Akinwande, B.A., Uzo-Peters, P.I., 2003. Effects of color and flavor changes on acceptability of ogi supplemented with okra seed meals. Plant Food Hum. Nutr. 58, 1–9.

Akintoye, H.A., Adebayo, A.G., Aina, O.O., 2011. Growth and yield response of okra intercropped with live mulches. Asian J. Agric. Res. 5, 146–153.

Akinyele, B.O., Temikotan, T., 2007. Effect of variation in soil texture on the vegetative and pod characteristics of okra (*Abelmoschus esculentus* (L.) Moench). Int. J. Agric. Res. 2, 165–169.

Alamri, M.S., Mohamed, A.A., Hussain, S., Almania, H.A., 2013. Legume starches and okra (*Abelmoschus esculentus*) gum blends: pasting, thermal, and viscous properties. Food Sci. Technol. Res. 19, 381–392.

Alba, K., Ritzoulis, C., Georgiadis, N., Kontogiorgos, V., 2013. Okra extracts as emulsifiers for acidic emulsions. Food Res. Int. 54, 1730–1737.

Amberg, G.C., Bonev, A.D., Rossow, C.F., Nelson, M.T., Santana, L.F., 2003. Modulation of the molecular composition of large conductance, Ca (2+) activated K(+) channels in vascular smooth muscle during hypertension. J. Clin. Invest. 112, 717–724.

Amran, H.A., Prasad, V.M., Saravanan, S., 2013. Effect of fym on growth, yield and fruits quality of okra (*Abelmoschus esculentus* L. Moench). IOSR J. Agric. Vet. Sci. 7, 7–12.

Anderson, J.W., Gilinsky, N.H., Deakins, D.A., 1991. Lipid responses of hypercholesterolemic men to oat-bran and wheat-bran intake. Am. J. Clin. Nutr. 54, 678–683.

Ando, K., Matsui, H., Fujita, M., Fujita, T., 2010. Protective effect of dietary potassium against cardiovascular damage in salt-sensitive hypertension: possible role of its antioxidant actions. Curr. Vasc. Pharmacol. 8, 59–63.

András, C.D., Simándi, B., Örsi, F., Lambrou, C., Missopolinou-Tatala, D., Panayiotou, C., et al., 2005. Supercritical carbon dioxide extraction of okra (*Hibiscus esculentus* L.) seeds. J. Sci. Food Agric. 85, 1415–1419.

Ansari, A.A., Sukhraj, K., 2010. Effect of vermiwash and vermicompost on soil parameters and productivity of okra (*Abelmoschus esculentus*) in Guyana. Afr. J. Agric. Res. 5, 1794–1798.

Antoniades, C., Antonopoulos, A.S., Tousoulis, D., Marinou, K., Stefanadis, C., 2009. Homocysteine and coronary atherosclerosis: from folate fortification to the recent clinical trials. Eur. Heart J. 30, 6–15.

Appel, L.J., 2010. ASH position paper: dietary approaches to lower blood pressure. J. Am. Soc. Hypertens. 4, 79–89.

Appel, L.J., Moore, T.J., Obarzanek, E., 1997. A clinical trial of the effects of dietary patterns on blood pressure. DASH collaborative research group. N. Engl. J. Med. 336, 1117–1124.

Arapitsas, P., 2008. Identification and quantification of polyphenolic compounds from okra seeds and skins. Food Chem. 110, 1041–1045.

Arlai, A., 2009. Effects of moisture heating and vacuum fry on organic and conventional okra quality. Asian J. Food Agro-Industry (Special Issue), S318–S324.

Arnaud, M.J., 2008. Update on the assessment of magnesium status. Br. J. Nutr. 99, S24–S36.

Arrigoni, O., De Tullio, M.C., 2002. Ascorbic acid: much more than just an antioxidant. Biochim. Biophys. Acta 1569, 1–9.

Ascherio, A., Rimm, E.B., Giovannucci, E.L., Colditz, G.A., Rosner, B., Willett, W.C., 1992. A prospective study of nutritional factors and hypertension among US men. Circulation 86, 1475–1484.

Aschner, J.L., Aschner, M., 2005. Nutritional aspects of manganese homeostasis. Mol. Aspects Med. 26, 353–362.

Awad, A.B., Barta, S.L., Fink, C.S., Bradford, P.G., 2008. β-sitosterol enhances tamoxifen effectiveness on breast cancer cells by affecting ceramide metabolism. Mol. Nutr. Food Res. 52, 419–426.

Awodoyin, R.O., Olubode, O.S., 2009. On field assessment of critical period of weed interference in okra [*Abelmoschus esculentus* (L.) Moench] field in Ibadan, a rainforest-savanna transition ecozone of Nigeria. Asian J. Food Agro-Industry (Special Issue), S288–S296.

Barbagallo, M., Dominguez, L.,J., Galioto, A., 2010. Oral magnesium supplementation improves vascular function in elderly diabetic patients. Magnes. Res. 23, 131–137.

Beaudin, A.E., Stover, P.J., 2009. Insights into metabolic mechanisms underlying folate-responsive neural tube defects: a minireview. Birth Defects Res. A Clin. Mol. Teratol. 85, 274–284.

Benjawan, C., Chutichudet, P., Kaewsit, S., 2007. Effect of green manures on growth yield and quality of green okra (*Abelmoschus esculentus* L.) har lium cultivar. Pakistan J. Biol. Sci. 10, 1028–1035.

Blom, H.J., Shaw, G.,M., den Heijer, M., Finnell, R.H., 2006. Neural tube defects and folate: case far from closed. Nat. Rev. Neurosci. 7, 724–731.

Boath, A.S., Grussu, D., Stewart, D., McDougall, G.J., 2012. Berry polyphenols inhibit digestive enzymes: a source of potential health benefits? Food Digest 3, 1–7.

Calisir, S., Özcan, M., Hacıseferoğulları, H., Yildiz, M.U., 2005. A study on some physico-chemical properties of Turkey okra (*Hibiscus esculenta*) seeds. J. Food Eng. 68, 73–78.

Chandra, J., 2010. Megaloblastic anemia: back in focus. Indian J. Pediatr. 77, 795–799.

Chaudhri, O.,B., Salem, V., 2008. Gastrointestinal satiety signals. Annu. Rev. Physiol. 70, 239–255.

Chauhan, D.V.S., 1972. Vegetable Production in India. RamPrasad and Sons, Agra, India.

Chen, C.P., 2008. Syndromes, disorders and maternal risk factors associated with neural tube defects (II). Taiwan J. Obstet. Gynecol. 47, 10–17.

Chen, Y., Zhang, J.-G., Sun, H.-J., Wei, Z.-J., 2014. Pectin from *Abelmoschus esculentus*: optimization of extraction and rheological properties. Int. J. Biol. Macromol. 70, 498–505.

Chisholm, M.J., Hopkins, C.Y., 1957. An oxygenated fatty acid from the seeds of *Hibiscus esculentus*. Can. J. Chem. 35, 358–364.

Chucktan, R., Fahey, G., Wright, W.L., McRorie, J., 2012. Viscous versus nonviscous soluble fiber supplements: mechanisms and evidence for fiber-specific health benefits. J. Am. Acad. Nurse Pract. 24, 476–487.

Comin-Anduix, B., Boren, J., Martinez, S., 2001. The effect of thiamine supplementation on tumour proliferation. A metabolic control analysis study. Eur. J. Biochem. 268, 4177–4182.

Crossley, A., Hilditch, T.P., 1951. The fatty acids and glycerides of okra seed oil. J. Sci. Food Agric. 2, 251–255.

Cumming, R.G., Mitchell, P., Smith, W., 2000. Diet and cataract: the Blue Mountains Eye Study. Ophthalmology. 107, 450–456.

Das, U.N., 2006. Essential fatty acids: biochemistry, physiology and pathology. Biotechnol. J. 1, 420–439.

Da Silva, V.R., Russell, K.A., Gregory 3rd, J.F., 2012. Vitamin B6. In: Erdman Jr, J.W., Macdonald, I.A., Zeisel, S.H. (Eds.), Present Knowledge in Nutrition, 10th ed. Wiley-Blackwell, Hoboken, NJ, pp. 307–320.

de Sousa Ferreira Soares, G., deMorais Gomes, V., dos Reis Albuquerque, A., Barbosa Dantas, Rosenhain, M.R., Gouveia de Souza, A., et al., 2012. Spectroscopic and thermooxidative analysis of organic okra oil and seeds from *Abelmoschus esculentus*. Sci. World J. Article ID 847471, 6 pages.

Dickinson, H.O., Nicolson, D.J., Campbell, F., 2006. Potassium supplementation for the management of primary hypertension in adults. Cochrane Database Syst. Rev. 3, CD004641.

Doijode, S.D., 2001. Seed Storage of Horticultural Crop. Food Product Press, New York.

Egert, S., Boesch-Saadatmandi, C., Wolffram, S., 2010. Serum lipid and blood pressure responses to quercetin vary in overweight patients by apolipoprotein E genotype. J. Nutr. 140, 278–284.

FAOSTAT, 2012. World Production of Okra. Statistics Division, Food and Agriculture Organization of the United Nations., http://faostat3.fao.org/download/Q/QC/E.

Faruque, O., 1995. Relationship between smoking and antioxidant status. Br. J. Nutr. 73, 625–632.

Ford, E.S., Mokdad, A.H., 2003. Dietary magnesium intake in a national sample of US adults. J. Nutr. 133, 2879–2882.

Freeland-Graves, J., Bose, T., Karbassian, A., 2005. Manganese metallotherapeutics. In: Gielen, M., Tiekink, E. (Eds.), Metallotherapeutic Drugs and Metal-Based Diagnostic Agents: The Use of Metals in Medicine, pp. 159–178. West Sussex, UK.

Fujiwara, N., Osanai, T., Kamada, T., Katoh, T., Takahashi, K., Okumura, K., 2000. Study on the relationship between plasma nitrite and nitrate level and salt sensitivity in human hypertension: modulation of nitric oxide synthesis by salt intake. Circulation 101, 856–861.

Gast, G.C.M., de Roos, N.M., Sluijs, I., Bots, M.L., Beulens, J.W., Geleijnse, J.M., 2009. A high menaquinone intake reduces the incidence of coronary heart disease. Nutr. Metab. Cardiovasc. Dis. 19, 504–510.

Gemede, H.F., Ratta, N., Haki, G.D., Ashagrie, Z., Beyene, W.D., 2014. Nutritional quality and health benefits of Okra (*Abelmoschus esculentus*): a review. Global J. Med. Res. 14, 29–37.

Gerhard, G.T., Duell, P.B., 1999. Homocysteine and atherosclerosis. Curr. Opin. Lipidol. 10, 417–428.

Gregory, J.F., 1997. Bioavailability of folate. Eur. J. Clin. Nutr. 51, 554–559.

Habib, N., Ashraf, M., Ali, Q., Perveen, R., 2012. Response of salt stressed okra (*Abelmoschus esculentus* Moench) plants to foliar-applied glycine betaine and glycine betaine containing sugarbeet extract. South Afr. J. Bot. 83, 151–158.

Haddy, F.J., Vanhoutte, P., M., Feletou, M., 2006. Role of potassium in regulating blood flow and blood pressure. Am. J. Physiol. Regul. Integr. Comp. Physiol. 290, R546–R552.

Haga, H., 1992. Effects of dietary magnesium supplementation on diurnal variations of blood pressure and plasma Na+, K+ -ATPase activity in essential hypertension. Jpn. Heart J. 33, 785–800.

Hatzistavri, L.S., Sarafidis, P.A., Georgianos, P.I., 2001. Oral magnesium supplementation reduces ambulatory blood pressure in patients with mild hypertension. Am. J. Hypertens. 22, 1070–1075.

He, J., Tell, G.S., Tang, Y.C., Mo, P.S., He, G., 1991. Relation of electrolytes to blood pressure in men. The Yi people study. Hypertension 17, 378–385.

Hedin, P.A., Lamar, P.L., Thompson, A.C., Minyard, J., 1968. Isolation and structural determination of 13 flavonoid glycosides in *Hibiscus esculentus* (okra). Am. J. Bot. 55, 431–437.

Howarth, N.C., Saltzman, E., Roberts, S.B., 2001. Dietary fiber and weight regulation. Nutr. Rev. 59, 129–139.

Hsu, C.L., Yen, G.C., 2006. Induction of cell apoptosis in 3T3-L1 pre-adipocytes by flavonoids is associated with their antioxidant activity. Mol. Nutr. Food Res. 50, 1072–1079.

Hussein, A.H., 2015. Formulation and evaluation of sustained release tablets of pentoxifylline using okra extract as a novel retardant. Int. J. Pharm. Pharm. Sci. 7, 204–208.

International Board for Plant Genetic Resources, 1990.

IOM: Institute of Medicine, 2005a. Dietary Reference Intakes for Energy, Carbohydrate, Fiber, Fat, Fatty Acids, Cholesterol, Protein, and Amino Acids. The National Academies Press, Washington, DC, <http://www.nap.edu/openbook.php?isbn=0309085373> (accessed 07.07.15.).

IOM: Institute of Medicine, 2005b. Dietary Reference Intakes for Vitamins and Minerals. The National Academies Press, Washington, DC, <http://www.nal.usda.gov/fnic/DRI/DRI_Tables/RDA_AI_vitamins_elements.pdf> (accessed 23.07.15.).

Ito, Y., Yamanaka, K., Susaki, H., Igata, A., 2012. A cross-investigation between thiamin deficiency and the physical condition of elderly people who require nursing care. J. Nutr. Sci. Vitaminol. 58, 210–216.

Jacques, P.F., Taylor, A., Moeller, S., 2005. Long-term nutrient intake and 5-year change in nuclear lens opacities. Arch. Ophthalmol. 123, 517–526.

Jain, N., 2012. A review on *Abelmoschus esculentus*. Pharmacacia 1, 1–8.

Jarret, R.L., Wang, M.L., Levy, I.J., 2011. Seed oil and fatty acid content in okra (*Abelmoschus esculentus*) and related species. J. Agric. Food Chem. 59, 4019–4024.

Jayaseelan, C., Ramkumar, R., Abdul Rahuman, A.A., Perumal, P., 2013. Green synthesis of gold nanoparticles using seed aqueous extract of *Abelmoschus esculentus* and its antifungal activity. Ind. Crops Prod. 45, 423–429.

Jenkins, D., J., Kendall, C.,W., Marchie, A., 2005. Direct comparison of a dietary portfolio of cholesterol-lowering foods with a statin in hypercholesterolemic participants. Am. J. Clin. Nutr. 81, 380–387.

Jenkins, D.J., Kendall, C.W., Marchie, A., Jenkins, A., L., Connelly, P.W., Jones, P.J., et al., 2003. The Garden of Eden-plant based diets, the genetic drive to conserve cholesterol and its implications for heart disease in the 21st century. Comp. Biochem. Physiol. A Mol. Integr. Physiol. 136, 141–151.

Katan, M.B., Grundy, S.,M., Jones, P., Law, M., Miettinen, T., Paoletti, R., 2003. Efficacy and safety of plant stanols and sterols in the management of blood cholesterol levels. Mayo Clin. Proc. 78, 965–978.

Kaur, K., Pathaki, M., Kaur, S., Pathak, D., Chawla, N., 2013. Assessment of morphological and molecular diversity among okra [*Abelmoschus esculentus* (L.) Moench.] germplasm. Afr. J. Biotechnol. 12, 3160–3170.

Keen, C.L., Ensunsa, J.L., Watson, M.H., Baly, D.L., Donovan, S.M., Monaco, M.H., et al., 1999. Nutritional aspects of manganese from experimental studies. Neurotoxicology 20, 213–223.

Kermath, B., Bennett, B.C., Pulsipher, L.M., 2014. Food Plants in the Americas. A Survey of the Domesticated, Cultivated, and Wild Plants Used for Human Food in North, Central, and South America and the Caribbean5.

Keum, N., Giovannucci, E.L., 2014. Folic acid fortification and colorectal cancer risk. Am. J. Prev. Med. 46, S65–S72.

Khan, A.M., Sullivan, L., McCabe, E., Levy, D., Vasan, R.S., Wang, T.J., 2010. Lack of association between serum magnesium and the risks of hypertension and cardiovascular disease. Am. Heart J. 160, 715–720.

Kim, J.H., Kang, M.J., Choi, H.N., 2011. Quercetin attenuates fasting and postprandial hyperglycemia in animal models of diabetes mellitus. Nutr. Res. Pract. 5, 107–111.

King, D.E., Mainous, A.G., Lambourne, C.A., 2012. Trends in dietary fiber intake in the United States, 1999–2008. J. Acad. Nutr. Diet. 112, 642–648.

Kobori, M., Masumoto, S., Akimoto, Y., Oike, H., 2011. Chronic dietary intake of quercetin alleviates hepatic fat accumulation associated with consumption of a Western-style diet in C57/BL6J mice. Mol. Nutr. Food Res. 55, 530–540.

Koren, G., 2011. Folic acid and colorectal cancer: unwarranted fears. Can. Fam. Physician 57, 889–890.

Kumar, D.S., Tony, D.E., Kumar, A.P., Kumar, K.A., Bramha, D., Rao, S., et al., 2013. A review on: *Abelmoschus esculentus* (okra). Int. Res. J. Pharm. Appl. Sci. (IRJPAS) 3, 129–132.

Kumar, R., Patil, M.B., Patil, S.R., Paschapur, M.S., 2009. Evaluation of *Abelmoschus esculentus* mucilage as suspending agent in paracetamol suspension. Int. J. PharmTech Res. 1 (3), 658–665.

Kuppusamy, U.R., Das, N.P., 1992. Effects of flavonoids on cyclic AMP phosphodiesterase and lipid mobilezation in rat adipocytes. Biochem. Pharma 44, 1307–1315.

Lamont, W.J., 1999. Okra–a versatile vegetable crop. Hortic. Technol. 9, 179–184.

Larkin, J.R., Zhang, F., Godfrey, L., 2012. Glucose-induced down regulation of thiamine transporters in the kidney proximal tubular epithelium produces thiamine insufficiency in diabetes. PLoS One 7, e53175.

Law, M.R., Wald, N.J., Thompson, S.G., 1994. By how much and how quickly does reduction in serum cholesterol concentration lower risk of ischaemic heart disease? BMJ 308, 367–372.

Li, Y., Schellhorn, H.E., 2007. New developments and novel therapeutic perspectives for vitamin C. J. Nutr. 137, 2171–2184.

Madisa, M.E., Mathowa, T., Mpofu, C., Oganne, T.A., 2015. Effects of plant spacing on the growth, yield and yield components of okra *(Abelmoschus esculentus L.)* in Botswana. Am. J. Exp. Agric. 6, 7–14.

Marineli, R.S., Marques, A.C., Furlan, C.P.B., Maróstica Jr., M.R., 2012. Antioxidant effects of the combination of conjugated linoleic acid and phytosterol supplementation in Sprague-Dawley rats. Food Res. Int. 49, 487–493.

Markose, B.L., Peter, K.V., 1990. Okra Review of Research on Vegetable and Tuber Crops. Kerala Agricultural University Press, Kerala, India.

Marlett, J.A., 2001. Dietary fiber and cardiovascular disease. In: Cho, S.S., Dreher, M.L. (Eds.), Handbook of Dietary Fiber Marcel Dekker, New York, pp. 17–30.

Mateus, R.F., 2011. Evaluation of Varieties and Cultural Practices of Okra (*Abelmoschus esculentus*) for Production in Massachusetts. Department of Plant, Soil and Insect Sciences, University of Massachusetts, Amherst42., Master of Science.

McCormick, D.B., 2006. Vitamin B6 In: Bowman, B.A. Russell, R.M. (Eds.), Present Knowledge in Nutrition, vol. I International Life Sciences Institute, Washington, DC, pp. 269–277.

Medagam, T.R., Kadiyala, H., Mutyala, G., Hameeddunnisa, B., 2012. Heterosis for yield and yield components in okra (*Abelmoschus esculentus* (L.) Moench). Chilean J. Agric. Res. 72, 316–325.

Meydani, S.N., Ribaya-Mercado, J.D., Russell, R.M., Sahyoun, N., Morrow, F.D., Gershoff, S.N., 1991. Vitamin B-6 deficiency impairs interleukin 2 production and lymphocyte proliferation in elderly adults. Am. J. Clin. Nutr. 53, 1275–1280.

Misawa, E., Tanaka, M., Nomaguchi, K., Yamada, M., Toida, T., Takase, M., et al., 2008. Administration of phytosterols isolated from Aloe vera gel reduce visceral fat mass and improve hyperglycemia in Zucker diabetic fatty (ZDF) rats. Obes. Res. Clin. Prac. 2, 239–245.

Moekchantuk, T., and Kumar, P. (2004). Export okra production in Thailand. Inter-country programme for vegetable IPM in South and SE Asia phase II. Food & Agriculture Organization of the United Nations, Bangkok, Thailand.

Monte, L.G., Santi-Gadelha, T., Reis, L.B., Braganhol, E., Prietsch, R.F., Dellagostin, O.A., et al., 2014. Lectin of *Abelmoschus esculentus* (okra) promotes selective antitumor effects in human breast cancer cells. Biotechnol. Lett. 36, 461–469.

Mota, W.F., Finger, F.L., Casali, V.W.D., 2000. Olericultura: Melhoramento Genético do Quiabeiro. UFV, Viçosa.144.

Motoyashiki, T., Morita, T., Ueki, H., 1996. Involvement of the rapid increase in cAMP content in the vanadate-stimulated release of lipoprotein lipase activity from rat fat pad. Biol. Pharm. Bull. 19, 1412–1416.

MRC Vitamin Study Research Group, 1991. Prevention of neural tube defects: results of the Medical Research Council Vitamin Study. Lancet 338, 131–137.

Nájera, M.O., Tinajero, I.S., Páez, L.I.R., Meza, S.E.T., Sánchez, J.L.M., 2013. Quercetin improves antioxidant response in diabetes through maintenance of reduced glutathione levels in blood. Afr. J. Pharm. Pharmacol. 7, 2531–2539.

Navarro, A., De las Heras, B., Villar, A., 2001. Anti-inflammatory and immunomodulating properties of a sterol fraction from *Sideritis foetens* Clem. Biol. Pharm. Bull. 24, 470–473.

Naz, A., Jamil, Y., ul Haq, Z., Iqbal, M., Ahmad, M.R., Ashraf, M.I., et al., 2012. Enhancement of the germination, growth, and yield of okra (*Abeslmoshus esculentus*) using pre-sowing magnetic treatment of seeds. Indian J. Biochem. Biophys. 49, 211–214.

Ndjouenkeu, R., Goycoolea, F.M., Morris, E.R., Akingbala, J.O., 1996. Rheology of okra (*Hibiscus esculentus* L.) and dika nut (*Irvingia gabonensis*) polysaccharides. Carbohydr Polym. 29, 263–269.

Ndunguru, J., Rajabu, A.C., 2004. Effect of okra mosaic virus disease on the above-ground morphological yield components of okra in Tanzania. Sci. Hortic. 99, 225–235.

Nwachukwu, E.C., Nulit, R.M., Go, R., 2014. Nutritional and biochemical properties of Malaysian okra variety. Adv. Med. Plant Res. 2, 16–19.

Ogundiran, O.A., 2013. The effect of combined application of poultry manure and sawdust on the growth and yield of okra. J. Agric. Sci. 5, 169–175.

Olivera, D.F., Mugridge, A., Chaves, A.R., Mascheroni, R.H., Viña, S.Z., 2012. Quality attributes of okra (*Abelmoschus esculentus* L. Moench) pods as affected by cultivar and fruit size. J. Food Res. 1, 224–235.

Ostlund Jr., R.E., 2002. Phytosterols in human nutrition. Annu. Rev. Nutr. 22, 533–549.

Ostlund Jr., R.E., McGill, J.B., Zeng, C.M., Covey, D.F., Stearns, J., Stenson, W.F., et al., 2002. Gastrointestinal absorption and plasma kinetics of soy Delta(5)-phytosterols and phytostanols in humans. Am. J. Physiol. Endocrinol. Metab. 282, E911–E916.

Palanuvej, C., Hokputsa, S., Tunsaringkarn, T., Ruangrungsi, N., 2009. *In vitro* glucose entrapment and alpha-glucosidase inhibition of mucilaginous substances from selected Thai medicinal plants. Sci. Pharm. 77, 837–849.

Paul, L., Ueland, P.M., Selhub, J., 2013. Mechanistic perspective on the relationship between pyridoxal 5′-phosphate and inflammation. Nutr. Rev. 71, 239–244.

Pawelec, G., Goldeck, D., Derhovanessian, E., 2014. Inflammation, ageing and chronic disease. Curr. Opin. Immunol. 29C, 23–28.

Piironen, V., Lindsay, D.G., Miettinen, T.A., Toivo, J., Lampi, A.-M., 2000. Plant sterols: biosynthesis, biological function and their importance to human nutrition. J. Sci. Food. Agric. 80, 939–966.

Preuss, H.G., 1997. Diet, genetics and hypertension. J. Am. Coll. Nutr. 16, 296–305.

Prvulovic, D., Hampel, H., 2011. Amyloid β (A-β) and phospho-τ (p-τ) as diagnostic biomarkers in Alzheimer's disease. Clin. Chem. Lab. Med. 49, 367–374.

Raji, Y.O., Abubakar, L., Giwa, S.O., Giwa, A., 2015. Assessment of coagulation efficiency of okra seed extract for surface water treatment. Int. J. Sci. Eng. Res. 6, 719–725.

Rattray, D., 2001. Okra, Roselle, Aibika and Kenaf (other edible *Hibiscus*), Okra, Recipes and Information. Okra Phtodisc, Inc.1–3

Rifaai, R.A., El-Tahawy N.F., Ali Saber E. and Ahmed, R. (2012) Effect of quercetin on the endocrine pancreas of the experimentally induced diabetes in male albino rats: a histological and immunohistochemical study. 1, 330. http://dx.doi.org/10.4172/scientificreports.330.

Romanchik-Cerpovicz, J.E., Tilmon, R.W., Baldree, K.A., 2002. Moisture retention and consumer acceptability of chocolate bar cookies prepared with okra gum as fat ingredient substitute. J. Am. Diet. Assoc. 102, 1301–1303.

Roy, A., Shrivastava, S.L., Mandal, S.M., 2014. Functional properties of okra *Abelmoschus esculentus* L. (Moench): traditional claims and scientific evidences. Plant Sci. Today 1, 121–130.

Sacks, F.M., Campos, H., 2010. Dietary therapy in hypertension. N. Engl. J. Med. 362, 2102–2112.

Sacks, F.M., Svetkey, L.P., Vollmer, W.M., Appel, L.J., 2001. For the DASH-sodium collaborative research group. Effects on blood pressure or reduced dietary sodium and the Dietary Approaches to Stop Hypertension (DASH) diet. N. Engl. J. Med. 344, 3–10.

Sahoo, P.K., Srivastava, A.P., 2002. Physical properties of okra seed. Biosyst. Eng. 83, 441–448.

Said, H.M., 2010. Thiamin. In: Paul, M.C., Joseph, M.B., Marc, R.B., Gordon, M.C., Mark, L., Joel, M., Jeffrey, D.W. (Eds.), Encyclopedia of Dietary Supplements, 2nd ed. Informa Healthcare, London and New York, pp. 748–753.

Sanderson, P., McNulty, H., Mastroiacovo, P., McDowell, I.F., Melse-Boonstra, A., Finglas, P.M., 2003. Folate bioavailability: UK Food Standards Agency Workshop Report. Br. J. Nutr. 90, 473–479.

Sarban, S., Isikan, U., Kocabey, Y., Kocyigit, A., 2007. Relationship between synovial fluid and plasma manganese, arginase, and nitric oxide in patients with rheumatoid arthritis. Biol. Trace. Elem. Res. 115, 97–106.

Savello, P.H., Martin, F.W., Hill, J.M., 1980. Nutritional composition of okra seed meal. J. Agric. Food Chem. 28, 1163–1166.

Sekhar, R.V., McKay, S.V., Patel, S.G., Guthikonda, A.P., Reddy, V.T., Balasubramanyam, A., et al., 2011. Glutathione synthesis is diminished in patients with uncontrolled diabetes and restored by dietary supplementation with cysteine and glycine. Diabetes Care 34, 162–167.

Selhub, J., Rosenberg, I.H., 2008. Public health significance of supplementation or fortification of grain products with folic acid. Food Nutr. Bull. 29, S173–S176.

Selhub, J., Bagley, L.C., Miller, J., Rosenberg, I.H., 2000. B vitamins, homocysteine, and neurocognitive function in the elderly. Am. J. Clin. Nutr. 71, 614S–620S.

Sengkhamparn, N., Sagis, L.M.C., Vries, R.D., Schols, H.A., Sajjaanantakul, T., Voragen, A.G.J., 2010. Physicochemical properties of pectins from okra (*Abelmoschus esculentus* (L.) Moench. Food Hydrocolloids 24, 35–41.

Sengkhamparn, N., Verhoef, R., Schols, H.A., Saijaanantakul, T., Voragen, A.G., 2009. Characterisation of cell wall polysaccharides from okra (*Abelmoschus esculentus* (L.) Moench). Carbohydr. Res. 344, 1824–1832.

Serot, J.M., Christmann, D., Dubost, T., Béne, M.C., Faure, G.C., 2001. CSF-folate levels are decreased in late-onset AD patients. J. Neural. Transm. 108, 93–99.

Sharma, N., Kulkarni, G.T., Sharma, A., Bhatnagar, A., Kumar, N., 2013. Natural mucoadhesive microspheres of *Abelmoschus esculentus* polysaccharide as a new carrier for nasal drug delivery. J. Microencapsul 30, 589–598.

Shearer, M.J., Newman, P., 2008. Metabolism and cell biology of vitamin K. Thromb. Haemost. 100, 530–547.

Shearer, M.J., Fu, X., Booth, S.L., 2012. Vitamin K nutrition, metabolism, and requirements: *current concepts and future research*. Adv. Nutr. 3, 182–195.

Shechter, M., 2010. Magnesium and cardiovascular system. Magnes. Res. 23, 60–72.

Slavin, J., Green, H., 2007. Dietary fibre and satiety. Nutr. Bull. 32, 32–42.

Sorapong, B., 2012. Okra (*Abelmoschus esculentus* (L.) Moench) as a valuable vegetable of the World. Ratar. Povrt. 49, 105–112.

Steward, L.K., Wang, Z., Ribnicky, D., 2009. Failure of dietary quercetin to alter the temporal progression of insulin resistance among tissues of C57BL/6J mice during the development of diet-induced obesity. Diabetologia 52, 514–523.

Stewart, L.K., Soileau, J.L., Ribnicky, D., 2008. Quercetin transiently increases energy expenditure but persistently decreases circulating markers of inflammation in C57BL/6J mice fed a high-fat diet. Metabolism 57 (Suppl. 1), S39–S46.

Sun, J., Chang, E.B., 2014. Exploring gut microbes in human health and disease: pushing the envelope. Genes Dis. 1, 132–139.

Surendra, P., Nawalagatti, C.M., Chetti, M.B., Hiremath, S.M., 2006. Effect of plant growth regulators and micronutrients on yield and yield components in okra. Karnataka J. Agric. Sci. 19, 264–267.

Taiye, O.A., Temitope, L.O., Igbokwe, C.C., Bolanle, A.A., 2013. Anti-*Helicobacter pylori* activity of *Abelmoschus esculentus* L. Moench (okra): an *in vitro* study. AJPAC 7, 330–336.

Talati, R., Sobieraj, D.M., Makanji, S.S., Phung, O.J., Coleman, C.I., 2010. The comparative efficacy of plant sterols and stanols on serum lipids: a systematic review and meta-analysis. J. Am. Diet Assoc. 110, 719–726.

Thornalley, P.J., Babaei-Jadidi, R., Al Ali, H., 2007. High prevalence of low plasma thiamine concentration in diabetes linked to a marker of vascular disease. Diabetologia 50, 2164–2170.

Thurnham, D.I., 1994. β-Carotene, are we misreading the signals in risk groups? Some analogies with vitamin C. Proc. Nutr. Soc. 53, 557–569.

Tindall, H.D., 1983. Vegetables in the Tropics. Macmillan Press Ltd., London and Basingstoke.25–328.

Trautwein, E.A., Kunath-Rau, A., Erbersdobler, H.F., 1999. Increased fecal bile acid excretion and changes in the circulating bile acid pool are involved in the hypocholesterolemic and gallstone-preventive actions of psyllium in hamsters. J. Nutr. 129, 896–902.

Uka, U.N., Chukwuka, K.S., Iwuagwu, M., 2013. Relative effect of organic and inorganic fertilizers on the growth of okra (*Abelmoschus esculentus* (L.) Moench). J. Agric. Sci. 58, 159–166.

Van Leer, E.M., Seidell, J.C., Kromhout, D., 1995. Dietary calcium, potassium, magnesium and blood pressure in the Netherlands. Int. J. Epidemiol. 24, 1117–1123.

Vaquero, M.P., 2002. Magnesium and trace elements in the elderly: intake, status and recommendations. J. Nutr. Health Aging 6, 147–153.

Wein, S., Behm, N., Petersen, R.K., 2010. Quercetin enhances adiponectin secretion by a PPARγ independent mechanism. Eur. J. Pharm. Sci. 41, 16–22.

Whelton, P.K., He, J., Cutler, J.A., 1997. Effects of oral potassium on blood pressure: meta-analysis of randomized controlled clinical trials. JAMA 277, 1624–1632.

Wilhelm, M., Fishman, J., Pontikis, R., Aubertin, A., Wilhelm, F., 2002. Susceptibility of recombinant porcine endogenous retrovirus reverse transcriptase to nucleoside and non-nucleoside inhibitors. Cell Mol. Life Sci. 59, 2184–2190.

Woolfe, M.L., Chaplin, M.F., Otchere, G., 1977. Studies on the mucilages extracted from okra fruits (*Hibiscus esculentus* L.) and baobab leaves (*Adansonia digitata* L.). J. Sci. Food Agric. 28, 519–529.

World Health Organization, 2012. Effect of Increased Potassium Intake on Cardiovascular Disease, Coronary Heart Disease and Stroke, Geneva, Switzerland.

World Health Organization, 2015. Fact sheet: obesity and overweight. <http://www.who.int/mediacentre/factsheets/fs311/en/> (accessed 16.07.15.).

Wu, K., Platz, E.A., Willett, W.C., Fuchs, C.S., Selhub, J., Rosner, B.A., 2009. A randomized trial on folic acid supplementation and risk of recurrent colorectal adenoma. Am. J. Clin. Nutr. 90, 1623–1631.

Wu, W., Kang, S., Zhang, D., 2013. Association of vitamin B6, vitamin B12 and methionine with risk of breast cancer: a dose–response meta-analysis. Br. J. Cancer 109, 1926–1944.

Ying, H., Jiang, H., Liu, H., Chen, F., Du, Q., 2014. Ethyl acetate-*n*-butanol gradient solvent system for high-speed countercurrent chromatography to screen bioactive substances in okra. J. Chromatogr. A 1359, 117–123.

Ying, W.Z., Aaron, K., Want, P.X., Sanders, P.W., 2009. Potassium inhibits dietary salt-induced transforming growth factor-beta production. Hypertension 54, 115.

Youssef, M.S., 2008. Studies on mycological status of sundried Jew's-mallow leaves and okra fruits in Egypt. Res. J. Microbiol. 3, 375–385.

Zhang, Q., Yang, G., Li, W., 2011. Thiamine deficiency increases beta-secretase activity and accumulation of beta-amyloid peptides. Neurobiol. Aging 32, 42–53.

Zodape, S.T., Kawarkhe, V.J., Patolia, J.S., Warade, A.D., 2008. Effect of liquid seaweed fertilizer on yield and quality of okra (*Abelmoschus esculentus* L.). J. Sci. Ind. Res. 67, 1115–1117.

Chapter 19

Fruit and vegetable consumption in the United States: patterns, barriers and federal nutrition assistance programs

Ming-Chin Yeh, Marian Glick-Bauer and Seren Wechsler
City University of New York, New York, NY, United States

CHAPTER OUTLINE

FRUIT AND VEGETABLE CONSUMPTION IN THE UNITED STATES

The Dietary Guidelines for Americans, 2010, lists among its key recommendations that individuals should increase fruit and vegetable intake and "eat a variety of vegetables, especially dark green and red and orange vegetables and beans and peas." These recommendations were based upon three key factors: (1) fruits and vegetables contribute to underconsumed nutrients in the United States, including folate, magnesium, potassium, dietary fiber, and vitamins A, C, and K; (2) consumption of fruits and vegetables is associated with a decrease in chronic diseases; (3) most fruits and vegetables are relatively low in calories when prepared without added sugar or fat (USDA and USDHHS, 2010).

Fruits, Vegetables, and Herbs.
DOI: http://dx.doi.org/10.1016/B978-0-12-802972-5.00019-6

However, most Americans over age 2 fail to meet the recommended 2.5 cups of vegetables per day, with usual consumption of only 1.6 cups. Americans over the age of 4 consume only 1 cup of fruit and juice per day, meeting only half of the USDA recommendations (USDA and USDHHS, 2010). According to the Healthy People 2020 Leading Health Indicators, the mean daily intake of total vegetables has remained unchanged between 2001–04 and 2007–10. Mean daily intake by persons age 2 and older was 0.8 cup equivalents of total vegetables per 1000 calories (age adjusted), or 37.5% below the 2020 target of 1.1 cup equivalents per 1000 calories (USDHHS, 2014). The Healthy Eating Index (HEI-2010) indicates that Americans are particularly deficient in consumption of dark green vegetables, beans, and peas. The 2010 USDA Food Patterns found that intakes of the "Greens and Beans" subgroup of vegetables were furthest from recommended levels (Guenther et al., 2013).

Intake of fruits and vegetables varies across regions and demographics. Among the American public, age, gender, income, and ethnic differences may influence consumption rates for fresh produce, with lower consumption among children than adults, and greater consumption by women and those living in higher income households (Hoelzer et al., 2012). Among children, no sociodemographic group met the Healthy People 2020 target for vegetable consumption between 2003 and 2010, while only children aged 2–5 years met the target for fruit intake (Kim et al., 2014). Adults living in the rural United States are less likely to consume five or more daily servings of fruits and vegetables than nonrural adults (Lutfiyya et al., 2012). In 2009, 32.5% of US adults consumed fruit two or more times per day and 26.3% consumed vegetables three or more times per day, but consumption varied considerably by consumer characteristics. Greatest fruit and vegetable intake was found for women, persons aged ≥65 years, college graduates, persons with annual household incomes ≥$50,000, and persons with a body mass index (BMI) in the healthy range of <25 kg/m^2 (Grimm et al., 2010).

VEGETARIAN DIETS IN THE UNITED STATES

A 2012 Gallup survey on consumption habits found that approximately 5% of the 1014 adults polled identified themselves as vegetarian, a rate that has remained steady since 1999 (Newport, 2012). As recently as the 1970s though, apprehensive, mainstream society believed that vegetarians held affiliations with underground sects and antiestablishment groups (Weinsier, 2000). Throughout the 1960s and 1970s, the overriding belief was that vegetarians faced an increased risk of developing nutritional deficiency diseases when compared to omnivores. A systematic review of relevant literature from 1966 to 1995 found that up until 1975, half of the published work on vegetarian diets documented nutritional insufficiencies. However, this percentage decreased substantially over the next two decades as articles increasingly focused on preventive and therapeutic applications of vegetarian diets (Sabate et al., 1999). Today the typical vegetarian is young, female, concerned with animal welfare, personal health, or both, and has followed a vegetarian diet for greater than 10 years (Hoffmann et al., 2013).

Vegetarianism is a generic term that encompasses a variety of distinct dietary patterns, each involving at least a relative avoidance of meat (Craig and Mangels, 2009). Vegetarianism in common usage may refer to any of these patterns, as well as to the exclusion of only red meat, often termed "semi-vegetarian." Pesco-vegetarianism refers to diets that allow fish but not other meat products. Lacto-ovo-vegetarianism permits the consumption of dairy products and eggs, while lacto-vegetarianism allows for dairy products but not eggs. Veganism is the strict avoidance of all animal products, including meat, fish eggs, dairy foods, and often honey (Craig and Mangels, 2009). Adherents of vegetarian diets may further distinguish themselves with additional food restrictions or philosophical tenets. For example, adherents of the macrobiotic diet follow a low-fat, high-fiber, high-complex carbohydrate diet that follows a spiritual philosophy of life (Lerman, 2010). Followers of the raw vegan diet, commonly referred to as the Living Food Movement, consume no foods that have been cooked, relying on a diet of germinated seeds, sprouts, cereals, vegetables, fruits, berries, and nuts (Hobbs, 2005).

A cross-sectional analysis of nearly 90,000 participants' food consumption patterns found that vegetarians consume comparatively more vegetables, fruits, avocados, legumes, whole grains, nonfried potatoes, soy foods, seeds, and nuts. Not surprisingly, vegetarians consumed lesser amounts of meats, dairy foods, and eggs but their intake was also characterized by attendant reductions in refined grains, added fats (particularly shortenings and margarines), snack foods, sweets, and nonwater beverages (Orlich et al., 2014). Thus vegetarian diets may differ from the typical American diet by more than just an avoidance of animal products.

Nutrient intake profiles vary among the categories of vegetarian diets. For example, a recent study found pesco-vegetarians have the highest intake of omega-3 fatty acids, as well as vitamins E and D, while vegans appear to have higher intakes of fiber, soy protein, folate, vitamins C and E, and β-carotene (Rizzo et al., 2013). Traditionally, low dietary intakes of iron, calcium, omega-3 fatty acids, zinc, and vitamins B12 and D, have been a concern for those following a vegan diet (Craig, 2009). However, the above study found that mean intake values for all of these nutrients exceed minimum requirements among vegan adherents, likely due to the modern practice of fortifying foods (Rizzo et al., 2013). A cross-sectional analysis of the nutritional profiles of 1475 omnivores, and four types of vegetarians, found very few differences among the vegetarian diets, with the exception of the vegan diet. For most nutrients, contrasts were most apparent between omnivores and vegans, with the latter having the lowest total energy and protein intake, but a better fat profile and the highest dietary fiber intake (Clarys et al., 2014).

The HEI-2010 and Mediterranean Diet Score both identify vegans as having the highest diet quality while omnivores received the lowest (Clarys et al., 2014). Nonetheless, strict dietary restrictions pose some risk of micronutrient deficiencies, including vitamin B12, iron, zinc, bone nutrients, and omega-3 fatty acids. Vitamin B12, or cobalamin, is a water-soluble vitamin necessary for DNA synthesis, red blood cell formation and neurologic function. Vitamin B12, which is synthesized by bacteria and Archaea, is found almost exclusively in animal products, and thus vegetarians, and particularly vegans, are at increased risk for developing deficiency. Low levels of serum B12 are associated with elevated levels of homocysteine, which is a risk factor for heart disease. A systematic literature review found that among vegetarians, vitamin B12 deficiency ranged from 0 to 86.5% with the highest prevalence among vegans who do not consume fortified foods (Pawlak et al., 2014). Biologically active vitamin B12 has been found in substantial amounts in dried seaweed, notably purple laver (Takenaka et al., 2001), which may be a suitable source of this vitamin for vegetarians, in addition to supplements.

Although plant foods contain less concentrated and less bioavailable sources of iron and zinc than does meat, these minerals can be obtained at satisfactory levels with a balanced and diverse vegetarian diet, especially when absorption is enhanced by concomitant intake of vitamin C (Gibson et al., 2014). Multiple foods may inhibit the absorption of iron, including the polyphenolic compounds in tea. The high phytate content of legumes, nuts, unrefined cereals, and oleaginous seeds may also act to inhibit both zinc and nonheme iron absorption. However, the high vitamin C content of vegetarian diets, along with leavened whole grains and fermented soy foods may further enhance absorption of both minerals (Gibson et al., 2014).

Dietary exclusion of all animal products may lead to inadequate intakes of calcium, vitamin D, vitamin B12, protein, and omega-3 fatty acids, leading to impaired bone health (Tucker, 2014). However, a plant-based diet that meets the Dietary Reference Intakes for calcium and protein, and includes fortified foods is sufficient for bone health (Mangels, 2014). Vitamin D is naturally present in very few foods, but needs can be met through exposure to sufficient sunlight or supplements (Biancuzzo et al., 2013). Preformed omega-3 polyunsaturated fatty acids (*n*-3 PUFA) can be found in marine sources as eicosapentaenoic acid (EPA) and docosahexaenoic acid (DHA), and in plant sources as α-linolenic acid (ALA). Dietary exclusion of fish may elevate the ratio of *n*-6 to *n*-3 PUFA, with potentially adverse cardiovascular effects (Mann et al., 2006; Sarter et al., 2015). However, vegetarians who do not consume fish can avoid an imbalance of essential fatty acids with the inclusion of soybeans, flaxseed, and walnuts, which are excellent sources of ALA, or algal-derived *n*-3 PUFA (Sarter et al., 2015). Thus carefully designed vegetarian diets can avoid nutrient deficiencies while promoting substantial health benefits (Craig and Mangels, 2009).

BARRIERS TO FRUIT AND VEGETABLE CONSUMPTION

Ironically, even as vegetarian diets have gained in acceptance in the United States, current fruit and vegetable consumption fails to meet the recommendations of The Dietary Guidelines for Americans, 2010 (USDA and USDHHS, 2010). Numerous factors impact the public's ability to meet the Health and Human Services recommendations for fruit and vegetable consumption. Even when there is awareness of the health benefits of a diet rich in fruits and vegetables, multiple impediments exist to reduce adequate intake including cost and time constraints, early home food environment, and limited access to fresh produce (Yeh et al., 2008), as well as psychosocial determinants such as limited health literacy (Speirs et al., 2012; Song et al., 2014; Colón-Ramos et al., 2014).

The most fundamental barrier to fulfilling goals for fruit and vegetable consumption may be that the US food supply is not aligned with healthy eating guidelines. An analysis of the food supply data from the past 40 years found that consumption of fruit, vegetables, greens and beans, whole grains, dairy, and sodium were below half of the optimal healthy eating goals, indicating that the quality of the US food supply may not be up to the standards set by the HEI-2010 (Miller et al., 2015). Thus the federal dietary guidelines are misaligned with the food supply available to the American public.

Neighborhood racial composition, income, and rurality all play a role in the availability of healthy food. Rural residents have lower rates of fruit and vegetable consumption than their urban counterparts, and consumption is lowest among low-income rural residents (McGuirt et al., 2014). Yet low-income urban neighborhoods also tend to lack available fresh produce. A study of food deserts in Leon County, FL found that neighborhoods characterized as primarily Black had no supermarkets and 16.7% of county neighborhoods had no Supplemental Nutrition Assistance Program (SNAP)-accepting stores (Rigby et al., 2012).

It is unclear whether simply providing grocery stores or access to fresh produce in urban "food deserts" will enhance fruit and vegetable consumption. A study of 19 corner stores in Hartford, CT found that increasing the variety of fruits and vegetables offered significantly increased the probability of produce purchase by food-insecure and low-income residents, most notably with SNAP customers (Cho and Blaser, 2012). However, a recent study of two high-need communities in the Bronx, NY found that the addition of a government-subsidized supermarket in one community produced no significant difference in the availability of healthful and unhealthful foods in the home or in children's dietary intake (Elbel et al., 2015).

The key to increasing fruit and vegetable consumption may be to shift focus away from traditional large-scale supermarkets as the sole source of produce for underserved customers, both urban and rural. Alternative sources of produce include not only farmers markets and curbside produce vendors, but convenience stores, dollar stores, mass merchandizers, and pharmacies (Sharkey et al., 2010; Brinkley et al., 2013). A study of produce availability in rural Texas found that although the supermarkets offered the greatest variety of fruits and vegetables, among nontraditional food outlets, dollar stores offered the greatest variety (Sharkey et al., 2010). Geographic information systems-based research on benefit usage of the SNAP in Minneapolis and St Paul indicate that in low-income neighborhoods, convenience stores and mid-sized grocers play a large role in resident's food shopping, though low-income residents often travel outside their neighborhood to get food (Shannon, 2014).

One approach to increasing access to fruits and vegetables in underserved neighborhoods has been to introduce curbside produce vendors. A study of curbside produce vendors in a low- and middle-income African American section of Philadelphia found that vendors provide culturally appropriate produce as well as common fruits and vegetables at lower cost than conventional food stores (Brinkley et al., 2013). Among SNAP participants of Fayette County, KY, living within a half mile of a farmers market or produce stand increased the odds of consuming one or more servings of vegetables daily (Gustafson et al., 2013).

Both food cost and "time poverty" may contribute toward a growing disparity in diet quality between affluent Americans and low-income households, the latter relying on convenience foods with a lower consumption of vegetables and fruit (Rehm et al., 2015; Drewnowski and Eichelsdoerfer, 2010). HEI-2010 scores from 11,181 adults in the 2007–10 NHANES were analyzed together with diet cost. Lower diet costs were positively associated with lower HEI-2010 scores, with lower consumption of produce, whole grains and seafood and greater consumption of refined grains, solid fat, alcohol, and added sugars (Rehm et al., 2015). Among low-income households, fruits and vegetables are often limited to iceberg lettuce, potatoes, canned corn, bananas, and frozen orange juice (Drewnowski and Eichelsdoerfer, 2010). Food price data similarly indicates that areas with higher costs for fresh fruits and vegetables are associated with higher BMI in local children (Morrissey et al., 2014). While some cost analyses find that healthy foods, including fresh produce, are affordable at any income bracket (Carlson and Frazão, 2014), there is the counter argument that low-income American households purchase a lower quality diet than do more affluent households, in part due to a lack of time to shop for and prepare fresh food (Drewnowski and Eichelsdoerfer, 2010). An analysis of 10,247 households found a significant relationship between food insecurity, SNAP participation, and the time devoted to meal preparation, eating, and grocery shopping (Beatty et al., 2014). Similarly, cost and travel time have been identified as barriers to fruit and vegetable consumption among low-income communities in North Carolina (Haynes-Maslow et al., 2013).

Lastly, nutrition knowledge, and health literacy in general, are important factors affecting fruit and vegetable intake. Surveys of SNAP-eligible adults found that 37–43.5% of the sample had adequate health literacy (Speirs et al., 2012; Song et al., 2014). The challenge is that populations with the lowest intake of fresh produce may also be the least likely to seek out nutrition or health information. An analysis of the 2007–08 US National Cancer Institute's Health Information National Trends Survey in the United States and in Puerto Rico found that respondents who reported never seeking information on health or medical topics also reported significantly lower fruit and vegetable intake and were less likely to follow dietary recommendations regarding adequate fruit and vegetable consumption (Colón-Ramos et al., 2014).

PROMOTING FRUIT AND VEGETABLE CONSUMPTION

In 2010, 14.5% of Americans were food insecure. The percent of households that were "... uncertain of having, or unable to acquire, enough food because had insufficient money or other resources" dramatically increased in 2008 and remained high throughout 2010 (Gundersen, 2013). Numerous federal nutrition assistance programs have been developed to help struggling Americans meet the Dietary Guidelines. The SNAP is the largest food assistance program in the United States. One in seven Americans participate in SNAP each month, which has been shown to reduce the percentage of participating households who report food insecurity and severe insecurity by up to 19% (Mabli and Ohls, 2015). Other programs include the Special Supplemental Nutrition Program for Women, Infants, and Children (WIC), and the National School Lunch and School Breakfast Programs (NSLP/SBP) (Yaktine and Murphy, 2013). Recent enhancements to these federal programs have sought to increase fruit and vegetable consumption.

In 2009, the US Department of Agriculture created a revision called The Special Supplemental Nutrition Program for WIC, mandating that WIC-certified vendors offer fresh produce, whole grains and reduced fat milk. The policy revision also made changes to the WIC food package, adding cash-value vouchers (CVVs) for women and children for the purchase of fruits and vegetables, including jarred baby foods (Agriculture, D.o., 2014). These significant revisions to the federal food and nutrition assistance program had an impact not only on participants' shopping habits, but on retail providers as well. With 49,000 authorized retailers affected nationwide, this policy had the potential to increase fruit and vegetable availability to neighborhoods previously lacking in healthy foods (Zenk et al., 2012, 2014).

A 2-year study of scanner data on grocery purchases in two New England states with 2137 WIC-participating households found that purchases of fresh and frozen fruits and vegetables increased up to 27.8% with the implementation of cash-value vouchers for produce. The participants allocated three times more vouchers to fruit purchases than to vegetables, adding almost 1 kg of fresh fruit per household per month (Andreyeva and Luedicke, 2014). A study of California WIC participants found that two-thirds of participants preferred to use the CVVs for fresh fruits and vegetables over jarred baby fruits and vegetables (Kim et al., 2013). Corner stores in Hartford, CT with WIC certification significantly increased their offering of these healthy foods compared to stores without certification (Havens et al., 2012). Similarly, improvements in fruit and vegetable availability were found in a study of seven Northern Illinois counties after implementation of the new policy (Zenk et al., 2012).

The National School Lunch Program expanded the Fresh Fruit and Vegetable Program (FFVP) in 2008 to provide free fruit and vegetables to students in participating elementary schools nationwide (Food and Nutrition Services, 2014). In 2009–10, 24.5% of public elementary schools were included in the expanded FFVP program, with participation associated with healthier food availability and greater fruit offerings at meals (Ohri-Vachaspati et al., 2012). In 2012, the 2010 Healthy, Hunger-Free Kids Act introduced a new school food menu pattern. The new menu included criteria for providing two servings of vegetables and one serving of fruit per lunch meal, including dark green and red/orange vegetables as well as legumes, in accordance with the Dietary Guidelines for Americans (USDA, 2012). A 2011 pilot study of Houston elementary schools found that students at schools with the new menu guidelines were selecting and consuming significantly more vegetables than students at control schools (Cullen et al., 2015). Thus federal programs have made significant strides in the past few years not only to help alleviate food insecurity, but to align America's eating habits with the Dietary Guidelines, and to encourage greater fruit and vegetable consumption among those most at nutritional risk.

CONCLUSION

Despite the consistent prevalence of vegetarianism in the United States since the 1990s, and the increased funding for federal programs to promote greater consumption of produce, the majority of the US population nonetheless fails to meet the recommendations for fruit and vegetable consumption set by the Dietary Guidelines for Americans, 2010 (USDA and USDHHS, 2010; USDHHS, 2014). Possible barriers to adequate fruit and vegetable consumption in the United States includes inadequacies in the US food supply, poor availability of fresh produce in rural areas and underserved urban neighborhoods, food costs and "time poverty," and poor health literacy. Federal programs including SNAP, the Special Supplemental Nutrition Program for WIC, and the FFVP have made strides in improving availability and consumption of fruits and vegetables for those most at risk of nutritional inadequacy. However, further efforts are needed to align Americans' eating habits with the USDA's goals for fruit and vegetable consumption.

REFERENCES

Agriculture, D.o., 2014. Special Supplemental Nutrition Program for Women, Infants and Children (WIC): Revisions in the WIC Food Packages; Final Rule. Federal Register.

Andreyeva, T., Luedicke, J., 2014. Incentivizing fruit and vegetable purchases among participants in the Special Supplemental Nutrition Program for Women, Infants, and Children. J. Public Health Nutr. 9, 1–9.

Beatty, T.K., Nanney, M.S., Tuttle, C., 2014. Time to eat? The relationship between food security and food-related time use. Public Health Nutr. 17 (1), 66–72.

Biancuzzo, R., et al., 2013. Serum concentrations of 1,25-dihydroxyvitamin D2 and 1,25-dihydroxyvitamin D3 in response to vitamin D2 and vitamin D3 supplementation. J. Clin. Endocrinol. Metab. 98, 973–979.

Brinkley, C., Chrisinger, B., Hillier, A., 2013. Tradition of healthy food access in low-income neighborhoods: price and variety of curbside produce vending compared to conventional retailers. J. Agric. Food Syst. Community Dev. 4 (1), 155–169.

Carlson, A., Frazão, E., 2014. Food costs, diet quality and energy balance in the United States. Physiol. Behav. 134, 20–31.

Cho, I., Blaser, M.J., 2012. The human microbiome: at the interface of health and disease. Nat. Rev. Genet. 13 (4), 260–270.

Clarys, P., et al., 2014. Comparison of nutritional quality of the vegan, vegetarian, semi-vegetarian, pesco-vegetarian and omnivorous diet. Nutrients 6 (3), 1318–1332.

Colón-Ramos, U., et al., 2014. The association between fruit and vegetable intake, knowledge of the recommendations, and health information seeking within adults in the U.S. mainland and in Puerto Rico. J. Health Commun., 1–7.

Craig, W.J., 2009. Health effects of vegan diets. Am. J. Clin. Nutr. 89 (Suppl.), 1627S–1633S.

Craig, W.J., Mangels, A.R., 2009. Position paper of the American Dietetic Association: vegetarian diets. J. Am. Diet. Assoc. 109 (7), 1266–1282.

Cullen, K., et al., 2015. Differential improvements in student fruit and vegetable selection and consumption in response to the new national school lunch program regulations: a pilot study. J. Acad. Nutr. Diet. 115 (5), 743–750.

Drewnowski, A., Eichelsdoerfer, P., 2010. Can low-income americans afford a healthy diet? Nutr. Today 44 (6), 246–249.

Elbel, B., et al., 2015. Assessment of a government-subsidized supermarket in a high-need area on household food availability and children's dietary intakes. Public Health Nutr. 26, 1–10.

Food and Nutrition Services, U., August 20, 2014. Fresh Fruit and Vegetable Program. Available from: <http://www.fns.usda.gov/sites/default/files/FFVPFactSheet.pdf>. Accessed May 3, 2015.

Gibson, R., Heath, A., Szymlek-Gay, E., 2014. Is iron and zinc nutrition a concern for vegetarian infants and young children in industralized countries? Am. J. Clin. Nutr. 100 (Suppl. 1), 459S–468S.

Grimm, K., Blanck, H., Scanlon, K., 2010. State-specific trends in fruit and vegetable consumption among adults—United States, 2000–2009. MMWR 59, 35.

Guenther, P., et al., 2013. Update of the Healthy Eating Index: HEI-2010. J. Acad. Nutr. Diet. 113 (4), 569–580.

Gundersen, C., 2013. Food insecurity is an ongoing national concern. Adv. Nutr. 4, 36–41.

Gustafson, A., et al., 2013. Neighbourhood and consumer food environment is associated with dietary intake among Supplemental Nutrition Assistance Program (SNAP) participants in Fayette County, Kentucky. Public Health Nutr. 16 (7), 1229–1237.

Havens, E., et al., 2012. Federal nutrition program changes and healthy food availability. Am. J. Prev. Med. 43 (4), 419–422.

Haynes-Maslow, L., et al., 2013. A qualitative study of perceived barriers to fruit and vegetable consumption among low-income populations, North Carolina, 2011. Prev. Chronic Dis. 10, E34.

Hobbs, S., 2005. Attitudes, practices, and beliefs of individuals consuming a raw foods diet. Explore 1 (4), 272–277.

Hoelzer, K., et al., 2012. Produce consumption in the United States: an analysis of consumption frequencies, serving sizes, processing forms, and high consuming population subgroups for microbial risk assessment. J. Food Prot. 75 (2), 328–340.

Hoffmann, S., et al., 2013. Differences between health and ethical vegetarians. Strength of conviction, nutrition knowledge, dietary restriction, and duration of adherence. Appetite 65, 139–144.

Kim, L., et al., 2013. Mothers prefer fresh fruits and vegetables over jarred baby fruits and vegetables in the new special supplemental nutrition program for women, infants, and children food pack. J. Nutr. Educ. Behav. 45 (6), 723–727.

Kim, S., Morre, L., Galuska, D., 2014. Vital signs: fruit and vegetable intake among children—United States, 2003–2010. MMWR 63 (31), 671–676.

Lerman, R., 2010. The macrobiotic diet in chronic disease. Nutr. Clin. Pract. 25 (6), 621–626.

Lutfiyya, M., Chang, L., Lipsky, M., 2012. A cross-sectional study of US rural adults' consumption of fruits and vegetables: do they consume at least five servings daily? BMC Public Health 12, 280.

Mabli, J., Ohls, J., 2015. Supplemental nutrition assistance program participation is associated with an increase in household food security in a national evaluation. J. Nutr. 145 (2), 344–351.

Mangels, A., 2014. Bone nutrients for vegetarians. Am. J. Clin. Nutr. 100 (Suppl. 1), 469S–475S.

Mann, N., et al., 2006. Fatty acid composition of habitual omnivore and vegetarian diets. Lipids 41 (7), 637–646.

McGuirt, J., et al., 2014. Factors influencing local food procurement among women of reproductive age in rural eastern and western North Carolina, USA. J. Agric. Food Syst. Community Dev. 4 (4), 143–154.

Miller, P., et al., 2015. The United States food supply is not consistent with dietary guidance: evidence from an evaluation using the Healthy Eating Index-2010. J. Acad. Nutr. Diet. 115 (1), 95–100.

Morrissey, T., Jacknowitz, A., Vinopal, K., 2014. Local food prices and their associations with children's weight and food security. Pediatrics 133 (3), 422–430.

Newport, F., 2012. In U.S., 5% consider themselves vegetarians.

Ohri-Vachaspati, P., Turner, L., Chaloupka, F., 2012. Fresh fruit and vegetable program participation in elementary schools in the United States and availability of fruits and vegetables in school lunch meals. J. Acad. Nutr. Diet. 112 (6), 921–926.

Orlich, M.J., Jaceldo-Siegl, K., Sabate, J., 2014. Patterns of food consumption among vegetarians and non-vegetarians. Br. J. Nutr. 112 (10), 1644–1653.

Pawlak, R., Lester, S., Babatunde, T., 2014. The prevalence of cobalamin deficiency among vegetarians assessed by serum vitamin B12: a review of literature. Eur. J. Clin. Nutr. 68, 541–548.

Rehm, C., Monsivais, P., Drewnowski, A., 2015. Relation between diet cost and Healthy Eating Index 2010 scores among adults in the United States 2007-2010. Prev. Med. 73C, 70–75.

Rigby, S., et al., 2012. Food deserts in Leon County, FL: disparate distribution of Supplemental Nutrition Assistance Program-accepting stores by neighborhood characteristics. J. Nutr. Educ. Behav. 44 (6), 539–547.

Rizzo, N., et al., 2013. Nutrient profiles of vegetarian and non vegetarian dietary patterns. J. Acad. Nutr. Diet. 113 (12), 1610–1619.

Sabate, J., Duk, A., Lee, C.L., 1999. Publication trends of vegetarian nutrition articles in biomedical literature, 1966-1995. Am. J. Clin. Nutr. 70 (Suppl.), 601S–607S.

Sarter, B., et al., 2015. Blood docosahexaenoic acid and eicosapentaenoic acid in vegans: associations with age and gender and effects of an algal-derived omega-3 fatty acid supplement. Clin. Nutr. 34 (2), 212–218.

Shannon, J., 2014. What does SNAP benefit usage tell us about food access in low-income neighborhoods? J. Soc. Sci. Med. 107, 89–99.

Sharkey, J., Horel, S., Dean, W., 2010. Neighborhood deprivation, vehicle ownership, and potential spatial access to a variety of fruits and vegetables in a large rural area in Texas. Int. J. Health Geogr. 25, 9–26.

Song, H., Grutzmacher, S., Kostenko, J., 2014. Personal weight status classification and health literacy among Supplemental Nutrition Assistance Program (SNAP) participants. J. Community Health 39 (3), 446–453.

Speirs, K., et al., 2012. Health literacy and nutrition behaviors among low-income adults. Health Care Poor Underserved 23 (3), 1082–1091.

Takenaka, S., et al., 2001. Feeding dried purple laver (nori) to vitamin B12-deficient rats significantly improves vitamin B12 status. Br. J. Nutr. 85, 699–703.

Tucker, K., 2014. Vegetarian diets and bone health. Am. J. Clin. Nutr. 100 (Suppl. 1), 329S–335S.

USDA, 2012. USDA Unveils Historic Improvements to Meals Served in America's Schools New Standards Will Improve the Health and Wellbeing of 32 Million Kids Nationwide, in Release No. 0023.12. USDA Office of Communications.

U.S. Department of Agriculture and U.S. Department of Health and Human Services, 2010. Dietary Guidelines for Americans, 2010. 7th Edition, Washington, DC: U.S. Government Printing Office.

USDHHS, May 2014. Healthy People 2020 Leading Health Indicators: Nutrition, Physical Activity, and Obesity. [cited May 2015]. Available from: <http://www.healthypeople.gov/sites/default/files/HP2020_LHI_Nut_PhysActiv_0.pdf> Accessed May 3, 2015.

Weinsier, R., 2000. Use of the term vegetarian. Am. J. Clin. Nutr. 71, 1211–1212.

Yaktine, A., Murphy, S., 2013. Aligning nutrition assistance programs with the Dietary Guidelines for Americans. Nutr. Rev. 71 (9), 622–630.

Yeh, M.-C., Ickes, S.B., Lowenstein, L.M., 2008. Understanding barriers and facilitators of fruit and vegetable consumption among a diverse multi-ethnic population in the USA. Health Promotion Int. 23 (1), 42–51.

Zenk, S., et al., 2012. Fruit and vegetable availability and selection: federal food package revisions, 2009. Am. J. Prev. Med. 43 (4), 423–428.

Zenk, S., et al., 2014. Impact of the revised Special Supplemental Nutrition Program for Women, Infants, and Children (WIC) food package policy on fruit and vegetable prices. J. Acad. Nutr. Diet. 114 (2).

Chapter 20

Dietary fiber and health: cardiovascular disease and beyond

Yikyung Park
Washington University School of Medicine, St. Louis, MO, United States

CHAPTER OUTLINE

INTRODUCTION

In the early twentieth century, there was little interest in the food constituents that are not digestible by human gastrointestinal enzymes. In 1953, Hipsley used the term "dietary fiber" to describe the nondigestible component of a human diet containing "lignin, cellulose, and the hemicelluloses" (Hipsley, 1953). Trowell et al. (1976) further defined dietary fiber

Fruits, Vegetables, and Herbs.
DOI: http://dx.doi.org/10.1016/B978-0-12-802972-5.00020-2

as plant polysaccharides and lignin that are resistant to hydrolysis by the digestive enzymes in humans. In 1970s, Burkitt and Trowell showed that diet, especially diet high in fiber, was accountable for lower rates of western diseases in Africa (Burkitt et al., 1972; Trowell, 1972; Burkitt, 1971), and the "dietary fiber hypothesis" was conceived. Since then, numerous epidemiologic studies tested the dietary fiber hypotheses. At the same time, experimental and clinical studies were initiated to understand physiologic mechanisms underlying the beneficial effects of dietary fiber on health.

Dietary fiber, mainly derived from fruit, vegetables, and grains, is composed of many constituents such as cellulose, hemicelluloses, inulin, gums, β-glucan, pectin, mucilage, lignin, and resistant starches. The Institute of Medicine defines that "dietary fiber consists of nondigestible carbohydrates and lignin that are intrinsic and intact in plants" and "total fiber is the sum of dietary fiber and added fiber that consists of isolated, nondigestible carbohydrates that have beneficial physiologic effects in humans" (National Research Council, 2001). Thus, fiber can be classified as dietary fiber that is naturally occurring in foods or functional fiber that is added during the food processing or consumed separately as a supplement. Dietary fiber has also been categorized as soluble and insoluble fiber. However, the classification of soluble and insoluble fiber is based on the chemical properties of fiber, which do not necessarily reflect the physiologic effects. As the physicochemical properties of dietary fiber such as viscosity, water-holding capacity, and fermentability account or contribute to the beneficial effects of dietary fiber on health, the Institute of Medicine recommended the terms soluble and insoluble fibers be phased out and replaced with the physicochemical property (National Research Council, 2001).

Epidemiologic studies have significantly contributed to the recognition of dietary fiber as an essential constituent of a healthy diet and promoted dietary fiber in dietary guidelines. In the United States, the recommended adequate intake of dietary fiber for adults is 25–38 g/day (14 g/1000 kcal) (USDA and USDHHS, 2010). However, the National Health and Nutrition Examination Survey in the United States showed that a mean daily intake of dietary fiber in adults was 15.9 g/day in 2007–2008, which indicated a majority of population did not meet the recommendation (King et al., 2012). In Europe, the recommend dietary fiber intake for adults is 25 g/day, and the average daily intake of dietary fiber in adults ranged from 15 to 30 g/day across European countries (EFSA Panel on Dietetic Products and Nutrition and Allergies, 2010). Diet low in fiber has been identified as one of the risk factors that causes the global burden of disease. The estimated 16.5 million disability-adjusted life-years were due to diet low in fiber (Murray and Lopez, 2013).

This chapter summarizes the existing as well as emerging epidemiologic evidence on dietary fiber and various diseases. When available, most recent reports from meta-analyses or pooled analyses that summarized existing evidence, especially from prospective cohort studies, are used.

TOTAL MORTALITY

Early studies conducted in various populations suggested an inverse association between dietary fiber intake and total mortality, but the evidence was weak. The Scottish Heart Health study (Todd et al., 1999) reported that dietary fiber intake was inversely related to total mortality in men (comparing the highest category of intake to the lowest, relative risk (RR) $_{H\ vs\ L}$ = 0.62, 95% confidence interval (CI): 0.42–0.92), but not in women ($RR_{H\ vs\ L}$ = 0.65, 95% CI: 0.35–1.22). The Zutphen study in the Netherlands (Streppel et al., 2008) observed a 9% (95% CI: 0–18%) lowered risk of total death per 10g/day of dietary fiber intake, whereas another study conducted in Israeli population observed a 43% lowered risk of total death in people consuming ≥25g/day of dietary fiber compared to those with <25g/day dietary fiber intake (Lubin et al., 2003). In contrast, a study using data from the National Health and Nutrition Examination Survey I Epidemiologic Follow-up Study (Bazzano et al., 2003) found no association between dietary fiber intake and total mortality.

Recent reports from two large prospective cohort studies, however, provide strong support for the inverse association between dietary fiber intake and total mortality. The National Institutes of Health (NIH)-AARP Diet and Health study (NIH-AARP study) conducted in the United States assessed diet of 388,122 men and women who were 50–71 years old and did not have a history of cancer, heart disease, stroke, or diabetes at baseline (Park et al., 2011). After following participants for an average of 9 years, the study found that both men and women in the highest quintile of dietary fiber intake compared to those in the lowest quintile had a 22% lower risk of total mortality ($RR_{H\ vs\ L}$ = 0.78, 95% CI: 0.73–0.82 in men; $RR_{H\ vs\ L}$ = 0.78, 95% CI: 0.73–0.85 in women). When fiber from food sources was examined, the inverse association was more evident for fiber from grains ($RR_{H\ vs\ L}$ = 0.77, 95% CI: 0.73–0.81 in men; $RR_{H\ vs\ L}$ = 0.81, 95% CI: 0.76–0.86 in women). Fiber from vegetables showed a weaker, but significant association with total mortality ($RR_{H\ vs\ L}$ = 0.95, 95% CI: 0.91–0.99 in men; $RR_{H\ vs\ L}$ = 0.95, 95% CI: 0.89–1.01 in women), whereas fiber from fruit showed no association ($RR_{H\ vs\ L}$ = 1.03, 95% CI: 0.99–1.09 in men; $RR_{H\ vs\ L}$ = 1.02, 95% CI: 0.95–1.09 in women).

Similarly, the European Prospective Investigation into Cancer and Nutrition Cohort (EPIC) study with 452,717 men and women in 10

European countries found that higher dietary fiber intake was related to a lower risk of total mortality (Chuang et al., 2012). The risk of total mortality was reduced by 30% in men ($RR_{H\ vs\ L}$ = 0.70, 95% CI: 0.68–0.79) and 20% in women ($RR_{H\ vs\ L}$ = 0.80, 95% CI: 0.71–0.82). This study also found that the association was stronger for fiber from grains (per 5 g/day increase RR = 0.93, 95% CI: 0.91–0.95 in men; RR = 0.92, 95% CI: 0.89–0.95 in women) and for fiber from vegetables (RR = 0.91, 95% CI: 0.87–0.95 in men; RR = 0.97, 95% CI: 0.94–1.01 in women) than that of fiber from fruit (RR = 1.01, 95% CI: 0.97–1.05 in men; RR = 0.96, 95% CI: 0.93–1.00 in women).

Because people who consumed higher amount of dietary fiber tended to have higher education level and healthier lifestyle such as lower body mass index, being physically active, and not smoke, higher dietary fiber intake could be a marker of healthier lifestyle and the association observed in these studies could be due to confounding. However, both NIH-AARP and EPIC studies carefully controlled for lifestyle and other dietary factors in statistical analyses and found that the association was independent of lifestyle and dietary factors. Besides, both studies performed stratified analyses by smoking and body mass index and found that the inverse association between dietary fiber intake and total mortality persisted across subgroups of these lifestyle factors. Interestingly, both studies found that fiber from grains had a stronger association with total mortality than fiber from vegetables did, and fiber from fruit was not related to the risk of total mortality.

A meta-analysis of seven prospective cohort studies with general population, including studies mentioned above, summarized that dietary fiber was associated with a 23% lower risk of total mortality ($RR_{H\ vs\ L}$ = 0.77, 95% CI: 0.74–0.80) (Kim and Je, 2014). Another meta-analysis of 17 studies conducted in both general and patient populations also found a 16% lower risk of total death ($RR_{H\ vs\ L}$ = 0.84, 95% CI: 0.80–0.87) (Yang et al., 2015). The inverse association between dietary fiber intake and mortality was also observed across strata of body mass index, smoking, and physical activity.

HEART DISEASE AND STROKE

Since Trowell (1972) hypothesized that dietary fiber intake lowered the risk of ischemic heart disease, possible through lowering serum cholesterol levels, in early 1970s, numerous epidemiologic studies have supported the hypothesis. A pooled analysis of 10 prospective cohort studies from the United States and Europe found that every 10 g/day increase in dietary fiber intake was associated with a 14% lower risk of all coronary events (fatal and nonfatal) and a 27% lower risk of coronary heart disease deaths (Pereira et al., 2004). Fiber from grains (per 10 g/day increase, RR = 0.75, 95% CI: 0.63–0.91) and fiber from fruit (RR = 0.70, 95% CI: 0.55–0.89) showed strong inverse associations with coronary heart disease deaths, but fiber from vegetables did not show an association (RR = 1.00, 95% CI: 0.82–1.23).

Two large prospective cohort studies, the NIH-AARP study (Park et al., 2011) and the EPIC study (Chuang et al., 2012), both were larger than the earlier pooled analysis (Pereira et al., 2004), also added further evidence supporting the beneficial effect of dietary fiber on cardiovascular disease. In the NIH-AARP study (Park et al., 2011), the risk of cardiovascular disease death was reduced by 24% ($RR_{H\ vs\ L}$ = 0.76, 95% CI: 0.68–0.85) in men and 34% ($RR_{H\ vs\ L}$ = 0.66, 95% CI: 0.55–0.79) in women. The EPIC study (Chuang et al., 2012) also found that dietary fiber intake was related to a 17% ($RR_{H\ vs\ L}$ = 0.83, 95% CI: 0.71–0.98) and a 33% ($RR_{H\ vs\ L}$ = 0.67, 95% CI: 0.55–0.82) lower risk of cardiovascular disease death in men and women, respectively. When examining fiber from food sources separately, both studies consistently found that fiber from grains, but not from fruit, was related to a lower risk of cardiovascular disease death. Comparing the highest quintile of fiber from grains intake to the lowest quintile, the RR of cardiovascular disease death was 0.77 (95% CI: 0.71–0.85) in men and 0.72 (95% CI: 0.63–0.82) in women in the NIH-AARP study. In the EPIC study, the RR of cardiovascular disease death for every 5 g/day increase in fiber from grains was 0.95 (95% CI: 0.91–1.00) in men and 0.93 (95% CI: 0.87–1.00) in women. The NIH-AARP study did not find an association with fiber from vegetables, but the EPIC study observed an inverse association with fiber from vegetables in men, but not in women.

Recently a meta-analysis reviewed findings from 22 studies published between 1990 and 2013, which examined the association between dietary fiber intake and incidence or mortality of coronary heart disease or cardiovascular disease (Threapleton et al., 2013a). The study found that every 7 g/day increase in dietary fiber intake was associated with a 9% decrease in the risk of coronary heart disease (0.91, 95% CI: 0.87–0.94) and cardiovascular disease (RR = 0.91, 95% CI: 0.88–0.94) (Table 20.1). A 4–16% decreased risk of coronary heart disease or cardiovascular diseases were found for fiber from fruit, vegetables, and grains. Another meta-analysis of studies on dietary fiber and coronary heart disease also found that higher dietary fiber intake was associated with a lower risk of both coronary heart disease incidence and mortality (Wu et al., 2014).

Several physiologic mechanisms support the findings of the inverse association between dietary fiber and heart disease from the epidemiologic

Table 20.1 Relative Risks (95% Confidence Intervals) for the Association Between Dietary Fiber Intake and Heart Disease and Diabetes: Summary Risks Reported in Meta-Analyses

Disease	No. of Studies Included in the Meta-Analysis	Total Dietary Fiber	Fiber from Fruit	Fiber from Vegetables	Fiber from Grains
Coronary heart disease[a] (Threapleton et al., 2013a)	12	0.91 (0.87–0.94)	0.92 (0.83–1.01)	0.94 (0.89–1.00)	0.84 (0.76–0.94)
Cardiovascular disease[a] (Threapleton et al., 2013a)	10	0.91 (0.88–0.94)	0.96 (0.93–1.00)	0.92 (0.87–0.96)	0.92 (0.84–1.00)
Coronary heart disease incidence[b] (Wu et al., 2014)	16	0.93 (0.91–0.96)	0.92 (0.86–0.98)	0.95 (0.89–1.01)	0.92 (0.85–0.99)
Coronary heart disease mortality[b] (Wu et al., 2014)	15	0.83 (0.76–0.91)	0.68 (0.43–1.07)	0.91 (0.74–1.12)	0.81 (0.72–0.92)
Stroke[a] (Threapleton et al., 2013b)	7	0.93 (0.88–0.98)	–	–	–
Type-2 Diabetes[c] (Consortium, 2015)	19	0.91 (0.87–0.96)	0.95 (0.87–1.03)	0.93 (0.82–1.05)	0.75 (0.65–0.86)

[a]Per 7 g/day increase for total dietary fiber and fiber from grains; per 4g/day increase for fiber from fruit and from vegetables.
[b]Comparing the highest intake category to the lowest category.
[c]Per 10 g/day increase.

studies. Experimental studies and clinical trials of a high fiber diet showed that dietary fiber lowered cholesterol levels. Dietary fiber increased excretion of cholesterol binding fecal bile acids, which may result in a higher rate of cholesterol synthesis and reduced serum cholesterol concentrations and change the activity of 3-hydroxy-3-methylglutaryl-Co A that is a rate-limiting enzyme of cholesterol synthesis (Garcia-Diez et al., 1996). In addition, short-chain fatty acids, products of dietary fiber fermentation by intestinal bacteria, inhibit hepatic cholesterol synthesis and lower serum cholesterol levels (Hara et al., 1999). A meta-analysis of 67 controlled clinical trials summarized that diets high in soluble fiber (2–10 g/day) were associated with a significant decrease in total cholesterol (−0.045 mmol/L, 95% CI: −0.054 to −0.035 mmol/L) and LDL cholesterol (−0.057 mmol/L, 95% CI: −0.070 to −0.044 mmol/L) (Brown et al., 1999). Also, higher intake of dietary fiber lowered blood pressure in people with hypertension (Whelton et al., 2005; Streppel et al., 2005). In a quantitative review of studies on dietary fiber and blood pressure, dietary fiber lowered systolic blood pressure by 0.9 mmHg (95% CI: −2.5 to 0.6 mmHg) and diastolic blood pressure by 0.7 mmHg (95% CI: −1.9 to 0.5 mmHg) (Evans et al., 2015). The cholesterol-lowering and antihypertensive properties of dietary fiber have also been postulated to lower risk of stroke.

Stroke is the second leading cause of death in the world in 2012 (World Health Organization, 2015) and the third leading cause of the global burden of the disease in 2010 (Murray and Lopez, 2013). Epidemiologic studies that examined the association between dietary fiber intake and risk of stroke reported inconsistent results. Some studies found an inverse association (Ascherio et al., 1998; Kokubo et al., 2011; Oh et al., 2005; Larsson and Wolk, 2014), whereas others found no association (Bazzano et al., 2003; Larsson et al., 2009). When seven cohort studies conducted around the world were summarized in a meta-analysis, a 7% decrease in the risk of stroke per 7 g/day increase in dietary fiber intake was found (RR = 0.93, 95% CI: 0.88–0.98) (Table 20.1) (Threapleton et al., 2013b). Another meta-analysis of six cohort studies with 314,864 participants and 8920 stroke cases also found the inverse association (Chen et al., 2013). Studies conducted in Japan (Kokubo et al., 2011) and Sweden (Wallstrom et al., 2012) reported dietary fiber intake was related to a lower risk of ischemic stroke.

TYPE-2 DIABETES

The evidence for a beneficial effect of dietary fiber on type-2 diabetes is consistent although the inverse association was confined to fiber from grains. A previous meta-analysis of nine studies on dietary fiber and type-2 diabetes found intake of dietary fiber from grains, but not from fruit and vegetables, was associated with significantly lowered risk of type-2 diabetes (Schulze et al., 2007). Comparing the highest category of fiber intake to the lowest, RRs for fiber from grains, fruit, and vegetables were 0.67 (95% CI: 0.62–0.72), 0.96 (95% CI: 0.88–1.04), and 1.04 (95% CI: 0.94–1.15), respectively. Another meta-analysis was conducted more recently with 19 studies and included 617,968 participants and 41,066 incident type-2 diabetes cases (InterAct Consortium, 2015) (Table 20.1). The risk of type-2 diabetes decreased by 9% per 10 g/day increase in dietary fiber intake (RR = 0.91, 95% CI: 0.87–0.96). The inverse association with type-2 diabetes was stronger for fiber from grain (RR = 0.75, 95% CI: 0.65–0.86) than for fiber from fruit (RR = 0.95, 95% CI: 0.87–1.03) and vegetables (RR = 0.93, 95% CI: 0.82–1.05).

The protective effect of dietary fiber on type-2 diabetes is also supported by clinical trials of high fiber diet or dietary supplements in people with type-2 diabetes (Post et al., 2012). The Finnish Diabetes Prevention Study provided an intensive lifestyle intervention—dietary and exercise counseling—to their overweight participants with impaired glucose tolerance. During a mean follow-up of 4.1 years, people with high fiber intake (>15.6 g/1000 kcal) compared to those with low intake (<10.9 g/1000 kcal) had a 62% lower risk of type-2 diabetes (RR = 0.38, 95% CI: 0.19–0.77) (Lindstrom et al., 2006). Furthermore, a meta-analysis of clinical trials showed that the intervention group with higher fiber intake either from diet or supplements lowered fasting blood glucose by 0.85 mmol/L (95% CI: 0.46–1.25 mmol/L) than the control group did (Post et al., 2012). The intervention group also lowered concentration of glycosylated hemoglobin (HbA1c) by 0.26% (95% CI: 0.02%–0.51%) over the control group. The reduction in postprandial glucose responses and improvement of insulin sensitivity with high dietary fiber intake have also been postulated to lower risk of type-2 diabetes (Weickert and Pfeiffer, 2008).

WEIGHT LOSS

Dietary fiber has been hypothesized to have effects on appetite and energy intake, thereby affects body weight or weight loss (Pereira and Ludwig, 2001; Anderson et al., 2009). Dietary fiber increases the viscosity of diets and stomach distension, and delays gastric emptying, which increase satiety. Also, foods high in dietary fiber often take longer to chew. Therefore, it may increase satiety, and high fiber content in food reduces the energy density of the food, thus may lower total energy intake. A food's energy density consists of the net quantity of calories in a particular weight of food (usually expressed as kcal/g). Taken all together, dietary fiber has been hypothesized to promote weight loss or prevent weight gain (Pereira and Ludwig, 2001).

An observational study followed 27,082 men aged 40–75 years over 8 years found that dietary fiber intake was inversely related to weight gain. Men who had the lowest quintile of fiber intake change (median = −5.2 g/day) gained 1.40 kg, whereas men in the highest quintile of change (8.5 g/day) gained 0.39 kg (Koh-Banerjee et al., 2004). Similarly, among 74,091 women aged 38–63 years, women with the greatest increase in dietary fiber intake during 12 years of follow-up gained an average of 1.52 kg less than those with the smallest increase in dietary fiber intake (P for trend <0.0001) (Liu et al., 2003). Women in the highest quintile of dietary fiber intake had a 49% lower risk of weight gain than women in the lowest quintile of intake (odds ratio, OR = 0.51; 95% CI: 0.39–0.67) (Liu et al., 2003).

A study conducted in Europe also reported that dietary fiber intake was inversely associated with subsequent weight and waist circumference change. For a 10 g/day higher fiber intake, the pooled estimate was −39 g/year

(95% CI: −71, −7 g/year) for weight change and −0.08 cm/year (95% CI: −0.11, −0.05 cm/year) for waist circumference change (Du et al., 2010).

Intervention studies with high fiber diet showed that a diet high in fiber promoted more weight loss than the control diet. In a weight loss intervention with high dietary fiber diet, the intervention group increased consumption of fruit, vegetables, and whole grains, which resulted in 16 g/day more intake of dietary fiber than the control group had (Esposito et al., 2004). After 2 years of intervention, the intervention group had 4.0 kg body weight loss while the control group lost 1.2 kg. Another dietary intervention study with 240 obese participants with metabolic syndrome used the American Heart Association's (AHA) dietary recommendations for the management of metabolic syndrome (with caloric restriction) and a high fiber diet (no caloric restriction) (Ma et al., 2015). After 12 months, weight loss was greater in the AHA diet group than in the high fiber group. However, there were no significant differences between two groups for changes in blood pressures, blood lipids, insulin resistance scores, and inflammation markers. This study showed that a simple high fiber diet was as effective as the multicomponent AHA diet.

COLORECTAL CANCER

Since Burkitt proposed that dietary fiber lowers the risk of colorectal cancer in early 1970s (Burkitt et al., 1972), numerous studies have rigorously tested the hypothesis. Recently, the expert report from the World Cancer Research Fund and American Institute for Cancer Research (2011) concluded that the evidence for a protective effect of foods containing dietary fiber on colorectal cancer is convincing. This was supported by findings from a meta-analysis that reviewed 25 prospective cohort studies conducted in Asia, Europe, and North America (Aune et al., 2011) (Table 20.2). Every 10 g/day increase in dietary fiber intake was associated with a 10% lower risk of colorectal cancer (RR = 0.90, 95% CI: 0.86–0.94, $I^2 = 0\%$). Among fiber from food sources, fiber from grains was inversely related to the risk of colorectal cancer (per 10 g/day increase RR = 0.90, 95% CI: 0.83–0.97). Fiber from fruit was also inversely associated with the risk of colorectal cancer (RR = 0.93, 95% CI: 0.82–1.05), but it was not statistically significant. Fiber from vegetables was not associated with the risk of colorectal cancer (RR = 0.98, 95% CI: 0.91–1.06).

Several plausible physiologic mechanisms support the preventive effect of dietary fiber on colorectal cancer (Lipkin et al., 1999). Dietary fiber increased excretion of fecal carcinogens and procarcinogens by binding to them. Dietary fiber reduces the transit time of feces through the bowel, thus, decreases the contact of fecal carcinogens and procarcinogens with colonic lumen. Fermented dietary fiber in colon produces short-chain fatty acids that promote anticarcinogenic actions. In addition, dietary fiber may provide a beneficial effect on colorectal cancer through indirect mechanisms such as improving insulin sensitivity and promoting weight loss.

Parkin and Boyd (2011) estimated that 12.2% of colorectal cancer in the United Kingdom in 2010 was due to failure to meet the recommended dietary fiber intake that was 23 g/day. Also, it is estimated that 4.9% of colorectal cancer cases could be avoidable if the population meets the recommended intake of dietary fiber by consuming five or more servings of fruit and vegetables per day, assuming that the benefit is exclusively due to dietary fiber in fruit and vegetables.

Dietary fiber intake was also associated with the risk of colorectal adenoma, a precursor of colorectal cancer (Ben et al., 2014). A meta-analysis of 20 studies, including both case–control studies and prospective cohorts, found that compared to people in the lowest category of dietary fiber intake, people in the highest intake category had 28% lowered risk of colorectal adenoma (RR = 0.72, 95% CI: 0.63–0.83). Fibers from fruit, vegetables, and grains were also related to 7–24% lower risk of colorectal adenoma. However, the inverse association was observed from the meta-analysis of case–control studies (RR = 0.66, 95% CI: 0.56–0.77), but not from prospective cohort studies (RR = 0.92, 95% CI: 0.76–1.10). In addition, clinical trials of high fiber diet or fiber supplement did not find the protective effect of fiber on the recurrence of colorectal adenoma (Schatzkin et al., 2000; Lanza et al., 2007; Alberts et al., 2000).

BREAST CANCER

A study showing that vegetarian women had increased fecal excretion of estrogens and decreased plasma concentration of estrogen compared with omnivorous women (Goldin et al., 1982) spiked the interest in the effect of dietary fiber on breast cancer. It has been postulated that dietary fiber may increase fecal excretion of estrogens and inhibit the intestinal reabsorption of estrogens, which result in lower plasma concentration of estrogen (Goldin et al., 1982; Rose et al., 1991). Dietary fiber's role in modulating insulin resistance and insulin-like growth factors also suggest a preventive effect against breast cancer (Lawlor et al., 2004; Yu and Rohan, 2000).

Epidemiologic studies that investigated the relation of dietary fiber to the risk of breast cancer have reported inconsistent findings. However, a recent comprehensive meta-analysis that summarized results from 16 prospective cohort studies found that dietary fiber intake was associated with a 7% lower risk of breast cancer overall ($RR_{H\ vs\ L}$ = 0.93, 95% CI: 0.89–0.98, I^2 = 0%) (Aune et al., 2012) (Table 20.2). The inverse association was found in postmenopausal women ($RR_{H\ vs\ L}$ = 0.93, 95% CI: 0.88–0.99, n = 13 studies) and premenopausal women ($RR_{H\ vs\ L}$ = 0.90, 95% CI: 0.73–1.10, n = 4 studies). Among fiber from food sources, fiber from grains (per 10 g/day increment RR = 0.91, 95% CI: 0.79–1.04) and fiber from fruit (RR= 0.88, 95% CI: 0.75–1.03) were associated with a lower risk of breast cancer, but fiber from vegetables was not (RR = 0.97, 95% CI: 0.85–1.12).

Only three cohort studies examined the association by hormone receptor status of breast cancer. The meta-analysis of three studies found statistically nonsignificant inverse association between dietary fiber intake and each subtype of breast cancer (Aune et al., 2012). The $RR_{H\ vs\ L}$ for dietary fiber intake was 0.91 (95% CI: 0.79–1.06) for ER+/PR+ (estrogen receptor positive and progesterone receptor positive) tumors, 0.89 (95% CI: 0.67–1.19) for ER+/PR− tumors, and 0.76 (95% CI: 0.52–1.11) for ER−/PR− tumors.

Interestingly, a recent Canadian case–control study reported that dietary fiber intakes during adolescent (ages 10–15 years old) were related to a significantly lower risk of breast cancer later in adulthood ($OR_{H\ vs\ L}$ = 0.66, 95% CI: 0.55–0.78) (Liu et al., 2014). The reduced risk for adolescent intakes of dietary fiber was more evident for postmenopausal breast cancer (OR = 0.58, 95% CI: 0.47–0.72) than premenopausal breast cancer (OR = 0.84, 95% CI: 0.64–1.12).

Although limited, studies of breast cancer survivors also suggested that higher intake of dietary fiber improved overall survival after breast cancer diagnosis (McEligot et al., 2006; Holmes et al., 2009; Buck et al., 2011). A study with postmenopausal breast cancer survivors in California (n = 516) found that dietary fiber intake was related to a lower risk of death from any causes ($RR_{H\ vs\ L}$ = 0.48, 95% CI: 0.27–0.86) (McEligot et al., 2006). Similarly, breast cancer survivors with higher intake of fiber from grains in the Nurses' Health Study (n = 3846) had a 29% lowered risk of death from any causes ($RR_{H\ vs\ L}$ = 0.71, 95% CI: 0.53–0.96) (Holmes et al., 2009). In a study of 2653 postmenopausal breast cancer survivors in Germany, dietary fiber intake before cancer diagnosis was significantly related to lower risk of death from any causes ($RR_{H\ vs\ L}$ = 0.52, 95% CI: 0.32–0.82) and death from breast cancer ($RR_{H\ vs\ L}$ = 0.64, 95% CI: 0.37–1.11) (Buck et al., 2011). However, a Canadian study that followed women with

Table 20.2 Relative Risks (95% Confidence Intervals) for the Association Between Dietary Fiber Intake and Cancer: Summary Risks Reported in Meta-Analyses

Cancer	No. of Studies Included in the Meta-Analysis	Total Dietary Fiber	Fiber from Fruit	Fiber from Vegetables	Fiber from Grains
Colorectal[a] (Aune et al., 2011)	25 cohort studies	0.90 (0.86–0.94)	0.93 (0.82–1.05)	0.98 (0.91–1.06)	0.90 (0.83–0.97)
Breast[a] (Aune et al., 2012)	16 cohort studies	0.95 (0.91–0.98)	0.83 (0.75–1.03)	0.97 (0.85–1.12)	0.91 (0.79–1.04)
Breast cancer survival[b] (Yang et al., 2015)	4 cohort studies	0.68 (0.54–0.84)	–	–	–
Esophageal adenocarcinoma[b] (Coleman et al., 2013)	8 case–control	0.66 (0.44–0.98)	–	–	–
Esophageal squamous cell carcinoma[b] (Coleman et al., 2013)	5 case–control	0.61 (0.31–1.20)	–	–	–
Stomach[b] (Zhang et al., 2013)	19 case–control and 2 cohorts	0.58 (0.49–0.67)	0.67 (0.46–0.99)	0.72 (0.57–0.90)	0.58 (0.41–0.82)
Kidney[b] (Huang et al., 2014)	5 case–control and 2 cohorts	0.84 (0.74–0.96)	0.92 (0.80–1.05)	0.70 (0.49–1.00)	1.04 (0.91–1.18)
Pancreas[b] (Wang et al., 2015)	13 case–control	0.52 (0.43–0.63)	–	–	–
Endometrium[b] (Bandera et al., 2007)	9 case–control	0.71 (0.59–0.85)	–	–	–

[a]Per 10g/day increase.
[b]Comparing the highest intake category to the lowest category.

breast cancer for 10 years did not find a significant association between dietary fiber intake and death from breast cancer ($RR_{H\ vs\ L}$ = 0.7, 95% CI: 0.4–1.3). The Health, Eating, Activity, and Lifestyle study with breast cancer survivors also found no significant association between dietary fiber intake and death from any causes ($RR_{H\ vs\ L}$ = 0.75, 95% CI: 0.43–1.31) and death from breast cancer ($RR_{H\ vs\ L}$ = 0.85, 95% CI: 0.46–1.59) (Belle et al., 2011). When the results of these studies on dietary fiber intake and survival among breast cancer survivors were meta-analyzed, dietary fiber intake was related to a 32% lower risk of death ($RR_{H\ vs\ L}$ = 0.68, 95% CI: 0.54–0.84) (Yang et al., 2015).

ESOPHAGEAL CANCER

Esophageal cancer is the fifth and eighth leading cause of cancer death in men and women, respectively, in the world (Jemal et al., 2011). Two distinct histologic types of esophageal cancer—squamous cell carcinoma and adenocarcinoma—exist. Esophageal squamous cell carcinoma is the predominant form of esophageal cancer, but recently the incidence of esophageal adenocarcinoma that often occurs in the lower third of the esophagus has increased sharply in Europe and in the United States (Pennathur et al., 2013). Smoking and alcohol are risk factors for esophageal squamous cell carcinoma, whereas gastroesophageal reflux disease, Barrett esophagus, and obesity are known risk factors for esophageal adenocarcinoma.

High consumption of fruit and vegetables has been linked to a lower risk of esophageal cancer (World Cancer Research Fund and American Institute for Cancer Research, 2007). Dietary fiber has been proposed as a contributor to the protective effect of fruit and vegetables against esophageal cancer. However, epidemiologic studies have reported inconsistent results. When findings from 10 case–control studies that examined an association with dietary fiber intake were summarized in a meta-analysis, a significant inverse association was found for both esophageal squamous cell carcinoma ($OR_{H\ vs\ L}$ = 0.61, 95% CI: 0.31–1.20) and esophageal adenocarcinoma ($OR_{H\ vs\ L}$ = 0.66, 95% CI: 0.44–0.98) (Coleman et al., 2013) (Table 20.2). However, there was a significant heterogeneity in the summary estimates, and the sources of the heterogeneity were not identified in this meta-analysis.

When evaluating the evidence from case–control studies on diet and disease, several inherent methodologic limitations should be taken into account. The retrospective evaluation of diet after disease diagnosis is prone to recall bias that will distort the association between diet and a disease. In addition, a selection of an appropriate control group for the study of diet and disease is particularly challenging. A hospital-based case–control study selects people with diseases that are not related to exposures of interest as controls. However, it is hardly possible to identify a disease that is not related to diet. A population-based case–control study also suffers from methodologic limitations because people who are health conscious and have good health tend to participate in a study. These biases in case–control studies may result in incorrect associations. More prospective investigations on diet and esophageal cancer are needed.

STOMACH CANCER

Stomach cancer, also called gastric cancer, is the fourth most common cancer in men and fifth most common cancer in women in the world

(Jemal et al., 2011). High intake of salt-preserved foods and dietary nitrite were related to increased risk of stomach cancer, while high intakes of fruit and vegetables were linked to a lower risk of stomach cancer. Dietary fiber's beneficial effect on stomach cancer has been supported by an experimental study demonstrating that dietary fiber may scavenge nitrite, a precursor for carcinogenic N-nitroso compounds and a risk factor for stomach cancer (Moller et al., 1988).

Numerous case–control studies found that dietary fiber intake was associated with lower risk of stomach cancer. In contrast, cohort studies found no association between dietary fiber intake and risk of stomach cancer. The Netherlands Cohort Study that followed 120,852 men and women, aged 55–69 years, for about 6 years and identified 282 incident cases of gastric carcinoma. This study found that dietary fiber intake was not related to gastric carcinoma ($RR_{H\ vs\ L}$ = 0.90, 95% CI: 0.60–1.40) (Botterweck et al., 2000). Another cohort study, EPIC (*n* = 435,366, gastric cancer cases = 312), also found no association between dietary fiber intake and gastric cancer ($RR_{H\ vs\ L}$ = 0.89, 95% CI: 0.63–1.26) (Mendez et al., 2007). However, fiber from grains was associated with a lower risk of stomach cancer ($RR_{H\ vs\ L}$ = 0.69, 95% CI: 0.48–0.99).

A meta-analysis of 19 case–control studies and two cohort studies (Zhang et al., 2013) found that dietary fiber intake was related to a significantly lowered risk of gastric cancer ($OR_{H\ vs\ L}$ = 0.58, 95% CI: 0.49–0.67) (Table 20.2). However, the association was limited to case–control studies ($OR_{H\ vs\ L}$ = 0.53, 95% CI: 0.45–0.62) and the meta-analysis of cohort studies generated $OR_{H\ vs\ L}$ = 0.89 (95% CI: 0.68–1.17). Dietary fiber intake was related to both cardia ($OR_{H\ vs\ L}$ = 0.66, 95% CI: 0.37–1.15) and noncardia cancers ($OR_{H\ vs\ L}$ = 0.55, 95% CI: 0.36–0.83). The inverse association was observed for fiber from fruit ($OR_{H\ vs\ L}$ = 0.67, 95% CI: 0.46–0.99), fiber from vegetables ($OR_{H\ vs\ L}$ = 0.72, 95% CI: 0.57–0.90), and fiber from grains ($OR_{H\ vs\ L}$ = 0.58, 95% CI: 0.41–0.82).

KIDNEY CANCER

Kidney cancer is more prevalent in Europe and North America than in Asia and South America (Chow et al., 2010). Kidney cancer incidence rate increased until the mid-1990s and then plateaued or declined for some countries in worldwide. However, kidney cancer incidence has been steadily increasing in the United States, in accordance with the growing epidemic of obesity and hypertension, which are known risk factors for renal cell carcinoma. Several physiologic effects of dietary fiber such as lowering blood pressure and systemic inflammation, improving insulin sensitivity, and promoting weight loss have postulated to link to renal health. Also, dietary fiber may decrease the production of potentially toxic uremic retention molecules, which are produced by gut bacteria and either excreted or metabolized by the kidney (Evenepoel et al., 2009).

Several case–control studies suggested that dietary fiber intake was related to a lower risk of renal cell carcinoma, the most common type of kidney cancer (Brock et al., 2012; Hu et al., 2008; Lindblad et al., 1997). However, prospective cohort studies reported inconsistent results. The EPIC study conducted in Europe, which followed 435,293 participants for an average of 9 years and identified 507 renal cell carcinoma cases, found no association between dietary fiber intake and renal cell carcinoma ($RR_{H\ vs\ L}$ = 1.06, 95% CI: 0.73–1.53) (Allen et al., 2009). However, during 9 years of follow-up, the NIH-AARP study conducted in the United States (n = 491,841, 1816 renal cell cancer cases) found that dietary fiber intake was associated with a lower risk of renal cell carcinoma (Daniel et al., 2013). Compared to people in the lowest quintile of intake, people in the highest quintile had a 19% lower risk of renal cell carcinoma ($RR_{H\ vs\ L}$ = 0.81, 95% CI: 0.69–0.95).

A recent meta-analysis including five case–control studies and two prospective cohort studies found that dietary fiber intake was related to 16% lowered risk of renal cell carcinoma ($RR_{H\ vs\ L}$ = 0.84, 95% CI: 0.74–0.96) (Table 20.2) (Huang et al., 2014). The association was more apparent for fiber from vegetables ($RR_{H\ vs\ L}$ = 0.70, 95% CI: 0.49–1.00) than fiber from fruit ($RR_{H\ vs\ L}$ = 0.92, 95% CI: 0.80–1.05) and from grains ($RR_{H\ vs\ L}$ = 1.04, 95% CI: 0.91–1.18).

OTHER CANCER

Pancreatic cancer is one of the fatal cancers and has poor survival rate. Diabetes and chronic pancreatitis, which cause chronic inflammation, are known risk factors for pancreatic cancer. Anti-inflammatory properties of dietary fiber and its ability to improve insulin sensitivity postulated a beneficial effect of dietary fiber on pancreatic cancer. Several case–control studies reported a significant inverse association between dietary fiber intake and pancreatic cancer (Bidoli et al., 2012; Howe et al., 1990; Ji et al., 1995; Kalapothaki et al., 1993; Chan et al., 2007; Zhang et al., 2009). A meta-analysis of 13 case–control studies summarized that the high dietary fiber intake is inversely associated with the risk of pancreatic cancer ($OR_{H\ vs\ L}$ = 0.52, 95% CI: 0.43–0.63) (Table 20.2) (Wang et al., 2015). However, only one prospective cohort study examined dietary fiber intake in relation to pancreatic cancer and found no association (Stolzenberg-Solomon et al., 2002).

Recently, the EPIC study, a prospective cohort study that followed 477,206 participants for an average of 11 years, found that dietary fiber intake was inversely associated with the risk of hepatocellular carcinoma (Fedirko et al., 2013). Per 10 g/day increase of dietary fiber intake, the risk of hepatocellular carcinoma decreased by 30% (RR = 0.70, 95% CI: 0.52–0.93). As this is the first study to suggest a preventive role of dietary fiber on hepatocellular carcinoma, more studies are warranted.

An inverse association between dietary fiber intake and endometrial cancer was also summarized in a meta-analysis of case–control studies. High consumption of dietary fiber was related to a significantly lowered risk of endometrial cancer ($OR_{H\ vs\ L}$ = 0.71, 95% CI: 0.59–0.85) (Table 20.2) (Bandera et al., 2007). In contrast, three prospective cohort studies conducted in the United States, Canada, and Denmark found no association between dietary fiber intake and risk of endometrial cancer (Aarestrup et al., 2012; Cui et al., 2011; Jain et al., 2000). It is plausible that dietary fiber intake lowers the risk of endometrial cancer by controlling estrogen metabolism and improves insulin sensitivity and weight loss. However, limited evidence supports the potential protective effect of dietary fiber on endometrial cancer.

INFLAMMATORY DISEASES MORTALITY

An interesting finding that dietary fiber intake was related to a lower risk of death from infectious diseases was reported from two large prospective cohort studies. The NIH-AARP study (*n* = 388,122) found that the risk of death from infectious diseases was reduced by 56% in men ($RR_{H\ vs\ L}$ = 0.44, 95% CI: 0.26–0.74) and 59% in women ($RR_{H\ vs\ L}$ = 0.41, 95% CI: 0.23–0.73) (Park et al., 2011). The EPIC study (*n* = 452,717) also found dietary fiber intake was associated with significantly lowered risk of death from inflammatory diseases, including infectious diseases and other noncardiovascular noncancer diseases that have inflammation as a predominant pathophysiology. Comparing the highest quintile of dietary fiber intake to the lowest, the RR was 0.54 (95% CI: 0.41–0.70) in men and 0.62 (95% CI: 0.47–0.80) in women (Chuang et al., 2012). Both the NIH-AARP and the EPIC studies also found that the significant inverse association was more evident with fiber from grains than with fiber from fruit or vegetables. In contrast, the Blue Mountains Eye Study (*n* = 3654) conducted in Australia (Buyken et al., 2010) found no association between dietary fiber intake and death from inflammatory diseases ($RR_{H\ vs\ L}$ = 0.79, 95% CI: 0.42–1.49 in men; $RR_{H\ vs\ L}$ = 0.86, 95% CI: 0.47–1.58 in women). This small study did not find an association between dietary fiber intake and cardiovascular disease mortality, either, which has been established in other studies.

The inverse association between dietary fiber and inflammatory disease mortality is supported by accumulating evidence that dietary fiber has anti-inflammatory properties. A randomized crossover intervention trial of a high dietary fiber diet (mean intake = 28 g/day) or fiber supplemented diet (mean intake = 26 g/day) compared to baseline diet (mean intake = 12 g/day) found that concentration of C-reactive protein (CRP), an inflammatory marker, decreased by 13.7% and 18.1%, respectively, after 3 weeks of the diet (King et al., 2007). A review of clinical trials that examined the effect of high dietary fiber diet (13.8–32.6 g/1000 kcal) summarized that six out of seven trials found that high fiber diet was related to a weight loss and 25–54% decreased level of CRP in healthy men and women (North et al., 2009). Recently, another randomized crossover trial for 5 weeks of high fiber or low fiber diet also found that the decrease in CRP was significantly higher in high fiber diet than that in the low fiber diet ($P = 0.0017$) (Johansson-Persson et al., 2014).

A cross-sectional observation study also found that dietary fiber intake was associated with lower levels of other inflammation markers such as interleukin 6 (IL-6) and tumor necrosis factor-α receptor 2 in postmenopausal women (Ma et al., 2008). A lower level of CRP in people with high fiber diet was found in breast cancer survivors, too (Villasenor et al., 2011). Several others studies also found that dietary fiber intake was inversely related to CRP or IL-6 concentrations (Bo et al., 2006; Estruch et al., 2009; Herder et al., 2009; Kantor et al., 2013). Although specific mechanisms by which dietary fiber modulates inflammatory response are yet to be elucidated, it is plausible that anti-inflammatory properties of dietary fiber may provide beneficial effects on inflammatory diseases.

CHRONIC KIDNEY DISEASE

Recently several studies found that dietary fiber intake was associated with a lower risk of chronic kidney disease (CKD) (Gopinath et al., 2011; Fujii et al., 2013; Diaz-Lopez et al., 2013). The Blue Mountains Eye Study conducted in Australia followed 2600 participants of 50 years old and over for 5 years and found that people with high consumption of fiber from grains had a 50% lower risk of CKD defined as estimated glomerular filtration rate <60 mL/min per 1.73 m^2 ($OR_{H\ vs\ L} = 0.50$, 95% CI: 0.24–1.03) (Gopinath et al., 2011). Also, a Japanese study found that higher intake of dietary fiber was inversely associated with the prevalence of CKD in people with type-2 diabetes (Fujii et al., 2013). Another study conducted in Spain found that dietary fiber intake was related to a lower risk of CKD ($OR_{H\ vs\ L}$ = 0.68, 95% CI: 0.48–0.95) in people with no type-2 diabetes (Diaz-Lopez et al., 2013). Considering the preventive role of dietary fiber in hypertension, diabetes, obesity, and hyperlipidemia, which are risk factors for CKD, it is plausible that dietary fiber intake may be protective against CKD.

Moreover, some studies suggested that dietary fiber had beneficial effects on health of people with CKD. A study investigated whether dietary fiber intake was related to serum CRP concentration and total mortality in people with CKD and non-CKD in the National Health and Nutrition Examination Survey III (Krishnamurthy et al., 2012). After controlling for other risk factors of CKD, every 10 g/day increase in dietary fiber intake reduced the risk of elevated serum CRP (>3 mg/L) by 38% in people with CKD and also lowered risk of total mortality by 19% in people with CKD.

Furthermore, a summary of 14 trials of dietary fiber supplements among people with CKD supported the benefits of dietary fiber on improving kidney functions (Chiavaroli et al., 2014). Dietary fiber supplementation, ranged from 3.1 to 50 g/day across trials (median = 26.9 g/day), lowered serum urea concentration by −1.76 nmol/L (95% CI: −3.00 to −0.51 nmol/L) and creatinine levels by −22.83 mmol/L (95% CI: −42.63 to −3.02 mmol/L). People with CKD have been advised to limit their intakes on fruit and vegetables because a diet high in fruit and vegetables tend to have a higher amount of potassium and phosphorus. However, given the emerging evidence on the beneficial effects of dietary fiber on renal health, more studies are warranted. Also, studies to elucidate the mechanisms of how dietary fiber acts on kidney function are needed.

CHRONIC OBSTRUCTIVE PULMONARY DISEASE AND RESPIRATORY DISEASES MORTALITY

Chronic obstructive respiratory disease (COPD), which includes emphysema and chronic bronchitis, is the ninth common cause of the global burden of disease in 2010 (Murray and Lopez, 2013). COPD is the disease that involves abnormal pulmonary inflammatory responses and thickening of the airway, which cause limitations in lung airflow. As inflammation is one of the distinctive features of COPD and other respiratory diseases, it is plausible that anti-inflammatory properties of dietary fiber may play a role in the etiology of a respiratory disease.

The Singapore Chinese Health Study investigated whether dietary factors were related to the incidence of cough with phlegm among 45–74 years

Table 20.3 Results from Studies on Dietary Fiber Intake and Risk of Respiratory Diseases

Study	Outcome	Relative Risk (95% Confidence Intervals)			
		Total Dietary Fiber	Fiber from Fruit	Fiber from Vegetables	Fiber from Grains
SCHS (Butler et al., 2004)	Incident cough with phlegm	0.61 (0.47–0.78)	–	–	–
ARCS (Kan et al., 2008)	COPD	0.80 (0.63–1.02)	0.81 (0.64–1.03)	–	0.79 (0.64–0.98)
Japanese case–control (Hirayama et al., 2009)	COPD	0.49 (0.26–0.95)	–	–	–
NHS & HPFS (Varraso et al., 2010)	COPD	0.67 (0.50–0.90)	0.77 (0.59–1.01)	0.92 (0.71–1.18)	0.77 (0.59–0.99)
NIH-AARP (men) (Park et al., 2011)	Respiratory disease death	0.69 (0.54–0.87)	0.95 (0.79–1.15)	0.85 (0.71–1.02)	0.74 (0.62–0.89)
NIH-AARP (women) (Park et al., 2011)	Respiratory disease death	0.54 (0.40–0.72)	0.84(0.67–1.06)	0.72 (0.58–0.89)	0.83 (0.68–1.02)
EPIC (men) (Chuang et al., 2012)	Respiratory disease death	0.47 (0.30–0.75)	1.01 (0.81–1.25)	0.88 (0.68–1.14)	0.90 (0.78–1.03)
EPIC (women) (Chuang et al., 2012)	Respiratory disease death	0.40 (0.25–0.64)	0.79 (0.64–0.97)	0.76 (0.60–0.96)	0.77 (0.66–0.90)

SCHS, Singapore Chinese Health Study; ARCS, Atherosclerosis Risk in Communities Study; NHS, Nurses' Health Study; HPFS, Health Professionals Follow-up Study; NIH-AARP, NIH-AARP Diet and Health Study; EPIC, European Prospective Investigation into Cancer and Nutrition.

old men and women (Table 20.3) (Butler et al., 2004). This study found that intake of nonstarch polysaccharides, a major component of dietary fiber, was related to a lower risk of cough with phlegm ($OR_{H\ vs\ L} = 0.61$, 95% CI: 0.47–0.78). In the Atherosclerosis Risk in Communities Study, higher dietary fiber intake was related to better lung function and lower risks of COPD (Kan et al., 2008). Compared to people in the lowest quintile of dietary fiber intake, people in the highest quintile had a 60.2 mL higher forced expiratory volume in 1 s (FEV_1), 55.2 mL higher forced vital capacity (FVC), and 0.4% higher FEV_1/FVC ratio after controlling for potential confounders. Also, people in the highest quintile of dietary fiber intake had a 20% lower risk of spirometry-defined COPD ($OR_{H\ vs\ L} = 0.80$, 95% CI: 0.63–1.02). The inverse association was more apparent with fiber from grains ($OR_{H\ vs\ L} = 0.79$, 95% CI: 0.64–0.98) and from fruit ($OR_{H\ vs\ L} = 0.81$, 95% CI: 0.64–1.03), but not with fiber from vegetables.

A Japanese case–control study also found that high intake of dietary fiber was associated with significantly lower risk of COPD ($OR_{H\ vs\ L} = 0.49$,

95% CI: 0.26–0.95) (Hirayama et al., 2009). Findings from two prospective cohort studies also support the inverse association between dietary fiber intake and the risk of COPD. A combined analysis of the Nurses' Health Study and Health Professionals Follow-up Study that carefully controlled for other COPD risk factors also found that dietary fiber intake was inversely associated with the risk of incident COPD (Varraso et al., 2010). Comparing the highest quintile of intake to the lowest, the RR was 0.67 (95% CI: 0.50–0.90) for dietary fiber, 0.77 (95% CI: 0.59–1.01) for fiber from fruit, 0.92 (95% CI: 0.71–1.18) for fiber from vegetables, and 0.77 (95% CI: 0.59–0.99) for fiber from grains.

Recent reports from the NIH-AARP study (Park et al., 2011) and the EPIC study (Chuang et al., 2012) also provided evidence on a potential beneficial effect of dietary fiber on respiratory diseases. Both the NIH-AARP and the EPIC studies found that dietary fiber, especially fiber from grains, lowered the risk of death from respiratory diseases. The NIH-AARP study found dietary fiber intake was related to a 31% ($RR_{H\ vs\ L}$ = 0.69, 95% CI: 0.54–0.87) and 46% ($RR_{H\ vs\ L}$ = 0.54, 95% CI: 0.40–0.72) reduction of death from respiratory diseases in men and women, respectively. Fiber from fruit was not related to the risk of death from respiratory diseases, whereas fibers from vegetables and grains were associated with a lower risk of death from respiratory diseases. The $RR_{H\ vs\ L}$ for fiber from vegetables was 0.85 (95% CI: 0.71–1.02) in men and 0.72 (95% CI: 0.58–0.89) in women. The $RR_{H\ vs\ L}$ for fiber from grains was 0.74 (95% CI: 0.62–0.89) in men and 0.83 (95% CI: 0.68–1.02) in women.

Similarly, the EPIC study found that the risk of death from respiratory diseases was reduced by 53% in men ($RR_{H\ vs\ L}$ = 0.47, 95% CI: 0.30–0.75) and 60% in women ($RR_{H\ vs\ L}$ = 0.40, 95% CI: 0.25–0.64) with high dietary fiber intake. Fibers from fruit and vegetables were associated with the risk of death from respiratory diseases in women (per 5 g/day increase RR = 0.79, 95% CI: 0.64–0.97 for fiber from fruit; RR = 0.76, 95% CI: 0.60–0.96 for fiber from vegetables), but not in men. For every 5 g/day increase in fiber from grains, the RR was 0.90 (95% CI: 0.78–1.03) in men and 0.77 (95% CI: 0.66–0.90) in women.

CONCLUSIONS

Epidemiologic studies have significantly contributed to the recognition of dietary fiber as an essential constituent of a healthy diet. Numerous epidemiologic studies consistently found that high intake of dietary fiber was associated with a lower risk of cardiovascular disease, type-2 diabetes, and colorectal cancer. Accumulating evidence suggested that dietary fiber intake was inversely related to the risk of death from any causes and cancer in breast, esophagus, stomach, and kidney. Recently, interesting new evidence has emerged that dietary fiber was related to a lower risk of infectious and respiratory diseases, including CKD and COPD. These epidemiologic findings on the benefits of dietary fiber on various health conditions were supported by plausible physiologic mechanisms provided by numerous clinical studies. Recent development in studies on gut microbiome may provide new approaches to study the role of dietary fiber and its physiologic mechanisms in health (Flint et al., 2012). More prospective studies on dietary fiber and infectious, respiratory, and renal diseases are needed.

REFERENCES

Aarestrup, J., Kyro, C., Christensen, J., Kristensen, M., Wurtz, A.M., Johnsen, N.F., et al., 2012. Whole grain, dietary fiber, and incidence of endometrial cancer in a Danish cohort study. Nutr. Cancer 64, 1160–1168.

Alberts, D.S., Martinez, M.E., Roe, D.J., Guillen-Rodriguez, J.M., Marshall, J.R., van Leeuwen, J.B., et al., 2000. Lack of effect of a high-fiber cereal supplement on the recurrence of colorectal adenomas. Phoenix Colon Cancer Prevention Physicians' Network. N. Engl. J. Med. 342, 1156–1162.

Allen, N.E., Roddam, A.W., Sieri, S., Boeing, H., Jakobsen, M.U., Overvad, K., et al., 2009. A prospective analysis of the association between macronutrient intake and renal cell carcinoma in the European Prospective Investigation into Cancer and Nutrition. Int. J. Cancer 125, 982–987.

Anderson, J.W., Baird, P., Davis Jr., R.H., Ferreri, S., Knudtson, M., Koraym, A., et al., 2009. Health benefits of dietary fiber. Nutr. Rev. 67, 188–205.

Ascherio, A., Rimm, E.B., Hernan, M.A., Giovannucci, E.L., Kawachi, I., Stampfer, M.J., et al., 1998. Intake of potassium, magnesium, calcium, and fiber and risk of stroke among US men. Circulation 98, 1198–1204.

Aune, D., Chan, D.S., Greenwood, D.C., Vieira, A.R., Rosenblatt, D.A., Vieira, R., et al., 2012. Dietary fiber and breast cancer risk: a systematic review and meta-analysis of prospective studies. Ann. Oncol. 23, 1394–1402.

Aune, D., Chan, D.S., Lau, R., Vieira, R., Greenwood, D.C., Kampman, E., et al., 2011. Dietary fibre, whole grains, and risk of colorectal cancer: systematic review and dose–response meta-analysis of prospective studies. BMJ 343, d6617.

Bandera, E.V., Kushi, L.H., Moore, D.F., Gifkins, D.M., McCullough, M.L., 2007. Association between dietary fiber and endometrial cancer: a dose–response meta-analysis. Am. J. Clin. Nutr. 86, 1730–1737.

Bazzano, L.A., He, J., Ogden, L.G., Loria, C.M., Whelton, P.K., 2003. Dietary fiber intake and reduced risk of coronary heart disease in US men and women: the National Health and Nutrition Examination Survey I Epidemiologic Follow-up Study. Arch. Intern. Med. 163, 1897–1904.

Belle, F.N., Kampman, E., McTiernan, A., Bernstein, L., Baumgartner, K., Baumgartner, R., et al., 2011. Dietary fiber, carbohydrates, glycemic index, and glycemic load in relation to breast cancer prognosis in the HEAL cohort. Cancer Epidemiol. Biomarkers Prev. 20, 890–899.

Ben, Q., Sun, Y., Chai, R., Qian, A., Xu, B., Yuan, Y., 2014. Dietary fiber intake reduces risk for colorectal adenoma: a meta-analysis. Gastroenterology 146 689–699.e6.

Bidoli, E., Pelucchi, C., Zucchetto, A., Negri, E., Dal Maso, L., Polesel, J., et al., 2012. Fiber intake and pancreatic cancer risk: a case–control study. Ann. Oncol. 23, 264–268.

Bo, S., Durazzo, M., Guidi, S., Carello, M., Sacerdote, C., Silli, B., et al., 2006. Dietary magnesium and fiber intakes and inflammatory and metabolic indicators in middle-aged subjects from a population-based cohort. Am. J. Clin. Nutr. 84, 1062–1069.

Botterweck, A.A., van den Brandt, P.A., Goldbohm, R.A., 2000. Vitamins, carotenoids, dietary fiber, and the risk of gastric carcinoma: results from a prospective study after 6.3 years of follow-up. Cancer 88, 737–748.

Brock, K.E., Ke, L., Gridley, G., Chiu, B.C., Ershow, A.G., Lynch, C.F., et al., 2012. Fruit, vegetables, fibre and micronutrients and risk of US renal cell carcinoma. Br. J. Nutr. 108, 1077–1085.

Brown, L., Rosner, B., Willett, W.W., Sacks, F.M., 1999. Cholesterol-lowering effects of dietary fiber: a meta-analysis. Am. J. Clin. Nutr. 69, 30–42.

Buck, K., Zaineddin, A.K., Vrieling, A., Heinz, J., Linseisen, J., Flesch-Janys, D., et al., 2011. Estimated enterolignans, lignan-rich foods, and fibre in relation to survival after postmenopausal breast cancer. Br. J. Cancer 105, 1151–1157.

Burkitt, D.P., 1971. Epidemiology of cancer of the colon and rectum. Cancer 28, 3–13.

Burkitt, D.P., Walker, A.R., Painter, N.S., 1972. Effect of dietary fibre on stools and the transit-times, and its role in the causation of disease. Lancet 2, 1408–1412.

Butler, L.M., Koh, W.P., Lee, H.P., Yu, M.C., London, S.J., 2004. Dietary fiber and reduced cough with phlegm: a cohort study in Singapore. Am. J. Respir. Crit. Care Med. 170, 279–287.

Buyken, A.E., Flood, V., Empson, M., Rochtchina, E., Barclay, A.W., Brand-Miller, J., et al., 2010. Carbohydrate nutrition and inflammatory disease mortality in older adults. Am. J. Clin. Nutr. 92, 634–643.

Chan, J.M., Wang, F., Holly, E.A., 2007. Whole grains and risk of pancreatic cancer in a large population-based case–control study in the San Francisco Bay Area, California. Am. J. Epidemiol. 166, 1174–1185.

Chen, G.C., Lv, D.B., Pang, Z., Dong, J.Y., Liu, Q.F., 2013. Dietary fiber intake and stroke risk: a meta-analysis of prospective cohort studies. Eur. J. Clin. Nutr. 67, 96–100.

Chiavaroli, L., Mirrahimi, A., Sievenpiper, J.L., Jenkins, D.J., Darling, P.B., 2014. Dietary fiber effects in chronic kidney disease: a systematic review and meta-analysis of controlled feeding trials. Eur. J. Clin. Nutr. 69 (7), 761–768.

Chow, W.H., Dong, L.M., Devesa, S.S., 2010. Epidemiology and risk factors for kidney cancer. Nat. Rev. Urol. 7, 245–257.

Chuang, S.C., Norat, T., Murphy, N., Olsen, A., Tjonneland, A., Overvad, K., et al., 2012. Fiber intake and total and cause-specific mortality in the European Prospective Investigation into Cancer and Nutrition cohort. Am. J. Clin. Nutr. 96, 164–174.

Coleman, H.G., Murray, L.J., Hicks, B., Bhat, S.K., Kubo, A., Corley, D.A., et al., 2013. Dietary fiber and the risk of precancerous lesions and cancer of the esophagus: a systematic review and meta-analysis. Nutr. Rev. 71, 474–482.

Cui, X., Rosner, B., Willett, W.C., Hankinson, S.E., 2011. Dietary fat, fiber, and carbohydrate intake in relation to risk of endometrial cancer. Cancer Epidemiol. Biomarkers Prev. 20, 978–989.

Daniel, C.R., Park, Y., Chow, W.H., Graubard, B.I., Hollenbeck, A.R., Sinha, R., 2013. Intake of fiber and fiber-rich plant foods is associated with a lower risk of renal cell carcinoma in a large US cohort. Am. J. Clin. Nutr. 97, 1036–1043.

Diaz-Lopez, A., Bullo, M., Basora, J., Martinez-Gonzalez, M.A., Guasch-Ferre, M., Estruch, R., et al., 2013. Cross-sectional associations between macronutrient intake and chronic kidney disease in a population at high cardiovascular risk. Clin. Nutr. 32, 606–612.

Du, H., van der, A.D., Boshuizen, H.C., Forouhi, N.G., Wareham, N.J., Halkjaer, J., et al., 2010. Dietary fiber and subsequent changes in body weight and waist circumference in European men and women. Am. J. Clin. Nutr. 91, 329–336.

EFSA Panel on Dietetic Products, Nutrition and Allergies, 2010. Scientific opinion on dietary reference values for carbohydrates and dietary fibre. EFSA J., 1462–1539.

Esposito, K., Marfella, R., Ciotola, M., Di Palo, C., Giugliano, F., Giugliano, G., et al., 2004. Effect of a Mediterranean-style diet on endothelial dysfunction and markers of vascular inflammation in the metabolic syndrome: a randomized trial. JAMA 292, 1440–1446.

Estruch, R., Martinez-Gonzalez, M.A., Corella, D., Basora-Gallisa, J., Ruiz-Gutierrez, V., Covas, M.I., et al., 2009. Effects of dietary fibre intake on risk factors for cardiovascular disease in subjects at high risk. J. Epidemiol. Community Health 63, 582–588.

Evans, C.E., Greenwood, D.C., Threapleton, D.E., Cleghorn, C.L., Nykjaer, C., Woodhead, C.E., et al., 2015. Effects of dietary fibre type on blood pressure: a systematic review and meta-analysis of randomized controlled trials of healthy individuals. J. Hypertens. 33, 897–911.

Evenepoel, P., Meijers, B.K., Bammens, B.R., Verbeke, K., 2009. Uremic toxins originating from colonic microbial metabolism. Kidney Int. Suppl., S12–S19.

Fedirko, V., Lukanova, A., Bamia, C., Trichopolou, A., Trepo, E., Nothlings, U., et al., 2013. Glycemic index, glycemic load, dietary carbohydrate, and dietary fiber intake and risk of liver and biliary tract cancers in Western Europeans. Ann. Oncol. 24, 543–553.

Flint, H.J., Scott, K.P., Louis, P., Duncan, S.H., 2012. The role of the gut microbiota in nutrition and health. Nat. Rev. Gastroenterol. Hepatol. 9, 577–589.

Fujii, H., Iwase, M., Ohkuma, T., Ogata-Kaizu, S., Ide, H., Kikuchi, Y., et al., 2013. Impact of dietary fiber intake on glycemic control, cardiovascular risk factors and chronic kidney disease in Japanese patients with type 2 diabetes mellitus: the Fukuoka Diabetes Registry. Nutr. J. 12, 159.

Garcia-Diez, F., Garcia-Mediavilla, V., Bayon, J.E., Gonzalez-Gallego, J., 1996. Pectin feeding influences fecal bile acid excretion, hepatic bile acid and cholesterol synthesis and serum cholesterol in rats. J. Nutr. 126, 1766–1771.

Goldin, B.R., Adlercreutz, H., Gorbach, S.L., Warram, J.H., Dwyer, J.T., Swenson, L., et al., 1982. Estrogen excretion patterns and plasma levels in vegetarian and omnivorous women. N. Engl. J. Med. 307, 1542–1547.

Gopinath, B., Harris, D.C., Flood, V.M., Burlutsky, G., Brand-Miller, J., Mitchell, P., 2011. Carbohydrate nutrition is associated with the 5-year incidence of chronic kidney disease. J. Nutr. 141, 433–439.

Hara, H., Haga, S., Aoyama, Y., Kiriyama, S., 1999. Short-chain fatty acids suppress cholesterol synthesis in rat liver and intestine. J. Nutr. 129, 942–948.

Herder, C., Peltonen, M., Koenig, W., Sutfels, K., Lindstrom, J., Martin, S., et al., 2009. Anti-inflammatory effect of lifestyle changes in the Finnish Diabetes Prevention Study. Diabetologia 52, 433–442.

Hipsley, E.H., 1953. Dietary "fibre" and pregnancy toxaemia. Br. Med. J. 2, 420–422.

Hirayama, F., Lee, A.H., Binns, C.W., Zhao, Y., Hiramatsu, T., Tanikawa, Y., et al., 2009. Do vegetables and fruits reduce the risk of chronic obstructive pulmonary disease? A case–control study in Japan. Prev. Med. 49, 184–189.

Holmes, M.D., Chen, W.Y., Hankinson, S.E., Willett, W.C., 2009. Physical activity's impact on the association of fat and fiber intake with survival after breast cancer. Am. J. Epidemiol. 170, 1250–1256.

Howe, G.R., Jain, M., Miller, A.B., 1990. Dietary factors and risk of pancreatic cancer: results of a Canadian population-based case–control study. Int. J. Cancer 45, 604–608.

Hu, J., La Vecchia, C., DesMeules, M., Negri, E., Mery, L., 2008. Nutrient and fiber intake and risk of renal cell carcinoma. Nutr. Cancer 60, 720–728.

Huang, T.B., Ding, P.P., Chen, J.F., Yan, Y., Zhang, L., Liu, H., et al., 2014. Dietary fiber intake and risk of renal cell carcinoma: evidence from a meta-analysis. Med. Oncol. 31, 125.

InterAct Consortium, 2015. Dietary fibre and incidence of type 2 diabetes in eight European countries: the EPIC-InterAct Study and a meta-analysis of prospective studies. Diabetologia 58 (7), 1394–1408.

Jain, M.G., Rohan, T.E., Howe, G.R., Miller, A.B., 2000. A cohort study of nutritional factors and endometrial cancer. Eur. J. Epidemiol. 16, 899–905.

Jemal, A., Bray, F., Center, M.M., Ferlay, J., Ward, E., Forman, D., 2011. Global cancer statistics. CA Cancer J. Clin. 61, 69–90.

Ji, B.T., Chow, W.H., Gridley, G., McLaughlin, J.K., Dai, Q., Wacholder Jr., S., et al., 1995. Dietary factors and the risk of pancreatic cancer: a case–control study in Shanghai China. Cancer Epidemiol. Biomarkers Prev. 4, 885–893.

Johansson-Persson, A., Ulmius, M., Cloetens, L., Karhu, T., Herzig, K.H., Onning, G., 2014. A high intake of dietary fiber influences C-reactive protein and fibrinogen, but not glucose and lipid metabolism, in mildly hypercholesterolemic subjects. Eur. J. Nutr. 53, 39–48.

Kalapothaki, V., Tzonou, A., Hsieh, C.C., Karakatsani, A., Trichopoulou, A., Toupadaki, N., et al., 1993. Nutrient intake and cancer of the pancreas: a case–control study in Athens, Greece. Cancer Causes Control 4, 383–389.

Kan, H., Stevens, J., Heiss, G., Rose, K.M., London, S.J., 2008. Dietary fiber, lung function, and chronic obstructive pulmonary disease in the atherosclerosis risk in communities study. Am. J. Epidemiol. 167, 570–578.

Kantor, E.D., Lampe, J.W., Kratz, M., White, E., 2013. Lifestyle factors and inflammation: associations by body mass index. PLoS One 8, e67833.

Kim, Y., Je, Y., 2014. Dietary fiber intake and total mortality: a meta-analysis of prospective cohort studies. Am. J. Epidemiol. 180, 565–573.

King, D.E., Egan, B.M., Woolson, R.F., Mainous 3rd, A.G., Al-Solaiman, Y., Jesri, A., 2007. Effect of a high-fiber diet vs a fiber-supplemented diet on C-reactive protein level. Arch. Intern. Med. 167, 502–506.

King, D.E., Mainous 3rd, A.G., Lambourne, C.A., 2012. Trends in dietary fiber intake in the United States, 1999–2008. J. Acad. Nutr. Diet. 112, 642–648.

Koh-Banerjee, P., Franz, M., Sampson, L., Liu, S., Jacobs Jr., D.R., Spiegelman, D., et al., 2004. Changes in whole-grain, bran, and cereal fiber consumption in relation to 8-y weight gain among men. Am. J. Clin. Nutr. 80, 1237–1245.

Kokubo, Y., Iso, H., Saito, I., Yamagishi, K., Ishihara, J., Inoue, M., et al., 2011. Dietary fiber intake and risk of cardiovascular disease in the Japanese population: the Japan Public Health Center-based study cohort. Eur. J. Clin. Nutr. 65, 1233–1241.

Krishnamurthy, V.M., Wei, G., Baird, B.C., Murtaugh, M., Chonchol, M.B., Raphael, K.L., et al., 2012. High dietary fiber intake is associated with decreased inflammation and all-cause mortality in patients with chronic kidney disease. Kidney Int. 81, 300–306.

Lanza, E., Yu, B., Murphy, G., Albert, P.S., Caan, B., Marshall, J.R., et al., 2007. The polyp prevention trial continued follow-up study: no effect of a low-fat, high-fiber, high-fruit, and -vegetable diet on adenoma recurrence eight years after randomization. Cancer Epidemiol. Biomarkers Prev. 16, 1745–1752.

Larsson, S.C., Wolk, A., 2014. Dietary fiber intake is inversely associated with stroke incidence in healthy Swedish adults. J. Nutr. 144, 1952–1955.

Larsson, S.C., Mannisto, S., Virtanen, M.J., Kontto, J., Albanes, D., Virtamo, J., 2009. Dietary fiber and fiber-rich food intake in relation to risk of stroke in male smokers. Eur. J. Clin. Nutr. 63, 1016–1024.

Lawlor, D.A., Smith, G.D., Ebrahim, S., 2004. Hyperinsulinaemia and increased risk of breast cancer: findings from the British Women's Heart and Health Study. Cancer Causes Control 15, 267–275.

Lindblad, P., Wolk, A., Bergstrom, R., Adami, H.O., 1997. Diet and risk of renal cell cancer: a population-based case–control study. Cancer Epidemiol. Biomarkers Prev. 6, 215–223.

Lindstrom, J., Peltonen, M., Eriksson, J.G., Louheranta, A., Fogelholm, M., Uusitupa, M., et al., 2006. High-fibre, low-fat diet predicts long-term weight loss and decreased type 2 diabetes risk: the Finnish Diabetes Prevention Study. Diabetologia 49, 912–920.

Lipkin, M., Reddy, B., Newmark, H., Lamprecht, S.A., 1999. Dietary factors in human colorectal cancer. Annu. Rev. Nutr. 19, 545–586.

Liu, S., Willett, W.C., Manson, J.E., Hu, F.B., Rosner, B., Colditz, G., 2003. Relation between changes in intakes of dietary fiber and grain products and changes in weight and development of obesity among middle-aged women. Am. J. Clin. Nutr. 78, 920–927.

Liu, Y., Colditz, G.A., Cotterchio, M., Boucher, B.A., Kreiger, N., 2014. Adolescent dietary fiber, vegetable fat, vegetable protein, and nut intakes and breast cancer risk. Breast Cancer Res. Treat. 145, 461–470.

Lubin, F., Lusky, A., Chetrit, A., Dankner, R., 2003. Lifestyle and ethnicity play a role in all-cause mortality. J. Nutr. 133, 1180–1185.

Ma, Y., Hebert, J.R., Li, W., Bertone-Johnson, E.R., Olendzki, B., Pagoto, S.L., et al., 2008. Association between dietary fiber and markers of systemic inflammation in the Women's Health Initiative Observational Study. Nutrition 24, 941–949.

Ma, Y., Olendzki, B.C., Wang, J., Persuitte, G.M., Li, W., Fang, H., et al., 2015. Single-component versus multicomponent dietary goals for the metabolic syndrome: a randomized trial. Ann. Intern. Med. 162, 248–257.

McEligot, A.J., Largent, J., Ziogas, A., Peel, D., Anton-Culver, H., 2006. Dietary fat, fiber, vegetable, and micronutrients are associated with overall survival in postmenopausal women diagnosed with breast cancer. Nutr. Cancer 55, 132–140.

Mendez, M.A., Pera, G., Agudo, A., Bueno-de-Mesquita, H.B., Palli, D., Boeing, H., et al., 2007. Cereal fiber intake may reduce risk of gastric adenocarcinomas: the EPIC-EURGAST study. Int. J. Cancer. 121, 1618–1623.

Moller, M.E., Dahl, R., Bockman, O.C., 1988. A possible role of the dietary fibre product, wheat bran, as a nitrite scavenger. Food Chem. Toxicol. 26, 841–845.

Murray, C.J., Lopez, A.D., 2013. Measuring the global burden of disease. N. Engl. J. Med. 369, 448–457.

National Research Council, 2001. Dietary Reference Intakes: Proposed Definition of Dietary Fiber. The National Academies Press, Washington, DC.

North, C.J., Venter, C.S., Jerling, J.C., 2009. The effects of dietary fibre on C-reactive protein, an inflammation marker predicting cardiovascular disease. Eur. J. Clin. Nutr. 63, 921–933.

Oh, K., Hu, F.B., Cho, E., Rexrode, K.M., Stampfer, M.J., Manson, J.E., et al., 2005. Carbohydrate intake, glycemic index, glycemic load, and dietary fiber in relation to risk of stroke in women. Am. J. Epidemiol. 161, 161–169.

Park, Y., Subar, A.F., Hollenbeck, A., Schatzkin, A., 2011. Dietary fiber intake and mortality in the NIH-AARP diet and health study. Arch. Intern. Med. 171, 1061–1068.

Parkin, D.M., Boyd, L., 2011. Cancers attributable to dietary factors in the UK in 2010. III. Low consumption of fibre. Br. J. Cancer 105 (Suppl. 2), S27–S30.

Pennathur, A., Gibson, M.K., Jobe, B.A., Luketich, J.D., 2013. Oesophageal carcinoma. Lancet 381, 400–412.

Pereira, M.A., Ludwig, D.S., 2001. Dietary fiber and body-weight regulation. Observations and mechanisms. Pediatr. Clin. North Am. 48, 969–980.

Pereira, M.A., O'Reilly, E., Augustsson, K., Fraser, G.E., Goldbourt, U., Heitmann, B.L., et al., 2004. Dietary fiber and risk of coronary heart disease: a pooled analysis of cohort studies. Arch. Intern. Med. 164, 370–376.

Post, R.E., Mainous 3rd, A.G., King, D.E., Simpson, K.N., 2012. Dietary fiber for the treatment of type 2 diabetes mellitus: a meta-analysis. J. Am. Board Fam. Med. 25, 16–23.

Rose, D.P., Goldman, M., Connolly, J.M., Strong, L.E., 1991. High-fiber diet reduces serum estrogen concentrations in premenopausal women. Am. J. Clin. Nutr. 54, 520–525.

Schatzkin, A., Lanza, E., Corle, D., Lance, P., Iber, F., Caan, B., et al., 2000. Lack of effect of a low-fat, high-fiber diet on the recurrence of colorectal adenomas. Polyp Prevention Trial Study Group. N. Engl. J. Med. 342, 1149–1155.

Schulze, M.B., Schulz, M., Heidemann, C., Schienkiewitz, A., Hoffmann, K., Boeing, H., 2007. Fiber and magnesium intake and incidence of type 2 diabetes: a prospective study and meta-analysis. Arch. Intern. Med. 167, 956–965.

Stolzenberg-Solomon, R.Z., Pietinen, P., Taylor, P.R., Virtamo, J., Albanes, D., 2002. Prospective study of diet and pancreatic cancer in male smokers. Am. J. Epidemiol. 155, 783–792.

Streppel, M.T., Arends, L.R., van't Veer, P., Grobbee, D.E., Geleijnse, J.M., 2005. Dietary fiber and blood pressure: a meta-analysis of randomized placebo-controlled trials. Arch. Intern. Med. 165, 150–156.

Streppel, M.T., Ocke, M.C., Boshuizen, H.C., Kok, F.J., Kromhout, D., 2008. Dietary fiber intake in relation to coronary heart disease and all-cause mortality over 40 y: the Zutphen Study. Am. J. Clin. Nutr. 88, 1119–1125.

Threapleton, D.E., Greenwood, D.C., Evans, C.E., Cleghorn, C.L., Nykjaer, C., Woodhead, C., et al., 2013a. Dietary fibre intake and risk of cardiovascular disease: systematic review and meta-analysis. BMJ 347, f6879.

Threapleton, D.E., Greenwood, D.C., Evans, C.E., Cleghorn, C.L., Nykjaer, C., Woodhead, C., et al., 2013b. Dietary fiber intake and risk of first stroke: a systematic review and meta-analysis. Stroke 44, 1360–1368.

Todd, S., Woodward, M., Tunstall-Pedoe, H., Bolton-Smith, C., 1999. Dietary antioxidant vitamins and fiber in the etiology of cardiovascular disease and all-causes mortality: results from the Scottish Heart Health Study. Am. J. Epidemiol. 150, 1073–1080.

Trowell, H., 1972. Ischemic heart disease and dietary fiber. Am. J. Clin. Nutr. 25, 926–932.

Trowell, H., Southgate, D.A., Wolever, T.M., Leeds, A.R., Gassull, M.A., Jenkins, D.J., 1976. Letter: dietary fibre redefined. Lancet 1, 967.

US Department of Agriculture and US Department of Health and Human Services, 2010. Dietary Guidelines for Americans, 2010. US Government Printing Office. December 2010.

Varraso, R., Willett, W.C., Camargo Jr., C.A., 2010. Prospective study of dietary fiber and risk of chronic obstructive pulmonary disease among US women and men. Am. J. Epidemiol. 171, 776–784.

Villasenor, A., Ambs, A., Ballard-Barbash, R., Baumgartner, K.B., McTiernan, A., Ulrich, C.M., et al., 2011. Dietary fiber is associated with circulating concentrations of C-reactive protein in breast cancer survivors: the HEAL study. Breast Cancer Res. Treat. 129, 485–494.

Wallstrom, P., Sonestedt, E., Hlebowicz, J., Ericson, U., Drake, I., Persson, M., et al., 2012. Dietary fiber and saturated fat intake associations with cardiovascular disease differ by sex in the Malmo Diet and Cancer Cohort: a prospective study. PLoS One 7, e31637.

Wang, C.H., Qiao, C., Wang, R.C., Zhou, W.P., 2015. Dietary fiber intake and pancreatic cancer risk: a meta-analysis of epidemiologic studies. Sci. Rep. 5, 10834.

Weickert, M.O., Pfeiffer, A.F., 2008. Metabolic effects of dietary fiber consumption and prevention of diabetes. J. Nutr. 138, 439–442.

Whelton, S.P., Hyre, A.D., Pedersen, B., Yi, Y., Whelton, P.K., He, J., 2005. Effect of dietary fiber intake on blood pressure: a meta-analysis of randomized, controlled clinical trials. J. Hypertens. 23, 475–481.

World Cancer Research Fund and American Institute for Cancer Research, 2007. Food, Nutrition, Physical Activity, and the Prevention of Cancer: A Global Perspective. AICR, Washington, DC.

World Cancer Research Fund and American Institute for Cancer Research, 2011. Continuous Update Project: Food, Nutrition, Physical Activity, and the Prevention of Cancer: A Global Perspective.

World Health Organization, 2015. The top 10 causes of death. <http://www.who.int/mediacentre/factsheets/fs310/en/> (accessed 05.15.).

Wu, Y., Qian, Y., Pan, Y., Li, P., Yang, J., Ye, X., et al., 2014. Association between dietary fiber intake and risk of coronary heart disease: a meta-analysis. Clin. Nutr.

Yang, Y., Zhao, L.G., Wu, Q.J., Ma, X., Xiang, Y.B., 2015. Association between dietary fiber and lower risk of all-cause mortality: a meta-analysis of cohort studies. Am. J. Epidemiol. 181, 83–91.

Yu, H., Rohan, T., 2000. Role of the insulin-like growth factor family in cancer development and progression. J. Natl. Cancer Inst. 92, 1472–1489.

Zhang, J., Dhakal, I.B., Gross, M.D., Lang, N.P., Kadlubar, F.F., Harnack, L.J., et al., 2009. Physical activity, diet, and pancreatic cancer: a population-based, case–control study in Minnesota. Nutr. Cancer 61, 457–465.

Zhang, Z., Xu, G., Ma, M., Yang, J., Liu, X., 2013. Dietary fiber intake reduces risk for gastric cancer: a meta-analysis. Gastroenterology 145, 113–120.e3.

Chapter 21

Fruits, vegetables, and herbs: bioactive foods promoting wound healing

Lawrence W. Sanchez and Ronald Ross Watson
University of Arizona, Tucson, AZ, United States

CHAPTER OUTLINE

INTRODUCTION

Postsurgery or after injury, it is very important to eat well in order to increase the rate of recovery. Essentially all vitamins, minerals, macronutrients, and fatty acids are going to aide in the healing process. However, certain nutrients are more beneficial than others. These nutrients include vitamin C, vitamin E, vitamin A, protein, and zinc. There are also many

Fruits, Vegetables, and Herbs.
DOI: http://dx.doi.org/10.1016/B978-0-12-802972-5.00021-4

dietary and nondietary plants, herbs, and other foods that increase wound healing recovery.

The body's process of healing wounds is very complex. The process is divided up into three phases: inflammatory, proliferative, and maturation (Wild et al., 2010). There is no set limit on the amount of time the body spends in each phase. It starts with the injury and can continue for years (Wild et al., 2010). The body is able to progress forward or backward in the phases depending on many other factors. Factors that negatively influence wound healing can be categorized into two groups: local factors and systemic factors. Local factors include scalds and burns, physical or chemical, local pressure, and neurologic defects. Systemic factors include trauma, immunodeficiency, malignancy, autoimmune diseases of connective tissue, metabolic diseases, malnutrition and our nutritional deficiencies, psychosocial stress, drug use, chronic diseases, and advanced age (Wild et al., 2010). The process of wound healing is a very demanding process that requires a lot of energy in order to build new cells (Wild et al., 2010).

STAGES OF HEALING

The first of three phases is the inflammatory phase. This phase occurs immediately after injury (Wild et al., 2010). Signs associated with this phase include redness, warmth, swelling, pain, and loss of function (Wild et al., 2010). Coagulation and vasoconstriction occur. Due to the many mediators associated with coagulation, inflammation processes also occur (Wild et al., 2010). During the inflammatory phase, the body creates a barrier to further prevent microbial invasion. Pain is important because it causes decreased activity in the injured area (Wild et al., 2010). The healing process starts to occur at the end of the inflammation phase. The second phase is the proliferative phase. The proliferative phase lasts for days to weeks (Wild et al., 2010). In this phase, fibroblasts migrate inward from the wound into the matrix. Fibroblasts are then stimulated by basic fibroblast growth factor and tumor growth factor beta to produce glycosaminoglycans, proteoglycans, and collagen (Wild et al., 2010).

The third phase is the maturation phase. The maturation phase, or remodeling phase, can last for weeks to years (Wild et al., 2010). During the maturation phase, the newly created collagen is randomly deposited into the tissue. The collagen fibers are then organized into a structure with increased tensile strength (Wild et al., 2010). Type III collagen is then replaced by type I collagen gradually. Once the ratio of type I to type III collagen is 4:1, the normal skin ratio, the replacement ceases (Wild et al., 2010) (Table 21.1).

Table 21.1 Nutrients Used in the Different Stages of Wound Healing

Stage of Healing	Events That Take Place in Stage	Nutrients Needed
Inflammatory	Vasoconstriction Coagulation Phagocytosis by macrophages Collagen synthesis initiated	Protein, carbohydrates, vitamin A, vitamin C, vitamin E, vitamin K
Proliferative	Angiogenesis	Protein, vitamin A, vitamin C, iron
Maturation	Continued collagen cross-linking Wound closure and contraction Maturation of scar tissue	Vitamin C, iron, protein, carbohydrates, zinc

Source: Todorovic, 2002.

VITAMIN A

Vitamin A benefits the healing process by stimulating epithelialization and aids in collagen synthesis and deposition (Arnold and Barbul, 2006). Vitamin A boosts the body's inflammatory response to wounds. Boosting the inflammatory response results in increased macrophage influx and also increases the stimulation of collagen synthesis (Arnold and Barbul, 2006). Although vitamin A is beneficial for wound healing, too much of the vitamin can be toxic to the body. The amount of vitamin A is dependent on the size and severity of the wound. A severe injury can require up to 5 times the amount of the recommended daily dose of vitamin A, but again too much of the vitamin can cause more damage than benefits (Arnold and Barbul, 2006). The recommended amount for vitamin A in adult males is 900 μg/day. The recommended amount of vitamin A in adult females is 700 μg/day (Trumbo et al., 2001). Vitamin A is found in beef liver, other organ meats, and some types of fish. Vitamin A is also found in vegetables, especially leafy green ones. Some specific types of vegetables include broccoli, carrots, and squash. Vitamin A is found in fruits like cantaloupe, mangos, and apricots. One of the major sources of vitamin A is dairy products (Vitamin A, 2013). Vitamin A can also be found in dietary supplements.

VITAMIN C

Vitamin C, also known as ascorbic acid, is critical for the synthesis of collagen. Ascorbic acid stabilizes the collagen triple helix structure (Wild et al., 2010). Ascorbic acid is also important for the synthesis of other organic components found in the extracellular matrix of bones, skin, and other connective tissues (MacKay and Miller, 2003). Vitamin C aids in angiogenesis, the formation of new blood and lymph vessels (Todorovic, 2002). Vitamin C is also critical for optimal immune response. Vitamin C is an antioxidant that facilitates the migration of white blood cells toward the wound; this increases the resistance against infection (Todorovic, 2002). More specifically, vitamin C has the ability to induce monocyte migration into the wound tissue. Monocytes differentiate into macrophages during the inflammatory phase (Wild et al., 2010). A scientific study conducted in 1974 illustrated that ascorbic acid, vitamin C, increased random migration of human leukocytes by 100–300% (Goetzel et al., 1974). The study also illustrated that enhanced mobility of isolated neutrophils, eosinophils, and mononuclear leukocytes occurred in the presence of ascorbic acid (Goetzel et al., 1974).

A deficiency of vitamin C leads to irregular formation of collagen fibers that cause poor adhesion of endothelium cells and decreased tensile strength (MacKay and Miller, 2003). Vitamin C is commonly found in fruit and fruit juices: citrus, strawberries, tomatoes, and cantaloupe. Vitamin C is also found in vegetables: Brussel sprouts, cauliflower, broccoli, sweet peppers, and potatoes (Wild et al., 2010). Vitamin C is also found in supplements that may be purchased at various drug stores and grocery stores. The recommended dietary intake of vitamin C for adult men and women under normal conditions is between 75 and 90 mg/day (Monsen, 2000). It is recommended to increase the amount of vitamin C consumed if recovering from surgery or injury.

VITAMIN E

Vitamin E is generally praised among consumers for skin care and to prevent scar formation. Vitamin E functions as an antioxidant that the body requires for cell membrane protection (Borhanuddin et al., 2012). Vitamin E has a very complex effect on wound healing. Vitamin E is extremely important in the process of bone repair. When a bone is fractured, free radicals are produced in the inflammatory phase and blood supply to the bone is compromised (Borhanuddin et al., 2012). Free radicals have been illustrated to reduce bone fracture healing by causing damage to the cell membranes eventually resulting in cell destruction (Borhanuddin et al., 2012). Vitamin E disrupts these radicals and does not allow them to react and cause cell membrane destruction or cell death (Borhanuddin et al., 2012). However, many scientific studies have only been done on animals, not many have been done on humans (Borhanuddin et al., 2012). Since not many experiments have been done on human subjects, the exact role of vitamin E in the process of bone healing is unclear. Besides the beneficial effects of vitamin E on healing bones, vitamin E is also beneficial for healing other wounds. Vitamin E is essential in maintaining cellular membranes. Vitamin E protects the membranes from oxidation, which would ultimately destroy the cell (Arnold and Barbul, 2006).

The recommended dietary intake for vitamin E for adult men and women under normal conditions is 15 mg/day (Monsen, 2000). Under abnormal conditions, like postsurgery or after an injury, it is recommended to increase dietary intake of vitamin E.

FAT AND CARBOHYDRATES

The body used carbohydrates and fats as the main source of energy. Energy is needed to create new cells and synthesize collagen in wound healing. Small wounds do not alter the body's metabolism very much, meaning the body does not need a ludicrous amount of excess carbohydrates to heal. However, large wounds and burns require more energy for repair (Arnold and Barbul, 2006). A surplus of carbohydrates and fats are needed to maximize the healing process. Fats are essential for wound healing. Components found in fats are precursors for phospholipids and prostaglandins (Arnold and Barbul, 2006). Phospholipids make up part of the cellular basement membrane; therefore, they are critical in the formation of new cells. Prostaglandins have key roles in inflammation and metabolism (Arnold and Barbul, 2006).

ZINC

Zinc is one of the most well-known micronutrient elements used in wound healing (Arnold and Barbul, 2006). Zinc plays an important role in the biosynthesis of RNA, DNA, and proteins. RNA, DNA, and proteins are key cofactors in creating new cells. Therefore, it is critical for all proliferating cells (Wild et al., 2010). Zinc is necessary for tissue regeneration and repair (MacKay and Miller, 2003). A deficiency in zinc leads to suppression of the inflammatory phase of wound healing (Wild et al., 2010). The suggested daily intake of zinc for men and women is 15 mg (Arnold and Barbul, 2006). It is also noted that patients given excess zinc did not have improved wound healing, only those who were zinc deficient did (Arnold and Barbul, 2006). It is important to continually intake at least 15 mg of zinc a day to maintain a healthy amount in case of injury.

PROTEIN

Protein is a very important macronutrient. Not only does it provide the body with energy, but it is also used by cells in the process of healing. Inadequate protein intake delays wound healing. More specifically, it delays the inflammatory phase of wound healing (MacKay and Miller, 2003). The immune system is composed of many proteins (Todorovic, 2002). When wounds are present, increased factors of the immune system are then produced and targeted toward the area needing repair (Todorovic, 2002). Common factors of the immune system include lymphocytes, leucocytes, phagocytes, and macrophages. Without protein the immune system will have an inadequate response. Not only does inadequate protein intake disrupt the immune system, it also alters fibroblast response and collagen formation (Todorovic, 2002). This will cause longer healing time and poor repairs.

IRON

Iron plays a huge role in the human body. Iron is found in hemoglobin which is used to transport oxygen in the body. Iron is crucial to transporting oxygen to new and regenerating tissue (Wild et al., 2010). A deficiency in iron not only affects regenerating tissues in the wound, but it also negatively affects the rest of the body. Besides transporting oxygen, iron is a cofactor of two enzymes, prolyl and lysyl, that are essential for synthesizing new collagen (Wild et al., 2010). Without iron, collagen formation will be impaired and not as effective. Collagen is an important tool in repairing wounds. The daily intake amount of iron suggested in females aged 19–50 is 18 mg. The daily intake amount of iron suggested in males aged 19–50 is 8 mg (Trumbo et al., 2001). The main sources of iron include red meats, beans, lentils, certain cereals and breads, and green vegetables (Todorovic, 2002) (Table 21.2).

Besides the micronutrients and macronutrients needed by the body to perform adequate wound healing, there are many other substances that can be used to accelerate the process. Plants, herbs, and other bioactive foods are commonly used.

HONEY

Honey has been generally recognized as a super food. Studies have shown that the application of honey on a cutaneous wound could cause clearing of infection and improve wound healing (Lusby, 2002). Honey has been used as a traditional wound healing agent for many years in the past. It is referred numerous times throughout literature from Egypt, Greece, and India (Lusby,

Table 21.2 Dietary Factors in the Role of Wound Healing

Nutrient	Role in Healing	Dietary Source
Protein	Needed for synthesis of new tissues	Meat, eggs, milk, fish, cereals, legumes, lentils
Fat and carbohydrates	Provides energy for synthesis Fatty acids have a key role in cell membrane synthesis	Fats: butter, margarine, oils Carbohydrates: bread, pasta, rice, noodles, potatoes, oats
Vitamin A	Antioxidant Aids in collagen synthesis and cross-linkage	Butter, margarine, oils, fats, milk, fish, eggs, carrots, tomatoes, red peppers
Vitamin C	Antioxidant Collagen synthesis Collagen cross-linkage Angiogenesis	Citrus, strawberries, Brussel sprouts, cauliflower, broccoli, sweet peppers, potatoes
Vitamin E	Antioxidant Enhances immune response	Vegetable oil, egg yolk, nuts, seeds
Vitamin K	Coagulation	Green vegetables, liver meats
Iron	Anemia prevention Promotes collagen synthesis	Red meat, certain cereals, green vegetables, lentils, beans
Zinc	Cell proliferation Maturation of collagen	Meat, milk, potatoes, bread

Source: Todorovic, 2002.

2002). In these texts, honey is described to heal wounds by itself or sometimes in combination of other ingredients (Lusby, 2002). Therapeutic honey is different then what is found on the shelf at the grocery store. Therapeutic honey is derived from a specific floral source and is treated with gamma irradiation to destroy any bacteria spores (Lusby, 2002). Honey found in grocery stores is treated with heat instead of gamma irradiation; the heat destroys an important enzyme that produces hydrogen peroxide (Lusby, 2002). The properties that make honey a beneficial healing agent include osmotic activity, pH, production of hydrogen peroxide, and the provision of a moist wound environment (Lusby, 2002). Honey contains a high sugar content that inhibits bacterial growth. The pH of honey is between 3.2 and 4.2, making it pretty acidic. The acidity of the honey also inhibits most pathogenic bacterial growth. The low amount of hydrogen peroxide produced is enough to kill bacteria without damaging tissues (Lusby, 2002). A moist environment protects the wound, reduces rates of infection, promotes tissue formation, and reduces pain (Lusby, 2002).

Honey must be applied to the wound topically. Ingesting honey does not provide its beneficial properties to wound healing. Besides inhibiting bacterial growth honey provides other healing capabilities. One of the most beneficial properties is the provision of a moist environment for the wound to heal. Moist wound environments allow new cells to grow on top of the wound rather than just under the scab in a dry environment (Lusby, 2002). This moist environment also permits deep pitted scars from forming. The viscosity of the honey provides a protective barrier on the wound by sealing it from the outside environment (Lusby, 2002). Although honey is very viscous, it does not adhere to the wound which allows the honey dressing to be changed easily (Lusby, 2002). The sugars such as levulose and fructose found in honey supply local nutrition to the wound, which also promotes rapid new cell growth (Lusby, 2002). The pH of honey provides optimal environment conditions for fibroblast migration, proliferation, and organization of collagen (Lusby, 2002). The types of wounds most beneficial for therapeutic honey is still uncertain, but there is a lot of potential for using honey as a source for healing wounds in the future.

BROMELAIN

Bromelain is the name of a group of enzymes derived from the pineapple plant (MacKay and Miller, 2003). It is found to be highly concentrated in the stems of mature pineapples (Orsini, 2006). Bromelain is closely related to various proteinases (Pavan et al., 2012). Eating these enzymes has shown reduction of edema, bruising, pain, and healing time after trauma or surgery. One important function of bromelain is its capability of reducing inflammation. Bromelain was found to alter leukocyte expression by removing types of cell surface molecules. Therefore, decreasing the amount of leukocyte activation and adhesion eventually decreases inflammation (Orsini, 2006). Another note of interest is bromelain's ability to increase reabsorption rate of hematomas, also known as bruises (MacKay and Miller, 2003). A study involving rabbits reported that rabbits who ingested a combination of bromelain, trypsin, and rutin observed reduced interstitial edema compared to rabbits who did not ingest the combination of supplements (Orsini, 2006).

There are many beneficial properties of Bromelain that are useful for healing wounds, burns, and for post- or presurgery. Ischemia is known as a restriction in blood supply to the tissues. Bromelain has shown to effectively prevent or minimize the effects of ischemia (Neumayer et al., 2006). Ischemia can cause serious complications in the process of wound healing. If the tissue is not receiving adequate blood supply, the wound will take longer to heal or not completely heal at all. Bromelain has also been illustrated to increase blood coagulation. The effect of increased blood coagulation is due to bromelain's influence on increasing the serum fibrinolytic ability. Recent studies suggest that bromelain stimulates plasminogen to convert to plasmin, which results in increased fibrinolysis (Taussig and Batkin, 1988). Another study indicated that a bromelain dressing on wound incisions accelerated blood perfusion, the ability to deliver blood to capillaries (Wu et al., 2012). This is beneficial considering blood brings nutrients and other supplies needed for recovery. Bromelain can be very effective in treating burns. Some second- and third-degree burns require the removal of damaged tissue. Applying bromelain as a dressing to the burn is beneficial for removing the necrotic, dead, tissue, and accelerating healing (Houck et al., 1983). The active component in bromelain is escharase, which is what causes the effect. Two different preparations of bromelain were created and applied to a burn, both displayed rapid removal of the necrotic layer of the dermis while not harming the unburned tissues (Rosenberg et al., 2012). Taking bromelain presurgery can reduce the number of days before complete pain disappearance and can decrease postsurgery inflammation (Tassman et al., 1964).

Achillea millefolium

The western yarrow, or *Achillea millefolium*, is a plant commonly found in North America (Species: *Achillea millefolium* (n.d.). Retrieved April 3, 2015). The flower tops of the plants can be very beneficial to the process of wound healing. On burn wounds specifically, contraction, granulation, epithelization, and arrangement of collagen fibers were enhanced (Farzaei et al., 2014). This was illustrated from a study conducted on animal models. Ten rabbits were acquired and a small burn wound was made on the dorsal side. The control rabbits were washed daily with saline solution while the other rabbits were washed daily with 5 mL of aqueous extracts from the yarrow. It was determined through histopathological evaluation and digital scanning software that granulation and epithelization was more evident and the collagen fibers were better arranged in the rabbits treated with aqueous extract from the yarrow (Jalali et al., 2007).

Achillea biebersteinii, a close relative of *A. millefolium*, displayed wound healing activity on excision wounds and incision wounds. An extract created from the flowering tops exhibited enhanced tensile strength and contraction rate. It also enhanced the formation of collagen and the growth of fibroblasts (Farzaei et al., 2014). Another animal study conducted on rats illustrated the potential benefits of the *A. biebersteinii* yarrow. A series of extracts were made and tested on rats with incisions or excisions.

The yarrow extract displayed increased contraction and increased tensile strength (Akkol et al., 2011). Contraction takes place during the final phase of wound healing and can often take years. By speeding up contraction rates, it would ultimately speed up the final stage of the wound healing process, resulting in a shorter period of wound healing.

Centella asiatica

Centella asiatica aka Gotu Kola has a variety of benefits for the body. It is used to repair nervous tissue due to spinal injury, neuromuscular disorders, and to increase general brain function and memory. Gotu Kola is also used in skin treatments for a wide spectrum of skin conditions. A study in 2012 conducted on the effects of Gotu Kola on burn and incision wounds in rats determined the beneficial effects on wound healing. The rats were separated first into two groups: incision and burn wounds. Then, within the selected group, they were placed in subgroups: untreated, control, and extract. It was concluded that *C. asiatica* facilitates the wound healing process in both incision and burn wounds (Somboonwong et al., 2012). The strength of the fibers in the incision wounded rats that were treated with extracts was stronger than that of the control and untreated rats. The degrees of healing in rats with burn wounds were significantly higher in the rats that received treatment of the extracts compared to the control group, which did not receive treatment from the extracts. Fourteen days after the initial treatment, all of the burn wounded rats that received treatment from the extracts of *C. asiatica* had fully developed epithelialization and keratinization (Somboonwong et al., 2012).

A more recent study conducted on rat models in 2015 concluded similar findings. The experiment tested the effects of *C. asiatica* extract on rat models with burn wounds. The study applied gelatin nanofibers containing *C. asiatica* extract on the burn wound of the rats (Yao et al., 2015). These rats had an extremely high recovery rate compared to rats that were treated with just gauze and commercial wound dressings. This study illustrated that *C. asiatica* extracts promote fibroblast proliferation, collagen synthesis, and displays antibacterial activity (Yao et al., 2015).

Arnebia densiflora

Arnebia densiflora is a wild plant that is commonly found in the Middle East. It flowers from June to August. However, its medicinal benefits are found in its roots (Akkol et al., 2009). The roots have been used for healing wounds in folk medicine: the extracts of the root applied to open wounds promote rapid wound healing (Akkol et al., 2009). A study conducted on rats and mice in 2009 illustrated the potential benefits. There were two groups of mice and rats, one for incision models and one for excision models. The *A. densiflora* root was extracted using four different solvents: hexane, chloroform, ethyl acetate, and methanol (Akkol et al., 2009). Out of the four extracts, hexane was the best followed closely by chloroform. By day 6, the hexane and chloroform extracts displayed 95.2% and 89.9% contractions on the wounds respectively, meaning the two extracts had a higher rate of healing compared to the other extracts (Akkol et al., 2009). The topical application of the hexane and chloroform extracts on incision wounds demonstrated a significant improvement of wound tensile strength. On day 10, the tensile strength was highest in the hexane extract at 47.5% and was second highest in the chloroform extract at 30.0% (Akkol et al., 2009). Upon histopathological examination of the extracts on wound segments, proliferation of fibroblasts was the main observation. In the excision wound models, the hexane extract produced the highest percent of reepithelization at a value of 100% (Akkol et al., 2009).

A close relative to the *A. densiflora*, called *Arnebia euchroma*, exhibits beneficial effects in healing burn wounds. A study conducted in 2009 on rat models with second-degree burns displayed beneficial effects of the plant (Ashkani-Esfahani et al., 2012). The leaves and roots of the plant were extracted and two topical creams with a concentration of 10% and 20% were produced. The rats were separated into four groups: untreated, topical cream with 10% concentration, topical cream with 20% concentration, and a silver sulfadiazine ointment (Ashkani-Esfahani et al., 2012). Reepithelization was higher than 50% in each of the groups except the untreated group, which was less than 50%. The topical cream with 20% concentration displayed slower wound contraction compared to the topical cream with 10% and the silver sulfadiazine ointment. The fibroblast proliferation rate was higher than the control; the silver sulfadiazine ointment had a rate of 42%, the topical cream with 10% concentration had a rate of 40%, and the topical cream with 20% concentration had a rate of 55%. The total collagen volume was significantly higher in the treated groups compared to the untreated group, but between the three treated groups they were very similar (Ashkani-Esfahani et al., 2012). There is not much information on the effects of *A. densiflora* on burn wounds, but its close relative *A. euchroma* provides many beneficial effects on healing burn wounds.

Aloe vera

Aloe vera is a commonly found household plant. It grows naturally in hot arid climates, like the desert (*Aloe vera* (aloe vera) (n.d.). Retrieved May 22, 2015). *Aloe vera* is a succulent plant, meaning parts of the plant are thicker in order to retain water. *Aloe vera* has a variety of uses and is found in many products. *Aloe vera* extracts are used cosmetically and medicinally (*Aloe vera* (aloe vera) (n.d.). Retrieved May 22, 2015). A glycoprotein found in the gel of the *A. vera* plant showed beneficial wound healing characteristics. The glycoproteins enhanced granulation and epithelialization in living organism models (Choi et al., 2001). In the laboratory setting, glycoproteins increased cell proliferation activity and enhanced epidermal tissue (Choi et al., 2001). *Aloe vera* extract also demonstrated anti-inflammatory activity. The mechanism of the anti-inflammatory activity was due to the inhibition of matrix metalloproteinase-9 on blood cells (Vijayalakshmi et al., 2012). The *A. vera* plant also demonstrated antioxidant activity; this is beneficial because antioxidants help destroy free radicals which can lead to cancerous cells. More specifically, the *A. vera* leaf skin and flower displayed antioxidant activity in the laboratory (López et al., 2013). The yellow substance found under the *A. vera* leaf's skin demonstrated antibacterial property (Pandey and Mishra, 2010). The antibacterial property is also very beneficial because it kills bacteria and helps lower the risk of infection in the wound.

Traditionally, *A. vera* has been used to treat burn wounds. A systemic review of multiple studies was conducted. It was concluded that out of the four studies and 371 patients, those treated with *A. vera* had an average of 9 days shorter healing time compared to the controls who did not receive *A. vera* treatment (Maenthaisong et al., 2006). A study conducted on second-degree burn wounds in rats concluded similar findings. Forty-eight rats were divided up into four groups: control, untreated burn wound rats, once-daily saline application, and once-daily application of *A. vera* gel. It was illustrated that *A. vera* potentially exhibits the actions of anti-inflammation and the action of wound healing promotion (Somboonwong et al., 2000), thus decreasing the time it takes to heal. Another study conducted in 2006 evaluated the effects of *A. vera* on excision wounds in rabbits (Subramanian et al., 2006). The rabbits were placed in two groups: control and *A. vera* treatment twice daily. The topical application of *A. vera* resulted in significant wound healing. The *A. vera* increased wound contraction and decreased the total healing time (Subramanian et al., 2006). Not only does *A. vera* produce beneficial characteristics in burn healing, but it also produced beneficial characteristics in other wounds, like excision wounds.

REFERENCES

Akkol, E., Koca, U., Peşin, I., Yılmazer, D., Toker, G., Yeşilada, E., 2009. Exploring the wound healing activity of *Arnebia densiflora* (Nordm.) Ledeb. by in vivo models. J. Ethnopharmacol., 137–141.

Akkol, E.K., Koca, U., Pesin, I., Yilmazer, D., 2011. Evaluation of the Wound Healing Potential of *Achillea biebersteinii* Afan. (Asteraceae) by *In Vivo* excision and incision models. Evid.-Based Complement. Altern. Med.: eCAM 2011, 474026. http://dx.doi.org/10.1093/ecam/nep039.

Aloe vera (aloe vera) (n.d.). Retrieved May 22, 2015. Available from <http://www.kew.org/science-conservation/plants-fungi/aloe-vera-aloe-vera>.

Arnold, M., Barbul, A., 2006. Nutrition and wound healing. Plastic Reconstr. Surg. 117 (7S), 42S–58S.

Ashkani-Esfahani, S., Imanieh, M., Khoshneviszadeh, M., Meshksar, A., Noorafshan, A., Geramizadeh, B., et al., 2012. The healing effect of *Arnebia euchroma* in second degree burn wounds in rat as an animal model. Iran. Red Crescent Med. J. 14, 70–74.

Borhanuddin, B., Mohd Fozi, N., Mohamed, I., 2012. Vitamin E and the healing of bone fracture: the current state of evidence. Evid. Based Complement. Altern. Med. Volume 2012, 1–26.

Choi, S.W., Son, B.W., Son, Y.S., Park, Y.I., Lee, S.K., Chung, M.H., 2001. The wound-healing effect of a glycoprotein fraction isolated from aloe vera. Br. J. Dermatol. 145 (4), 535–545.

Farzaei, M., Abbasabadi, Z., Ardekani, M., Abdollahi, M., Rahimi, R., 2014. A comprehensive review of plants and their active constituents with wound healing activity in traditional Iranian medicine. Wounds 26 (7), 197–206.

Goetzel, E., Wasserman, S., Gigli, I., Austen, F., 1974. Enhancement of random migration and chemotactic response of human leukocytes by ascorbic acid. J. Clin. Invest. Volume 53, 813–818.

Houck, J.C., Chang, C.M., Klein, G., 1983. Isolation of an effective debriding agent from the stems of pineapple plants. Int. J. Tissue React. vol. 5 (no. 2), 125–134.

Jalali, F.S.S., Tajik, H., Tehrani, A., 2007. Experimental evaluation of repair process of burn wound treated with aqueous extract of *Achillea millefolium* on animal model: clinical and histopathological study. J. Animal Vet. Adv. 6, 1357–1361.

López, A., de Tangil, M.S., Vega-Orellana, O., Ramírez, A.S., Rico, M., 2013. Phenolic constituents, antioxidant and preliminary antimycoplasmic activities of leaf skin and flowers of *Aloe vera* (L.) Burm. f. (syn. *A. barbadensis* Mill.) from the Canary Islands (Spain). Molecules 18 (5), 4942–4954.

Lusby, P., 2002. Honey: a potent agent for wound healing? J. WOCN 29 (6), 295–300.

MacKay, D., Miller, A., 2003. Nutritional support for wound healing. Altern. Med. Rev. Volume 8 (Number 4), 359–377.

Maenthaisong, R., Chaiyakunapruk, N., Niruntraporn, S., Kongkaew, C., 2006. The efficacy of *Aloe vera* used for burn wound healing: a systematic review. Burns 33 (6), 713–718.

Monsen, E., 2000. Dietary reference intakes for the antioxidant nutrients: vitamin C, vitamin E, selenium, and carotenoids. Am. Diet. Assoc. 100 (6), 637–640.

Neumayer, C., Fügl, A., Nanobashvili, J., et al., 2006. Combined enzymatic and antioxidative treatment reduces ischemia reperfusion injury in rabbit skeletal muscle. J. Surg. Res. vol. 133 (no. 2), 150–158.

Orsini, R., 2006. Bromelain safety and efficacy report. Plastic Reconstr. Surg. 118 (7), 1640–1644. Retrieved April 6, 2015. <http://dx.doi.org/10.1097/01.prs.0000242503.50548.ee>.

Pandey, R., Mishra, A., 2010. Antibacterial activities of crude extract of *Aloe barbadensis* to clinically isolated bacterial pathogens. Appl. Biochem. Biotechnol. 160 (5), 1356–1361.

Pavan, R., Jain, S., Kumar, A., 2012. Properties and therapeutic application of bromelain: a review. Biotechnol. Res. Int., 1–6.

Rosenberg, L., Krieher, Y., Silverstain, E., et al., 2012. Selectivity of a bromelain based enzymatic debridement agent: a porcine study. Elsevier.

Somboonwong, J., Thanamittramanee, S., Jariyapongskul, A., Patumraj, S., 2000. Therapeutic effects of *Aloe vera* on cutaneous microcirculation and wound healing in second degree burn model in rats. J. Med. Assoc. Thailand 83 (4), 417–425.

Somboonwong, J., Kankaisre, M., Tantisira, B., Tantisira, M., 2012. Wound healing activities of different extracts of *Centella asiatica* in incision and burn wound models: an experimental animal study. BMC Complement. Altern. Med 12, 103.

Species: Achillea millefolium. (n.d.). Retrieved April 3, 2015. Available from <http://www.fs.fed.us/database/feis/plants/forb/achmil/all.html>.

Subramanian, S., Kumar, D., Arulselvan, P., 2006. Wound healing potential of aloe vera leaf gel studied in experimental rabbits. Asian J. Biochem. 1, 178–185.

Tassman, G.C., Zafran, J.N., Zayon, G.M., 1964. Evaluation of a plate proteolytic enzyme for the control of inflammation and pain. J. Dental Med. vol. 19, 73–77.

Taussig, S.J., Batkin, S., 1988. Bromelain, the enzyme complex of pineapple (*Ananas comosus*) and its clinical application: an update. J. Ethnopharmacol. vol. 22 (no. 2), 191–203.

Todorovic, V., 2002. Food and wounds: nutritional factors in wound formation and healing. WoundCare 2002, 43–54.

Trumbo, P., Yates, A., Schlicker, S., Poos, M., 2001. Dietary reference intakes: vitamin A, vitamin K, arsenic, boron, chromium, copper, iodine, iron, manganese, molybdenum, nickel, silicon, vanadium, and zinc. J. Am. Diet. Assoc. 101 (3), 294–301.

Vijayalakshmi, D., Dhandapani, R., Jayaveni, S., Jithendra, P.S., Rose, C., Mandal, A.B., 2012. In vitro anti inflammatory activity of *Aloe vera* by down regulation of MMP-9 in peripheral blood mononuclear cells. J. Ethnopharmacol. 141 (1), 542–546.

Vitamin A. (2013). Retrieved May 27, 2015. Available from <http://ods.od.nih.gov/factsheets/VitaminA-Consumer/>.

Wild, T., Rahbarnia, A., Kellner, M., Sobotka, L., Eberlein, T., 2010. Basics in nutrition and wound healing. Nutrition, 862–866.

Wu, S.Y., Hu, W., Zhang, B., Liu, S., Wang, J.M., Wang, A.M., 2012. Bromelain ameliorates the wound microenvironment and improves the healing of firearm wounds. J. Surg. Res. vol. 176, 503–509.

Yao, C., Yeh, J., Chen, Y., Li, M., & Huang, C. (2015). Wound-healing effect of electrospun gelatin nanofibres containing *Centella asiatica* extract in a rat model. Retrieved from PubMed.

Chapter 22

Curcumin in hepatic stellate cell activation in health

Youcai Tang[1,2]
[1]*Zhengzhou University, Zhengzhou, Henan, China*
[2]*Saint Louis University School of Medicine, St. Louis, MO, United States*

CHAPTER OUTLINE

Fruits, Vegetables, and Herbs.
DOI: http://dx.doi.org/10.1016/B978-0-12-802972-5.00022-6

INTRODUCTION

Liver fibrosis is initiated by activation of hepatic stellate cell (HSC) and featured with the excessive accumulation of extracellular matrix (ECM) proteins including collagen in the extracellular spaces. Although it might occur in most types of chronic liver diseases, hepatic fibrosis is mainly resulted from chronic hepatitis C virus infection, alcoholic abuse, and nonalcoholic fatty liver disease (NAFLD) and nonalcoholic steatohepatitis (NASH). NASH is the advanced form of NAFLD that is commonly associated with obese and/or type II diabetes mellitus (T2DM) in patients. Approximately one-third of NASH patients develop hepatic fibrosis and even cirrhosis (Clark, 2006). Advanced liver fibrosis results in cirrhosis and even hepatocellular carcinoma, causing liver failure, portal hypertension, and even death. Currently, no approved agents for treatment and prevention of liver fibrosis in human beings are available.

HSCs, previously called Ito cells or perisinusoidal cells (earlier lipocytes or fat-storing cells), are pericytes located in the space of Disse (a small area between the sinusoids and hepatocytes) of the liver (Bataller and Brenner, 2005). The stellate cell is the major cell type involved in liver fibrosis, which is the formation of scar tissue in response to liver damage. During hepatic injury, quiescent HSCs undergo profound phenotypic changes, including enhanced cell proliferation, loss of lipid droplets, de novo expression of α-smooth muscle actin, and excessive production of collagen in extracellular space. This process is called HSC activation. Freshly isolated HSCs in culture gradually and spontaneously become fully activated, mimicking the process seen in vivo, which provides a good model for elucidating underlying mechanisms of HSC activation and studying potential therapeutic intervention of the process (Friedman, 2008; Kisseleva and Brenner, 2006).

The liver lobule consists of parenchymal cells, also called hepatocytes and made up 70–80% of the cytoplasmic mass of the livers, and nonparenchymal cells, including endothelial cells, kupffer cells, natural killer cells, dendritic cells, and HSCs (Senoo et al., 2010). Besides activated HSCs, portal fibroblasts and myofibroblasts of bone marrow origin also contribute to collagen production in the injured liver. These cells are activated by fibrogenic cytokines such as tissue growth factor-beta1 (TGF-β1), angiotensin II, and leptin (Bataller and Brenner, 2005), and regulated by proinflammatory cytokines such as nuclear factor kappa B (NF-κB), tumor necrosis factor alpha (TNF-α), and interleukin 6 (IL-6) (Bataller and Brenner, 2005; Luedde and Schwabe, 2011; Connolly et al., 2009), leading to the imbalance of formation and degradation of ECM in tissues.

Recent research demonstrated that advanced liver fibrosis in patients could be reversed, which has stimulated researchers to develop antifibrotic drugs (Bataller and Brenner, 2005; Ramachandran and Iredale, 2009). Potential antifibrotic therapies are aimed at inhibiting the activation and proliferation of fibrogenic cells, inducing the apoptosis of activated HSCs and/or ameliorating the deposition of ECM proteins.

The natural antioxidant curcumin is the polyphenol compound that is responsible for the yellow color in curry from turmeric. Besides its dietary use, turmeric has been historically used as a component of Chinese traditional medicine for thousands of years, especially for skin and gut diseases and wound healing. In the latter half of the 20th century, curcumin was identified as the agent responsible for most of the biological activity of turmeric, showing antitumor (Ströfer et al., 2011; Choi et al., 2006), antioxidant (Shukla et al., 2008), and anti-inflammatory properties (Stix, 2007) in both in vitro and in vivo studies. Since 2008, numerous clinical trials in humans are studying the effect of curcumin on various diseases, including multiple myeloma, pancreatic cancer, myelodysplastic syndromes, colon cancer, psoriasis, arthritis, major depressive disorder, and Alzheimer's disease (Sanmukhani et al., 2014).

Recent studies demonstrate that dietary administration of curcumin inhibits HSC activation by inhibiting cell proliferation, inducing endogenous peroxisome proliferator-activated receptor gamma (PPARγ) expression and suppressing expression of genes closely relevant to the activation of HSCs in vitro (O'Connell and Rushworth, 2008; Zheng and Chen, 2004; Tang et al., 2009) and protected the liver from chemical-caused fibrogenesis in vivo (Fu et al., 2008; Bruck et al., 2007), indicating that targeting HSC activation by curcumin might be a promising approach to fighting liver fibrosis. In this chapter, we will extensively discuss the inhibitory roles by which curcumin plays and elucidate its underlying mechanisms in HSC activation in vivo and in vitro.

CURCUMIN ALLEVIATES HEPATIC FIBROSIS BY AFFECTING BIOACTIVITIES OF HSCs

Curcumin inhibits the growth and proliferation and activation of HSC in vitro

Activation of HSCs initiates liver fibrogenesis, so targeting HSC activation might be an effective and direct way to fight hepatic fibrosis. Emerging data show that curcumin plays critical roles in inhibiting HSC activation in vitro. Xu et al. (2003) reported that curcumin inhibited rat HSC growth by activating PPARγ. Curcumin inhibited alcohol-induced HSC proliferation to exert its hepatoprotective effects against alcohol-induced hepatic fibrosis (Chen et al., 2014). Curcumin deactivates HSCs by suppressing the TGF-β signaling pathway (Chen et al., 2014; Zheng and Chen, 2007). Zhai et al. reported that curcumin inhibits HSC activation by regulating peroxisome PPARγ coactivator-1α (PGC-1α) expression by AMP-activated protein kinase (AMPK) pathway in an in vitro system (Zhai et al., 2015). The same team also reported that suppression of β-catenin by curcumin contributed to an inhibition of activation of the cultured HSCs (Abd El-Kader and El-Den Ashmawy, 2015). Lin et al. (2009a) reported that curcumin dose-dependently eliminated insulin-induced HSC activation by suppressing expression of type I collagen gene and other key genes relevant to HSC activation. Interestingly, recent report showed that curcumin downregulated patched and smoothened, two key elements in Hh signaling, but restored Hhip expression in rat liver with carbon tetrachloride-induced fibrosis and in cultured HSCs, and arrested the cell cycle, induced mitochondrial apoptosis, reduced fibrotic gene expression, restored lipid accumulation, and inhibited invasion and migration in cultured HSCs, suggesting that curcumin modulated cell fate and metabolism by disrupting the Hh pathway in HSCs, providing novel molecular insights into curcumin reduction of HSC activation (Lian et al., 2015).

Curcumin ameliorates HSC activation in animal models

It is well documented that curcumin plays a critical role to limit fibrogenic evolution in mouse and rat fibrotic models induced by carbon tetrachloride (CCl_4)(Fu et al., 2008; Hassan and Al-Olayan, 2012; Morsy et al., 2012; Reyes-Gordillo et al., 2008), thioacetamide (Bruck et al., 2007; Wang et al., 2012; Ali et al., 2014), alcohol (Zhao et al., 2012), bile duct ligation (Reyes-Gordillo et al., 2008), and NASH model induced by high-fat diet (Hasan et al., 2014; Vizzutti et al., 2010), suggesting an inhibitory role of curcumin in HSC activation in vivo, which is regarded as a direct and potential therapeutic approach. Curcumin reduced liver damage and lowered α-smooth muscle actin (α-SMA) and collagen expression in the livers in rat and mouse liver fibrosis models through different pathways, such as antioxidant activities and inflammatory cytokines (Fu et al., 2008; Bruck et al., 2007; Reyes-Gordillo et al., 2008; Wang et al., 2012; Ali et al., 2014; Zhao et al., 2012; Hasan et al., 2014), miRNAs (Hassan and Al-Olayan, 2012), TGF-β (Reyes-Gordillo et al., 2008; Bassiouny et al., 2011), PPARγ (Fu et al., 2008; Bassiouny et al., 2011), matrix metalloproteinases

(MMPs) (Ali et al., 2014), metalloproteinases (TIMPs) (Vizzutti et al., 2010), and apoptotic pathway (Wang et al., 2012). Additionally, curcumin ameliorates hepatic angiogenesis and sinusoidal capillarization in CCl_4-induced rat liver fibrosis through suppressing multiple proangiogenic factors (Yao et al., 2013). Bassiouny AR report that oral administration of curcumin was accompanied by a robust increase in APE1 protein and mRNA levels, and improved the histological architecture of rat liver (Bassiouny et al., 2011). Although the underlying mechanisms remain largely elusive, it is accepted that curcumin may target multiple pathways to stem HSC activation.

Curcumin induces apoptosis of activated HSC

Treatment of isolated HSCs in culture with curcumin-caused apoptosis during later stages confirming that curcumin-induced apoptosis of activated HSCs and not in unactivated quiescent HSCs (Priya and Sudhakaran, 2008). Administration of curcumin inhibited alcohol-induced HSC proliferation and even induced HSC apoptosis by stimulating endoplasmic reticulum (ER) stress (Chen et al., 2014). At higher concentrations (20, approximately 40 μM), curcumin exerted induction of apoptosis and cytochrome c release in HSC-T6 cells (Lin et al., 2009b). Chen N's results indicate the inducing role of curcumin in the apoptosis of HSCs by stimulating ER stress (Chen et al., 2014).

Curcumin suppresses accumulation of ECM

Liver fibrosis occurs because of imbalance of the formation and degradation of ECM proteins that are predominantly synthesized by activated HSCs in chronic liver damages. Excessive ECM is a characteristic of most types of chronic liver diseases and distorts the hepatic architecture by forming a fibrous scar, and the subsequent development of nodules of regenerating hepatocytes defines cirrhosis. Cirrhosis leads to hepatocellular dysfunction, hepatic insufficiency, and portal hypertension. In vivo studies showed that curcumin improved liver fibrosis via suppressing ECM accumulation in hamster (Pinlaor et al., 2010), mice (Vizzutti et al., 2010), and rats (Morsy et al., 2012; Rajagopalan et al., 2010). Zheng also reported that curcumin suppresses the expression of ECM genes in activated HSCs (Zheng and Chen, 2006). Administration of curcumin impaired the production of ECM proteins in alcohol-stimulated HSCs (Chen et al., 2014). Targeting ECM accumulation by curcumin might be a promising approach to improving hepatic fibrogenesis.

THE MECHANISMS BY WHICH CURCUMIN TARGETS IN ACTIVATED HSCs

Curcumin maintains redox homeostasis and antioxidant and suppresses inflammation in HSC

It has been reported that curcumin activates an intracellular antioxidant defense system through its stimulation of nuclear factor-erythroid-2-related factor 2, a transcription factor, which binds to the antioxidant response element in the regulatory region of several genes coding for intracellular antioxidants, cytoprotective and detoxification proteins, including heme oxygenase 1, NADPH (the reduced form of nicotinamide adenine dinucleotide phosphate)–quinone oxidoreductase, ferritin, and genes that regulate intracellular glutathione (Chen and Kunsch, 2004; Rushworth et al., 2006; O' Connell and Rushworth, 2008). Zheng et al. (2007) reported that de novo synthesis of glutathione is a prerequisite for curcumin to inhibit HSC activation. Curcumin is against metal-induced oxidative damage in cultured hepatocytes (Barreto et al., 2005). Fazal et al. (2014) reported that curcumin treatment reduced oxidative stress in animals by scavenging reactive oxygen species, protecting the antioxidant enzymes from being denatured and reducing the oxidative stress marker lipid peroxidation. Curcumin induces the apoptosis of HSCs by stimulating ER stress (Chen et al., 2014). In addition, curcumin attenuated oxidative stress by increasing the content of hepatic glutathione within normal values, leading to the reduction in the level of lipid hydroperoxide (Bassiouny et al., 2011). Curcumin remarkably suppressed inflammation by reducing levels of inflammatory cytokines, including TNF-α, NF-κB, and IL-6 (Bassiouny et al., 2011).

Curcumin activates PPARγ signaling pathway in activated HSCs

PPARs belong to the superfamily of nuclear receptors of which three subtypes exist in mammals: PPARα, PPARβ/δ, and PPARγ. PPARs physiologically act by binding to their ligands and regulate the downstream transcriptional factors, including various enzymes and proteins, which may potentially influence lipid metabolism, lipid accumulation, insulin resistance, inflammation, and fibrosis. PPARs form heterodimers with retinoid X receptors (RXRs) and these heterodimers regulate transcription of various genes. Fatty acids (FAs) and prostaglandins are the natural ligands of PPARs. Synthetic ligands of PPARα or PPARγ have been used in humans to treat hypertriglyceridemia or diabetes.

Among three isoforms of PPARs, PPARγ is the most well-documented one. PPARγ is involved in FA storage and glucose metabolism. The genes activated by PPARγ stimulate lipid uptake and adipogenesis by fat cells. PPARγ knockout mice fail to generate adipose tissue when fed a high-fat diet (Jones et al., 2005).

PPARγ is highly expressed in quiescent HSC with a large amount of lipid droplets in the normal livers. However, expression of PPARγ and its activity are dramatically reduced with HSC activation in vitro and in vivo (Galli et al., 2000), which is accompanied by an increase in cell growth and proliferation, loss of lipid droplet and vitamin A-storing capability, expression of α-SMA and type I collagen-α 1, and deposition of excessive ECM in extracellular space. Extensive data indicate that induction of PPARγ activity by its agonists reduces HSC proliferation and α1 (I) collagen production (Galli et al., 2002). Moreover, forced expression of PPARγ via adenoviral vector-mediated system draws the morphology of activated HSC back to the quiescent phenotype (Hazra et al., 2003). Additionally, PPARγ ligands inhibit cell proliferation and collagen-1(I) expression in primary HSCs. It is, therefore, implied that targeting PPARγ signaling is a potential therapeutic strategy in prevention and treatment of liver fibrosis.

Our data and others show that curcumin inhibits liver fibrosis through dramatically inducing the expression of PPARγ at levels of transcription and translation as well as revived PPARγ trans-activating activity in activated HSC. Furthermore, activation of PPARγ by curcumin resulted in inhibition of transcription factor NF-κB trans-activating activity. On the other hand, blockade of PPARγ by a specific PPARγ antagonist led to a marked increase of activated HSC proliferation. Zhai et al. reported that curcumin enhances PGC-1α expression through AMPK pathway, leading to the increases in PPARγ activity and superoxide dismutase 2 transcription and activity. These data might suggest a possible new explanation for the inhibitory effect of curcumin on HSC activation and on liver fibrogenesis in vitro (Zhai et al., 2015). Together, emerging data have indicated that PPARγ activation by curcumin plays critical and significant roles in an inhibition of activated HSC.

Curcumin blocks leptin signaling pathway in HSCs

Increasing evidence shows the role of leptin and its receptor in the progression of hepatic fibrosis that is initiated by HSC activation in animal models (Leclercq et al., 2002; Sakaida et al., 2003) and humans (García-Suárez et al., 2004; Cayón et al., 2006) with NASH. These observations collectively indicate the significance and essential of leptin and leptin receptor (Ob-R) in the activation of HSCs.

An abnormally enhanced level of leptin activates Ob-R and its downstream signaling pathways in HSCs, which induce oxidative stress (Tang et al.,

2009; Tang and Chen, 2014b; Abu-Tair et al., 2013), cell proliferation (Lang et al., 2004), and overproduction of ECM (Tang et al., 2009; García-Ruiz et al., 2012), leading to the activation of HSCs. In vitro study shows that curcumin abrogates the stimulatory effects of leptin by interrupting leptin signaling via inhibiting the phosphorylation of Ob-R and suppressing Ob-R gene expression (Tang et al., 2009). The latter is mediated by stimulating PPARγ activity and attenuating oxidative stress (Tang et al., 2009). Also, curcumin eliminated stimulatory effects of leptin on HSC activation via increasing AMPK activity and regulating intracellular lipids in HSCs (Tang and Chen, 2010b). Moreover, curcumin prevented leptin from elevating levels of intracellular glucose in activated HSCs, leading to the inhibition of HSC activation (Tang and Chen, 2010a). The same group recently reported that curcumin contributes to the inhibition of HSC activation by eliminating the advanced glycation end-products (AGE)-caused activation of leptin signaling in activated HSC (Tang and Chen, 2014a). Those observations provide novel insights into mechanisms of curcumin in inhibiting leptin-induced HSC activation in vitro. Further research needs to confirm the inhibitory roles of curcumin in leptin-induced HSC activation in vivo systems. It apparently indicates that curcumin may exert as a therapeutic candidate for the treatment and prevention of liver fibrogenesis induced by hyperleptinemia which was commonly accompanied with NASH, obesity, and/or T2DM.

Curcumin suppresses TGFβ and TGFβ-R signaling pathway in activated HSCs

TGFβ and TGFβ-R signaling pathway is also important target of curcumin in activated HSCs. Chen et al. (2014) reported that curcumin showed the hepatoprotective effects against alcohol-induced hepatic fibrosis via suppressing the TGF-β/Smad signaling pathway and inhibiting HSC proliferation. Moreover, it also inhibited hepatic HSC activation by elevating the level of PPARγ and reducing TGF-β (Bassiouny et al., 2011). Curcumin dose-dependently suppressed TGF-β1-induced α-SMA expression and collagen deposition in HSC-T6 cells, without cytotoxicity (Lin et al., 2009b). Interruption of TGF-β signaling by curcumin induces gene expression of PPARγ in activated HSC in vitro, leading to the inhibition of HSC activation (Zheng and Chen, 2007). Inhibition of alphaI(I)-collagen gene expression in HSCs by curcumin is mediated by interrupting TGF-β signaling and suppressing connective TGF gene expression (Zheng and Chen, 2006). Curcumin suppressed the gene expression of TGF-β receptors and interrupted the TGF-β signaling pathway in activated HSC by inducing PPARγ activation (Zheng and Chen, 2004). Taken together, curcumin exerts its hepatoprotective effects on hepatic fibrosis by suppressing the TGF-β and its receptor signaling pathway.

Curcumin blocks insulin signaling and regulates intracellular glucose and its derivatives in activated HSCs

NAFLD encompasses a spectrum of conditions, ranging from simple hepatocellular steatosis to inflammatory NASH, fibrosis, and cirrhosis (Abd El-Kader and El-Den Ashmawy, 2015). The prevalence of overt diabetes mellitus (DM) in liver cirrhosis is about 30%. T2DM is recognized as the etiology of over 80% of all DMs. T2DM and NASH are greatly associated with hepatic fibrosis. The correlation of hyperglycemia with the presence of liver fibrosis in NASH patients has been clinically described (Abd El-Kader and El-Den Ashmawy, 2015). Hyperglycemia is suggested as a harmful prognostic factor in the evolution of NASH toward fibrosis (Tsochatzis et al., 2008), which is a poorly studied complication of T2DM. T2DM is also thought as a predictor of worsening hepatic fibrosis.

It has been well known that NAFLD is consistently associated with obesity and insulin resistance. Hyperinsulinemia, that is, abnormally elevated levels of plasma insulin, is a feature of T2DM. Further data indicated that curcumin interrupted insulin signaling in HSCs by reducing the phosphorylation level of insulin receptor (InsR) and suppressing gene expression of InsR. Furthermore, curcumin attenuated insulin-induced oxidative stress in HSCs by inducing gene expression of glutamate-cysteine ligase, leading to de novo synthesis of glutathione and the suppression of gene expression of InsR. These results support our initial hypothesis that curcumin eliminates the effects of insulin on stimulating HSC activation by interrupting insulin signaling and attenuating oxidative stress (Lin et al., 2009a).

Glucose metabolism homeostasis is mainly maintained by glucose transporters (GLUTs) which are important molecular targets of antidiabetic drugs (Asano et al., 2004). Physiologically, glucose transporter-2 (GLUT2) and glucose transporter-4 (GLUT4) are the major GLUTs responsible for glucose transportation into hepatocytes (Leturque et al., 2005; Zhao and Keating, 2007). Due to its low affinity and high capacity, GLUT2 transports glucose in a large range of physiological concentrations of glucose, whereas GLUT4 action is extensively regulated by insulin-activated phosphoinositide 3-kinases (PI3K) (Leturque et al., 2005; Zhao and Keating, 2007). In the liver, GLUT2 is translocated from the cytoplasm to the plasma membrane in response to high levels of plasma glucose and is the primary carrier to transport plasma glucose into hepatocytes

(Leturque et al., 2005; Zhao and Keating, 2007). An abnormally high level of intracellular glucose could be a deleterious to cellular functions in some types of cells (Jellinger, 2007).

A research showed that hyperglycemia stimulated the activation of HSCs and curcumin reversed this action in vitro (Lin and Chen, 2011). Extensive studies suggested that curcumin decreased intracellular glucose level of HSCs by suppressing membrane translocation and gene expression of GLUT2 (Lin and Chen, 2011). Results from the same group also implied that curcumin blocked translocation of GLUT4 by interrupting the insulin receptor substrates/PI3K/AKT signaling pathway, a cross-link between leptin and insulin pathway, and increased glucokinase activity by increasing AMPK activity and suppressing protein kinase A activity, leading to increased conversion of glucose to glucose-6-phosphate and lowered glucose levels in HSCs (Tang and Chen, 2010a).

Hyperglycemia facilitates the nonenzymatic formation of AGEs, which are a heterogeneous group of molecules formed by nonoxidative and oxidative reactions of sugars with proteins and/or lipids (Gaens et al., 2013). Accumulation of AGEs in tissues and circulation during aging, diabetes, chronic renal failure, and liver fibrogenesis resulted in inflammation and pathogenesis. One of the mechanisms by which glycated proteins are converted into AGEs is involved in oxidation reaction. The formation of AGEs from Amadori products occurred, partially, due to oxidation. Therefore, agents with antioxidation properties can prevent further oxidation of Amadori products and decrease the accumulation of AGEs. Khan et al. (2014) reported that curcumin had the properties of anti-glycation. In vitro studies suggested that AGEs played a critical role in HSC activation, which can be diminished by curcumin (Tang and Chen, 2014b; Lin et al., 2012a,b).

Effects of AGEs are mediated by their receptor system, which could be generally divided into two categories, such as receptor for AGEs (RAGEs) and AGE receptors (AGE-Rs, also called OST-48). RAGE, a member of the immunoglobulin superfamily of cell surface molecules, mediates effects of AGEs and induces oxidative stress, cell growth, and inflammation. The interaction of AGEs and RAGE may stimulate the activation of a diverse array of signaling cascades, including mitogen-activated protein kinase, Janus kinase/signal transducer and activator of transcription, and PI3K (Ramasamy et al., 2009). RAGE was upregulated in cultured HSCs and AGEs stimulated the activation of HSCs in vitro by inducing cell proliferation and stimulating expression of genes relevant to HSC activation (Lin et al., 2012a; Iwamoto et al., 2008). The phytochemical curcumin eliminated the stimulating effects of AGEs and inhibited the gene expression of RAGE by attenuating oxidative stress and stimulating the activity of PPARγ in HSCs (Lin et al., 2012b).

AGE-Rs, for example, AGE-R1, are responsible for detoxification and clearance of AGEs. In contrast to a dramatic increase in expression of RAGE in diabetes with high levels of AGEs, the abundance of AGE-R1 is significantly reduced in diabetic organs, for example, kidney, suggesting a possible negative relationship between AGEs-mediated cell injury and low expression of AGE-R1. In addition to its participation in AGE removal, AGE-R1 negatively regulates AGE pro-inflammatory signal processing (Lu et al., 2004). Studies demonstrated that curcumin inhibited AGEs-caused HSC activation, at least partially, by inducing AGE-R1 gene expression. This process was likely mediated by inhibiting extracellular signal-regulated kinases activity, inducing gene expression of PPARγ and stimulating its transactivity (Lin et al., 2012a). Furthermore, curcumin eliminated the effects of AGEs on the divergent regulation of gene expression of RAGE and AGE-R1 in HSC by interrupting the AGE-caused activation of leptin signaling, leading to the inhibition of HSC activation (Tang and Chen, 2014b).

In summary, AGEs might be one of the mechanisms which HSCs are activated in high glucose conditions, which probably can, at least partially, explain why liver fibrosis is highly associated with T2DM. Curcumin has a potential to fight against AGE involved HSC activation. However, no evidence is available to show the role of curcumin in regulating gene expression of RAGE and AGE-R1 in vivo.

Curcumin modulates lipid metabolism in HSCs

As mentioned above, during hepatic injury, quiescent HSCs undergo profound phenotypic changes, including enhanced cell proliferation, loss of lipid droplets, de novo expression of α-SMA, and excessive production of ECM. Published evidence supports the proposal that recovering the accumulation of lipids could inhibit HSC activation (Tsukamoto et al., 2006).

Lipid homeostasis is tightly controlled by a group of proteins via biosynthesis and cellular uptake. Several transcription factors, including sterol regulatory element-binding protein-1c (SREBP-1c), PPARγ, and CCAAT/enhancer-binding protein-α (C/EBP α), have emerged as master regulators in lipogenesis as well as in lipid uptake and metabolism (Lefterova and Lazar, 2009). Interaction, cooperation, and cross talk have been observed among those regulators (Lefterova et al., 2008). It has been proposed that the process of HSC activation may be similar to that of adipocyte dedifferentiation, causally associated with transcriptional regulation of genes relevant to lipid accumulation (Tsukamoto et al., 2006). In vitro study demonstrated that curcumin could increase intracellular lipid accumulation in HSC via inducing expression of lipogenesis related genes, such as SREBP-1c, PPARγ, and C/EBP α, causing an inhibition of HSC activation (Tang and Chen, 2010b). Similarly, the effect of curcumin on lipid metabolism has been also observed in HepG2 cells (Peschel et al., 2007). Despite the observation that curcumin paradoxically promotes lipid accumulation and inhibits HSC activation in vitro, curcumin and its water-soluble derivative displays an effective improvement in the lipid metabolism and delays the progression of hepatic fibrosis in rats and mice with steatohepatitis (Hasan et al., 2014; Ejaz et al., 2009).

AMPK, a sensor of cellular energy homeostasis, is induced by rising AMP and falling ATP via a complex mechanism that results in an ultrasensitive response. The activation of AMPK by pharmacological agents presents a unique challenge, given the complexity of the biology, but holds a considerable potential to reverse the metabolic abnormalities. In skeletal muscles, AMPK mediates glucose transport and FA oxidation. In the liver, it decreases glucose output, leading to lowered blood glucose levels in hyperglycemic individuals (Gruzman et al., 2009). AMPK plays a key role in regulating the activation of SREBP-1 and lipogenesis (You et al., 2004). In vitro experiments demonstrated that curcumin inhibited HSC activation by activating AMPK activity, leading to the induction of the expression of genes relevant to lipid accumulation and to the elevation of the levels of intracellular FAs and triglycerides (Tang and Chen, 2010b). Interestingly, activation of AMPK by curcumin shows different functions in other cell types, such as hepatoma cells (Kim et al., 2009), HT-29 colon cancer cells (Lee et al., 2009), and 3T3-L1 adipocytes (Ejaz et al., 2009). These observations collectively suggested that curcumin might show distinct effects on regulating gene expression and on lipid accumulation depending on cell types. Therefore, additional experiments are necessary to elucidate the mechanisms by which curcumin activates AMPK and shows distinct effects in different cell types.

Additionally, Kang and Chen (2009c) reported that curcumin inhibited low-density lipoprotein (LDL)-induced activation of HSCs by suppressing expression of LDL receptor (LOX), removed the role of oxidized LDL in activating HSCs by lowering gene expression of lectin-like oxidized LOX-1 (Kang and Chen, 2009a), and attenuated expression of SREBP-2 by reducing the activity of specific protein-1, resulting in inhibition of HSC activation (Kang and Chen, 2009b). Recently, Kuo et al.

(2012) reported that curcumin protects hepatocytes from high free fatty acid–induced lipoapoptosis and mitochondrial dysfunction, which partially occurred through the regulation of mitochondrial biogenesis.

Curcumin balances formation and degradation of ECM via distinctively regulating TIMPs and MMPs

As well known, the accumulation of ECM is controlled by the rate of their synthesis and degradation. Physiologically, balance of ECM in liver is sustained by a group of enzymes, MMPs, and their specific inhibitors, TIMPs. Once secreted, MMP activity is regulated by the binding of TIMPs (Hemmann et al., 2007). Overall, all MMPs are inhibited by at least one of the specific endogenous TIMPs once they are activated.

Among 23 different members in the MMP family, only a few are expressed in liver tissue and associated with activation of HSCs. They are MMP-1, MMP-2 (Parsons et al., 2004), MMP-3 (Benyon and Arthur, 2001), MMP-7 (Pinlaor et al., 2010), MMP-9, and MMP-13 (Han et al., 2004; Roderfeld et al., 2006). Upregulation of the above MMPs may facilitate the activation of HSCs, leading to liver fibrosis.

So far, four subtypes of TIMPs have been identified, including TIMP-1, TIMP-2, TIMP-3, and TIMP-4. TIMP-1 and TIMP-2 are mainly produced by HSCs (Schuppan et al., 2001). TIMP-1 plays a putative role in tissue fibrosis and is capable of inhibiting programmed cell death of HSCs via inhibition of pro-MMP activation and MMP activity (Murphy et al., 2002). TIMP-2 is essential for MMP-2 activation in mice (Wang et al., 2000).

During chronic liver injury, HSCs are activated and differentiate into a fibroblast-like phenotype. The balance between MMPs and TIMPs is broken, leading to excessive ECM accumulation in the extracellular spaces. Accumulating data demonstrate that curcumin distinctively regulates the above two protein families that are responsible for fibrogenesis and fibrolysis, respectively, to balance formation and degradation of ECM in therapeutic intervention of fibrosis, for example, upregulation of MMP activity or downregulation of TIMP activity. Curcumin downregulates TIMP-1 and TIMP-2 (Pinlaor et al., 2010; Rajagopalan et al., 2010) and upregulates MMP-2 (Rajagopalan et al., 2010), MMP-7 (Pinlaor et al., 2010), MMP-9 (Rajagopalan et al., 2010), and MMP-13 (Pinlaor et al., 2010; Morsy et al., 2012) in vivo and in vitro, resulting in the degradation of fibrillar collagens, the main components in ECM, and inhibition of HSC activation. Taken together, curcumin balances formation and degradation of ECM via TIMPs and MMPs.

CLINICAL TRIALS AND FUTURE DIRECTION

Although some clinical trials are still ongoing to evaluate the efficacy of curcumin against human disorders, numerous ones have been completed and provide positive information. A search on www.clinicaltrials.gov (accessed in June 2015) indicated that among 114 clinical trials with curcumin, 39 are still ongoing. The most common human diseases for which curcumin are being evaluated are cancer, inflammatory conditions, arthritis, neurological conditions, and diabetes. Only one ongoing clinical trial with curcumin is for NAFLD and one for inflammation bowel disease. No clinical trial with curcumin is available for liver fibrosis. Therefore, these ongoing clinical trials are expected to provide a deeper understanding of curcumin's efficacy and mechanism of action against human diseases.

Since curcumin has shown beneficial properties in diverse experimental models of liver damage, including CCL4-induced fibrotic model, the following work should be encouraged in the future. Due to the development of its analogues, the bioavailability of curcumin has been greatly increased in the guts. Curcumin, as a promising therapeutic approach, is particularly suggested to treat chronic liver diseases. In addition, hepatic disorder has become one of the main causes of worldwide mortality and the number of studies of curcumin on liver diseases is still very low, clinical investigations are encouraged to perform in this area. Moreover, clinical trial with curcumin is encouraged to treat liver fibrosis.

CONCLUSIONS

HSCs are the major sources of collagen products during development of liver fibrosis, leading to an imbalance of formation and degradation of ECM in tissues. So far, no approved agents for treatment and prevention of liver fibrosis in human beings are available. Antifibrogenic agents that are involved in inhibiting HSC activation is of high priority and is urgently needed. Increasing evidence has shown that curcumin has antitumor, antioxidant, and anti-inflammatory properties. Our results and others, both in vitro and in vivo, demonstrate that curcumin plays a role in inhibiting HSC activation by blocking leptin and insulin signaling, inducing PPARγ signaling, suppressing TFG-β signaling, regulating intracellular glucose and its derivatives, and modulating lipid metabolism, as well as balancing formation and degradation of ECM. These results provide novel insights into therapeutic mechanisms of curcumin in inhibiting HSC activation and intervening liver fibrogenesis associated with NAFLD and/or NASH. Currently, however, no clinical trial with curcumin is particularly designed to treat liver fibrosis.

ABBREVIATIONS

AGEs advanced glycation end-products
AGE-Rs AGE receptors
AMPK AMP-activated protein kinase
CCL4 carbon tetrachloride
C/EBP α CCAAT/enhancer-binding protein-α
CTGF connective tissue growth factor
ECM extracellular matrix
ER endoplasmic reticulum
FA fatty acid
GLUTs glucose transporters
HSCs hepatic stellate cells
IL-6 interleukin 6
LOX-1 LDL receptor-1
MMPs matrix metalloproteinases
NAFLD nonalcoholic fatty liver disease
NASH nonalcoholic steatohepatitis
NF-κB nuclear factor kappa B
Ob-R leptin receptor
PI3K phosphoinositide 3-kinases
PPARs peroxisome proliferator-activated receptors
PGC-1α peroxisome proliferator-activated receptor-γ coactivator-1α
RAGE receptor for AGEs
SREBP-1c sterol regulatory element-binding protein-1c
T2DM type II diabetes mellitus
TGF-β tissue growth factor β
TIMPs metalloproteinases
TNF-α tumor necrosis factor alpha

ACKNOWLEDGMENT

This work is supported by NSFC (National Natural Science Foundation of China) granted to Dr. Youcai Tang (NSFC 31471330).

REFERENCES

Abd El-Kader, S.M., El-Den Ashmawy, E.M., 2015. Non-alcoholic fatty liver disease: the diagnosis and management. World J. Hepatol. 7, 846–858.

Abu-Tair, L., Doron, S., Mahamid, M., Amer, J., Safadi, R., 2013. Leptin modulates lymphocytes' adherence to hepatic stellate cells is associated with oxidative status alterations. Mitochondrion 13, 473–480.

Ali, S.O., Darwish, H.A., Ismail, N.A., 2014. Modulatory effects of curcumin, silybin-phytosome and alpha-R-lipoic acid against thioacetamide-induced liver cirrhosis in rats. Chem. Biol. Interact. 216, 26–33.

Asano, T., Ogihara, T., Katagiri, H., Sakoda, H., Ono, H., Fujishiro, M., et al., 2004. Glucose transporter and Na+/glucose cotransporter as molecular targets of anti-diabetic drugs. Curr. Med. Chem. 11, 2717–2724.

Barreto, R., Kawakita, S., Tsuchiya, J., Minelli, E., Pavasuthipaisit, K., Helmy, A., et al., 2005. Metal-induced oxidative damage in cultured hepatocytes and hepatic lysosomal fraction: beneficial effect of a curcumin/absinthium compound. Chin. J. Dig. Dis. 6, 31–36.

Bassiouny, A.R., Zaky, A., Kandeel, K.M., 2011. Alteration of AP-endonuclease1 expression in curcumin-treated fibrotic rats. Ann. Hepatol. 10, 516–530.

Bataller, R., Brenner, D.A., 2005. Liver fibrosis. J. Clin. Invest. 115, 209–218.

Benyon, R.C., Arthur, M.J., 2001. Extracellular matrix degradation and the role of hepatic stellate cells. Semin. Liver. Dis. 21, 373–384.

Bruck, R., Ashkenazi, M., Weiss, S., Goldiner, I., Shapiro, H., Aeed, H., et al., 2007. Prevention of liver cirrhosis in rats by curcumin. Liver. Int. 27, 373–383.

Cayón, A., Crespo, J., Mayorga, M., Guerra, A., Pons-Romero, F., 2006. Increased expression of Ob–Rb and its relationship with the overexpression of TGF-β1 and the stage of fibrosis in patients with nonalcoholic steatohepatitis. Liver. Int. 26, 1065–1071.

Chen, N., Geng, Q., Zheng, J., He, S., Huo, X., Sun, X., 2014. Suppression of the TGF-β/Smad signaling pathway and inhibition of hepatic stellate cell proliferation play a role in the hepatoprotective effects of curcumin against alcohol-induced hepatic fibrosis. Int. J. Mol. Med. 34, 1110–1116.

Chen, X.L., Kunsch, C., 2004. Induction of cytoprotective genes through Nrf2/antioxidant response element pathway: a new therapeutic approach for the treatment of inflammatory diseases. Curr. Pharm. Des. 10, 879–891.

Choi, H., Chun, Y.S., Kim, S.W., Kim, M.S., Park, J.W., 2006. Curcumin inhibits hypoxia-inducible factor-1 by degrading aryl hydrocarbon receptor nuclear translocator: a mechanism of tumor growth inhibition. Mol. Pharmacol. 70, 1664–1671.

Clark, J.M., 2006. The epidemiology of nonalcoholic fatty liver disease in adults. J. Clin. Gastroenterol. 40 (Suppl. 1), S5–10.

Connolly, M.K., Bedrosian, A.S., Mallen-St Clair, J., Mitchell, A.P., Ibrahim, J., Stroud, A., et al., 2009. In liver fibrosis, dendritic cells govern hepatic inflammation in mice via TNF-α. J. Clin. Invest. 119, 3213–3225.

Ejaz, A., Wu, D., Kwan, P., Meydani, M., 2009. Curcumin inhibits adipogenesis in 3T3-L1 adipocytes and angiogenesis and obesity in C57/BL mice. J. Nutr. 139, 919–925.

Fazal, Y., Fatima, S.N., Shahid, S.M., Mahboob, T., 2014. Effects of curcumin on angiotensin-converting enzyme gene expression, oxidative stress and anti-oxidant status in thioacetamide-induced hepatotoxicity. J. Renin. Angiotensin. Aldosterone. Syst. 1470320314545777. (Epub ahead of print).

Friedman, S.L., 2008. Mechanisms of hepatic fibrogenesis. Gastroenterology 134, 1655–1669.

Fu, Y., Zheng, S., Lin, J., Ryerse, J., Chen, A., 2008. Curcumin protects the rat liver from CCl4-caused injury and fibrogenesis by attenuating oxidative stress and suppressing inflammation. Mol. Pharmacol. 73, 399–409.

Gaens, K.H., Stehouwer, C.D., Schalkwijk, C.G., 2013. Advanced glycation endproducts and its receptor for advanced glycation endproducts in obesity. Curr. Opin. Lipidol. 24, 4–11.

Galli, A., Crabb, D., Price, D., Ceni, E., Salzano, R., Surrenti, C., et al., 2000. Peroxisome proliferator-activated receptor gamma transcriptional regulation is involved in platelet-derived growth factor-induced proliferation of human hepatic stellate cells. Hepatology 31, 101–108.

Galli, A., Crabb, D.W., Ceni, E., Salzano, R., Mello, T., Svegliati-Baroni, G., et al., 2002. Antidiabetic thiazolidinediones inhibit collagen synthesis and hepatic stellate cell activation in vivo and in vitro. Gastroenterology 122, 1924–1940.

García-Ruiz, I., Gómez-Izquierdo, E., Díaz-Sanjuán, T., Grau, M., Solís-Muñoz, P., Muñoz-Yagüe, T., et al., 2012. Sp1 and Sp3 transcription factors mediate leptin-induced collagen α1(I) gene expression in primary culture of male rat hepatic stellate cells. Endocrinology 153, 5845–5856.

García-Suárez, C., Crespo, J., Fernández-Gil, P.L., Amado, J.A., García-Unzueta, M.T., Pons-Romero, F., 2004. Plasma leptin levels in patients with primary biliary cirrhosis and their relationship with degree of fibrosis. Gastroenterol. Hepatol. 27, 47–50.

Gruzman, A., Babai, G., Sasson, S., 2009. Adenosine monophosphate activated protein kinase (AMPK) as a new target for antidiabetic drugs: a review on metabolic, pharmacological and chemical considerations. Rev. Diabet. Stud. 6, 13–36.

Han, Y.P., Zhou, L., Wang, J., Xiong, S., Garner, W.L., French, S.W., et al., 2004. Essential role of matrix metalloproteinases in interleukin-1-induced myofibroblastic activation of hepatic stellate cell in collagen. J. Biol. Chem. 279, 4820–4828.

Hasan, S.T., Zingg, J.M., Kwan, P., Noble, T., Smith, D., Meydani, M., 2014. Curcumin modulation of high fat diet-induced atherosclerosis and steatohepatosis in LDL receptor deficient mice. Atherosclerosis 232, 40–51.

Hassan, Z.K., Al-Olayan, E.M., 2012. Curcumin reorganizes miRNA expression in a mouse model of liver fibrosis. Asian. Pac. J. Cancer. Prev. 13, 5405–5408.

Hazra, S., Xiong, S., Wang, J., Rippe, R.A., Krishna, V., Chatterjee, K., et al., 2003. PPARgamma induces a phenotypic switch from activated to quiescent hepatic stellate cells. J. Biol. Chem. 279, 11392–11401.

Hemmann, S., Graf, J., Roderfeld, M., Roeb, E., 2007. Expression of MMPs and TIMPs in liver fibrosis—a systematic review with special emphasis on anti-fibrotic strategies. J. Hepatol. 46, 955–975.

Iwamoto, K., Kanno, K., Hyogo, H., Yamagishi, S., Takeuchi, M., Tazuma, S., et al., 2008. Advanced glycation end products enhance the proliferation and activation of hepatic stellate cells. J. Gastroenterol. 43, 298–304.

Jellinger, P.S., 2007. Metabolic consequences of hyperglycemia and insulin resistance. Clin. Cornerstone. 8 (Suppl. 7), S30–S42.

Jones, J.R., Barrick, C., Kim, K.A., Lindner, J., Blondeau, B., Fujimoto, Y., et al., 2005. Deletion of PPARγ in adipose tissues of mice protects against high fat diet-induced obesity and insulin resistance. Proc. Natl. Acad. Sci. U.S.A. 102, 6207–6212.

Kang, Q., Chen, A., 2009a. Curcumin eliminates oxidized LDL roles in activating hepatic stellate cells by suppressing gene expression of lectin-like oxidized LDL receptor-1 (LOX-1). Lab. Invest. 89, 1275–1290.

Kang, Q., Chen, A., 2009b. Curcumin inhibits srebp-2 expression in activated hepatic stellate cells in vitro by reducing the activity of specificity protein-1. Endocrinology 150, 5384–5394.

Kang, Q., Chen, A., 2009c. Curcumin suppresses expression of low-density lipoprotein (LDL) receptor, leading to the inhibition of LDL-induced activation of hepatic stellate cells. Br. J. Pharmacol. 157, 1354–1367.

Khan, I., Ahmad, H., Ahmad, B., 2014. Anti-glycation and anti-oxidation properties of *Capsicum frutescens* and *Curcuma longa* fruits: possible role in prevention of diabetic complication. Pak. J. Pharm. Sci. 27, 1359–1362.

Kim, T., Davis, J., Zhang, A.J., He, X., Mathews, S.T., 2009. Curcumin activates AMPK and suppresses gluconeogenic gene expression in hepatoma cells. Biochem. Biophys. Res. Commun. 388, 377–382.

Kisseleva, T., Brenner, D.A., 2006. Hepatic stellate cells and the reversal of fibrosis. J. Gastroenterol. Hepatol. 21 (Suppl. 3), S84–S87.

Kuo, J.J., Chang, H.H., Tsai, T.H., Lee, T.Y., 2012. Curcumin ameliorates mitochondrial dysfunction associated with inhibition of gluconeogenesis in free fatty acid-mediated hepatic lipoapoptosis. Int. J. Mol. Med. 30, 643–649.

Lang, T., Ikejima, K., Yoshikawa, M., Enomoto, N., Iijima, K., Kitamura, T., et al., 2004. Leptin facilitates proliferation of hepatic stellate cells through up-regulation of platelet-derived growth factor receptor. Biochem. Biophys. Res. Commun. 323, 1091–1095.

Leclercq, I.A., Farrell, G.C., Schriemer, R., Robertson, G.R., 2002. Leptin is essential for the hepatic fibrogenic response to chronic liver injury. J. Hepatol. 37, 206–213.

Lee, Y.K., Park, S.Y., Kim, Y.M., Park, O.J., 2009. Regulatory effect of the AMPK-COX-2 signaling pathway in curcumin-induced apoptosis in HT-29 colon cancer cells. Ann. N. Y. Acad. Sci. 1171, 489–494.

Lefterova, M.I., Lazar, M.A., 2009. New developments in adipogenesis. Trends. Endocrinol. Metab. 20, 107–114.

Lefterova, M.I., Zhang, Y., Steger, D.J., Schupp, M., Schug, J., Cristancho Jr., A., et al., 2008. PPARγ and C/EBP factors orchestrate adipocyte biology via adjacent binding on a genome-wide scale. Genes Dev. 22, 2941–2952.

Leturque, A., Brot-Laroche, E., Le Gall, M., Stolarczyk, E., Tobin, V., 2005. The role of GLUT2 in dietary sugar handling. J. Physiol. Biochem. 61, 529–537.

Lian, N., Jiang, Y., Zhang, F., Jin, H., Lu, C., Wu, X., et al., 2015. Curcumin regulates cell fate and metabolism by inhibiting hedgehog signaling in hepatic stellate cells. Lab. Invest. http://dx.doi.org/10.1038/labinvest.2015.59. (Epub ahead of print).

Lin, J., Chen, A., 2011. Curcumin decrease intracellular glucose level of HSCs by cells by suppressing membrane translocation and gene expression of glucose transporter-2. Mol. Cell. Endocrinol. 333, 160–171.

Lin, J., Tang, Y., Kang, Q., Chen, A., 2012a. Curcumin eliminates the inhibitory effect of advanced glycation end-products (AGEs) on gene expression of AGE receptor-1 in hepatic stellate cells in vitro. Lab. Invest. 92, 827–841.

Lin, J., Tang, Y., Kang, Q., Feng, Y., Chen, A., 2012b. Curcumin inhibits gene expression of receptor for advanced glycation end-products (RAGE) in hepatic stellate cells in vitro by elevating PPARγ activity and attenuating oxidative stress. Br. J. Pharmacol. 166, 2212–2227.

Lin, J., Zheng, S., Chen, A., 2009a. Curcumin attenuates the effects of insulin on stimulating hepatic stellate cell activation by interrupting insulin signaling and attenuating oxidative stress. Lab. Invest. 89, 1397–1409.

Lin, Y.L., Lin, C.Y., Chi, C.W., Huang, Y.T., 2009b. Study on antifibrotic effects of curcumin in rat hepatic stellate cells. Phytother. Res. 23, 927–932.

Lu, C., He, J.C., Cai, W., Liu, H., Zhu, L., Vlassara, H., 2004. Advanced glycation end-product (AGE) receptor 1 is a negative regulator of the inflammatory response to AGE in mesangial cells. Proc. Natl. Acad. Sci. U.S.A. 101, 11767–11772.

Luedde, T., Schwabe, R.F., 2011. NF-κB in the liver—linking injury, fibrosis and hepatocellular carcinoma. Nat. Rev. Gastroenterol. Hepatol. 8, 108–118.

Morsy, M.A., Abdalla, A.M., Mahmoud, A.M., Abdelwahab, S.A., Mahmoud, M.E., 2012. Protective effects of curcumin, α-lipoic acid, and *N*-acetylcysteine against carbon tetrachloride-induced liver fibrosis in rats. J. Physiol. Biochem. 68, 29–35.

Murphy, F.R., Issa, R., Zhou, X., Ratnarajah, S., Nagase, H., Arthur, M.J., et al., 2002. Inhibition of apoptosis of activated hepatic stellate cells by tissue inhibitor of metalloproteinase-1 is mediated via effects on matrix metalloproteinase inhibition: implications for reversibility of liver fibrosis. J. Biol. Chem. 277, 11069–11076.

O'Connell, M.A., Rushworth, S.A., 2008. Curcumin: potential for hepatic fibrosis therapy? Br. J. Pharmacol. 153, 403–405.

Parsons, C.J., Bradford, B.U., Pan, C.Q., Cheung, E., Schauer, M., Knorr, A., et al., 2004. Antifibrotic effects of a tissue inhibitor of metalloproteinase-1 antibody on established liver fibrosis in rats. Hepatology 40, 1106–1115.

Peschel, D., Koerting, R., Nass, N., 2007. Curcumin induces changes in expression of genes involved in cholesterol homeostasis. J. Nutr. Biochem. 18, 113–119.

Pinlaor, S., Prakobwong, S., Hiraku, Y., Pinlaor, P., Laothong, U., Yongvanit, P., 2010. Reduction of periductal fibrosis in liver fluke-infected hamsters after long-term curcumin treatment. Eur. J. Pharmacol. 638, 134–141.

Priya, S., Sudhakaran, P.R., 2008. Curcumin-induced recovery from hepatic injury involves induction of apoptosis of activated hepatic stellate cells. Indian. J. Biochem. Biophys. 45, 317–325.

Rajagopalan, R., Sridharana, S., Menon, V.P., 2010. Hepatoprotective role of bis-demethoxy curcumin analog on the expression of matrix metalloproteinase induced by alcohol and polyunsaturated fatty acid in rats. Toxicol. Mech. Methods 20, 252–259.

Ramachandran, P., Iredale, J.P., 2009. Reversibility of liver fibrosis. Ann. Hepatol. 8, 283–291.

Ramasamy, R., Yan, S.F., Schmidt, A.M., 2009. RAGE: therapeutic target and biomarker of the inflammatory response—the evidence mounts. J. Leukoc. Biol. 86, 505–512.

Reyes-Gordillo, K., Segovia, J., Shibayama, M., Tsutsumi, V., Vergara, P., Moreno, M.G., et al., 2008. Curcumin prevents and reverses cirrhosis induced by bile duct obstruction or CCl4 in rats: role of TGF-beta modulation and oxidative stress. Fundam. Clin. Pharmacol. 22, 417–427.

Roderfeld, M., Geier, A., Dietrich, C.G., Siewert, E., Jansen, B., Gartung, C., et al., 2006. Cytokine blockade inhibits hepatic tissue inhibitor of metalloproteinase-1 expression and up-regulates matrix metalloproteinase-9 in toxic liver injury. Liver. Int. 26, 579–586.

Rushworth, S.A., Ogborne, R.M., Charalambos, C.A., O'Connell, M.A., 2006. Role of protein kinase C delta in curcumin-induced antioxidant response element-mediated gene expression in human monocytes. Biochem. Biophys. Res. Commun. 341, 1007–1016.

Sakaida, I., Jinhua, S., Uchida, K., Terai, S., Okita, K., 2003. Leptin receptor-deficient Zucker (fa/fa) rat retards the development of pig serum-induced liver fibrosis with Kupffer cell dysfunction. Life. Sci. 73, 2491–2501.

Sanmukhani, J., Satodia, V., Trivedi, J., Patel, T., Tiwari, D., Panchal, B., et al., 2014. Efficacy and safety of curcumin in major depressive disorder: a randomized controlled trial. Phytother. Res. 28, 579–585.

Schuppan, D., Ruehl, M., Somasundaram, R., Hahn, E.G., 2001. Matrix as a modulator of hepatic fibrogenesis. Semin. Liver. Dis. 21, 351–372.

Senoo, H., Yoshikawa, K., Morii, M., Miura, M., Imai, K., Mezaki, Y., 2010. Hepatic stellate cell (vitamin A-storing cell) and its relative—past, present and future. Cell. Biol. Int. 34, 1247–1272.

Shukla, P.K., Khanna, V.K., Ali, M.M., Khan, M.Y., Srimal, R.C., 2008. Anti-ischemic effect of curcumin in rat brain. Neurochem. Res. 33, 1036–1043.

Stix, G., 2007. Spice healer. Sci. Am. 296, 54–67.

Ströfer, M., Jelkmann, W., Depping, R., 2011. Curcumin decreases survival of Hep3B liver and MCF-7 breast cancer Cells. Strahlenther Onkol. 187, 393–400.

Tang, Y., Chen, A., 2010a. Curcumin block translocation of glucose transporter-4 by interrupting the IRS/PI3K/AKT signalling pathway and increase glucokinase activity by increasing AMPK activity and suppressing PKA activity, leading to increased conversion of glucose to G-6-P. Br. J. Pharmacol. 161, 1137–1149.

Tang, Y., Chen, A., 2010b. Curcumin protects hepatic stellate cells against leptin-induced activation in vitro by accumulating intracellular lipids. Endocrinology 151, 4168–4177.

Tang, Y., Chen, A., 2014. Curcumin eliminates the effect of advanced glycation end-products (AGEs) on the divergent regulation of gene expression of receptors of AGEs by interrupting leptin signaling. Lab Invest. 94, 503–516.

Tang, Y., Zheng, S., Chen, A., 2009. Curcumin eliminates leptin's effects on hepatic stellate cell activation via interrupting leptin signaling. Endocrinology 150, 3011–3020.

Tsochatzis, E., Papatheodoridis, G.V., Manesis, E.K., Kafiri, G., Tiniakos, D.G., Archimandritis, A.J., 2008. Metabolic syndrome is associated with severe fibrosis in chronic viral hepatitis and non-alcoholic steatohepatitis. Aliment. Pharmacol. Ther. 27, 80–89.

Tsukamoto, H., She, H., Hazra, S., Cheng, J., Miyahara, T., 2006. Antiadipogenic regulation underlies hepatic stellate cell transdifferentiation. J. Gastroenterol. Hepatol. 21 (Suppl. 3), S102–S105.

Vizzutti, F., Provenzano, A., Galastri, S., Milani, S., Delogu, W., Novo, E., et al., 2010. Curcumin limits the fibrogenic evolution of experimental steatohepatitis. Lab. Invest. 90, 104–115.

Wang, M.E., Chen, Y.C., Chen, I.S., Hsieh, S.C., Chen, S.S., Chiu, C.H., 2012. Curcumin protects against thioacetamide-induced hepatic fibrosis by attenuating the inflammatory response and inducing apoptosis of damaged hepatocytes. J. Nutr. Biochem. 23, 1352–1366.

Wang, Z., Juttermann, R., Soloway, P.D., 2000. TIMP-2 is required for efficient activation of proMMP-2 in vivo. J. Biol. Chem. 275, 26411–26415.

Xu, J., Fu, Y., Chen, A., 2003. Activation of peroxisome proliferatoractivated receptor-gamma contributes to the inhibitory effects of curcumin on rat hepatic stellate cell growth. Am. J. Physiol. Gastrointest. Liver. Physiol. 285, G20–G30.

Yao, Q., Lin, Y., Li, X., Shen, X., Wang, J., Tu, C., 2013. Curcumin ameliorates intrahepatic angiogenesis and capillarization of the sinusoids in carbon tetrachloride-induced rat liver fibrosis. Toxicol. Lett. 222, 72–82.

You, M., Matsumoto, M., Pacold, C.M., Cho, W.K., Crabb, D.W., 2004. The role of AMP-activated protein kinase in the action of ethanol in the liver. Gastroenterology 127, 1798–1808.

Zhai, X., Qiao, H., Guan, W., Li, Z., Cheng, Y., Jia, X., et al., 2015. Curcumin regulates peroxisome proliferator-activated receptor-γ coactivator-1α expression by AMPK pathway in hepatic stellate cells in vitro. Eur. J. Pharmacol. 746, 56–62.

Zhao, F.Q., Keating, A.F., 2007. Functional properties and genomics of glucose transporters. Curr. Genomics. 8, 113–128.

Zhao, H.L., Song, C.H., Chai, O.H., 2012. Negative effects of curcumin on liver injury induced by alcohol. Phytother. Res. 26, 1857–1863.

Zheng, S., Chen, A., 2004. Activation of PPARγ is required for curcumin to induce apoptosis and to inhibit the expression of extracellular matrix genes in hepatic stellate cells in vitro. Biochem. J. 384, 149–157.

Zheng, S., Chen, A., 2006. Curcumin suppresses the expression of extracellular matrix genes in activated hepatic stellate cells by inhibiting gene expression of connective tissue growth factor. Am. J. Physiol. Gastrointest. Liver. Physiol. 290, G883–G893.

Zheng, S., Chen, A., 2007. Disruption of transforming growth factor-beta signaling by curcumin induces gene expression of peroxisome proliferator-activated receptor-gamma in rat hepatic stellate cells. Am. J. Physiol. Gastrointest. Liver. Physiol. 292, G113–G123.

Zheng, S., Yumei, F., Chen, A., 2007. De novo synthesis of glutathione is a prerequisite for curcumin to inhibit hepatic stellate cell (HSC) activation. Free. Radic. Biol. Med. 43, 444–453.

Chapter 23

Curcumin against amyloid pathology in mental health and brain composition

Ikuo Tooyama[1], Nor Faeizah Ibrahim[1,2], Lina Wati Durani[1,2], Hamizah Shahirah Hamezah[1,2], Mohd Hanafi Ahmad Damanhuri[2], Wan Zurinah Wan Ngah[2], Hiroyasu Taguchi[1] and Daijiro Yanagisawa[1]

[1]*Shiga University of Medical Science, Otsu, Japan*

[2]*Universiti Kebangsaan Malaysia, Kuala Lumpur, Malaysia*

CHAPTER OUTLINE

INTRODUCTION

Turmeric, also known as *Curcuma longa*, is an Indian spice with a long history of use in traditional Asian medicine and is also used in preparation of curries (Hatcher et al., 2008; Goel et al., 2008). The active medicinal components of turmeric are curcuminoids, which consist of a mixture of curcumin (75–80%), demethoxycurcumin (15–20%), and bisdemethoxycurcumin (3–5%) (Fig. 23.1) (Aggarwal et al., 2007; Hamaguchi et al., 2010).

Fruits, Vegetables, and Herbs.
DOI: http://dx.doi.org/10.1016/B978-0-12-802972-5.00023-8

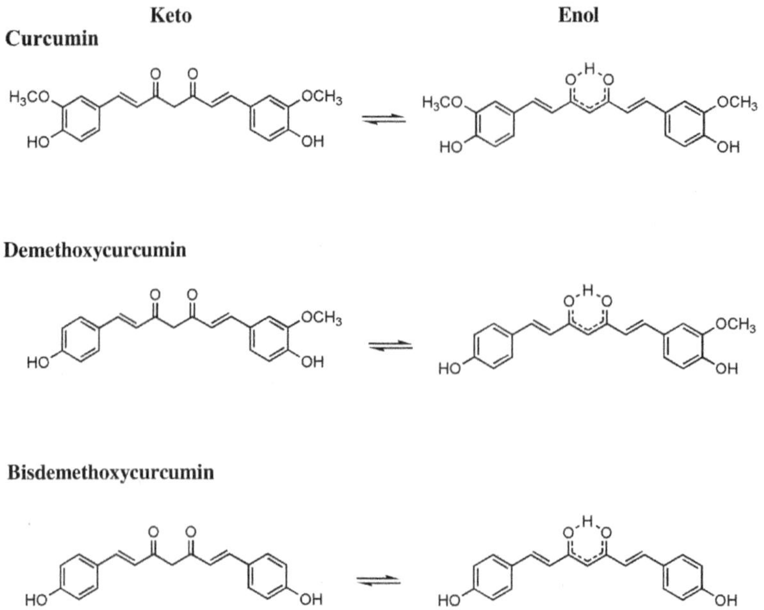

■ FIGURE 23.1 Tautomeric structures of curcumin, demethoxycurcumin, and bis-demethoxycurcumin.

Curcuminoids exist in an equilibrium of keto–enol tautomerism, and these tautomeric structures are involved in the binding of amyloid-β (Aβ) aggregates (Yanagisawa et al., 2010).

Curcumin has various pharmacological properties, including antitumor, antioxidative, antiinflammatory, and antiamyloid effects (Goel et al., 2008). Therefore, curcumin has been applied to the prevention and treatment of a wide variety of chronic inflammatory diseases (Ghosh et al., 2015; He et al., 2015). These include inflammatory bowel disease, pancreatic disease, diabetes, cardiovascular disease, asthma, rheumatoid arthritis, and various neurological diseases.

The keto–enol tautomerism property of curcuminoids has led to curcumin receiving attention as a potential therapeutic agent for Alzheimer's disease (AD). This is supported by several epidemiological studies that have reported the incidence of AD to be lower in India than in the United States, United Kingdom, and other developing countries (Chandra et al., 2001; Shaji et al., 2005; Vas et al., 2001; Ganguli et al., 2000). The levels of Aβ in the cerebrospinal fluid in healthy Indian people without dementia are lower than in those reported for other developing countries. Another report showed that curry consumption in the elderly population is associated with higher Mini-Mental State Examination (MMSE) scores (Ng et al., 2006).

Therefore, these studies suggest that the lower incidence of AD could be due to differences in environmental and dietary factors, supporting a potential role for curcumin.

AD is characterized by progression from episodic memory problems to a slow decline in global cognitive functions. The neuropathological hallmarks are senile plaques and neurofibrillary tangles (Braak and Braak, 1996), with the main component of senile plaques and neurofibrillary tangles being Aβ peptides and hyperphosphorylated tau protein (Braak and Braak, 1996). The first genetic mutations shown to be associated with familial AD were discovered in the amyloid precursor protein (APP) gene (Goate et al., 1991). These findings led to the proposal of the amyloid hypothesis, which states that the deposition of Aβ is the primary pathological event in AD (Hardy and Selkoe, 2002; Hardy and Higgins, 1992). In addition to APP gene, mutations have also been found in presenilin I (Sherrington et al., 1995) and presenilin II (Rogaev et al., 1995; Levy-Lahad et al., 1995), which are also involved in familial AD; APP generates Aβ by β-site APP cleaving with β-secretase and γ-secretase (Nunan and Small, 2000), and presenilin is a component of the γ-secretase complex (De Strooper, 2003; Selkoe and Wolfe, 2007). The mutations of these three genes cause increased production of Aβ (Hardy and Selkoe, 2002).

Recent evidence shows that amyloid pathology occurs 10–20 years before the clinical onset of AD (Bateman et al., 2012; Jack et al., 2013). When cognitive decline occurs in a patient with AD, they already show senile plaques, neurofibrillary tangles, and neuronal loss in the brain. Therefore, Aβ-targeting drugs need to be applied at very early stages of AD, including when patients are preclinical or have only mild cognitive impairment. Although several clinical trials have been employed for preclinical AD (Sperling et al., 2014), it is important to remember that people with preclinical AD are clinically normal and that treatment should have minimal side effects. From this point of view, the ability to develop therapeutic drugs from natural food products would be of great interest. Therefore, in this review, we focus on the effect of curcumin on the neuropathology of AD.

Aβ OLIGOMERS ARE THE MAIN THERAPEUTIC TARGETS FOR PRECLINICAL AD

According to the amyloid cascade hypothesis, deposition of Aβ is the first pathological event in AD (Fig. 23.2) (Hardy and Selkoe, 2002; Hardy and Higgins, 1992). Consequently, researchers have looked to reduce Aβ production, increase Aβ clearance, and inhibit Aβ aggregation as therapeutic targets. However, more than 100 drugs directed at the Aβ pathway in

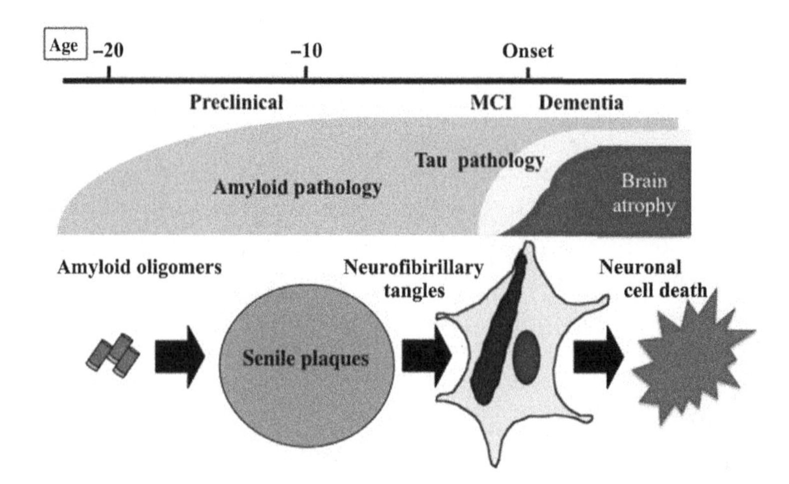

■ FIGURE 23.2 Schematic drawing of the progression of neuropathology in Alzheimer's disease. *MCI*, mild cognitive impairment; age is represented in years.

AD have failed to show any success in clinical trials (Becker et al., 2008; Giacobini and Becker, 2007). In addition, although the number of neurofibrillary tangles correlate well with cognitive decline, the number of senile plaques does not correlate (Braak and Braak, 1996; Arriagada et al., 1992). Moreover, while tau-targeting therapy might be more effective (Giacobini and Gold, 2013), tau pathology is not significant in the preclinical stages of AD (Fig. 23.2) (Jack et al., 2013; Handoko et al., 2013).

Interestingly, cognitive disturbance in transgenic mouse models of AD occurs without tau pathology (Morgan et al., 2000). Recent studies have indicated that the brains of patients with AD contain soluble Aβ assemblies, including Aβ oligomers, and that the degree of cognitive impairment correlates well with the amount of soluble Aβ oligomers but not with the total Aβ burden (Kuo et al., 1996; Lue et al., 1999; McLean et al., 1999; Naslund et al., 2000; Wang et al., 1999). Thus, Aβ oligomers, rather than monomers or insoluble Aβ fibrils, may be responsible for neuronal and synaptic dysfunction in AD (Ferreira and Klein, 2011; Walsh and Selkoe, 2004; Cleary et al., 2005). This is supported by a report showing that Alzheimer-type dementia occurred in a patient with a novel mutation of the APP gene that caused Aβ oligomers but not senile plaques (Tomiyama et al., 2008). These results suggest that Aβ oligomers are appropriate as the main therapeutic targets for AD.

In the brains of patients with AD, Aβ can efficiently generate reactive oxygen species (ROS) in the presence of the transition metals copper and iron in vitro. Under oxidative conditions, Aβ will form stable dityrosine cross-linked dimers through free radical attack on the tyrosine residue at position 10 (Smith et al., 2007). Butterfield and Sultana (2011) reported that methionine at position 35 of Aβ was critical to Aβ-induced oxidative stress and neurotoxicity. In this process, methionine undergoes two-electron oxidation to form methionine sulfoxide. Then, Aβ oligomers enter the lipid bilayer of the cell membrane where methionine interacts with the carboxyl oxygen of isoleucine at position 31 and undergoes one-electron oxidation to form a sulfonyl-free radical (Butterfield et al., 2013).

Murakami et al. proposed an interesting hypothesis for Aβ. They found that Aβ42 showed a conformational change with a turn at position 22 (glutamic acid) and position 23 (aspartic acid) (Izuo et al., 2013). If this conformational change occurs, methionine at position 35 reaches tyrosine at position 10 and can undergo one-electron oxidation to form the sulfonyl-free radical, which is stable in the c-terminal core of Aβ oligomers (Izuo et al., 2013). When they examined amyloid depositions in APP transgenic mice with and without superoxide dismutase (SOD) knockout, Aβ depositions were increased in the transgenic mice with SOD1 deletion (Murakami et al., 2011). Therefore, inhibition of Aβ oligomerization appears to protect against oxidative stress and could be of particular importance when seeking to protect the brain against toxicity from Aβ oligomers.

More recently, several studies have reported that Aβ oligomers promote tau phosphorylation. ROS generated from Aβ oligomers activate p38 mitogen-activated protein kinases that phosphorylate the tau protein (Giraldo et al., 2014) as well as the regulator of calcineurin 1 (RCAN1) proteins that inhibit the phosphatase activity of calcineurin (Lloret et al., 2011). In addition, Aβ oligomers inhibit the insulin-signaling pathway and activate glycogen synthase kinase-3β that is involved in tau phosphorylation (Lloret et al., 2015). Thus, inhibition of Aβ oligomers could inhibit progression from amyloid to tau pathology in AD.

These studies indicate that inhibition of Aβ oligomerization and protection of neurons against oxidative stress are of particular importance for preclinical therapy in AD.

CURCUMIN DISPLAYS ANTIOXIDANT EFFECTS AND CAN INHIBIT Aβ AGGREGATIONS

Curcumin is known to be a potent antioxidant that protects cells against oxidative stress. Kim et al. (2001) reported that curcumin, demethoxycurcumin, and bisdemethoxycurcumin protected PC12 cells (half-maximal

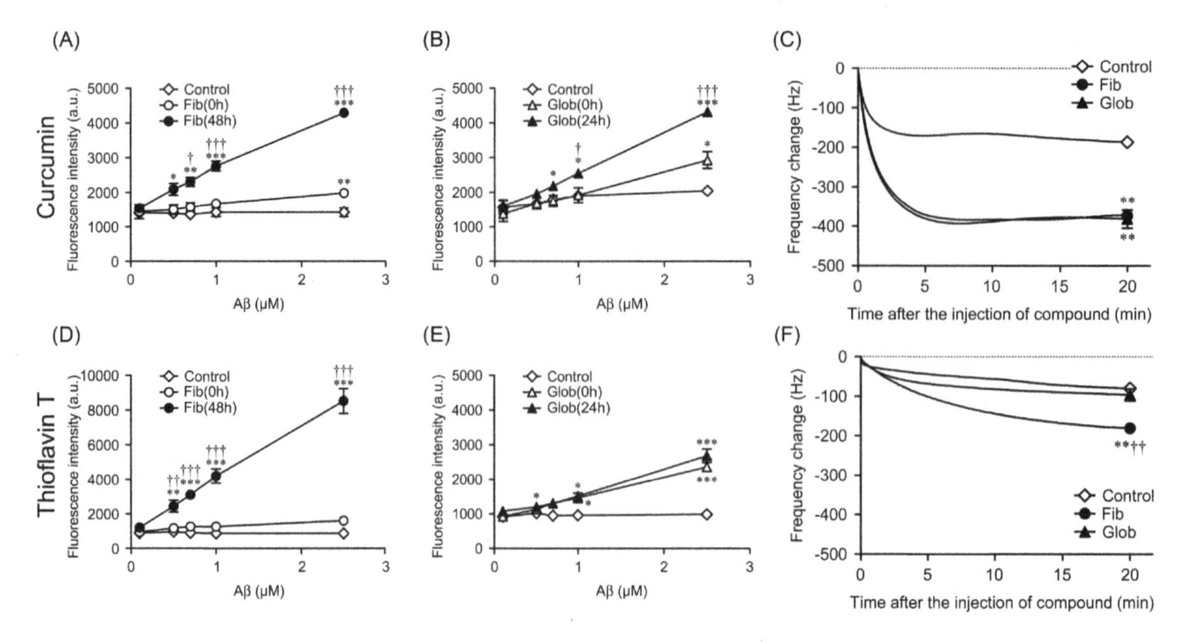

■ **FIGURE 23.3** Analysis of curcumin and thioflavin T in the presence of amyloid β (Aβ) samples by fluorescence and quartz crystal microbalance analysis. (A, B, D, and E): Fluorescence of curcumin (A and B) and thioflavin T (D and E) was measured after the addition of fibril (A and D) and globulomer (B and D). (C and F): Frequency of the fibril-immobilized electrode (*closed circle*) or globulomer-immobilized electrode (*closed triangle*) was recorded for 20 min after injection. The final concentrations were 10 μM for curcumin (C) and 30 μM for thioflavin T (F). Control (rhombus) indicates frequency change using the electrode that was not immobilized by Aβ peptide. Data were recorded every second for 20 min and represent the mean collected from four or five experiments. Data at the end point represent mean±SEM, and statistical comparisons were performed. *$P < 0.05$; **$P < 0.01$; ***$P < 0.001$ compared with control. †$P < 0.05$; ††$P < 0.01$; †††$P < 0.001$ compared with unaggregated Aβ sample.

effective concentration (EC_{50}) = 19.3 μM) and normal human umbilical vein endothelial cells (EC_{50} = 18.5 μM) from Aβ42 insult. In addition, curcumin was shown to inhibit oxidative damage and tau phosphorylation (Park et al., 2008).

Curcumin inhibits the formation of both Aβ fibrils (Hamaguchi et al., 2010; Ono et al., 2004; Ono et al., 2006; Hamaguchi et al., 2006; Kim et al., 2005) and Aβ oligomerization (Necula et al., 2007). We previously investigated the interaction between curcumin and Aβ oligomers using fluorescence analysis and quartz crystal microbalance (QCM) analysis (Yanagisawa et al., 2011a). Curcumin was analyzed using thioflavin T as a control. The fluorescence intensities of curcumin and thioflavin T significantly increased in the presence of Aβ fibrils (Fig. 23.3A and D). Curcumin showed increased fluorescence when mixed with globulomer Aβ (Fig. 23.3B) compared with that when mixed with nonaggregated Aβ samples, while thioflavin T did not show a significant increase in fluorescence in the presence of globulomer Aβ (Fig. 23.3E). Competition curves for curcumin against thioflavin T were plotted and the half-maximal inhibitory concentrations (IC_{50}) were estimated; the IC_{50} of curcumin was 0.20 μM (Yanagisawa et al., 2010).

Next, we used a 27-MHz QCM analyzer (AffinixQ; Initium, Tokyo, Japan) to monitor interactions between curcumin and thioflavin T with Aβ aggregates or oligomers. The QCM analysis revealed significant frequency decreases in both globulomer- and fibril-immobilized electrodes compared with the control when curcumin was injected into the vessel at a final concentration of 10 μM (Fig. 23.3C). In contrast, QCM analysis with thioflavin T at a final concentration of 30 μM resulted in a significant frequency decrease in the fibril-immobilized electrode but showed no difference between control and globulomer-immobilized electrode (Fig. 23.3F).

These results indicate that curcumin directly associates with Aβ oligomers and fibrils, suggesting that curcumin could alter the property of soluble Aβ oligomers through this association, thereby exerting a therapeutic effect by removing Aβ oligomers from the system and attenuating their toxicity.

KETO–ENOL TAUTOMERISM OF CURCUMIN IS A KEY TO ITS Aβ-BINDING ACTIVITY

Curcuminoids exist in equilibrium between keto and enol tautomers (Fig. 23.1). To assess the relationship between the tautomeric structures of curcumin and their Aβ-binding activity, we synthesized a wide variety of curcumin derivatives. Curcumin derivatives with keto–enol tautomerism showed high affinity for Aβ aggregates but not for Aβ monomers. Among them, we found an interesting chemical, 1,7-bis(4′-hydroxy-3′-trifluoromethoxyphenyl)-4-methoxycarbonylethyl-1,6-heptadiene-3,5-dione, which was named FMeC1 (Fig. 23.4). FMeC1 was shown to exist in physiological saline with a yellow color; when an Aβ aggregate was added, but not a monomer, the color of the FMeC1 solution changed from yellow to orange within 30 min (Yanagisawa et al., 2010). In addition, FMeC1 displayed intense fluorescence, and the intensity of the red color measured using absorbance at 550 nm correlated well with the ratio of the enol form of FMeC1 in the solution (Fig. 23.4). An analysis of ultraviolet-visible spectra showed that almost all of the FMeC1 existed as the keto form in the physiological solution but 75% of the FMeC1 was converted to its enol form when it bound Aβ aggregates (Yanagisawa et al., 2010). When we synthesized a curcumin derivative with two substituents at C-4 position which has no enolizability, its affinity to Aβ aggregates was much weaker than the corresponding enolizable derivatives.

Enolization of curcumin appears to be crucial for binding to Aβ aggregates, with the enol form predominantly existing when binding to Aβ aggregates (Fig. 23.5). Therefore, the keto–enol tautomerism of curcumin derivatives may represent a novel target for amyloid-binding agents that can be used for both therapy and amyloid imaging in AD.

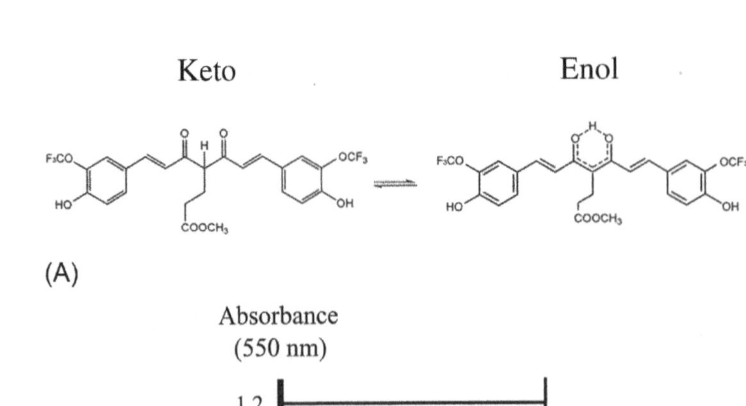

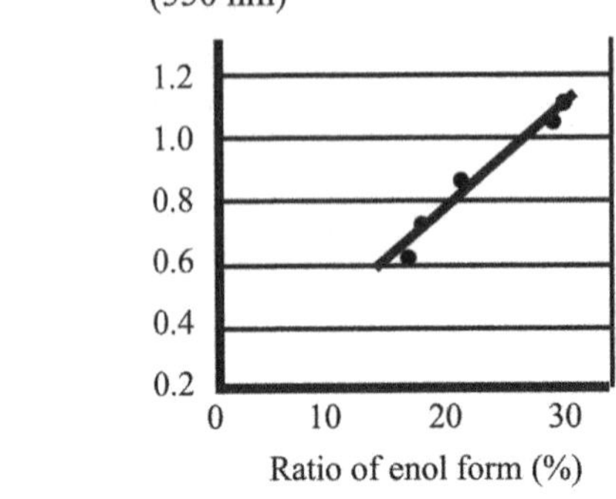

■ **FIGURE 23.4** (A) Tautomeric structures of 1,7-bis(4′-hydroxy-3′-trifluoromethoxyphenyl)-4-methoxycarbonylethyl-1,6-heptadiene-3,5-dione (ie, FMeC1) and (B) the absorbance at 550 nm of solutions containing different ratios of the enol form of FMeC1.

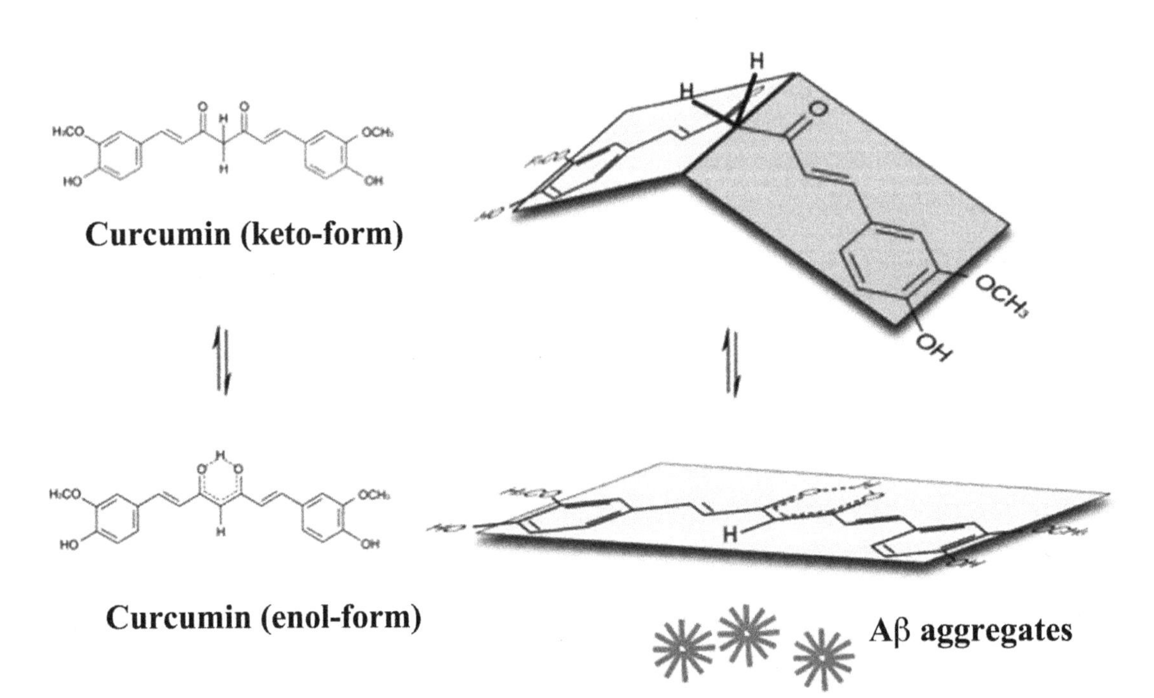

■ **FIGURE 23.5** Schematic drawings of the tautomeric structures of curcumin and their binding to amyloid β aggregates.

CURCUMIN INHIBITS β-SECRETASE ACTIVITY

In addition to antioxidant and anti-amyloid activities, curcumin has other therapeutic effects in AD. Aβ is generated from APP by β-site APP cleaving enzyme-1 (BACE-1) (β-secretase) and γ-secretases. The inhibition of these enzymes is one of the therapeutic targets for AD, and curcumin can inhibit both Aβ- and metal-induced BACE-1 upregulation (Shimmyo et al., 2008; Lin et al., 2008). Zhang et al. (2010) reported that curcumin treatment significantly increased the retention of immature APP in the endoplasmic reticulum and simultaneously attenuated APP endocytosis from the plasma membrane. Thus, curcumin was shown to lower Aβ levels by attenuating the maturation of APP in the secretory pathway.

CURCUMIN AND NEUROINFLAMMATION

Curcumin has potent antiinflammatory effects that have been applied to the prevention and treatment of several chronic inflammatory diseases (Ghosh et al., 2015; He et al., 2015). These include inflammatory bowel disease, pancreatic disease, diabetes, cardiovascular disease, asthma, rheumatoid arthritis, and neurological diseases, such as AD. Pathologically vulnerable regions of the AD brain show massive inflammation, with evidence of microglial activation, compliment deposition, and upregulation of proinflammatory cytokines (Akiyama et al., 2000). Studies using transgenic mouse models of AD (eg, Tg2576 mice expressing the Swedish familial AD double mutation K670N–M671L; Hsiao et al., 1996) have reported that curcumin inhibited the inflammatory responses in the brain. Lim et al. (2001) reported that curcumin lowered IL-1β expression, glial fibrillary acidic protein levels, phosphotyrosine-positive microglia, and oxidative proteins. In addition, Begum et al. (2008) reported that curcumin inhibited lipopolysaccharide-induced expression of inducible nitric oxide synthase, interleukin (IL)-1β, and F2 isoprostane (a marker of lipid peroxidation).

In vitro, curcumin has been shown to protect primary microglia from lipopolysaccharide toxicity (Parada et al., 2015). Under lipopolysaccharide conditions, curcumin reduced the levels of inducible nitric oxide synthase and tumor necrosis factor (TNF), which are microglial proinflammatory markers but increased the levels of IL-4, an anti-inflammatory cytokine (Parada et al., 2015). Shi et al. (2015) also reported that curcumin inhibited Aβ42-induced IL-1β, IL-6, and TNF-α production in cultured microglia. Since blockage of extracellular signal-regulated kinase (ie, ERK1/2) and p38 pathways can reduce inflammatory cytokine production by microglia, the authors suspected that curcumin suppressed ERK1/2 and p38 signaling, thereby attenuating the inflammatory response (Shi et al., 2015). Interestingly, Giri et al. (2004) reported that curcumin also suppressed the activation of DNA binding by early growth response 1 (EGR-1) in a human acute monocytic leukemia cell line (THP-1). EGR-1 activation was shown to induce production of cytokines and chemokines, while curcumin abrogated Aβ-induced expression of TNF-α, IL-1β, and other chemokines (eg, macrophage inflammatory protein 1β, monocyte chemotactic protein 1, and IL-8) (Giri et al., 2004).

ANIMAL STUDIES WITH CURCUMIN

When curcumin was intravenously injected into a transgenic mouse model of AD, it was shown to cross the blood–brain barrier, enter the brain, and bind to senile plaques (Garcia-Alloza et al., 2007). When fluorine atom is added to curcumin derivatives, we can monitor the distribution of fluorine-labeled curcumin derivatives in the mouse brain in vivo using fluorine MRI (Yanagisawa et al., 2011b). For example, when FMeC1 was injected into the tail vein of Tg2576, it passed through the blood–brain barrier and bound to senile plaques (Yanagisawa et al., 2011b). Interestingly, FMeC1 tended to be quickly removed from the brain (Yanagisawa et al., 2011b) when compared with other plaque-binding chemicals, such as styrylbenzoxazole (Yanagisawa et al., 2014). The relatively rapid clearance may be caused by the keto–enol tautomerism (Yanagisawa et al., 2010). In the case of FMeC1, the estimated half-lives in the brains of AD model and wild-type mice were 2 and 4h, respectively (Yanagisawa et al., 2011b). In contrast with intravenous administration, curcumin has shown very poor bioavailability when administered orally (Yang et al., 2007). When 500mg/kg of curcumin was administered orally to rats, the maximum concentration (C_{max}) and time to reach maximum concentration (T_{max}) were 0.06μg/mL and 41.7min, respectively, and the elimination half-life was 44.5min. Yang et al. (2007) reported that the oral bioavailability of curcumin was approximately 1%.

Because oral curcumin has low bioavailability, a relatively high dose is needed to achieve efficacy in transgenic mouse models. However, an appropriate dose of curcumin may still exist. Lim et al. (2001) orally administered curcumin to Tg2576 mice at low doses (160 parts per million (ppm); 0.43μmol/g) or high doses (5000ppm, 13.6μmol/g) for 6 months In mice given the low-dose treatment, significant decreases in the insoluble Aβ, soluble Aβ, and Aβ plaque burdens occurred. Interestingly, the outcomes were unchanged by the high-dose treatment (Lim et al., 2001). Table 23.1 shows a summary of the in vivo studies of oral curcumin for AD model mice, with slight modification from a previous report (Hamaguchi et al., 2010). According to Yang et al. (2005), Tg2576 mice

Table 23.1 Summary of the Effects of Oral Curcumin on Pathology in Alzheimer's Disease

Authors	Model Animal	Dose and Duration of Oral Curcumin	Neuropathological and Biochemical Effects	Behavioral Investigation
Lim et al. (2001)	Tg 2576	160 ppm for 6 months	Reduced insoluble Aβ, soluble Aβ, and Aβ plaque burden. Oxidative proteins and IL-1β in the brain were lowered	Not described
		5000 ppm for 6 months	Insoluble Aβ, soluble Aβ, and Aβ plaques were unchanged Oxidative proteins and IL-1β in the brain were lowered	Not described
Yang et al. (2005)	Tg2576	500 ppm for 5 months	Reduced amyloid levels and Aβ plaque burden	Not described
Begum et al. (2008)	Tg2576	500 ppm for 5 months	Reduced insoluble Aβ and Aβ plaque burden	
Ma et al. (2009)	3xTg-AD	500 ppm for 4 months	Reduced phosphorylated tau in the detergent lysis-buffer-extracted in hippocampal Membrane pellet fractions	Improvement in Y-maze performance
Hamaguchi et al. (2009)	Tg2576	5000 ppm for 10 months	Aβ depositions were unchanged TBS-soluble Aβ monomers were increased A11-positive Aβ were decreased	Not described
Cheng et al. (2013)	Tg2576	23 mg/kg (curcumin/body weight) once every week for 3 months	Reduced amyloid plaque burden	Improved cue memory in the contextual fear conditioning test
Yanagisawa et al. (2015)	APPswe/PS1dE9	500 ppm for 6 months	Aβ depositions were unchanged Insoluble Aβ40 and Aβ42 were unchanged Soluble Aβ40 monomers were increased (FMeC1 reduced insoluble Aβ40 and Aβ42)	Curcumin showed no effect in water-maze test (while, FMeC1 improved memory)

Modified from Table 1 of Hamaguchi et al., (2009).
Aβ, *amyloid* β; *FMeC1, 1,7-Bis(4′-hydroxy-3′-trifluoromethoxyphenyl)-4-methoxycarbonylethyl-1,6-heptadiene-3,5-dione; IL, interleukin; ppm, parts per million.*

were orally given curcumin for 5 months (dose, 500 ppm; 1.36 μmol/g) and the Aβ burden reduced. Begum et al. (2008) also reported a similar effect on the Aβ burden of Tg2576 mice when using 500 ppm (1.36 μmol/g) of curcumin. Meanwhile, Hamaguchi et al. (2009) reported that 5000 ppm (13.6 μmol/g) of oral curcumin did not reduce Aβ depositions in the brains of Tg2576 mice but that it did increase Aβ monomers soluble in tris-buffered saline (TBS) and decreased Aβ oligomers. The increase of TBS-soluble Aβ monomers with oral curcumin was also observed in our recent study using APPswe–PS1dE9 double transgenic mice (Yanagisawa et al., 2015). As pointed out by Hamaguchi et al. (2010), this was probably because curcumin mainly inhibits the pathway from Aβ monomers to oligomers but not the pathway from Aβ oligomers to fibrils (Necula et al., 2007).

Recently, Cheng et al. reported interesting results associated with nanocurcumin. They mixed a nanoprecipitation of curcumin, polyethylene glycol–polylactic acid coblock polymer, and polyvinylpyrrolidone before freeze drying the mixture with beta-cyclodextrin. Nanocurcumin improved the bioavailability of curcumin when they administered nanocurcumin powder, unformulated curcumin, or placebo orally to Tg2576 mice for 3 months. Nanocurcumin produced significantly higher curcumin concentration in plasma, improved cognitive function, and suppressed amyloid pathology in the brain (Cheng et al., 2013).

Several studies have also reported that curcumin improved not only amyloid pathology but also tau pathology. Treatment of triple-transgenic AD mice fed a high-fat diet with fish oil, curcumin, or a combination of both for 4 months was shown to reduce phosphorylated c-Jun N-terminal kinase, insulin receptor substrate 1, and tau (Ma et al., 2009). When 500 ppm of curcumin was administered to aged human transgenic tau mice, curcumin selectively suppressed the levels of soluble tau dimers but not those of insoluble tau or monomeric phospho-tau (Ma et al., 2013). In addition, curcumin corrected behavioral, synaptic, and heat-shock protein deficits (Ma et al., 2013).

CLINICAL TRIALS OF CURCUMIN FOR AD

To date, only few clinical trials have been completed and reported. According to the clinical trial website https://clinicaltrials.gov, the search term "Alzheimer+ and + curcumin," yielded seven clinical trials.

Baum et al. (2008) reported the results of a randomized, double-blind, placebo-controlled study of curcumin on AD in 2008. In that study, each participant randomly received either curcumin at two different doses (1 g/day or 4 g/day) or placebo (4 g/day) for 6 months. All participants also received 120 mg/day of standardized ginkgo biloba leaf extract. The authors then examined the change in MMSE scores and serum Aβ40 levels between 0 and 6 months, but they did not detect any significant difference between the curcumin- and placebo-treated groups.

Ringman et al. (2012) reported the results of another randomized, double-blind, placebo-controlled study. Thirty-six patients with mild-to-moderate AD were randomized to receive either placebo or Curcumin C3 Complex at 2 g/day or 4 g/day for 24 weeks. After 24 weeks, the trial was extended to 48 weeks as an open-label trial in which patients who received placebo were randomly assigned to receive either 2 g/day or 4 g/day of the Curcumin C3 Complex, while patients already receiving treatment continued with the same dose. There were no significant differences between groups on the cognitive component of the Alzheimer's Disease Assessment Scale (ADAScog), the Neuropsychiatric Inventory (NPI), the Alzheimer's Disease Cooperative Study Activities of Daily Living (ADCS-ADL) scale, or the MMSE. Plasma and cerebrospinal fluid levels of Aβ40–Aβ42 or tau were also not different between the treatment groups.

NEW APPROACHES OF CURCUMIN

The negative results of early clinical trials for AD could be attributable to the low bioavailability of oral curcumin due to low absorption and rapid metabolism (Mancuso et al., 2011). To increase the bioavailability of curcumin, several approaches have been proposed. Piperine is a known inhibitor of hepatic and intestinal glucuronidation. Therefore, Shoba et al. (1998) examined the effect of adding piperine on the bioavailability of curcumin in rats and healthy human volunteers and showed increased bioavailabilities of 154% and 2000%, respectively. Maiti et al. (2007) also reported that a novel formulation of curcumin in combination with the phospholipids (curcumin phospholipids) increased bioavailability, but carbon tetrachloride induced acute liver damage in rats. Another interesting approach was proposed by Sasaki et al. (2011) who developed a highly absorptive curcumin dispersed with colloidal nanoparticles called Theracurmin. The absorption efficacy of Theracurmin was more than 40- and 27-fold higher than that of curcumin powder in rats and humans, respectively (Sasaki et al., 2011). Nanoliposomes decorated with a curcumin derivative have also been shown to increase bioavailability (Matloob et al., 2014). Finally, we have proposed the inhalation of curcumin. In a recent report, we described a novel technique for aerosolizing the curcumin derivative

FMeC1 that can facilitate its safe delivery to the brain (McClure et al., 2015). Using this approach, curcumin reaches the brain directly via a non-blood pathway.

CONCLUSION

Recent advances show that amyloid pathology occurs 10–20 years before the clinical onset of AD; therefore, earlier treatment might be appropriate in the disease process. However, people with preclinical AD are clinically normal and may not progress to full AD, making it particularly important to treat them without causing serious side effects. Developing therapeutic drugs from natural food products could fulfill this requirement. In preclinical AD, amyloid pathology has been shown to precede tau pathology, with Aβ oligomers showing the most potent neurotoxicity. Curcumin can bind not only Aβ fibrils but also Aβ oligomers and can inhibit Aβ oligomerization, oxidative stress, and inflammation. When administered to transgenic mouse models of AD, curcumin can also suppress amyloid pathology in the mouse brain. However, to date, the results of early clinical trials of curcumin for AD in humans have been negative or inconclusive. This is probably because of its low bioavailability when taken orally; therefore, further research is needed using methods that can improve the bioavailability of curcumin.

ACKNOWLEDGMENTS

This study was supported by Grants-in-Aid for Scientific Research (Grant Number 26290022, I.T.; and 15K01282, H.T.) from the Japan Society for the Promotion of Science, and a Long Term Research Grant Scheme (Grant Number LRGS/BU/2012/UKM-UKM/K/04) from Ministry of Education Malaysia.

REFERENCES

Aggarwal, B.B., Sundaram, C., Malani, N., Ichikawa, H., 2007. Curcumin: the Indian solid gold. Adv. Exp. Med. Biol. 595, 1–75.

Akiyama, H., Barger, S., Barnum, S., Bradt, B., Bauer, J., Cole, G.M., et al., 2000. Inflammation and Alzheimer's disease. Neurobiol. Aging 21, 383–421.

Arriagada, P.V., Growdon, J.H., Hedley-Whyte, E.T., Hyman, B.T., 1992. Neurofibrillary tangles but not senile plaques parallel duration and severity of Alzheimer's disease. Neurology 42, 631–639.

Bateman, R.J., Xiong, C., Benzinger, T.L., Fagan, A.M., Goate, A., Fox, N.C., et al., 2012. Clinical and biomarker changes in dominantly inherited Alzheimer's disease. N. Engl. J. Med. 367, 795–804.

Baum, L., Lam, C.W., Cheung, S.K., Kwok, T., Lui, V., Tsoh, J., et al., 2008. Six-month randomized, placebo-controlled, double-blind, pilot clinical trial of curcumin in patients with Alzheimer disease. J. Clin. Psychopharmacol. 28, 110–113.

Becker, R.E., Greig, N.H., Giacobini, E., 2008. Why do so many drugs for Alzheimer's disease fail in development? Time for new methods and new practices? J. Alzheimers Dis. 15, 303–325.

Begum, A.N., Jones, M.R., Lim, G.P., Morihara, T., Kim, P., Heath, D.D., et al., 2008. Curcumin structure-function, bioavailability, and efficacy in models of neuroinflammation and Alzheimer's disease. J. Pharmacol. Exp. Ther. 326, 196–208.

Braak, H., Braak, E., 1996. Evolution of the neuropathology of Alzheimer's disease. Acta Neurol. Scand. Suppl. 165, 3–12.

Butterfield, D.A., Sultana, R., 2011. Methionine-35 of abeta(1-42): importance for oxidative stress in Alzheimer disease. J. Amino Acids 2011, 198430.

Butterfield, D.A., Swomley, A.M., Sultana, R., 2013. Amyloid beta-peptide (1-42)-induced oxidative stress in Alzheimer disease: importance in disease pathogenesis and progression. Antioxid. Redox Signal. 19, 823–835.

Chandra, V., Pandav, R., Dodge, H.H., Johnston, J.M., Belle, S.H., DeKosky, S.T., et al., 2001. Incidence of Alzheimer's disease in a rural community in India: the Indo-US study. Neurology 57, 985–989.

Cheng, K.K., Yeung, C.F., Ho, S.W., Chow, S.F., Chow, A.H., Baum, L., 2013. Highly stabilized curcumin nanoparticles tested in an in vitro blood-brain barrier model and in Alzheimer's disease Tg2576 mice. AAPS J. 15, 324–336.

Cleary, J.P., Walsh, D.M., Hofmeister, J.J., Shankar, G.M., Kuskowski, M.A., Selkoe, D.J., et al., 2005. Natural oligomers of the amyloid-beta protein specifically disrupt cognitive function. Nat. Neurosci. 8, 79–84.

De Strooper, B., 2003. Aph-1, Pen-2, and Nicastrin with Presenilin generate an active gamma-secretase complex. Neuron 38, 9–12.

Ferreira, S.T., Klein, W.L., 2011. The Abeta oligomer hypothesis for synapse failure and memory loss in Alzheimer's disease. Neurobiol. Learn. Mem. 96, 529–543.

Ganguli, M., Chandra, V., Kamboh, M.I., Johnston, J.M., Dodge, H.H., Thelma, B.K., et al., 2000. Apolipoprotein E polymorphism and Alzheimer disease: the Indo-US Cross-National Dementia Study. Arch. Neurol. 57, 824–830.

Garcia-Alloza, M., Borrelli, L.A., Rozkalne, A., Hyman, B.T., Bacskai, B.J., 2007. Curcumin labels amyloid pathology in vivo, disrupts existing plaques, and partially restores distorted neurites in an Alzheimer mouse model. J. Neurochem. 102, 1095–1104.

Ghosh, S., Banerjee, S., Sil, P.C., 2015. The beneficial role of curcumin on inflammation, diabetes and neurodegenerative disease: a recent update. Food Chem. Toxicol. 83, 111–124.

Giacobini, E., Becker, R.E., 2007. One hundred years after the discovery of Alzheimer's disease. A turning point for therapy? J. Alzheimers Dis. 12, 37–52.

Giacobini, E., Gold, G., 2013. Alzheimer disease therapy—moving from amyloid-beta to tau. Nat. Rev. Neurol. 9, 677–686.

Giraldo, E., Lloret, A., Fuchsberger, T., Vina, J., 2014. Abeta and tau toxicities in Alzheimer's are linked via oxidative stress-induced p38 activation: protective role of vitamin E. Redox Biol. 2, 873–877.

Giri, R.K., Rajagopal, V., Kalra, V.K., 2004. Curcumin, the active constituent of turmeric, inhibits amyloid peptide-induced cytochemokine gene expression and

CCR5-mediated chemotaxis of THP-1 monocytes by modulating early growth response-1 transcription factor. J. Neurochem. 91, 1199–1210.

Goate, A., Chartier-Harlin, M.C., Mullan, M., Brown, J., Crawford, F., Fidani, L., et al., 1991. Segregation of a missense mutation in the amyloid precursor protein gene with familial Alzheimer's disease. Nature 349, 704–706.

Goel, A., Kunnumakkara, A.B., Aggarwal, B.B., 2008. Curcumin as "Curecumin": from kitchen to clinic. Biochem. Pharmacol. 75, 787–809.

Hamaguchi, T., Ono, K., Yamada, M., 2006. Anti-amyloidogenic therapies: strategies for prevention and treatment of Alzheimer's disease. Cell. Mol. Life Sci. 63, 1538–1552.

Hamaguchi, T., Ono, K., Murase, A., Yamada, M., 2009. Phenolic compounds prevent Alzheimer's pathology through different effects on the amyloid-beta aggregation pathway. Am. J. Pathol. 175, 2557–2565.

Hamaguchi, T., Ono, K., Yamada, M., 2010. Review: curcumin and Alzheimer's disease. CNS Neurosci. Ther. 16, 285–297.

Handoko, M., Grant, M., Kuskowski, M., Zahs, K.R., Wallin, A., Blennow, K., et al., 2013. Correlation of specific amyloid-beta oligomers with tau in cerebrospinal fluid from cognitively normal older adults. JAMA Neurol. 70, 594–599.

Hardy, J., Selkoe, D.J., 2002. The amyloid hypothesis of Alzheimer's disease: progress and problems on the road to therapeutics. Science 297, 353–356.

Hardy, J.A., Higgins, G.A., 1992. Alzheimer's disease: the amyloid cascade hypothesis. Science 256, 184–185.

Hatcher, H., Planalp, R., Cho, J., Torti, F.M., Torti, S.V., 2008. Curcumin: from ancient medicine to current clinical trials. Cell. Mol. Life Sci. 65, 1631–1652.

He, Y., Yue, Y., Zheng, X., Zhang, K., Chen, S., Du, Z., 2015. Curcumin, inflammation, and chronic diseases: how are they linked? Molecules 20, 9183–9213.

Hsiao, K., Chapman, P., Nilsen, S., Eckman, C., Harigaya, Y., Younkin, S., et al., 1996. Correlative memory deficits, Abeta elevation, and amyloid plaques in transgenic mice. Science 274, 99–102.

Izuo, N., Murakami, K., Sato, M., Iwasaki, M., Izumi, Y., Shimizu, T., et al., 2013. Non-toxic conformer of amyloid beta may suppress amyloid beta-induced toxicity in rat primary neurons: implications for a novel therapeutic strategy for Alzheimer's disease. Biochem. Biophys. Res. Commun. 438, 1–5.

Jack Jr., C.R., Knopman, D.S., Jagust, W.J., Petersen, R.C., Weiner, M.W., Aisen, P.S., et al., 2013. Tracking pathophysiological processes in Alzheimer's disease: an updated hypothetical model of dynamic biomarkers. Lancet Neurol. 12, 207–216.

Kim, D.S., Park, S.Y., Kim, J.K., 2001. Curcuminoids from Curcuma longa L. (Zingiberaceae) that protect PC12 rat pheochromocytoma and normal human umbilical vein endothelial cells from betaA(1-42) insult. Neurosci. Lett. 303, 57–61.

Kim, H., Park, B.S., Lee, K.G., Choi, C.Y., Jang, S.S., Kim, Y.H., et al., 2005. Effects of naturally occurring compounds on fibril formation and oxidative stress of beta-amyloid. J. Agric. Food Chem. 53, 8537–8541.

Kuo, Y.M., Emmerling, M.R., Vigo-Pelfrey, C., Kasunic, T.C., Kirkpatrick, J.B., Murdoch, G.H., et al., 1996. Water-soluble Abeta (N-40, N-42) oligomers in normal and Alzheimer disease brains. J. Biol. Chem. 271, 4077–4081.

Levy-Lahad, E., Wasco, W., Poorkaj, P., Romano, D.M., Oshima, J., Pettingell, W.H., et al., 1995. Candidate gene for the chromosome 1 familial Alzheimer's disease locus. Science 269, 973–977.

Lim, G.P., Chu, T., Yang, F., Beech, W., Frautschy, S.A., Cole, G.M., 2001. The curry spice curcumin reduces oxidative damage and amyloid pathology in an Alzheimer transgenic mouse. J. Neurosci. 21, 8370–8377.

Lin, R., Chen, X., Li, W., Han, Y., Liu, P., Pi, R., 2008. Exposure to metal ions regulates mRNA levels of APP and BACE1 in PC12 cells: blockage by curcumin. Neurosci. Lett. 440, 344–347.

Lloret, A., Badia, M.C., Giraldo, E., Ermak, G., Alonso, M.D., Pallardo, F.V., et al., 2011. Amyloid-beta toxicity and tau hyperphosphorylation are linked via RCAN1 in Alzheimer's disease. J. Alzheimers Dis. 27, 701–709.

Lloret, A., Fuchsberger, T., Giraldo, E., Vina, J., 2015. Molecular mechanisms linking amyloid beta toxicity and Tau hyperphosphorylation in Alzheimers disease. Free Radic. Biol. Med. 83, 186–191.

Lue, L.F., Kuo, Y.M., Roher, A.E., Brachova, L., Shen, Y., Sue, L., et al., 1999. Soluble amyloid beta peptide concentration as a predictor of synaptic change in Alzheimer's disease. Am. J. Pathol. 155, 853–862.

Ma, Q.L., Yang, F., Rosario, E.R., Ubeda, O.J., Beech, W., Gant, D.J., et al., 2009. Beta-amyloid oligomers induce phosphorylation of tau and inactivation of insulin receptor substrate via c-Jun N-terminal kinase signaling: suppression by omega-3 fatty acids and curcumin. J. Neurosci. 29, 9078–9089.

Ma, Q.L., Zuo, X., Yang, F., Ubeda, O.J., Gant, D.J., Alaverdyan, M., et al., 2013. Curcumin suppresses soluble tau dimers and corrects molecular chaperone, synaptic, and behavioral deficits in aged human tau transgenic mice. J. Biol. Chem. 288, 4056–4065.

Maiti, K., Mukherjee, K., Gantait, A., Saha, B.P., Mukherjee, P.K., 2007. Curcumin-phospholipid complex: Preparation, therapeutic evaluation and pharmacokinetic study in rats. Int. J. Pharm. 330, 155–163.

Mancuso, C., Siciliano, R., Barone, E., 2011. Curcumin and Alzheimer disease: this marriage is not to be performed. J. Biol. Chem. 286, le3. author reply le4.

Matloob, A.H., Mourtas, S., Klepetsanis, P., Antimisiaris, S.G., 2014. Increasing the stability of curcumin in serum with liposomes or hybrid drug-in-cyclodextrin-in-liposome systems: a comparative study. Int. J. Pharm. 476, 108–115.

McClure, R., Yanagisawa, D., Stec, D., Abdollahian, D., Koktysh, D., Xhillari, D., et al., 2015. Inhalable curcumin: offering the potential for translation to imaging and treatment of Alzheimer's disease. J. Alzheimers Dis. 44, 283–295.

McLean, C.A., Cherny, R.A., Fraser, F.W., Fuller, S.J., Smith, M.J., Beyreuther, K., et al., 1999. Soluble pool of Abeta amyloid as a determinant of severity of neurodegeneration in Alzheimer's disease. Ann. Neurol. 46, 860–866.

Morgan, D., Diamond, D.M., Gottschall, P.E., Ugen, K.E., Dickey, C., Hardy, J., et al., 2000. A beta peptide vaccination prevents memory loss in an animal model of Alzheimer's disease. Nature 408, 982–985.

Murakami, K., Murata, N., Noda, Y., Tahara, S., Kaneko, T., Kinoshita, N., et al., 2011. SOD1 (copper/zinc superoxide dismutase) deficiency drives amyloid beta protein oligomerization and memory loss in mouse model of Alzheimer disease. J. Biol. Chem. 286, 44557–44568.

Naslund, J., Haroutunian, V., Mohs, R., Davis, K.L., Davies, P., Greengard, P., et al., 2000. Correlation between elevated levels of amyloid beta-peptide in the brain and cognitive decline. JAMA 283, 1571–1577.

Necula, M., Kayed, R., Milton, S., Glabe, C.G., 2007. Small molecule inhibitors of aggregation indicate that amyloid beta oligomerization and fibrillization pathways are independent and distinct. J. Biol. Chem. 282, 10311–10324.

Ng, T.P., Chiam, P.C., Lee, T., Chua, H.C., Lim, L., Kua, E.H., 2006. Curry consumption and cognitive function in the elderly. Am. J. Epidemiol. 164, 898–906.

Nunan, J., Small, D.H., 2000. Regulation of APP cleavage by alpha-, beta- and gamma-secretases. FEBS Lett. 483, 6–10.

Ono, K., Hasegawa, K., Naiki, H., Yamada, M., 2004. Curcumin has potent anti-amyloidogenic effects for Alzheimer's beta-amyloid fibrils in vitro. J. Neurosci. Res. 75, 742–750.

Ono, K., Hamaguchi, T., Naiki, H., Yamada, M., 2006. Anti-amyloidogenic effects of antioxidants: implications for the prevention and therapeutics of Alzheimer's disease. Biochim. Biophys. Acta 1762, 575–586.

Parada, E., Buendia, I., Navarro, E., Avendano, C., Egea, J., Lopez, M.G., 2015. Microglial HO-1 induction by curcumin provides antioxidant, antineuroinflammatory, and glioprotective effects. Mol. Nutr. Food Res.

Park, S.Y., Kim, H.S., Cho, E.K., Kwon, B.Y., Phark, S., Hwang, K.W., et al., 2008. Curcumin protected PC12 cells against beta-amyloid-induced toxicity through the inhibition of oxidative damage and tau hyperphosphorylation. Food Chem. Toxicol. 46, 2881–2887.

Ringman, J.M., Frautschy, S.A., Teng, E., Begum, A.N., Bardens, J., Beigi, M., et al., 2012. Oral curcumin for Alzheimer's disease: tolerability and efficacy in a 24-week randomized, double blind, placebo-controlled study. Alzheimers Res. Ther. 4, 43.

Rogaev, E.I., Sherrington, R., Rogaeva, E.A., Levesque, G., Ikeda, M., Liang, Y., et al., 1995. Familial Alzheimer's disease in kindreds with missense mutations in a gene on chromosome 1 related to the Alzheimer's disease type 3 gene. Nature 376, 775–778.

Sasaki, H., Sunagawa, Y., Takahashi, K., Imaizumi, A., Fukuda, H., Hashimoto, T., et al., 2011. Innovative preparation of curcumin for improved oral bioavailability. Biol. Pharm. Bull. 34, 660–665.

Selkoe, D.J., Wolfe, M.S., 2007. Presenilin: running with scissors in the membrane. Cell 131, 215–221.

Shaji, S., Bose, S., Verghese, A., 2005. Prevalence of dementia in an urban population in Kerala, India. Br. J. Psychiatry 186, 136–140.

Sherrington, R., Rogaev, E.I., Liang, Y., Rogaeva, E.A., Levesque, G., Ikeda, M., et al., 1995. Cloning of a gene bearing missense mutations in early-onset familial Alzheimer's disease. Nature 375, 754–760.

Shi, X., Zheng, Z., Li, J., Xiao, Z., Qi, W., Zhang, A., et al., 2015. Curcumin inhibits Abeta-induced microglial inflammatory responses in vitro: involvement of ERK1/2 and p38 signaling pathways. Neurosci. Lett. 594, 105–110.

Shimmyo, Y., Kihara, T., Akaike, A., Niidome, T., Sugimoto, H., 2008. Epigallocatechin-3-gallate and curcumin suppress amyloid beta-induced beta-site APP cleaving enzyme-1 upregulation. Neuroreport 19, 1329–1333.

Shoba, G., Joy, D., Joseph, T., Majeed, M., Rajendran, R., Srinivas, P.S., 1998. Influence of piperine on the pharmacokinetics of curcumin in animals and human volunteers. Planta Med. 64, 353–356.

Smith, D.G., Cappai, R., Barnham, K.J., 2007. The redox chemistry of the Alzheimer's disease amyloid beta peptide. Biochim. Biophys. Acta 1768, 1976–1990.

Sperling, R.A., Rentz, D.M., Johnson, K.A., Karlawish, J., Donohue, M., Salmon, D.P., et al., 2014. The A4 study: stopping AD before symptoms begin? Sci. Transl. Med. 6 228fs213.

Tomiyama, T., Nagata, T., Shimada, H., Teraoka, R., Fukushima, A., Kanemitsu, H., et al., 2008. A new amyloid beta variant favoring oligomerization in Alzheimer's-type dementia. Ann. Neurol. 63, 377–387.

Vas, C.J., Pinto, C., Panikker, D., Noronha, S., Deshpande, N., Kulkarni, L., et al., 2001. Prevalence of dementia in an urban Indian population. Int. Psychogeriatr 13, 439–450.

Walsh, D.M., Selkoe, D.J., 2004. Deciphering the molecular basis of memory failure in Alzheimer's disease. Neuron 44, 181–193.

Wang, J., Dickson, D.W., Trojanowski, J.Q., Lee, V.M., 1999. The levels of soluble versus insoluble brain Abeta distinguish Alzheimer's disease from normal and pathologic aging. Exp. Neurol. 158, 328–337.

Yanagisawa, D., Shirai, N., Amatsubo, T., Taguchi, H., Hirao, K., Urushitani, M., et al., 2010. Relationship between the tautomeric structures of curcumin derivatives and their Abeta-binding activities in the context of therapies for Alzheimer's disease. Biomaterials 31, 4179–4185.

Yanagisawa, D., Taguchi, H., Yamamoto, A., Shirai, N., Hirao, K., Tooyama, I., 2011a. Curcuminoid binds to amyloid-beta1-42 oligomer and fibril. J. Alzheimers Dis. 24 (Suppl. 2), 33–42.

Yanagisawa, D., Amatsubo, T., Morikawa, S., Taguchi, H., Urushitani, M., Shirai, N., et al., 2011b. In vivo detection of amyloid beta deposition using 19F magnetic resonance imaging with a 19F-containing curcumin derivative in a mouse model of Alzheimer's disease. Neuroscience 184, 120–127.

Yanagisawa, D., Taguchi, H., Ibrahim, N.F., Morikawa, S., Shiino, A., Inubushi, T., et al., 2014. Preferred features of a fluorine-19 MRI probe for amyloid detection in the brain. J. Alzheimers Dis. 39, 617–631.

Yanagisawa, D., Ibrahim, N.F., Taguchi, H., Morikawa, S., Hirao, K., Shirai, N., et al., 2015. Curcumin derivative with the substitution at C-4 position, but not curcumin, is effective against amyloid pathology in APP/PS1 mice. Neurobiol. Aging 36, 201–210.

Yang, F., Lim, G.P., Begum, A.N., Ubeda, O.J., Simmons, M.R., Ambegaokar, S.S., et al., 2005. Curcumin inhibits formation of amyloid beta oligomers and fibrils, binds plaques, and reduces amyloid in vivo. J. Biol. Chem. 280, 5892–5901.

Yang, K.Y., Lin, L.C., Tseng, T.Y., Wang, S.C., Tsai, T.H., 2007. Oral bioavailability of curcumin in rat and the herbal analysis from Curcuma longa by LC-MS/MS. J. Chromatogr. B Analyt. Technol. Biomed. Life Sci. 853, 183–189.

Zhang, C., Browne, A., Child, D., Tanzi, R.E., 2010. Curcumin decreases amyloid-beta peptide levels by attenuating the maturation of amyloid-beta precursor protein. J. Biol. Chem. 285, 28472–28480.

Chapter 24

Recent developments in using plant-derived natural products as tubulin inhibitors for the management of cancer

Yogesh A. Kulkarni[1], Mayuresh S. Garud[1], R.S. Gaud[1] and Anil B. Gaikwad[2]

[1]*Shobhaben Pratapbhai Patel School of Pharmacy & Technology Management, SVKM's NMIMS, Mumbai, Maharashtra, India*

[2]*Birla Institute of Technology and Science, Pilani, Rajasthan, India*

CHAPTER OUTLINE

INTRODUCTION

Cancer contributes a large share in deaths caused by diseases worldwide and the number is increasing in exponential way. According to "Word Cancer Report 2014" which was prepared by "The International Agency for Research on Cancer (IARC)," 8.2 million deaths were estimated annually in 2012, which is expected to increase up to 13 million in next years. In 2012, 14 million new cases were identified and this number is expected to reach 22 million per annum in next 20 years (Stewart and Wild, 2014). Defeating the cancer has become a global battle which has called urgency for developing new weapons to tackle with it.

Fruits, Vegetables, and Herbs.

DOI: http://dx.doi.org/10.1016/B978-0-12-802972-5.00024-X

Better understanding of molecular mechanisms involved in development of cancer has now opened numerous ways to treat the cancer. Targeting the microtubule dynamics and hence the tubulin is one of such promising ways which have developed into numerous antitumor agents. Drugs under this category have enjoyed a great clinical success and newer agents are on their way to clinical use. Plants have played an important role in development of modern medicines and anticancer agents are the one of the marked example of this.

In this chapter, we have explained the involvement of microtubule dynamics in cancer development with focus on various aspects of the natural tubulin inhibitors and their role in development of newer chemotherapeutic agents.

MICROTUBULES

Cytoskeleton is made up of three components: microtubules, actin microfilaments, and intermediate filaments (Risinger et al., 2009). Diverse cellular functions like mitosis, cell signaling, intracellular transport, and maintenance of cell integrity and shape have involvement of microtubules as an important factor (Perez, 2009; Garnham and Roll-Mecak, 2012). As microtubules have key role in cell division, targeting them is one of the promising ways for development of chemotherapeutic agent against the cancer.

Structurally microtubules are noncovalent dynamic polymers formed by association of α- and β-tubulin heterodimers. These heterodimers are assembled to form protofilaments and normally 13 such protofilaments are allied laterally to form the characteristic hollow and cylindrical microtubule having internal and external diameters of 12 and 25 nm, respectively. The heterodimers are structured in a polar manner where the α-tubulin subunit is exposed at one end called as the minus end and the β-tubulin subunit is exposed at the other called as the plus end (Fig. 24.1) (Garnham and Roll-Mecak, 2012).

The α-subunit has nonhydrolyzable GTP-binding site while the β-subunit has a hydrolyzable GTP-binding site. Stability of the microtubule polymer is largely controlled by hydrolysis on β-tubulin plus end. It is necessary to bind the GTP at the hydrolyzable site of the β-tubulin subunit to get assembled into microtubules. After getting arranged in microtubules, in short time, the GTP gets irreversibly hydrolyzed to GDP (Risinger et al., 2009).

Polymerization dynamics of microtubules

Dynamics of the microtubules polymerization define and regulate various biological functions of microtubules in all cells (Brouhard and

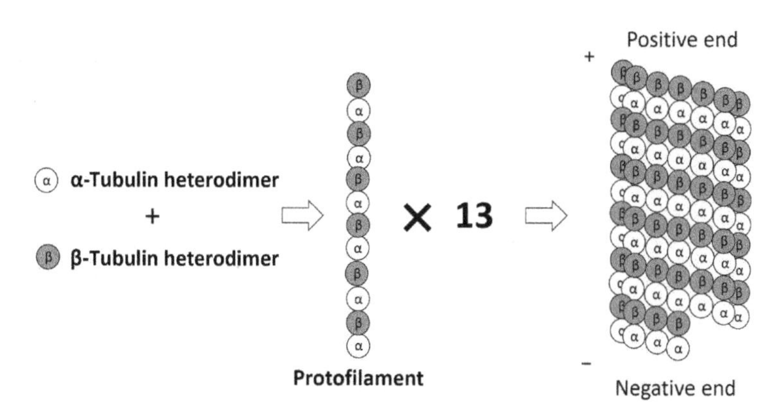

■ **FIGURE 24.1** Structure of microtubules.

Rice, 2014). The polymerization of microtubules occurs by a nucleation–elongation mechanism. Two types of nonequilibrium dynamics are observed in polymerization of microtubules. Most observed dynamic behavior termed as "dynamic instability," is process in which plus end grows or shrinks at a greater rate than the minus end that is, rate of addition or removal of β-tubulin subunits at plus end is more than that for α-tubulin subunits at minus end (Risinger et al., 2009; Matov et al., 2010). The rate of microtubule growth and the rate of shortening are involved in characterization of dynamic instability. 'Catastrophe', is the frequency of transition from the growth or paused state to shortening and a 'rescue', is the frequency of transition from shortening to growth or pause. The catastrophe frequency is ratio of the number of transitions from growth or pause to shortening and the total time growing and paused for each individual microtubule. The rescue frequency based on time was inversely calculated, dividing the total number of transitions from shortening to pause or growth by the time spent shortening (Jordan and Wilson, 2004; Bazaa et al., 2010). Drugs interacting with microtubule and microtubule-associated proteins can uphold or inhibit microtubule catastrophe as well as they affect the rate of microtubule growth and shortening (Jordan and Kamath, 2007).

Second type of dynamics is termed as "treadmilling" where plus and minus end grow/shrink at the same rate in controlled manner that is, removal of α-tubulin subunits from the minus end and addition of β-tubulin subunits to the plus end is equilibrated so that there is no net change in microtubule mass (Margolis and Wilson, 1978; Kueh et al., 2009). "Treadmilling" is supposed to be created by differences in the critical subunit concentrations at the opposite microtubule ends, and this dynamic behavior might be particularly important in mitosis (Chen and Zhang, 2004).

Microtubule dynamics has key role in mitosis. An interphase intracellular lattice-like network structure is formed by microtubules during the cell cycle. After entering the phase of mitosis, this structure is rearranged into the mitotic spindle. Highly coordinated microtubule dynamics is needed for the processes of depolymerization of the interphase microtubule structure, formation of the mitotic spindle, and step of finding, attaching, and separating chromosomes (Preciado Lopez et al., 2014).

Hence compounds having potential to interfere with the microtubule dynamics directly affect successfully completion of mitosis, and thus limiting proliferation and cell division.

Tubulin inhibitors as anticancer agents

The drugs that interfere with the dynamic stability of microtubules bind to tubulin subunits and leads to an increase or decrease in microtubule mass at the interphase. Depending on their mechanism of action, these compounds can be classified under two categories as microtubule stabilizers or destabilizers. These compounds act as antimitotic agents by inhibiting cell proliferation by interfering the polymerization and dynamics of spindle microtubules which are important for proper spindle function. Though there is difference in behavior of the agents under these classes at high concentration, at clinically relevant low concentrations, both classes of drugs inhibit mitosis through similar mechanism of slowing microtubule dynamics, resulting in mitotic arrest and apoptosis (Okouneva et al., 2003; Kelling et al., 2003).

Molecular-binding domains for anticancer drugs

There is a large chemical diversity among the substances that bind to the tubulin. All anticancer agents do not bind at the same site on the microtubules. These drugs either bind to soluble tubulin and/or directly to tubulin in the microtubules. Depending on the domain of the tubulin on which these drugs binds, they are further divided under different classes as vinca site–binding domain, colchicine site–binding domain, and taxane site–binding domain, which are named after the first drugs in that category (Fig. 24.2).

Researchers have also reported binding of few of the tubulin inhibitors to thiol groups on cysteine residues of tubulin. Agents binding to vinca domain, colchicine domain, and at thiol groups fall under microtubule destabilizers; and those binding to taxane domain fall under microtubule stabilizers. A large number of analogues of the natural tubulin inhibitors have been synthesized and explored for their anticancer activity.

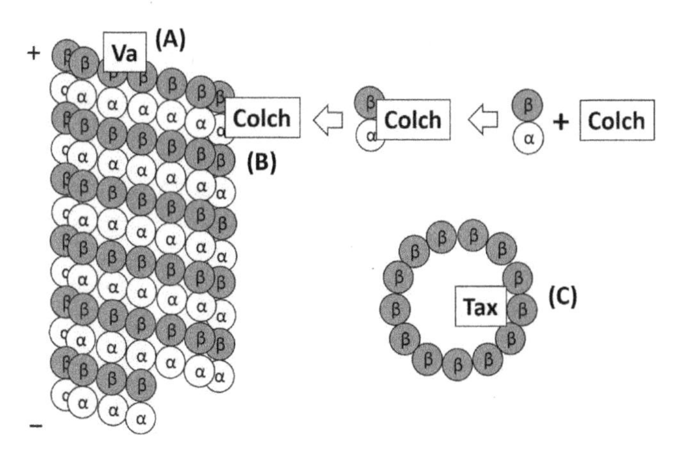

■ **FIGURE 24.2** Tubulin inhibitors–binding domains: (A) vinca domain, (B) colchicine domain, (C) taxane domain. *Va*, vinca alkaloid; *Colch*, colchicine; *Tax*, taxane.

Microtubule destabilizers

Microtubule destabilizing agents inhibit microtubule formation by inhibiting depolymerization which are reported to bind at two different domains on the microtubules.

Vinca domain

A distinct binding domain was recognized for vinca alkaloids where it binds to the β-subunit of tubulin dimers. This binding domain also shows affinity for various other novel chemotherapeutic agents.

The "vinca domain" is composed of the vinca-binding site and the peptide-binding site (Bai et al., 1990).

Vinca site–binding agents

The vinca alkaloids The era of using the plant materials for treatment of cancer was started with vinblastine and vincristine, which are the bisindole alkaloids first isolated from the leaves of the periwinkle plant *Catharanthus roseus* (L.) G. Don. (Apocynaceae), which were then obtained totally by synthetic route.

Vinca alkaloid, vinblastine, binds to soluble tubulin rapidly and reversibly (Wilson et al., 1982). This carries out conformational change in tubulin and increase the affinity of tubulin for binding of itself (Na and Timasheff, 1980).

Vinblastine reduces dynamic instability as well as treadmilling by nearly 50% at very low concentration of one or two molecules of per microtubule plus end and this involves no significant depolymerization of microtubule (Brouhard and Rice, 2014). This prevent normal assembling of the mitotic spindle and results in blocking of mitotic progression (Risinger et al., 2009). A series of the semisynthetic analogues of the two vinca alkaloids were synthesized by the researchers.

Vindesine (Eldisine) and vinorelbine (Navelbine) Vindesine is a first semisynthetic analogue of vinblastine which was succeeded to enter the clinical trials and has been approved for treatment of melanoma; and vinorelbine is second vinca analogue, which is approved for the treatment of nonsmall-cell lung (Ishikawa et al., 2009) (Fig. 24.3).

Vinflunine Vinflunine is a dihydrofluoro derivative of vinorelbine (Bennouna et al., 2008). Vinflunine similar to other vinca alkaloids inhibits the microtubule polymerization, which arrests the mitotic phase of cell division and results in apoptosis (Lobert and Puozzo, 2008).

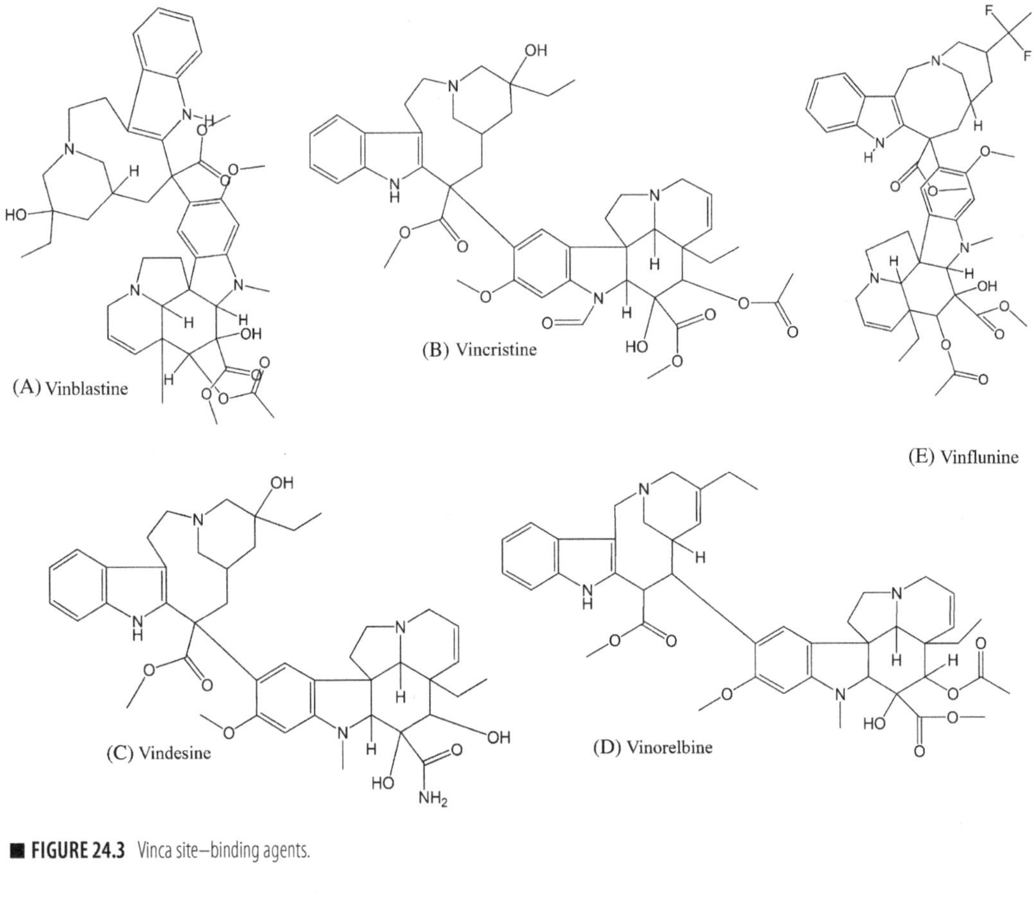

(A) Vinblastine

(B) Vincristine

(E) Vinflunine

(C) Vindesine

(D) Vinorelbine

■ **FIGURE 24.3** Vinca site–binding agents.

Peptide site–binding agents

A number of naturally occurring peptides have been found to bind at or near the vinca-binding site. These agents destabilize the microtubule.

Halichondrin B

Halichondrin B is a macrolide lactone polyether present in various species of marine sponges. Though the halichondrin B differs structurally from the vinca alkaloids, it noncompetitively inhibits binding of these alkaloids to tubulin through an allosteric interaction (Dabydeen et al., 2006).

Hemiasterlin

Hemiasterlins are the group of naturally occurring tripeptides derived from marine sponges like *Cymbastela* species, *Hemiasterella minor*, *Siphonochalina* species, and *Auletta* species (Loganzo et al., 2003). It is proposed that hemiasterlins binds to the vinca-peptide binding site and noncompetitively inhibits binding of other vinca alkaloid analogue (Bai et al., 1999).

Dolastatins 10 and 15

Dolastatins are isolated from the sea hare *Dolabella auricularia* which are potent inhibitors of tubulin which disturbs the microtubule assembly. Opposite to halichondrin B, dolastatins competitively inhibits binding of vinca alkaloid to tubulin (Bai et al., 1990).

Cryptophycin

Cryptophycin is a depsipeptide obtained from cyanobacteria found in fresh water. It has found to have very potent microtubule depolymerizing activity (Smith et al., 1994; Smith and Zhang, 1996).

Rhizoxin

Rhizoxin is a 16-membered antifungal macrocyclic lactone isolated from a potent pathogen of rice seedling blight *Rhizopus chinensis*. It binds to tubulin and inhibits mitosis by avoiding microtubule formation (Takahashi et al., 1987a; Hendriks et al., 1992; Kaplan et al., 1996). Binding of the rhizoxin is competitively inhibited by vinblastine (Takahashi et al., 1987b).

Spongistatins

The spongipyrans is a family of natural products of marine origin isolated from the sponges *Spirastrella spinispirulifera* and *Hyrtios erecta*. These are complex macrocyclic lactones having unique bis-spiroketal subunits. It demolishes microtubule dynamics and inhibits of mitotic spindle formation after binding to the tubulin (Uckun et al., 2001; Xu et al., 2011) (Fig. 24.4).

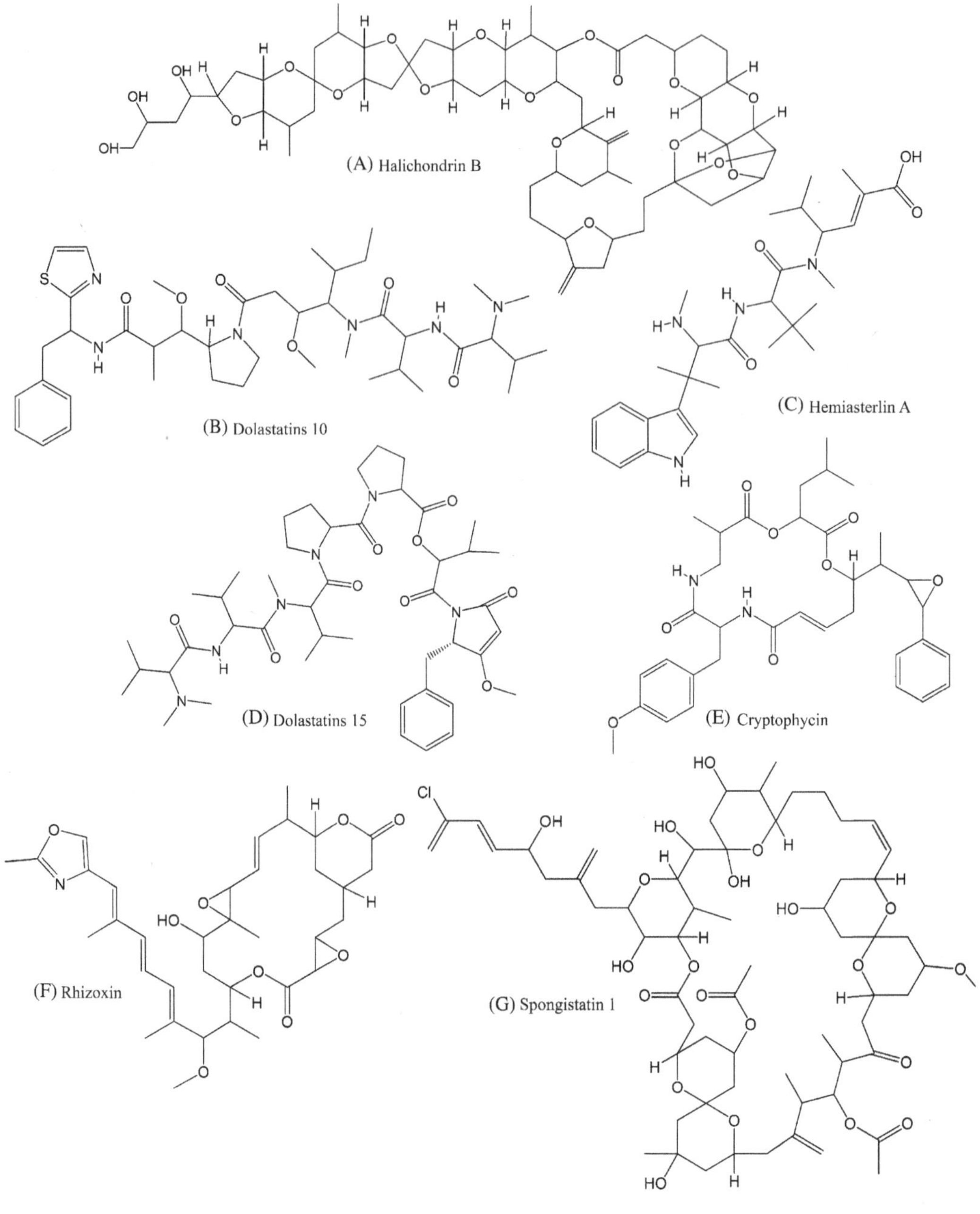

(A) Halichondrin B

(B) Dolastatins 10

(C) Hemiasterlin A

(D) Dolastatins 15

(E) Cryptophycin

(F) Rhizoxin

(G) Spongistatin 1

■ **FIGURE 24.4** Peptide site–binding agents.

Colchicine domain

Colchicine was first isolated by Pelletier and Caventou in 1820 from *Colchicum autumnale* L. which is also known as the poisonous meadow saffron (Lu et al., 2012). At high concentration, colchicine depolymerizes the microtubules while at low concentration it stabilizes microtubule dynamics. Colchicine substoichiometrically inhibits the microtubule polymerization (Wilson and Jordan, 1995). Colchicine does not bind directly to the microtubule. It forms a stable complex with unpolymerized tubulin heterodimers in solution, which further binds to microtubule ends and disturbs microtubule dynamics (Wilson and Jordan, 1995; Brossi et al., 1988; Hastie, 1991). Colchicine binding avoids the lateral contacts between protofilaments (Bhattacharyya et al., 2008).

Combretastatin

Combretastatin is a dihydrostilbenoid which was first isolated in 1989 by Pettit and coworkers from bark of the South African willow tree *Combretum caffrum* (Pettit et al., 1989; Mondal et al., 2012). In same year, Lin et al. (1989) proved that combretastatin binds to colchicine site and disturb the microtubule domain.

Combretatropone

Combretatropone is an amalgamation of colchicine and combretastatin (Janika and Bane, 2002). A series of combretatropone derivatives were synthesized and evaluated for their tubulin inhibitory activity.

It was found that combretatropone and its derivatives were less active than the corresponding derivatives of colchicine.

2-Methoxyestradiol

2-Methoxyestradiol is a natural end-metabolite of estradiol which was found to interrupt microtubule dynamics which arrests mitosis without depolymerizing microtubules (Kamath et al., 2006).

Centaureidin

Centaureidin is an *O*-methylated flavonol which is present in plants like *Tanacetum microphyllum*, *Brickellia veronicaefolia*, *Bidens pilosa*, and *Polymnia fruticosa* (Dalyot-Herman et al., 2009) (Fig. 24.5).

Centaureidin is the first known example of a flavone with antimitotic activity. It was found to compete the colchicine to bind with the tubulin (Beutler et al., 1993).

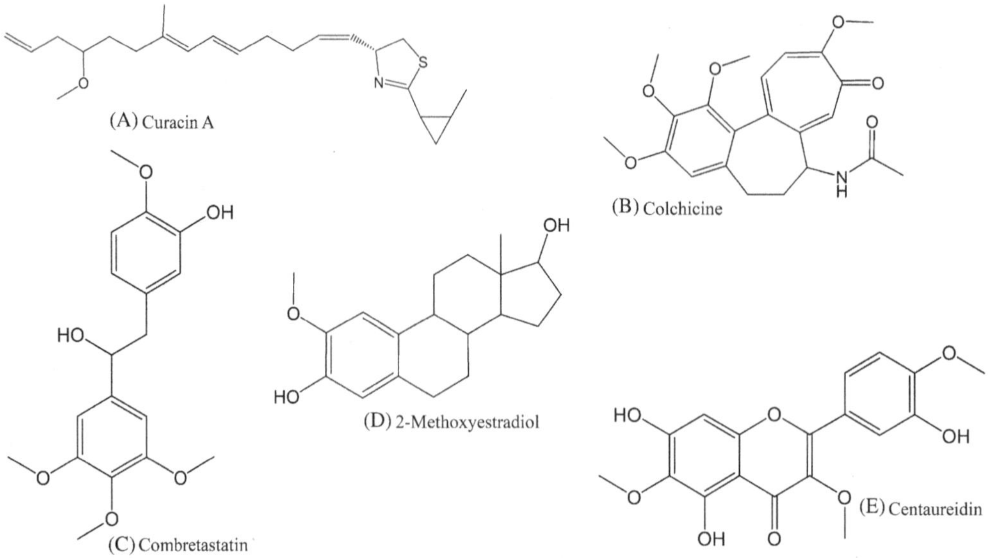

■ **FIGURE 24.5** Colchicine domain–binding agents.

Curacin A

Curacin A is also a natural product of marine origin which was isolated from the blue-green cyanobacterium *Lyngbya majuscula* first by Gerwick et al. (1994). Curacin A binds to the colchicine site and inhibits polymerization of tubulin (Wipf et al., 2004).

Thiol group on cysteine residues

Tubulin has 20 cysteine residues, 12 in α-tubulin and 8 in β-tubulin. These cysteine residues present thiol groups for the binding of few of the tubulin inhibitors (Krauhs et al., 1981). The mechanism is not fully uncovered but it is reviled that drugs which bind to these residues react with the nucleophilic thiols and this covalent interaction seems to prevent the formation of stable microtubules, which further prevents cell division (Nagle et al., 2006).

Calvatic acid

Calvatic acid isolated from *Calvatia lilacina* shows cytostatic properties as it prevents assembling of microtubules. In the presence of cysteine, the inhibition of assembly is prevented which suggests that tubulin sulfhydryl groups are the biological targets for the compound (Umezawa et al., 1975). Calvatic acid causes structural alteration of the protein structure

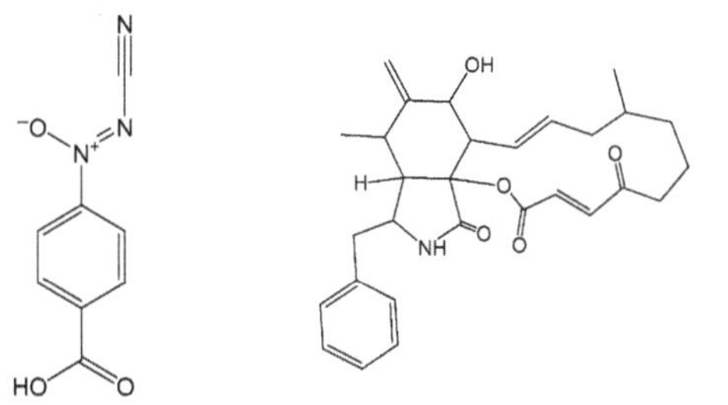

(A) Calvatic acid (B) Cytochalasin A

■ **FIGURE 24.6** Thiol group–binding agents.

and prevents the binding of colchicine to tubulin at colchicine-binding site (Gadoni et al., 1995) (Fig. 24.6).

Cytochalasin A

Cytochalasin A is a fungal metabolite having potential to inhibit the assembling of microtubules. It was also found to inhibit the binding of colchicine to tubulin. Studies have demonstrated that cytochalasin A covalently binds with tubulin thiol groups to obstruct microtubule assembly (Himes and Himes, 1980).

Microtubule stabilizers

Microtubule stabilizers prevent the depolymerization of the microtubules which binds to a well characterized site called as taxane-binding domain. This domain is present on lumen of the microtubules.

Taxane domain

Taxane domain–binding agents

Paclitaxel Paclitaxel, a prime compound in the taxane group was first isolated by Monroe Wall and Mansukh Wani in 1967 from the bark of the yew tree, *Taxus brevifolia* (Wani et al., 1971). Paclitaxel after binding to its domain on polymerized microtubules induces conformational change in the tubulin which increases its affinity for neighboring tubulin molecules and stabilizes the microtubule by increasing its polymerization (Nogales, 2001). This increases concentration of polymerized form of tubulin heterodimers which results in bundling of interphase microtubules (Rao et al., 1999). Suppression of the microtubule depolymerization blocks the mitotic phase and arrests the cell cycle (Yvon et al., 1999). It has been shown that paclitaxel induces the formation of microtubules containing 12 protofilaments which is different than from 13 protofilaments observed typically

(Andru et al., 1992). Its principal side effects, like the vinca alkaloids, are neurotoxicity and myelosuppression (Markman, 2003).

At clinically relevant lower concentrations, taxanes found to show similar activity as that of vinca and colchicine where they decrease microtubule dynamicity and cause mitotic spindle formation, mitotic arrest, and starts apoptosis (Okouneva et al., 2003; Kelling et al., 2003).

Docetaxel Docetaxel was the first semisynthetic derivatives of the paclitaxel which was synthesized in 1980 by researchers. It is more potent, having wide range of antitumors with less toxicity than that of paclitaxel (Gelmon, 1994; Bissery et al., 1995).

Abraxane Poor solubility is a major issue with the taxanes which imposed their formulation in cremophor which causes hypersensitivity reactions. To solve this problem, researchers have come up with a paclitaxel derivative Abraxane (Abraxis), which has increased intrinsic solubility compared to paclitaxel. This has avoided the requirement for cremophor and has dramatically decreases the time required for drug administration from 3 h to 30 min (Gradishar et al., 2005).

Epothilones Epothilone A and B are 16-membered macrolides which were first isolated by Höfle and coworkers from soil myxobacterium *Sorangium cellulosum* (Höfle et al., 1996). It was reported that epothilones and paclitaxel have some similarity in binding site and the mechanism of action. Molecular modeling studies reviled that paclitaxel and epothilone B share a common pharmacophore for tubulin binding (Petrylak et al., 2004) and epothilones also produce cell-cycle arrest at the G2-M transition similar to that of paclitaxel (Bollag et al., 1995; Kowalski et al., 1997a). Beside these similarities, epothilone showed lesser neurotoxicity compared to that of taxale (Rubin et al., 2001).

Taccalonolides The taccalonolides are novel class of microtubule stabilizers obtained from natural sources (Tinley et al., 2003). Taccalonolide was isolated from *Tacca plantaginea.* Taccalonolide A was first isolated by Chen et al. (1987). While Taccalonolide E and F were isolated by Shen et al. (1991).

Laulimalide Laulimalide (fijianolide) is a polyketide obtained from marine source. It stabilizes microtubule by binding to a novel microtubule-binding site on tubulin. It was found to synergies the activity of taxanes (Hamel et al., 2006) (Fig. 24.7).

Peloruside A Peloruside A was first isolated from *Mycale hentscheli*, a marine sponge. Peloruside A is a macrolide which is now chemically

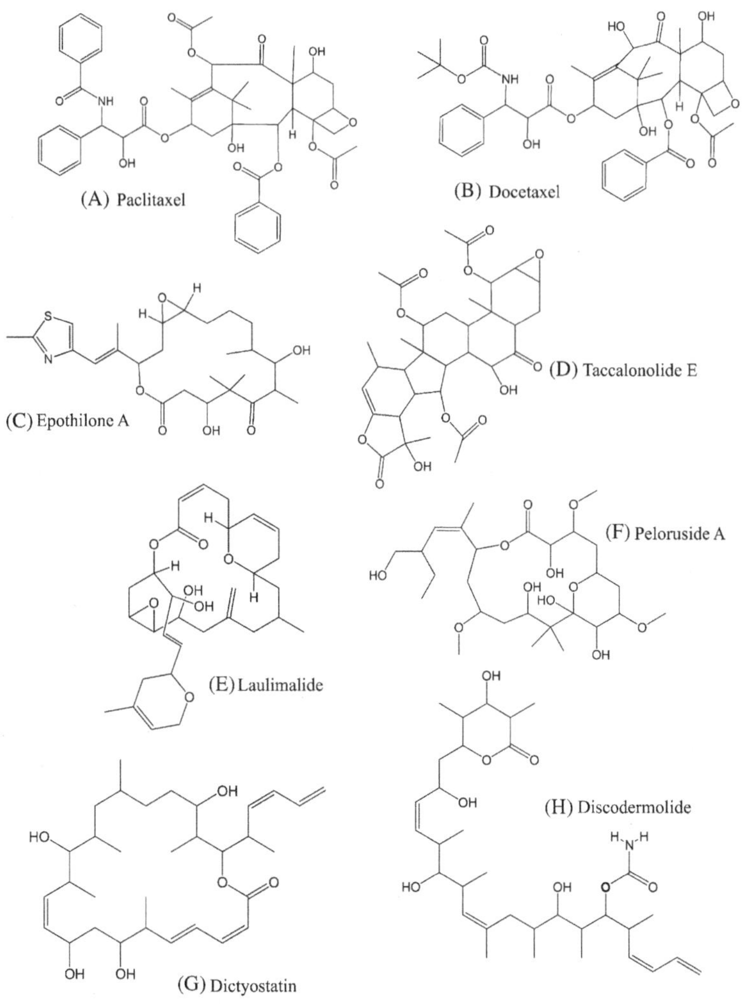

■ **FIGURE 24.7** Taxane domain–binding agents.

synthesized (Evans et al., 2009). This compound has potent microtubule-stabilizing activity and similar to that of epothilones, it induces G2-M cell-cycle arrest in cancer (Hood et al., 2002).

Discodermolide Discodermolide was first isolated Gunasekera and coworkers (1990) from the marine sponge *Discodermia dissoluta.* Discodermolide potentially acts as microtubule stabilizer by binding at taxane site with high affinity. It competitively inhibits the binding of the taxanes (Kowalski et al., 1997b).

Dictyostatin Dictyostatin was first isolated by Pettit from a deep-sea sponge in 1994 (Pettit et al., 1994). It is a 22-membered macrolide having microtubule-stabilizing potential (Isbrucker et al., 2003).

SUMMARY

Compounds obtained from natural sources have served as important leads for development of more potent, semisynthetic and synthetic drugs which are now being used widely for treatment of cancer. There is a large diversity of plants on the planet which is a hidden treasure for such compounds and researchers are trying to find them. Researchers are now equipped with highly developed and sophisticated techniques which have made them possible to scan a large library of compounds within short span. Manipulating the structures of mother compounds to increase their potency and resolve the problems like low solubility, high toxicity and resistance is now a well-established approach for discovery of anticancer drugs. Many of these compounds are now being screened for their anticancer activity and are in preclinical or clinical phase of study. In future, we can expect a magic drug which may have a wide range of activity with increased potency and least toxicity and is originated from a natural compound.

REFERENCES

Andru, J.M., Bordas, J., Diaz, J.F., Garcia de Ancos, J., Gil, R., Medrano, F.J., et al., 1992. Low resolution structure of microtubules in solution. Synchrotron X-ray scattering and electron microscopy of taxol-induced microtubules assembled from purified tubulin in comparison with glycerol and MAP-induced microtubules. J. Mol. Biol. 226 (1), 169–184.

Bai, R., Durso, N.A., Sackett, D.L., Hamel, E., 1999. Interactions of the sponge-derived antimitotic tripeptide hemiasterlin with tubulin: comparison with dolastatin 10 and cryptophycin 1. Biochemistry 38, 14302–14310.

Bai, R.B., Pettit, G.R., Hamel, E., 1990. Binding of dolastatin 10 to tubulin at a distinct site for peptide antimitotic agents near the exchangeable nucleotide and Vinca alkaloid sites. J. Biol. Chem. 265, 17141–17149.

Bazaa, A., Pasquier, E., Defilles, C., Limam, I., Kessentini-Zouari, R., Kallech-Ziri, O., et al., 2010. MVL-PLA2, a snake venom phospholipase A2, inhibits angiogenesis through an increase in microtubule dynamics and disorganization of focal adhesions. PLoS One 5 (4), e10124.

Bennouna, J., Delord, J.P., Campone, M., Nguyen, L., 2008. Vinflunine: a new microtubule inhibitor agent. Clin. Cancer Res. 14, 1625–1632.

Beutler, J.A., Cardellina II, J.H., Lin, C.M., Hamel, E., Cragg, G.M., Boyd, M.R., 1993. Centaureidin, a cytotoxic flavone from *Polymnia fruticosa*, inhibits tubulin polymerization. Bioorg. Med. Chem. Lett. 3, 581–584.

Bhattacharyya, B., Panda, D., Gupta, S., Banerjee, M., 2008. Anti-mitotic activity of colchicine and the structural basis for its interaction with tubulin. Med. Res. Rev. 28 (1), 155–183.

Bissery, M.C., Nohynek, G., Sanderink, G.J., Lavelle, F., 1995. Docetaxel (Taxotere): a review of preclinical and clinical experience, part 1—preclincial experience. Anticancer Drugs 6, 339–368.

Bollag, D.M., McQueney, P.A., Zhu, J., Hensens, O., Koupal, L., Liesch, J., et al., 1995. Epothilones, a new class of microtubule-stabilizing agents with a taxol-like mechanism of action. Cancer Res. 55 (11), 2325–2333.

Brossi, A., Yeh, H.J., Chrzanowska, M., Wolff, J., Hamel, E., Lin, C.M., et al., 1988. Colchicine and its analogues: recent findings. Med. Res. Rev. 8 (1), 77–94.

Brouhard, G.J., Rice, L.M., 2014. The contribution of αβ-tubulin curvature to microtubule dynamics. J. Cell Biol. 207 (3), 323–334.

Chen, W., Zhang, D., 2004. Kinetochore fibre dynamics outside the context of the spindle during anaphase. Nat. Cell Biol. 6, 227–231.

Chen, Z.L., Wang, B.D., Chen, M.Q., 1987. Steroidal bitter principles from *Tacca plantaginea*. Structures of taccalonolide A and B. Tetrahedron Lett. 28, 1673–1678.

Dabydeen, D.A., Burnett, J.C., Bai, R., Verdier-Pinard, P., Hickford, S.J., Pettit, G.R., et al., 2006. Comparison of the activities of the truncated halichondrin B analog NSC 707389 (E7389) with those of the parent compound and a proposed binding site on tubulin. Mol. Pharmacol. 70 (6), 1866–1875.

Dalyot-Herman, N., Delgado-Lopez, F., Gewirtz, D.A., Gupton, J.T., Schwartz, E.L., 2009. Interference with endothelial cell function by JG-03-14, an agent that binds to the colchicine site on microtubules. Biochem. Pharmacol. 78, 1167–1177.

Evans, D.A., Welch, D.S., Speed, A.W.H., Moniz, G.A., Reichelt, A., Ho, S., 2009. An aldol-based synthesis of (+)-Peloruside A, a potent microtubule stabilizing agent. J. Am. Chem. Soc. 131 (11), 3840–3841.

Gadoni, E., Gabriel, L., Olivero, A., Bocca, C., Miglietta, A., 1995. Antimicrotubular effect of calvatic acid and of some related compounds. Cell Biochem. Funct. 13 (4), 231–238.

Garnham, C.P., Roll-Mecak, A., 2012. The chemical complexity of cellular microtubules: tubulin post-translational modification enzymes and their roles in tuning microtubule functions. Cytoskeleton 69 (7), 442–463.

Gelmon, K.A., 1994. The taxoids: paclitaxel and docetaxel. Lancet 344, 1267–1272.

Gerwick, W.H., Proteau, P.J., Nagle, D.G., Hamel, E., Blokhin, A., Slate, D., 1994. Structure of curacin A, a novel antimitotic, antiproliferative, and brine shrimp toxic natural product from the marine cyanobacterium *Lyngbya majuscula*. J. Org. Chem. 59, 1243–1245.

Gradishar, W.J., Tjulandin, S., Davidson, N., Shaw, H., Desai, N., Bhar, P., et al., 2005. Phase III trial of nanoparticle albumin-bound paclitaxel compared with polyethylated castor oil-based paclitaxel in women with breast cancer. J. Clin. Oncol. 23 (31), 7794–7803.

Gunasekera, S.P., Gunasekera, M., Longley, R.E., Schulte, G.K., 1990. Discodermolide: a new bioactive polyhydroxylated lactone from the marine sponge *Discodermia dissolute*. J. Org. Chem. 55 (16), 4912–4915.

Hamel, E., Day, B.W., Miller, J.H., Jung, M.K., Northcote, P.T., Ghosh, A.K., et al., 2006. Synergistic effects of peloruside A and laulimalide with taxoid site drugs, but not with each other, on tubulin assembly. Mol. Pharmacol. 70 (5), 1555–1564.

Hastie, S.B., 1991. Interactions of colchicine with tubulin. Pharmacol. Ther. 512, 377–401.

Hendriks, H.R., Plowman, J., Berger, D.P., Paull, K.D., Fiebig, H.H., Fodstad, O., et al., 1992. Preclinical antitumour activity and animal toxicology studies of rhizoxin, a novel tubulin-interacting agent. Ann. Oncol. 3 (9), 755–763.

Himes, R.H., Himes, V.B., 1980. Inhibition of tubulin assembly by ethylacetylacrylate, a sulfhydryl reagent and potential analog of cytochalasin A. Biochim. Biophys. Acta 621 (2), 338–342.

Höfle, G., Bedorf, N., Steinmetz, H., Schomburg, D., Gerth, K., Hans, H., 1996. Reichenbach Epothilone A and B—novel 16-membered macrolides with cytotoxic activity: isolation, crystal structure, and conformation in solution. Angew. Chem. Int. Ed. Engl. 35 (13/14), 1567–1569.

Hood, K.A., West, L.M., Rouwe, B., Northcote, P.T., Berridge, M.V., Wakefield, S.J., et al., 2002. A novel antimitotic agent with paclitaxel-like microtubule-stabilizing activity. Cancer Res. 62 (12), 3356–3360.

Isbrucker, R.A., Cummins, J., Pomponi, S.A., Longley, R.E., Wright, A.E., 2003. Tubulin polymerizing activity of dictyostatin-1, a polyketide of marine sponge origin. Biochem. Pharmacol. 66 (1), 75–82.

Ishikawa, H., Colby, D.A., Seto, S., Va, P., Tam, A., Kakei, H., et al., 2009. Total synthesis of vinblastine, vincristine, related natural products, and key structural analogues. Am. Chem. Soc. 131 (13), 4904–4916.

Janika, M.E., Bane, S.L., 2002. Synthesis and antimicrotubule activity of combretatropone derivatives. Bioorg. Med. Chem. 10, 1895–1903.

Jordan, M.A., Wilson, L., 2004. Microtubules as a target for anticancer drugs. Nat. Rev. Cancer 4, 253–265.

Jordan, M.A., Kamath, K., 2007. How do microtubule-targeted drugs work? An overview. Curr. Cancer Drug Targets 7 (8), 730–742.

Kamath, K., Okouneva, T., Larson, G., Panda, D., Wilson, L., Jordan, M.A., 2006. 2-Methoxyestradiol suppresses microtubule dynamics and arrests mitosis without depolymerizing microtubules. Mol. Cancer Ther. 5 (9), 2225–2233.

Kaplan, S., Hanauske, A.R., Pavlidis, N., Bruntsch, U., te Velde, A., Wanders, J., et al., 1996. Single agent activity of rhizoxin in non-small-cell lung cancer: a phase II trial of the EORTC Early Clinical Trials Group. Br. J. Cancer 73 (3), 403–405.

Kelling, J., Sullivan, K., Wilson, L., Jordan, M.A., 2003. Suppression of centromere dynamics by Taxol in living osteosarcoma cells. Cancer Res. 63 (11), 2794–2801.

Kowalski, R.J., Giannakakou, P., Hamel, E., 1997a. Activities of the microtubule-stabilizing agents epothilones A and B with purified tubulin and in cells resistant to paclitaxel (Taxol(R)). J. Biol. Chem. 272 (4), 2534–2541.

Kowalski, R.J., Giannakakou, P., Gunasekera, S.P., Longley, R.E., Day, B.W., Hamel, E., 1997b. The microtubule-stabilizing agent discodermolide competitively inhibits the binding of paclitaxel (Taxol) to tubulin polymers, enhances tubulin nucleation reactions more potently than paclitaxel, and inhibits the growth of paclitaxel-resistant cells. Mol. Pharmacol. 52 (4), 613–622.

Krauhs, E., Little, M., Kempf, T., Hofer-Warbinek, R., Ade, W., Ponstingl, H., 1981. Complete amino acid sequence of beta-tubulin from porcine brain. Proc. Natl. Acad. Sci. 78 (7), 4156–4160.

Kueh, H.Y., Timothy, J., Mitchison, T.J., 2009. Structural plasticity in actin and tubulin polymer dynamics. Science 325 (5943), 960–963.

Lin, C.M., Ho, H.H., Pettit, G.R., Hamel, E., 1989. Antimitotic natural products combretastatin A-4 and combretastatin A-2: studies on the mechanism of their inhibition of the binding of colchicine to tubulin. Biochemistry 28, 6984–6991.

Lobert, S., Puozzo, C., 2008. Pharmacokinetics, metabolites, and preclinical safety of vinflunine. Semin. Oncol. 35 (3), S28–S33.

Loganzo, F., Discafani, C.M., Annable, T., Beyer, C., Musto, S., Hari, M., et al., 2003. HTI-286, a synthetic analogue of the tripeptide hemiasterlin, is a potent antimicrotubule agent that circumvents P-glycoprotein-mediated resistance in vitro and in vivo. Cancer Res. 63 (8), 1838–1845.

Lu, Y., Chen, J., Xiao, M., Li, W., Miller, D.D., 2012. An overview of tubulin inhibitors that interact with the colchicine binding site. Pharm. Res. 29 (11), 2943–2971.

Margolis, R.L., Wilson, L., 1978. Opposite end assembly and disassembly of microtubules at steady state in vitro. Cell 13, 1–8.

Markman, M., 2003. Managing taxane toxicities. Support Care Cancer 11, 144–147.

Matov, A., Applegate, K., Kumar, P., Thoma, C., Krek, W., Danuser, G., et al., 2010. Analysis of microtubule dynamic instability using a plus-end growth marker. Nat. Methods 7 (9), 761–768.

Mondal, S., Bandyopadhyay, S., Ghosh, M.K., Mukhopadhyay, S., Roy, S., Mandal, C., 2012. Natural products: promising resources for cancer drug discovery. Anticancer Agents Med. Chem. 12 (1), 49–75.

Na, G.C., Timasheff, S.N., 1980. Thermodynamic linkage between tubulin self-association and the binding of vinblastine. Biochemistry 19, 1347–1354.

Nagle, A., Hur, W., Gray, N.S., 2006. Antimitotic agents of natural origin. Curr. Drug Targets 7 (3), 305–326.

Nogales, E., 2001. Structural insights into microtubule function. Annu. Rev. Biophys. Biomol. Struct. 30, 397–420.

Okouneva, T., Hill, B.T., Wilson, L., Jordan, M.A., 2003. The effects of vinflunine, vinorelbine, and vinblastine on centromere dynamics. Mol. Cancer Ther. 2 (5), 427–436.

Perez, E.A., 2009. Microtubule inhibitors: differentiating tubulin-inhibiting agents based on mechanisms of action, clinical activity, and resistance. Mol. Cancer Ther. 8 (8), 2086–2095.

Petrylak, D.P., Tangen, C.M., Hussain, M.H., Lara Jr., P.N., Jones, J.A., Taplin, M.E., et al., 2004. Docetaxel and estramustine compared with mitoxantrone and prednisone for advanced refractory prostate cancer. N. Engl. J. Med. 351 (15), 1513–1520.

Pettit, G.R., Singh, S.B., Hamel, E., Lin, C.M., Alberts, D.S., Garcia-Kendall, D., 1989. Isolation and structure of the strong cell growth and tubulin inhibitor combretastatin A-4. Experientia 45 (2), 209–211.

Pettit, G.R., Cichacz, Z.A., Gao, F., Boyd, M.R., Schmidt, J.M., 1994. Isolation and structure of the cancer cell growth inhibitor dictyostatin 1. J. Chem. Soc. Chem. Commun. 9, 1111–1112.

Preciado Lopez, M., Huber, F., Grigoriev, I., Steinmetz, M.O., Akhmanova, A., Koenderink, G.H., et al., 2014. Actin-microtubule coordination at growing microtubule ends. Nat. Commun. 5, 47–78.

Rao, S., Chakravarty, S., Ojima, I., Orr, G.A., Horwitz, S.B., 1999. Characterization of the Taxol binding site on the microtubule. Identification of Arg(282) in beta-tubulin as the site of photoincorporation of a 7-benzophenone analogue of Taxol. J. Biol. Chem. 274 (53), 37990–37994.

Risinger, A.L., Giles, F.J., Mooberry, S.L., 2009. Microtubule dynamics as a target in oncology. Cancer Treat. Rev. 35 (3), 255–261.

Rubin, E.H., Siu, L.L., Beers, S., Moore, M.J., Thompson, C., 2001. A phase I and pharmacologic trial of weekly epothilone B in patients with advanced malignancies. Proc. Am. Soc. Clin. Oncol. 20, 270.

Shen, J., Chen, Z., Gao, Y., 1991. The pentacyclic steroidal constituents of *Tacca plantaginea*: taccalonolide E and F. Chin. J. Chem. 9, 92–94.

Smith, C.D., Zhang, X., 1996. Mechanism of action cryptophycin. Interaction with the vinca alkaloid domain of tubulin. J. Biol. Chem. 271 (11), 6192–6198.

Smith, C.D., Zhang, X., Mooberry, S.L., Patterson, G.M., Moore, R.E., 1994. Cryptophycin: a new antimicrotubule agent active against drug-resistant cells. Cancer Res. 54 (14), 3779–3784.

Stewart, B.W., Wild, C.P., 2014. World Cancer Report. International Agency for Research on Cancer, Lyon, France.

Takahashi, M., Iwasaki, S., Kobayashi, H., Okuda, S., Murai, T., Sato, Y., et al., 1987a. Studies on macrocyclic lactone antibiotics. XI. Anti-mitotic and anti-tubulin activity of new antitumor antibiotics, rhizoxin and its homologues. J. Antibiot. 40 (1), 66–72.

Takahashi, M., Iwasaki, S., Kobayashi, H., Okuda, S., Murai, T., Sato, Y., 1987b. Rhizoxin binding to tubulin at the maytansine-binding site. Biochim. Biophys. Acta 926, 215–223.

Tinley, T.L., Randall-Klubek, D.A., Leal, R.M., Jackson, E.M., Cessac, J.W., Quada, J.C., et al., 2003. Taccalonolides E and A: plant-derived steroids with microtubule-stabilizing activity. Cancer Res. 63, 3211–3220.

Uckun, F.M., Mao, C., Jan, S.T., Huang, H., Vassilev, A.O., Navara, C.S., et al., 2001. Spongistatins as tubulin targeting agents. Curr. Pharm. Des. 7 (13), 1291–1296.

Umezawa, H., Takeuchi, T., Iinuma, H., Ito, M., Ishizuka, M., 1975. A new antibiotic, calvatic acid. J. Antibiot. 28 (1), 87–90.

Wani, M.C., Taylor, H.L., Wall, M.E., Coggon, P., McPhail, A.T., 1971. Plant antitumor agents. VI. The isolation and structure of taxol, a novel antileukemic and antitumor agent from Taxus brevifolia. J. Am. Chem. Soc. 93 (9), 2325–2327.

Wilson, L., Jordan, M.A., 1995. Microtubule dynamics: taking aim at a moving target. Chem. Biol. 2 (9), 569–573.

Wilson, L., Jordan, M.A., Morse, A., Margolis, R.L., 1982. Interaction of vinblastine with steady-state microtubules in vitro. J. Mol. Biol. 159, 129–149.

Wipf, P., Reeves, J.T., Day, B.W., 2004. Chemistry and biology of curacin A. Curr. Pharm. Des. 10 (12), 1417–1437.

Xu, Q., Huang, K.C., Tendyke, K., Marsh, J., Liu, J., Qiu, D., et al., 2011. In vitro and in vivo anticancer activity of (+)-spongistatin 1. Anticancer Res. 31 (9), 2773–2779.

Yvon, A.M., Wadsworth, P., Jordan, M.A., 1999. Taxol suppresses dynamics of individual microtubules in living human tumor cells. Mol. Biol. Cell 10, 947–949.

Chapter 25

Medicinal and nutritional qualities of *Zingiber officinale*

Saima Khan, Pankaj Pandotra, Asif Khurshid Qazi, Sajad A Lone, Malik Muzafar, Ajai P Gupta and Suphla Gupta
CSIR-Indian Institute of Integrative Medicine, Jammu, India

CHAPTER OUTLINE

INTRODUCTION

The word "nutraceuticals" was coined by Stephan L. De Felice for the bioactive compounds that are found in foods, dietary supplements, and herbal products having health benefits. The word encompasses nutrition and pharmaceutical properties of the plant/molecule. Therefore, nutraceuticals are those molecules/plants which have health-promoting, disease-preventing medicinal properties. They are accredited to improve health, delay

Fruits, Vegetables, and Herbs.
DOI: http://dx.doi.org/10.1016/B978-0-12-802972-5.00025-1

age progression, prevent persistent diseases, and increase life expectancy by supporting the structure or function of the body. However, they differ from pharmaceutics in having a natural origin. Nowadays, considerable interest is being generated in nutraceuticals because of their potential nutritional, safety, and therapeutic effects with no/less side effects, as compared to modern system of medicine. Traditional systems of medicine of several Asian countries have been using plant as a source of medicines for general well-beings (Afzal et al., 2001). Not only whole plant but plant-derived bioactives including phytoestrogens, terpenoids, carotenoids, limonoids, phytosterols, glucosinolates, polyphenols, flavonoids, isoflavonoids, and anthocyanidins are also being used as nutraceuticals (Gupta and Sharma, 2014). Modern science has demonstrated that these phytochemicals/extracts have a specific pharmacological role in promoting human health. It could be as antiinflammatory, antiallergic, antioxidants, antibacterial, antifungal, antispasmodic role, or they may have chemopreventive, hepatoprotective, hypolipidemic, neuroprotective, hypotensive, and antiaging properties (Afzal et al., 2001). Literature cites several examples of plants having antidiabetic, antiosteoporotic, anticancer, and apoptosis-inducing properties (Gupta and Sharma, 2014). In the present chapter, we extend our focus to highlight the medicinal and nutritional qualities of *Zingiber officinale* (ginger) in the prevention and treatment of diseases. Ginger has a distinction of being among those few herbs that are used as food, culinary, and also as medicine (Badreldin et al., 2008). According to USFDA, it is categorized as GRAS (generally regarded as safe). Ginger is among the 20 top selling herbal supplements in the United States. Its retail sales in mainstream US market (including food stores, drug stores, and mass market retail sales) in 2001 amounted to US$1.2 million. In Germany, ginger products are marketed for the treatment of dyspepsia and prophylaxis of motion sickness. Today, pharmacopoeias of a number of different countries list ginger extract for various diseases (World Health Organization (WHO), 2000a). This chapter also underlines the related pharmacological research to give an insight of the scientific background to the traditional medicinal applications.

Ginger (*Z. officinale* Rosc.), a member of Zingiberaceae family, is grown in tropical and subtropical regions for spice and medicinal purposes, since decades. With 53 genera and over 1200 species, the Zingiberaceae is the largest of the eight families of the order (Kress, 1990). It is a member of a plant family that includes highly valued premium spices like cardamom and turmeric. The plant has long history of cultivation in the Asian subcontinent, probably originating from South East Asia (Ravindran and Nirmal, 2005) It is cultivated on a large scale in India, China, Bangladesh, Taiwan, Jamaica, and Nigeria from where it is exported to other countries of the world (Dedov et al., 2002). The plant is cultivated throughout the humid tropics, with India being the largest producer (Pandotra et al., 2013). Indians and Chinese are believed to have produced ginger as a tonic root for over 5000 years to treat several ailments. Ginger was an important article of trade and was exported from India to the Roman Empire over 2000 years ago, where it was especially valued for its medicinal properties. Ginger continued to be a highly sought after commodity in Europe even after the fall of the Roman Empire, with Arab merchants controlling the trade in ginger and other spices for centuries. In the 13th and 14th centuries, the value of a pound of ginger was equivalent to the cost of a sheep (Ravindran and Nirmal, 2005). By medieval times, it was being imported in preserved form to be used in sweets. The importance of ginger can be summarized in the invention of the "gingerbread man" by Queen Elizabeth I of England, which became a popular Christmas treat.

Morphologically, ginger plant has a perennial, tuberous root, or rhizome having erect annual stem invested by smooth sheaths of leaves, 2–3 ft in height. The rhizome, which is the horizontal stem from which the roots grow, is the main portion of ginger that is consumed as a spice in dried, preserved, and green forms (Pandotra et al., 2013). Dried-ginger-derived products (oil and oleoresins) are used in nutraceuticals and pharmaceuticals and are valued more in international trade than either of the other two forms. Its spicy aroma is mainly due to presence of ketones, especially the gingerols, which appear to be the primary component of ginger studied in much of the health-related scientific research. It is widely used as flavoring agent in great variety of food preparations. The roots contain polyphenolic compounds (gingerol homologs and shogaols), which have a high antioxidant activity (Bartley and Jacobs, 2000). In addition, ginger is also reported as detoxifying agent against alcohol abuse (Stoilova et al., 2007) and bromobenzene intoxication. The rhizome is also known to have antidiabetic, antihyperlipidemic, and hepatic anticancer effects (Hamed et al., 2012; Bordia et al., 1997; Akimoto et al., 2015).

GINGER IN TRADITIONAL USE

Ginger is an important plant with several medicinal, ethnomedicinal, and nutritional attributes. Traditionally, in Indian, Chinese, and Tibetan system of medicines, ginger is being used since ancient times, for the treatment of catarrh, rheumatism, nervous diseases, gingivitis, toothache, asthma, stroke, constipation, diabetes, cough and cold, motion sickness, menstrual cramps, cancer, and many more (Shukla and Singh, 2007). In *Ayurveda*, ginger is called "*maha aushadhi*," meaning the "great medicine" and recommended for use as carminative, diaphoretic, expectorant, peripheral circulatory stimulant, astringent, appetite stimulant, and diuretic and digestive aid (Ghosh et al., 2011). Studies have shown that ginger induces increase in the pancreatic and intestine lipase, when given in animal diets (Patel and Srinivasan, 2000). Some active components of ginger have been reported to increase the muscular activity of the digestive tract, thereby stimulating digestion, absorption, and relieving constipation and flatulence (Wu et al., 1990, 2008). It has been observed that ginger and its metabolites accumulate in the gastrointestinal tract; therefore, many of its effects are manifested in the gastrointestinal areas.

Compositional analysis has revealed the presence of carbohydrates, fats, vitamins, minerals, and extractable oleoresins (Shukla and Singh, 2007). Ginger contains 9% of lipids or glycolipids and 5–8% of oleoresin (Chrubasik et al., 2005). Literature survey divulged that, as seen in several medicinal herbs, most of the information on uses of ginger has been handed down by word of mouth with little demonstrable scientific evidence to support the numerous claims. However, in the last few years, more organized scientific investigations have focused on the mechanisms and targets of ginger and its various components. To comprehend the evident medicinal and nutritional qualities of ginger rhizome, understanding of the underlying scientific mechanism will provide a better insight of its qualities. Here, we will be discussing few of them in the later part of the chapter.

Essential oil

The aroma and flavor of ginger are determined by the composition of its steam volatile essential oil (1–2.5%), which is primarily comprised of monoterpene hydrocarbons, oxygenated monoterpenes, and sesquiterpene hydrocarbons. The major essential oil components are zingiberene (30–70%), β-sesquiphellandrene (15–20%), β-bisabolene (10–15%), and α-farmesene (Govindarajan, 1982). However, camphene, β-phellandrene, curcumene, geranyl acetate, borneol, geraniol, limonene, and linalool were also found in appreciable quantity (Gupta et al., 2011). Many of these volatile oil constituents contribute to the distinct aroma and taste of ginger. Both oil and oleoresins are used in many food items, soft drinks, beverages, pickles, and many types of medicinal preparations (Gurdip et al., 2008). Experiments have shown that ginger essential oil enhanced improvement in humoral immune response in immune suppressed mice (Carrasco et al., 2009).

NUTRIENT COMPOSITION

Ginger rhizome is a rich source of minerals like, iron, calcium, phosphorous, and vitamins such as thiamine, riboflavin, niacin, and vitamin C. Not only the rhizome-derived components, but the powdered rhizome also has nutritional components like fatty oil (3–6%), protein (9%), carbohydrates (60–70%), crude fiber (3–8%), and about 8% ash. Ginger rhizomes also contain a potent proteolytic enzyme called zingibain. Their composition varies with the type, variety, agronomic conditions, curing methods, and drying and storage conditions (Agrahari, 2015). Vitamin C and total carotenoids content were found to be 10.97 and 92.96mg per 100g, respectively, in ginger rhizome. Jeevani Osadee Wijekoon et al. (2011) evaluated the nutritional quality of torch ginger (*Etlingera elatior* Jack.) inflorescence and found the presence of high amounts of dietary fiber, unsaturated fatty acids (palmitoleic acid, linoleic acid, and oleic acid), and essential amino acids (leucine and lysine) (Jeevani Osadee Wijekoon et al., 2011). The study revealed that inflorescence of torch ginger is a rich source of essential minerals such as K (1589mg/100g), Ca (775mg/100g), Mg (327mg/100g), P (286mg/100g), and S (167mg/100g) with lower levels of heavy metal contaminants (Cd, As, Pb, Hg, Ni). This was also corroborated by Pandotra et al. (2015) in ginger germplasm, collected from north western Himalayan India (World Health Organization (WHO), 2000a). In this study, the ionome of the ginger rhizome suggested raw ginger to be a good source of beneficial elements/minerals like Mg, Ca, Mn, Fe, Cu, and Zn (Gupta et al., 2010). Evaluation of Malaysian ginger rhizome and ginger sourced from Nigeria revealed higher moisture (90.9% vs 76.9%), crude fiber (3.8g/100g), and lower carbohydrate content (6.3g/100g sample) than the USDA database (USDA Nutrient Database, 2013). An inductively coupled plasma-mass spectrometry based multielemental profiling to assess the quantitative complement of elements and nutritional quality in ginger rhizome showed abundance of 18 elements quantified (Gupta et al., 2010). The acid digested rhizomes was having K > Mg > Fe > Ca > Na > Mn > Zn > Ba > Cu > Cr > Ni > Pb > Co > Se > As > Be > Cd metals in that order of abundance. Chemometric of the data showed positive correlation among most of the elements. It is generally believed that paradol, formed on hydrogenation of shogoal, in ginger plant possess considerable antioxidant content which produces protective health benefits in various diseases (Badreldin et al., 2008).

BIOACTIVE COMPONENTS OF GINGER

Gingerol homologues

At least 115 constituents in fresh and dried ginger varieties have been identified by a variety of analytical processes. Chemical profiling of the methanolic crude extracts of fresh ginger rhizome has revealed at least 31 gingerol-related compounds (Jiang et al., 2005); homologs were found to be the major constituents (%) present in the solvent extract of ginger rhizome and attribute pungency to the rhizome. The concentrations of gingerols were found to be reduced in dried ginger, whereas the concentrations of shogaols, which are the major gingerol dehydration products, are more abundant (Jolad et al., 2004) in dried ginger. Ginger homologs are the biologically active pungent principles of ginger that significantly contributes toward medicinal applications of ginger (Sanwal et al., 2010). Ginger has been fractionated into at least 14 bioactive compounds, including [4]-gingerol, [6]-gingerol, [8]-gingerol, [10]-gingerol, [6]-paradol, [14]-shogaol, [6]-shogaol, 1-dehydro-[10]-gingerdione, [10]-gingerdione, hexahydrocurcumin, tetrahydrocurcumin, gingerenone A, 1,7-bis-(4′ hydroxyl-3′ methoxyphenyl)-5-methoxyhepthan-3-one, and methoxy-[10]-gingerol (Koh et al., 2009). Their proportion in the ginger depends on the habitat, processing mechanism, and the harvest stage of the ginger (Singh and Gupta, 2013). Of the four main bioactive pungent components of Jamaican ginger, including [6]-, [8]-, and [10]-gingerols and [6]-shogaol, [6]-gingerol appears to be the most abundant compound, in most of the oleoresin samples studied (Bailey-Shaw et al., 2008). Although phylogenetic analysis has shown that all the *Z. officinale* samples, from widely different geographical origins, are genetically indistinguishable, their metabolic profiling showed quantitative variation. 6-Gingerol has been shown to have a number of pharmacological activities such as antipyretic, antitussive, hypotensive (Suekawa et al., 1986), cardiotonic (Kobayashi et al., 1988), antiplatelet (Guh et al., 1995), neural protectant (Kim et al., 2014), antiinflammatory, analgesic (Lantz et al., 2007), cytotoxic, apoptotic (We et al., 2005), antitumor (Chan et al., 2012), anticancer (Yusof et al., 2008), antioxidant (Masuda et al., 2004), antihepatotoxic (Haniadka et al., 2013), antifungal (Ficker et al., 2003a), vanilloid receptor agonistic (Dedov et al., 2002), cholagogic (Yamahara et al., 1985), and antiemetic activities (Micklefield et al., 1999). Ginger is good for the respiratory system to fight against colds and flu (Langmead and Rampton, 2001). It relieves headaches, pains, and helps to clear sore throats (Gupta and Sharma, 2014). It is very effective as a cleansing agent through the bowels and kidneys and also through the skin (Uz et al., 2009).

It has been observed that consuming ginger regularly leads to decreased pain levels in people suffering from osteoarthritis or rheumatoid arthritis along with improvements in their mobility. The antiinflammatory property of gingerols is thought to have a role in these joint problems (Funk et al., 2009). One of the mechanisms by which ginger exerts its ameliorative effects could be related to inhibition of prostaglandin and leukotriene biosynthesis. Ginger not only stimulates the muscles of the gastric tract, but consumption of ginger is seen to stimulate heart muscles also, resulting in better blood circulation throughout the body and increased cellular metabolic activity. It also helps to reduce blood pressure and cardiac workload (Shoji et al., 1982).

Ginger has been found to be anticarcinogenic mediated by multiple pathways (Yusof et al., 2008; Chen et al., 2007) and reported to have colon cancer chemopreventive activity (Bode, 2003). Gingerols, the active phytonutrients in ginger, kill ovarian cancer cells by inducing apoptosis (programmed cell death) and autophagocytosis (self-digestion) (Rhode et al., 2006). A pro-inflammatory state is considered to be an important contributing factor in the development of ovarian cancer. In the presence of ginger, a number of key indicators of inflammation (vascular endothelial growth factor, interleukin-8 (IL-8), and prostaglandin E2) were found in lesser amount in the ovarian cancer cells (Rhode et al., 2006). It has been observed that the combined treatment with 6-shogaol and tumor necrosis factor (TNF)-related apoptosis-inducing ligand induces apoptosis in various cancer cells like renal carcinoma Caki cells, breast carcinoma MDA-MB-231 cells, and glioma U118MG cells, but not in normal mesangial cells and normal mouse kidney cells. 6-Shogaol also has the capability to reduce the mitochondrial membrane potential and released cytochrome c from mitochondria to cytosol via Bax activation. It is also involved in down-regulation of c-FLIP(L) expression at the posttranslational levels (Qazi et al., 2014). Gingerol also inhibited the growth of human colorectal cancer cells (Bode, 2003). The efficacy of ginger in mice was found to be significant in both cases, when the mice were fed with ginger before and after tumor cells were injected. The effects of chronic treatment with hot water extract of ginger rhizome on spontaneous mammary tumorigenesis in mice demonstrated that when mice had ginger extract (0.125%) in drinking water, the development of mammary tumors was significantly inhibited (Rhode et al., 2006). Tumor development and progressions are multistep processes incorporating genetic and metabolic changes (Qazi et al., 2014). The extract of ginger (*Z. officinale* Rosc.) and its major pungent components, that is 6-shogaol and 6-gingerol, have shown antiproliferative effect on several tumor cell lines in vitro. Moreover, a cytotoxic or cytostatic effect, mediated by apoptosis, was found for 6-gingerol and 6-paradol in human promyelocytic leukemia HL-60 cells (Lee and Surh, 1998), and also for four diarylheptanoids and two shogaols (We et al., 2005). On the basis of molecular target-based virtual screening of phytochemicals, several ingredients of ginger, including 6-shogaol, 6-paradol, and 6-gingerol, have been found as potential candidates for the prevention and therapy of nonsmall cell lung carcinoma (NSCLC).

Among the above mentioned compounds, 6 gingerols were found to be most effective in suppressing the proliferation of NSCLC cells (Yusof et al., 2008). Ginger and its constituents are also effective against pancreatic cancer (Akimoto et al., 2015). Besides, ginger extract inhibited cell proliferation and subsequently induced the autotic death of pancreatic cancer. It has been found that whole ginger extract or its constituents may have clinical implications for therapeutic intervention against pancreatic cancer (Patel and Srinivasan, 2000). Importantly, ginger has attracted attention for the chemoprevention of colorectal cancer. The suppression of tumor growth in colon cancer was found to be linked with the inhibition of leukotriene A4 hydrolase activity. Hexahydrocurcumin extracted from ginger was also found to be cytotoxic to colorectal cancer cells. It has been observed that treatment of SW480 colon cancer cells with hexahydrocurcumin (100 μM) resulted in apoptosis indicating its potential as anticancer agent (Lee and Surh, 1998). Besides ginger rhizome, treatment with ginger leaves induce apoptosis and reduction of cell viability, followed by the increased ATF3 expression via activating ATF3 promoter in human colorectal cancer cells (Park et al., 2014). Furthermore, in vitro studies revealed that ginger components are effective against liver cancer. In a study, 6-shogaol has been reported to induce apoptotic cell death of Mahlavu hepatoma cells via an oxidative stress-mediated caspase-dependent mechanism (Chen et al., 2011). The major components of ginger, 6-shogaol and 6-gingerol, have shown to exert antiinvasive activity against hepatoma cells. In animal model, ginger suppresses ethionine-induced liver carcinogenesis by scavenging the free radical formation and by reducing lipid peroxidation, thus preventing rat hepatocarcinogenesis (Mansour et al., 2010). An ethanolic ginger extract applied topically to mouse skin provided a highly significant protective effect against the development of skin tumors. This was found to be associated with the inhibition of 12-*O*-tetradecanoylphorbol-13-acetate-caused induction of epidermal ornithine decarboxylase, cyclooxygenase (COX), and lipoxygenase activities (Katiyar et al., 1996).

Drug resistance is growing worldwide and it is consider as a main offender in the failure of treatment. The use of antibiotics against microorganism is effective mode of treatment but also causes adverse complications. Consumption of ginger produces heat in body that promotes healthy sweating, which assists detoxification of the body through skin and conferring protection against invading microorganisms. Ginger has been traditionally exploited for having broad range of antimicrobial activity against both gram-positive and gram-negative bacteria and fungi. In vitro studies have shown that active constituents of ginger inhibit multiplication of colon bacteria. These bacteria are responsible for fermentation of undigested carbohydrates causing flatulence which can be counteracted with ginger (Habsah et al., 2000). It inhibits the growth of *Escherichia coli*, *Proteus* sp., *Staphylococci*, *Streptococci*, and *Salmonella* (Azu and Onyeagba, 2007). Earlier investigators have shown that ginger and its constituents play a vital role in the prevention of microbial growth or act as antimicrobial agents (Kumar et al., 2011). Ginger rhizome contains several constituents which have antibacterial and antifungal effects. The gingerol and shogaol are identified as more active agents (Atai et al., 2009). 10-Gingerol from Ginger extracts has demonstrated antimicrobial activity against a wide range of pathogenic microorganisms including gram-positive and gram-negative bacteria and the yeast *Candida albicans* (Chairgulprasert et al., 2005). Of particular interest is an in vitro study showing that a crude methanolic extract (minimum inhibitory concentration (MIC) 6–50 μg/mL) and a gingerol-containing fraction significantly inhibited the growth of 19 strains of *Helicobacter pylori*, the microorganism associated with peptic ulcer disease as well as gastric and colon cancers (Mahady et al., 2003). Various studies demonstrating time-dependent anthelmintic activity of crude powder and crude aqueous extract of dried ginger (1–3 g/kg) in sheep naturally infected with mixed species of gastrointestinal nematodes are reported (Iqbal et al., 2006). Ginger inhibits *Aspergillus* sp., a fungus known for the production of carcinogenic aflatoxin (Ficker et al., 2003a). Study on ginger rhizome afforded three lipophilic analogues: 6-gingerol, 8-gingerol, and 10-gingerol that exhibited antimicrobial activity (Ficker et al., 2003a). The lipophilic analogues (8-gingerol and 10-gingerol) were more active, with MIC values of 25–50 μg/mL exhibiting toward *Mycobacterium tuberculosis* H37Rv and *Mycobacterium avium*. Besides, 6-gingerol and 12-gingerol, isolated from ginger rhizome, showed antibacterial activity against periodontal bacteria (Miri et al., 2008). Thus, ginger which is a normal ingredient of our routine food preparations can provide protection against our natural enemies like bacterial and fungal pathogens.

Limited studies have observed the possible immunomodulatory action of ginger. Experiments have shown that mice fed a 50% ethanolic ginger extract (25 mg/kg) for 7 days had higher hemagglutinating antibody titer and plaque-forming cell counts and improved humoral immunity (Puri et al., 2000). In vitro study found that ginger suppressed lymphocyte proliferation mediated by decreased IL-2 and IL-10 production (Wilasrusmee et al., 2002) and aqueous ginger extract significantly increased the production of IL-1β, IL-6, and TNF-α in activated peritoneal mouse macrophages (Ryu and Kim, 2004). Aqueous ginger extract also stimulated splenocyte proliferation and cytokine production in a concentration-dependent manner in mice. Recently, study has shown the immunomodulatory effects of zerumbone on antigen-presenting dendritic cells in vitro and antiallergic effect via modulation of Th1/Th2 cytokines in an asthmatic mouse model (Shieh et al., 2015).

ANALGESIC EFFECT

Various studies have assessed for the analgesic effect of ginger and its constituents. It has a vigorous analgesic action and act by COX-1 inhibition. Gingerol and its derivatives, particularly 8-paradol, have been reported to be more effective antiplatelet and COX-1 inhibitors than aspirin (Nurtjahja-Tjendraputra et al., 2003). Inhibition of the arachidonic acid (AA) metabolism cascade via the COX-1/thromboxane synthase system by these phenolic compounds may highlight the mechanism of their action for peripheral and possible antiinflammatory action. Besides, 6-shogaol inhibits the release of substance P by stimulation of the primary afferents from their central terminal and hence shares this site of action with capsaicin (Onogi et al., 1992) while gingerols act as vanilloid receptor (VR1) agonists (Dedov et al., 2002). The VR1 has been shown to integrate chemical and thermal nociceptive stimuli (Ma and Quirion, 2007). This finding bears significance as direct activation or deactivation of the VR1 at the painful site recommends a new strategy for the development of a new class of peripheral analgesics devoid of the well-characterized side effects of currently available analgesics and antiinflammatory drugs.

The polyphenols present in ginger roots extracts contain compounds which possess high antioxidant activity. The antioxidants inhibit the reactive oxygen species, which are capable of causing damage to DNA, coronary heart disease, and many other health problems related to advancing age (Patel and Srinivasan, 2000). Antioxidant compounds are commonly used to counter the free-radical-mediated oxidative stress in the cell. The free radical assembly is stabilized by the antioxidative defense system of our body (Shyur et al., 2005). [6]-Gingerol is recognized as a strong antioxidant component comparable with its antiinflammatory and antiapoptotic action both in vivo and in vitro studies (Kim et al., 2007) Experiment performed on rats indicated extracts of red and white ginger protect the brain through their antioxidant activity, Fe^{2+} chelating and OH*- scavenging ability and prevents oxidative stress (Oboh et al., 2012a). Ginger provides number of antioxidants helping in the reduction of the lipid oxidation and inhibiting the pathogenesis of diseases. The polyphenolic compounds show high antioxidant activity due to the presence of secondary metabolites that includes flavones, flavonoids, coumarin, lignans, isoflavones, anthocyanin, catechins, and isocatechins (El-Ghorab et al., 2010). Experimentally, the total phenolic content in the alcoholic extract of the dried rhizome of ginger has been found 870.1 mg/g extract exhibiting 90.1% of 2,2-diphenyl-1-picrylhydrazyl (DPPH) radical scavenging activity with the IC_{50} value of 0.64 μg/mL (Bartley and Jacobs, 2000). Recently, there are growing evidences displaying ginger leaves have higher antioxidant activity than rhizomes and flowers (Eric Chan et al., 2011). The antioxidant property of ginger is an extremely significant activity being used as a preventive agent against a number of diseases. More than 50 compounds with antioxidant activity from ginger rhizome have been identified (Masuda et al., 2004). They belonged to either related to gingerols or diarylheptanoids. Structure–activity relationship studies of the gingerol-like compounds proposed that substitution on and the length of the alkyl chain contribute to the antioxidant activity. A glucoside of 6-gingerdiol has also been reported to exhibit strong antioxidant activity in vitro (Sekiwa et al., 2000). Several in vivo studies have also established the antioxidant activity of ginger on animal models, where lipid peroxidation was significantly lowered in rats fed on ginger (1%). Here, it was observed that the activities of the antioxidant enzymes, that is superoxide dismutase (SOD), catalase (CAT), and glutathione peroxidase were insistent, with significantly increased blood glutathione content. Besides, it was found that rats on a high fat diet complemented with ginger at 35 and 70 mg/kg had lowered levels of tissue thiobarbituric acid reactive substances and hydroperoxides, higher SOD and CAT activities, and raised levels of reduced glutathione in the kidney, intestine, and liver, compared with controls group (Jeyakuma et al., 1999). Also, rats noshed with dried ginger (1%) showed significant attenuated oxidative stress and lipid peroxidation when exposed to the organophosphorous pesticide malathion for 4 weeks (20 ppm) (Ahmed et al., 2000). Furthermore, atherosclerotic, apolipoprotein E-deficient mice fed on ginger extract showed a significant drop in the low-density lipoprotein (LDL) basal oxidative state, with reduced susceptibility to oxidation and aggregation (Fuhrman et al., 2000). Curcumin, another active component present in ginger, was found to be an antioxidant and an antiinflammatory agent and induced heme oxygenase-1 and protect endothelial cells against oxidative stress (Gurdip et al., 2008; Habsah et al., 2000; Kim et al., 2007). Antioxidants act as free radical scavengers and inhibit lipid peroxidation and other free radical–mediated processes; thereby helping to protect the human body from several diseases attributed to the reactions of radicals. Ginger is a good source of antioxidant and most of the antioxidant components exhibit higher activities in alcoholic media (Fuhrman et al., 2000; Ojewole, 2006). Hence, apart from its medicinal properties, ginger can also be used as an antioxidant supplement for preventive agent against a number of diseases.

In traditional system of medicine, ginger has been used for hyperglycemia and dyslipidemia (Bordia et al., 1997; Ojewole, 2006; Mascolo et al., 1989). Modern science has confirmed the role of ginger as antidiabetic (Hamed et al., 2012). Experiments have shown that ginger has the potential protective effect of oxidative damage to pancreatic β cells in rats. Studies have shown that, the long-term dietary intake of ginger has hypoglycemic and hypolipidemic effects (Akhani et al., 2004). Experiments have proved that fresh juice of ginger (4 mL/kg body weight) produced a significant time-dependent decrease in blood glucose level in streptozotocin-induced diabetic rats. The juice of ginger was also reported to control type I diabetes (Srivastava, 1984). Treatment with aqueous extract (500 mg/kg body weight) for a period of 7 weeks significantly decreased the serum glucose, cholesterol, and triacylglycerol levels in the treated diabetic rats compared with the control diabetic rats (Bordia et al., 1997). Reports point to the therapeutic usefulness of ginger extracts also with regard to diabetes and diabetic complications (Lantz et al., 2007; Mascolo et al., 1989). This was confirmed in a pilot study which was done to investigate the protective potential of *ginger* in a model of cytotoxic conditions imposed by diabetes in β cells.

CARDIOVASCULAR EFFECTS

Ginger, in traditional Chinese medicine, is used to monitor the movement of body fluids. It exhibited a dominant stimulatory effect on the heart muscles by diluting blood and thereby exciting blood circulation all over the body (Shoji et al., 1982). Enhanced circulation improved the cellular metabolic activity thereby relieving cramps and tension (Kobayashi et al., 1988). Besides, reports from Japanese group have shown that the blood pressure and cardiac workload could be declined due to certain active constituents in ginger. Additionally, ginger reduced the formation of pro-inflammatory prostaglandins and thromboxane thereby lowering the clotting ability of the blood (Bordia et al., 1997). The inhibition of platelet aggregation by ginger is more than the alike effects studied with garlic and onion (Pancho et al., 1989). One of the most important properties of ginger is that it be capable of averting increased cholesterol levels, following intake of cholesterol-rich diet (Haniadka et al., 2013). The ginger extracts as well as 6- and 8-gingerols have been shown to modulate eicosanoid responses in smooth vascular muscles ex vivo (Suekawa et al., 1986). These analogues were found to inhibit AA-induced serotonin release by human platelets in a dose range similar to the effective dose of aspirin and their aggregation. Importantly, 6-gingerol and 6-shogaol, at the doses of 10–100 μg/kg, not only lowered systemic blood pressure in anesthetized rats but also caused bradycardia when administered intravenously (Gayur and Gilani, 2005). Several evidences, mostly from experiments performed on rats, have suggested that ginger exerts many direct and indirect effects on blood pressure and heart rate (Afzal et al., 2001) showing a dose-dependent (0.3–3 mg/kg) fall in the arterial blood pressure of anesthetized rats. The Ca^{2+} channel-blocking activity of gingerols was found to be similar to the effect of verapamil, indicating that it acts at both the membrane-bound and the intracellular Ca^{2+} channels. Recent study has also confirmed the blood pressure lowering effect of ginger is mediated through blockade of voltage-dependent calcium channels (White, 2007) through a dual inhibitory effect mediated via stimulation of both muscarinic receptors and blockade of Ca^{2+} channels. This group noted that the different constituents of ginger might have opposing actions on the reactivity of blood vessels. For example, an atropine-resistant and L-NAME (NG-nitro-L-arginine methyl ester)-sensitive vasodilator activity was also noted for the ginger phenolic constituents 6-, 8-, and 10-gingerols, while 6-shogaol showed a mild vasodilator effect (Gayur et al., 2005). Experiments have shown inconclusive and contradictory results in anticoagulating potential of ginger. Lumb (1994) and Bordia et al. (1997) found no effect of ginger on platelet count, bleeding time, platelet aggregation, fibrinolytic activity, or fibrinogen levels. Ginger has been shown to inhibit platelet aggregation (Mahady et al., 2003) and to decrease platelet thromboxane production in vitro (Guh et al., 1995). 8-Gingerol, 8-shogaol, 8-paradol, and gingerol analogues exhibited antiplatelet activities (Nurtjahja-Tjendraputra et al., 2003), but Verma et al. (1993) found ginger to decrease platelet aggregation. Similarly, Janssen et al. (1996) showed no effect of oral ginger on platelet thromboxane B2 production, while Srivastava (1989) found thromboxane levels to be decreased by ginger ingestion in a small study. These studies demand a thorough evaluation of activity with respect to anticoagulant effect.

GASTROINTESTINAL EFFECTS

Peptic ulcer is a major health problem worldwide in both males and females having several factors triggering its effect including food ingredients, stress, *H. pylori*, and drugs. In traditional system of medicine, medicinal plants and its constituents have shown antiulcer effect in various ways, but their exact mechanism is not fully understood (Akhani et al., 2004). Ginger and its constituents show a vital role in ulcer prevention via increasing mucin secretion. Earlier findings have shown antiulcerative effects of ginger in experimental gastric ulcer models (Yamahara et al., 1988). Studies have demonstrated 6-gingerol and 6-shogaol suppressed gastric contraction in situ, with 6-shogaol having more intensive effect (Suekawa et al., 1986). It was found that acetone, 50% ethanolic extracts (100–500 mg/kg), and ginger juice (2–4 mL/kg) reversed cisplatin-induced delay in gastric emptying in rats when given orally (Sharma and Gupta, 1998). The effect on gastric motility may be partially explained by the antiemetic properties of ginger. Several experiments on the effect of ginger on gastric motility have supported this observation. Ginger is found to stimulate bile secretion, intestinal lipase, trypsin, chymotrypsin, amylase, sucrase, and maltase activities in rats, with 6- and 10-gingerols being chiefly responsible for this activity (Patel and Srinivasan, 2000). These findings support the traditional use of ginger as a digestive stimulant. Traditionally, ginger is probably best utilized in alleviating symptoms of nausea and vomiting, and several controlled studies have reported that ginger is generally effective as an antiemetic (Quimby, 2007). But its mechanism of action remains uncertain. However, there are several proposed mechanisms. The components in ginger that are responsible for the antiemetic effect are thought to be the gingerols, shogaols, and galanolactone, a diterpenoid of ginger (Mascolo et al., 1989). Animal models and in vitro studies have demonstrated that ginger extract possesses antiserotoninergic and 5-HT3 receptor antagonism effects, which play an important role in postoperative nausea and vomiting (Lumb, 1993). The effectiveness of ginger as an antiemetic has been attributed to its carminative effect, which helps to break up and expel intestinal gas. This idea was supported by the results of a randomized, double-blind trial in which healthy volunteers reported ginger effectively accelerated gastric emptying and stimulated antral contractions (Wu et al., 2008). Contrary to this in another randomized, placebo-controlled, crossover trial of 16 healthy volunteers, ginger (1 g orally) had no effect on gastric emptying (Phillips et al., 1993). However, this is also true that nausea and vomiting during pregnancy affects most pregnant women, and over the years, ginger has been used to alleviate the condition (Tripathi et al., 2007). At least one survey indicated that the overall use of dietary supplements in pregnant women appears to be low, but ginger is commonly recommended and used to prevent nausea (Tsui et al., 2001). Several double-blind, randomized, placebo-controlled clinical trials have indicated that ginger consumption is effective and safe in helping to prevent nausea and vomiting during pregnancy (Willetts et al., 2003; Yamahara et al., 1990).

Ginger may also increase the conversion of cholesterol into bile acids by increasing the activity of hepatic cholesterol-7-α-hydroxylase, the rate-limiting enzyme of bile acid biosynthesis (Sambaiah and Srinivasan, 1991). There is evidence that ginger rhizome (root) increases stomach acid production thereby interfering with antacids, sucralfate (Carafate),

H2 antagonists, or proton pump inhibitors. Interestingly (Ravindran and Nirmal, 2005), shogaol, generally being more potent than (6)-gingerol, has shown inhibitory intestinal motility in intravenous preparations and facilitatory gastrointestinal motility in oral preparations. A number of animal studies have demonstrated hypocholesterolemic action of ginger and ginger extracts by decreased lipid peroxidation and increased fibrinolytic activity. These studies have shown decreased levels of total cholesterol, LDL-cholesterol, very low-density-lipoprotein-cholesterol and triglycerides, and increased levels in high-density-lipoprotein-cholesterol (Fuhrman et al., 2000). In a more recent study, air-dried ginger powder (100 mg/kg orally daily) fed to rabbits with experimentally induced atherosclerosis for 75 days, inhibited atherosclerotic changes in the aorta and coronary arteries by about 50% (Verma et al., 1993). It is evident from these findings that ginger has demonstrated potential of being an antiatherosclerotic agent in animal studies, but as yet this promise has not been confirmed in human trials. Experimentally, it has found that ethanolic extract of ginger show antipyretic effect comparable to that of acetylsalicylic acid at the same dose (Akhani et al., 2004). This antipyretic activity may be mediated by COX inhibition. Furthermore, studies have shown that the ginger crude extract and the paracetamol drug have the same level of efficacy in lowering body temperature (Magdale et al., 2014). Further studies on this aspect will be a welcome step.

EFFECT ON MIGRAINE/RETINOPATHY

Migraine is considered as a neurological disorder with little convincing evidence of the involvement of some vascular phenomenon. Recent understanding of the mechanisms behind migraine pain generation and perception has considerably helped the development of modern migraine drugs. Evidences of ginger manifesting relief from migraine was shown when ginger powder, at dose of 500–600 mg, was administered for 3–4 days (Mustafa and Srivastava, 1990). Ginger is reported in Ayurvedic and Tibetan systems of medicine to be useful in neurological disorders. It is proposed that administration of ginger may exert abortive and prophylactic effects in migraine headache without any side effects. Considering the role of ginger in diabetes management, effect of ginger on retinopathy, a diabetes associated disease was investigated. It was found that ginger lowers intraocular pressure (IOP) in rabbits' eyes and could be useful in reducing IOP in humans as well. It has been proposed that ginger could be a useful medication for the prevention of blindness due to diabetes, as IOP increase is the major predisposing factor for the manifestation of glaucoma which is the second major cause of blindness in the world (Saraswat et al., 2009). Report has shown that an extract of ginger with dose 0.1 and 1.0 mg/mL reduced carboxymethyllysine-keyhole limpet haemocyanin (CML-KLH) and methylglyoxal (MGO)-derived advanced glycation end products (AGE) by 60–80% and glucose-derived AGE products by 50–60% (Akpalaba et al., 2009). Further evidences in this area may lead to ginger as medicine. It will be highly beneficial as ginger is cheap, readily available, and relatively nontoxical.

METABOLISM OF GINGER

Very limited information is available on the metabolism or metabolites of ginger. Evaluation of the bioactivity of ginger becomes obligatory for completely understanding its mechanism of action and potential therapeutic effects, as it is widely consumed. For investigating the fate of a metabolite, in blood plasma, method for identification and quantification of the desired molecule is a critical step. Several methods for the simultaneous quantification of [6]-, [8]-, and [10]-gingerols and [6]-shogaol in rat plasma are available in literature. The investigators were able to identify a glucuronide of [6]-gingerol following hydrolysis of β-glucuronidase and the intestinal glucuronidation (Wang et al., 2009a). The study facilitated pharmacokinetics, tissue distribution, and excretion of 6-gingerol, after oral or intraperitoneal administration in rats (Wang et al., 2009b). This type of experiments provides insight into the pharmacokinetic of the molecules, which in turn present the connecting link between traditional medicinal properties and scientific proof of concept. Several studies demonstrating maximum absorption time, site of absorption, and amount absorbed of the target molecule give insight to site of action and its mechanism. For example, several metabolites of [6]-gingerol, following its oral administration (50 mg/kg) in rats, have been identified (Nakazawa and Ohsawa, 2002). A primary metabolite, (S)-[6]-gingerol-4′-0-β-glucuronide, was detected in the bile and several minor metabolites were found in β-glucuronidase-treated urine, suggesting conjugation and oxidation of phenolic side chain of [6]-gingerol (Nakazawa and Ohsawa, 2002). Studies have shown that gingerol is rapidly cleared from rat plasma following intravenous administration (3 mg/kg) and it was reported to be metabolized enzymatically in a stereospecific reduction to gingerdiol (Chan et al., 2012). Studies have also demonstrated that oral intake of ginger extract in rats, having approximately 53% [6]-gingerol, revealed its maximum absorption into the plasma, with a maximal concentration (4.23 μg/mL) being reached after 10 min (Jiang et al., 2008). Also, it was found distributed in various tissues, but gastrointestinal tract had the maximum concentration. Its peak concentrations, in most tissues, were after about 30 min, and the concentration in tissues was higher than that in plasma (Jiang et al., 2008). Based on the success of several experiments, at least one clinical trial focusing on the pharmacokinetics of [6]-, [8]-, and [10]-gingerols and [6]-shogaol along with their respective conjugate metabolites (Zick et al., 2008), was conducted. In this case, human volunteers were given ginger at doses ranging from 100 mg to 2 g and blood samples were taken at 15 min to 72 h after a single oral dose. Results indicated that the free forms of [6]-, [8]-, and [10]-gingerols or [6]-shogaol were not detectable, whereas the respective glucuronide of each compound was detected, suggesting that these ginger components are readily absorbed after oral consumption and can be detected as glucuronide conjugates (Zick et al., 2008). Although progress in determining the active components and metabolites of ginger and understanding their pharmacokinetics has been made, however, more work is required in this direction.

Several in vitro and animal studies and one in vitro study employing human hepatic and intestinal microsomes have investigated the metabolism of the major pungent compound in ginger, 6-gingerol. The pharmacology and therapeutic use of ginger has been the subject of several recent reviews (Grzanna et al., 2005). Studies conducted in vitro have shown gingerols act as agonists of the vanilloid receptor (VR1) (Dedov et al., 2002), which are also activated by capsaicin, the major pungent principle in cayenne and chilli pepper, probably because of being structurally similar to the gingerols. Herbal products are extensively used in many Asian, African, and western countries in the complementary and alternative systems of medicine. According to a survey conducted by the World Health Organization (WHO), 60–80% of the world population relies on nonconventional or alternative medicines, mainly of botanical origin, as their primary form of health care (Chrubasik et al., 2005). However, not all herbal sources are safe. Rapid industrialization, population explosion, ineffective and insufficient pollution control, and indiscriminate use of chemical fertilizers and pest control agents have led to heavy metal contamination in agricultural soils and environment. Plants are being grown in the contaminated soil, most of the time unknowingly; toxic heavy metals from these polluted soil may accumulate in the plant and vegetables grown in them (especially underground part) thereby entering into the human food chain. It is a well-known fact that human health is directly affected by the food they consume and environment they live in. Thus monitoring of toxic heavy metals in the rhizome of ginger becomes important for protecting public health against the hazards of metal toxicity. Reports of heavy metal contaminations from Asia, Africa, and western countries have illustrated the presence of toxic metals in the plant-derived products. The WHO has also emphasized the need for safety assessment and quality assurance of plant products using modern techniques with suitable standards (World Health Organization, 2000b). Measurement of toxicity and lethal dose level is important before using herbs in health management. Several studies were performed to check the safe dose in animal model study. The dose and toxicity of ginger has been checked and recommended by various earlier investigators. Most of the studies have found that ginger extract was nontoxic in mice in different dosages (100, 333, and 1000 mg/kg) in pregnant rats (Weidner and Sigwart, 2001). Further, no teratogenicity effect of ginger on pregnant rats could be seen but embryo toxicity was detected when 20 or 50 g/L ginger tea via their drinking water was administered (Wilkinson, 2000). A patented ginger extract, when tested for teratogenic potential in pregnant rats (Weidner and Sigwart, 2001), caused neither maternal nor developmental toxicity at daily doses of up to 1 g/kg body weight. However, few earlier studies did find adverse effects of ginger-like involuntary contractions of skeletal muscle, gastrointestinal spasm, hypothermia, diarrhea, and anorexia (Akhani et al., 2004). Norethandrolone and oxandrolone were investigated for their genotoxic effect on human lymphocyte chromosomes using chromosomal aberrations and sister chromatid exchanges as parameters and subsequently Genistein and 6-gingerol were used as antigenotoxic agents to ameliorate the genotoxicity induced by the steroids. Genistein and 6-gingerol proved to be effective in reducing genotoxic damage at appropriate doses (Wilkinson, 2000). Studies have shown that 6-shogoal was much less mutagenic than 6-gingerol (Nakamura and Yamamoto, 1983). Besides, 6-gingerol and to a far lesser extent 6-shogaol were shown to have mutagenic properties in an assay using *E. coli* Hs30 as an indicator strain of mutagenesis (Nakamura and Yamamoto, 1983). Despite this pronouncement, ginger is not considered a mutagenic substance, apparently due to its long history of harmless use.

It is clear from the above that the current state of knowledge of the pharmacokinetics of ginger compounds in humans is embryonic. Expanding this knowledge and including information about oral bioavailability of compounds with known pharmacological activity should be a priority and ought to precede further clinical trials of ginger for inflammatory conditions.

FUTURE PROSPECTS

The use of ginger in human health has been documented since ancient times and they provide a useful source of new therapeutics. Scientific evidences have further confirmed its importance, not only as food, nutraceutical, spice but also as medicine. Now the time has come that time-tested traditionally employed herbs backed by scientific inputs should take a front seat as herbal nutraceuticals. These will not only alleviate the disease but also avoid it with no aftereffects.

REFERENCES

Afzal, M., Al-Hadidi, D., Menon, M., Pesek, J., Dhami, M.S., 2001. Ginger: an ethnomedical, chemical and pharmacological review. Drug Metabol. Drug interact. 18, 159–190.

Agrahari, P., 2015. A brief study on *Zingiber officinale*—a review. J. Drug Discov. Ther. 3 (28).

Ahmed, R.S., Seth, V., Pasha, S.T., Baneriee, B.D., 2000. Influence of dietary ginger (*Zingiber officinale* Rosc) in oxidative stress induced by malathion in rats. Food Chem. Toxicol. 38 (5), 443–450.

Akhani, S.P., Vishwakarma, S.L., Goyal, R.K., 2004. Anti-diabetic activity of *Zingiber officinale* in streptozotocin-induced type I diabetic rats. J. Pharm. Pharmacol. 56, 101–105.

Akimoto, M., Iizuka, M., Kanematsu, R., Yoshida, M., Takenaga, K., 2015. Anticancer effect of ginger extract against pancreatic cancer cells mainly through reactive oxygen species-mediated autotic cell death. PLoS One 10 (5), e0126605.

Akpalaba, R.U.E., Agu, C.G., Adeleke, O.O., Asonye, C.C., 2009. Effect of orally administered *Zingiber officinale* on the intra ocular pressure of experimental rabbits. Int. J. Health Res. 2 (3), 273–278.

Atai, Z., Atapour, M., Mohseni, M., 2009. Inhibitory effect of ginger extract on *Candida albicans*. Am. J. Appl. Sci. 6, 1067–1069.

Azu, N., Onyeagba, R., 2007. Antimicrobial properties of extracts of *Allium cepa* (onions) and *Zingiber officinale* (ginger) on *Escherichia coli*, *Salmonella typhi* and *Bacillus subtilis*. Internet J. Trop. Med. 3, 1–10.

Badreldin, H.A., Blunden, G., Tanira, M.O., Nemmar, A., 2008. Some phytochemical, pharmacological and toxicological properties of ginger (*Zingiber officinale* Roscoe): a review of recent research. Food Chem. Toxicol. 46, 409–420.

Bailey-Shaw, Y., Williams, L.A., Junor, G.A., Green, C.E., Hibbert, S.L., Salmon, C.N., et al., 2008. Changes in the contents of oleoresin and pungent bioactive principles of Jamaican ginger (*Zingiber officinale* Roscoe.) during maturation. J. Agric. Food Chem. 56 (14), 5564–5571.

Bartley, J.P., Jacobs, A.L., 2000. Effects of drying on flavour compounds in Australian-grown ginger (*Zingiber officinale*). J. Sci. Food Agric. 80, 209–215.

Bode, A., 2003. Ginger is an effective inhibitor of HCT 116 human colorectal carcinoma *in vivo*. Paper presented at the Frontiers in Cancer Prevention Research Conference, Phoenix, AZ.

Bordia, A., Verma, S.K., Srivastava, K.C., 1997. Effect of ginger (*Zingiber officinale* Rosc.) and fenugreek (*Trigonella foenumgraecum* L.) on blood lipids, bloodsugar and platelet aggregation in patients with coronary artery disease. ProstaglandinsLeukotEssent Fatty Acids 56 (5), 379–384.

Carrasco, F.R., Schmidt, G., Romero, A.L., Sartoretto, J.L., Caparroz-Assef, S.M., Bersani-Amado, C.A., et al., 2009. Immunomodulatory activity of *Zingiber officinale* Roscoe, *Salvia officinalis* L. and *Syzygium aromaticum* L. essential oils: evidence for humor- and cell-mediated responses. J. Pharm. Pharmacol. 61, 961–967.

Chairgulprasert, V., Prasertsongskun, S., Wicha-porn, W., 2005. Chemical constituents of the essential oil and antibacterial activity of *Zingiberwrayi var. halabala*. Songklanakarin. J. Sci. Technol. 27, 813–818.

Chan, A., Lin, T.H., Shih, V., Ching, T.H., Chiang, J., 2012. Clinical outcomes for cancer patients using complementary and alternative medicine. Altern. Ther. Health Med. 18, 12–17.

Chen, C.Y., Liu, T.Z., Liu, Y.W., 2007. 6-Shogaol (alkanone from ginger) induces apoptotic cell death of human hepatoma p53 mutant mahlavusubline via an oxidative stress-mediated caspase-dependent mechanism. J. Agric. Food Chem. 55, 948–954.

Chen, C.Y., Yang, W.L., Kuo, S.Y., 2011. Cytotoxic activity and cell cycle analysis of hexahydrocurcumin on SW 480 human colorectal cancer cells. Nat. Prod. Commun. 6, 1671–1672.

Chrubasik, S., Pittler, M.H., Roufogalis, B.D., 2005. *Zingiberis rhizoma*: a comprehensive review on the ginger effect and efficacy profiles. Phytomed 12, 684–701.

Dedov, V.N., Tran, V.H., Duk, C.C., Connor, M., Christie, M.J., Mandadi, S., et al., 2002. Gingerols: a novel class of vanilloid receptor (VR1) agonists. Br. J. Pharmacol. 137, 793–798.

El-Ghorab, A.H., Nauman, M., Anjum, F.M., Nadeem, M., Hussain, S., 2010. A comparative study on chemical composition and antioxidant activity of ginger (*Zingiber officinale*) and cumin (*Cuminum cyminum*). J. Agric. Food Chem. 58, 8231–8237.

Eric Chan, W.C., Lim, Y.Y., Wong, S.K., 2011. Antioxidant properties of ginger leaves: an overview. Free Radic. Res. 1, 6–16.

Ficker, C., Smith, M.L., Akpagana, K., Gbeassor, M., Zhang, J., Durst, T., et al., 2003a. Bioassay-guided isolation and identification of antifungal compounds from ginger. Phytother. Res. 17, 897–902.

Fuhrman, B., Rosenblat, M., Hayek, T., Coleman, R., Aviram, M., 2000. Ginger extract consumption reduces plasma cholesterol, inhibits LDL oxidation and attenuates development of atherosclerosis in atherosclerotic, apolipoprotein E-deficient mice. J. Nutr. 130 (5), 1124–1131.

Funk, J.L., Frye, J.B., Oyarzo, J.N., Timmermann, B.N., 2009. Comparative effects of two gingerol-containing *Zingiber officinale* extracts on experimental rheumatoid arthritis. J. Nat. Prod. 72, 403–407.

Gayur, M.N., Gilani, A.H., 2005. Ginger lowers blood pressure through blockage of voltage-dependent calcium channels. J. Cardiovasc. Pharmacol. 45, 74–80.

Gayur, M.N., Gilani, A.H., Afridi, M.B., Houghton, P.J., 2005. Cardiovascular effects of ginger aqueous extract and its phenolic constituents are mediated through multiple pathways. Vascul. Pharmacol. 43, 234–241.

Ghosh, A.K., Banerjee, S., Mullick, H.I., Banerjee, J., 2011. *Zingiber officinale*: a natural gold. Int. J. Pharma. Bio Sci. 2, 283–294.

Govindarajan, V., 1982. Ginger-chemistry technology and quality evaluation: Part-I CRC. Crit. Rev. Food Sci. Nutr. 17, 1–96.

Grzanna, R., Lindmark, L., Frondoza, C.G., 2005. Ginger—an herbal medicinal product with broad anti-inflammatory actions. J. Med. Food 8 (2), 125–132.

Guh, J.H., Ko, F.N., Jong, T.T., Teng, C.M., 1995. Antiplatelet effect of gingerol isolated from *Zingiber officinale*. J. Pharm. Pharmacol. 47 (4), 329–332.

Gupta, S., Pandotra, P., Gupta, A.P., Dhar, J.K., Sharma, G., Ram, G., et al., 2010. Volatile (As and Hg) and non-volatile (Pb and Cd) toxic heavy metals analysis in rhizome of *Zingiber officinale* collected from different locations of North Western Himalayas by atomic absorption spectroscopy. Food Chem. Toxicol. 48, 2966–2971.

Gupta, S., Pandotra, P., Ram, G., Anand, R., Gupta, A.P., Husain, M.K., et al., 2011. Composition of a monoterpenoid-rich essential oil from the rhizome of *Zingiber officinale* from North Western Himalayas. Nat. Pro. Commun. 6, 93–96.

Gupta, S.K., Sharma, S., 2014. Medicinal properties of *Zingiber officinale* Roscoe—a review. IOSR J. Pharma. Biol. Sci. 9, 124–129.

Gurdip, S., Kapoor, I.P.S., Prativa, S., Heluani, C.S.D., Marina, P.L., Cesar, A.N.C., 2008. Chemistry, antioxidant and antimicrobial investigations on essential oil and oleoresins of *Zingiber officinale*. Food Chem. Toxicol. 46, 3295–3302.

Habsah, M., Amran, M., Mackeen, M.M., Lajis, N.H., Kikuzaki, H., Nakatani, N., et al., 2000. Screening of Zingiberaceae extracts for antimicrobial and antioxidant activities. J. Ethnopharmacol. 72, 403–410.

Hamed, M.A., Ali, S.A., El-Rigal, N.S., 2012. Therapeutic potential of ginger against renal injury induced by carbon tetrachloride in rats. Scientific-World J. 2012, 1–12.

Haniadka, R., Saxena, A., Shivashankara, A.R., Fayad, R., Palatty, P.L., Nazreth, N., et al., 2013. Ginger protects the liver against the toxic effects of xenobiotic compounds: preclinical observations. J. Nutr. Food Sci. 3, 5.

Iqbal, Z., Lateef, M., Akhtar, M.S., Ghayur, M.N., Gilani, A.H., 2006. In vivo anthelmintic activity of ginger against gastrointestinal nematodes of sheep. J. Ethnopharmacol. 106, 285–287.

Janssen, P.L., Meyboom, S., Van Staveren, W.A., De Vegt, F., Katan, M.B., 1996. Consumption of ginger (*Zingiber officinale* Roscoe) does not affect exvivo platelet thromboxane production in humans. Eur. J. Clin. Nutr. 50 (11), 772–774.

Jeevani Osadee Wijekoon, M.M., Karim, A.A., Bhat, R., 2011. Evaluation of nutritional quality of torch ginger (*Etlingera elatior* Jack.) inflorescence. Int. Food Res. J. 18 (4), 1415–1420.

Jeyakuma, S., Nalini, N., Venugopal, M., 1999. Antioxidant activity of ginger in rats fed a high fat diet. Med. Sci. Res. 27, 341–344.

Jiang, S.Z., Wang, N.S., Mi, S.Q., 2008. Plasma pharmacokinetics and tissue distribution of [6]-gingerol in rats. Biopharm. Drug Dispos. 29 (9), 529–537.

Jiang, H., Solyom, A.M., Timmermann, B.N., Gang, D.R., 2005. Characterization of gingerol related compounds in ginger rhizome (*Zingiber officinale* Rosc.) by high performance liquid chromatography/electrospray ionization mass spectrometry. Rapid Commun. Mass Spectr. 19 (20), 2957–2964.

Jolad, S.D., Lantz, R.C., Solyom, A.M., Guan, J.C., Bates, R.B., Timmermann, B.N., 2004. Fresh organically grown ginger (*Zingiber officinale*): composition and effects on LPS-induced PGE2 production. Phytochemistry 65, 1937–1954.

Katiyar, S.K., Agarwal, R., Mukhtar, H., 1996. Inhibition of tumor promotion in SENCAR mouse skin by ethanol extract of *Zingiber officinale* rhizome. Cancer Res. 56, 1023–1030.

Kim, J.K., Kim, Y., Na, K.M., Surh, Y.J., Kim, T.Y., 2007. [6]-Gingerol prevents UVB-induced ROS production and COX-2 expression in vitro and in vivo. Free Radic. Res. 41, 603–614.

Kim, M.O., Lee, M.H., Oi, N., Kim, S.H., Bae, K.B., et al., 2014. [6]-Shogaol inhibits growth and induces apoptosis of non-small cell lung cancer cells by directly regulating Akt1/2. Carcinogenesis 35 (5), 1193.

Kobayashi, M., Tshida, Y., Shoji, N., Okizumi, Y., 1988. Cardiotonic action of [8]-gingerol, an activator of the Ca++ pumping adenosine triphosphatase of sarcoplasmic reticulum, in guinea pigatrial muscle. J. Pharmacol. Exp. Ther. 246, 667.

Koh, E.M., Kim, H.J., Kim, S., Choi, W.H., Choi, Y.H., Ryu, S.Y., et al., 2009. Modulation of macrophage functions by compounds isolated from *Zingiber officinale*. Planta Med. 75 (2), 148–151.

Kress, W.J., 1990. The phylogeny and classification of the Zingiberales. Ann. Mo. Bot. Gard. 77, 698–721.

Kumar, G., Kathie, L., Rao, K.V.B., 2011. A review on pharmacological and phytochemical properties of *Zingiber officinale* Roscoe (Zingiberaceae). J. Pharm. Res. 4 (9), 2963–2966.

Langmead, L., Rampton, D.S., 2001. Review article: herbal treatment in gastrointestinal and liver disease-benefits and dangers. Aliment. Pharmacol. Ther. 15 (9), 1239–1252.

Lantz, R.C., Chen, G.J., Sarihan, M., Solyom, A.M., Jolad, S.D., 2007. The effect of extract from ginger rhizome on inflammatory mediator production. Phytomed 14, 123–128.

Lee, E., Surh, Y.J., 1998. Induction of apoptosis in HL-60 cells by pungent vanilloids, [6]-gingerol and [6]-paradol. Cancer Lett. 134 (2), 163–168.

Lumb, A.B., 1993. Mechanism of antiemetic effect of ginger. Anaesthesia 48 (12), 1118.

Lumb, A.B., 1994. Effect of dried ginger on human platelet function. Thromb. Haemost. 71 (1), 110–111.

Ma, W., Quirion, R., 2007. Inflammatory mediators modulating the transient receptor potential vanilloid 1 receptor: therapeutic targets to treat inflammatory and neuropathic pain. Expert Opin. Ther. Targets 11, 307–320.

Magdale, C.D., Bargo, R., Caumban, J.C., Devibar, S.J., Ebajay, J., Requerme, J.K., et al., 2014. The effect of *Zingiber officinale* (Ginger) rhizome crude extract on the body temperature level of Brewer's yeast–induced male albino rabbits. Adv. Pharm. Res. 1 (1).

Mahady, G.B., Pendland, S.L., Yun, G.S., Lu, Z.Z., Stoia, A., 2003. Ginger (*Zingiber officinale* Roscoe) and the gingerols inhibit the growth of Cag A+ strains of *Helicobacter pylori*. Anticancer Res. 23 (5A), 3699–3702.

Mansour, M.A., Bekheet, S.A., Al-Rejaie, S.S., Al-Shabanah, O.A., Al-Howiriny, T.A., Al-Rikabi, A.C., et al., 2010. Ginger ingredients inhibit the development of diethylnitrosoamine induced premalignant phenotype in rat chemical hepatocarcinogenesis model. Biofactors 36 (6), 483–490.

Mascolo, N., Jain, R., Jain, S.C., Capasso, F., 1989. Ethnopharmacologic investigation of ginger (*Zingiber officinale*). J. Ethnopharmacol. 27 (1–2), 129–140.

Masuda, Y., Kikuzaki, H., Hisamoto, M., Nikatani, N., 2004. Antioxidant properties of gingerol related compounds from ginger. BioFactors 21, 293–296.

Micklefield, G.H., Redeker, Y., Meister, V., Jung, O., Greving, I., May, B., 1999. Effects of ginger on gastroduodenal motility. Int. J. Clin. Pharmacol. Ther. 37 (7), 341–346.

Miri, P., Bae, J., Lee, D.S., 2008. Antibacterial activity of [10]-gingerol and [12]-gingerol isolated from ginger rhizome against periodontal bacteria. Phytother. Res. 22, 1446–1449.

Mustafa, T., Srivastava, K.C., 1990. Ginger (*Zingiber officinale*) in migraine headache. J. Ethno-Pharmacol. 29, 267–273.

Nakamura, H., Yamamoto, T., 1983. The active part of the [6]-gingerol molecule in mutagenesis. Mutat. Res. Lett. 122, 87–940.

Nakazawa, T., Ohsawa, K., 2002. Metabolism of [6]-gingerol in rats. Life Sci. 70 (18), 2165–2175.

Nurtjahja-Tjendraputra, E., Ammit, A.J., Roufogalis, B.D., Tran, V.H., Duke, C.C., 2003. Effective anti-platelet and COX-1 enzyme inhibitors from pungent constituents of ginger. Thromb. Res. 111, 259–265.

Oboh, G., Akinyemi, A.J., Ademiluyi, A.O., 2012a. Antioxidant and inhibitory effect of red ginger (*Zingiber officinale* var. Rubra) and white ginger (*Zingiber officinale* Roscoe) on Fe2+ induced lipid peroxidation in rat brain—in vitro. Exp. Toxicol. Pathol. 64, 31–36.

Ojewole, J.A.O., 2006. Analgesic, antiinflammatory and hypoglycaemic effects of ethanol extract of *Zingiber officinale* (Roscoe) rhizomes (Zingiberaceae) in mice and rats. Phytother. Res. 20, 764–772.

Onogi, T., Minami, M., Kuraishi, Y., Satoh, M., 1992. Capsaicin-like effect of (6)-shogaol on substance P-containing primary afferents of rats: a possible mechanism of its analgesic action. Neuropharmacology 31 (11), 1165–1169.

Pancho, L.R., Kimura, I., Unno, R., Kurono, M., Kimura, M., 1989. Reversed effects between crude and processed ginger extracts on PGF2 alpha-induced contraction in mouse mesenteric veins. Jpn. J. Pharmacol. 50 (2), 243–246.

Pandotra, P., Gupta, A.P., Khan, S., Ram, G., Gupta, S., 2015. A comparative assessment of ISSR, RAPD, IRAP, & REMAP molecular markers in Zingiber officinale germplasm characterization. Scientia Horti. 194, 201–207.

Pandotra, P., Gupta, A.P., Ram, G., Husain, M.K., Gupta, S., 2013. Genetic and chemodivergence in eighteen core collection of *Zingiber officinale* from North-West Himalayas. Sci. Hortic. 160, 283–291.

Park, J., Park, H., Song, 2014. Anti-cancer activity of Ginger (*Zingiber officinale*) leaf through the expression of activating transcription factor 3 in human colorectal cancer cells. BMC Complement. Altern. Med. 14, 408.

Patel, K., Srinivasan, K., 2000. Influence of dietary spices and their active principles on pancreatic digestive enzymes in albino rats. Nahrung 44 (1), 42–46.

Phillips, S., Hutchinson, S., Ruggier, R., 1993. *Zingiber officinale* does not affect gastric emptying rate. Anaesthesia 48 (5), 393–395.

Puri, A., Sahai, R., Singh, K.L., Saxena, R.P., Tandon, J.S., Saxena, K.C., 2000. Immunostimulant activity of dry fruits and plant materials used in Indian traditional medical system for mothers after child birth and invalids. J. Ethnopharmacol. 71, 89–92.

Qazi, A.K., Hussain, A., Aga, M.A., Ali, S., Taneja, S.C., Sharma, P.R., et al., 2014. Cell specific apoptosis by RLX is mediated by NFκB in human colon carcinoma HCT-116 cells. BMC Cell Biol. 15, 36.

Quimby, E.L., 2007. The use of herbal therapies in pediatric oncology patients: treating symptoms of cancer and side effects of standard therapies. J. PediatrOncol. Nurs. 24 (1), 35–40.

Ravindran, P.N., Nirmal, B.K., 2005. Ginger: The Genus *Zingiber*. Medicinal and Aromatic Plant-Industrial Profile. CRC Press, Boca Raton, FL.

Rhode, J.M., Huang, J., Fogoros, S., Tan, L., Zick, S., Liu, J.R., 2006. Ginger induces apoptosis and autophagocytosis in ovarian cancer cells. Abstract no. 4510, presented April 4, 2006 at the 97th AACR Annual Meeting, April 1–5, 2006, Washington, DC.

Ryu, H.S., Kim, H.S., 2004. Effect of *Zingiber officinale* Roscoe extracts on mice immune cell activation. Korean J. Nutr. 37, 23–30.

Sambaiah, K., Srinivasan, K., 1991. Effect of cumin, cinnamon, ginger, mustard and tamarind in induced hyper cholesterolemic rats. Nahrung 35 (1), 47–51.

Sanwal, S.K., Rai, N., Singh, J., Buragohain, J., 2010. Antioxidant phytochemicals and gingerol content in diploid and tetraploid clones of ginger (*Zingiber officinale* Roscoe). Sci. Hortic. 124, 280.

Saraswat, M., Reddy, P.Y., Muthenna, P., Reddy, G.B., 2009. Prevention of non-enzymic glycation of proteins by dietary agents: prospects for alleviating diabetic complications. Brit. J. Nutr. 101, 1714–1721.

Sekiwa, Y., Kubota, K., Kobayashi, A., 2000. Isolation of novel glucosides related to gingerdiol from ginger and their antioxidative activities. J. Agric. Food Chem. 48 (2), 373–377.

Sharma, S.S., Gupta, Y.K., 1998. Reversal of cisplatin-induced delay in gastric emptying in rats by ginger (*Zingiber officinale*). J. Ethnopharmacol. 62 (1), 49–55.

Shieh, Y.H., Huang, H.M., Wang, C.C., Lee, C.C., Fan, C.K., Lee, Y.L., 2015. Zerumbone enhances the Th1 response and ameliorates ovalbumin-induced Th2 responses and airway inflammation in mice. Int. Immunopharmacol. 24 (2), 383–391.

Shoji, N., Iwasa, A., Takemoto, T., Ishida, Y., Ohizumi, Y., 1982. Cardiotonic principles of ginger (*Zingiber officinale* Roscoe). J. Pharm. Sci. 71 (10), 1174–1175.

Shukla, Y., Singh, M., 2007. Cancer preventive properties of zinger: a brief review. Food Chem. Toxicol. 45 (5), 683–690.

Shyur, L.F., Tsung, J.H., Chen, J.H., Chiu, C.Y., Lo, C.P., 2005. Antioxidant properties of extracts from medicinal plants popularly used in Taiwan oxidative stress play a significant effect in the pathogenesis of various types of disease. Int. J. Appl. Sci. Eng. 3, 195–202.

Singh, S., Gupta, A.K., 2013. Evaluation of phenolics content, flavonoids and antioxidant activity of *Curcuma amada* (mango ginger) and *Zingiber officinale*(ginger). Res. Rev. J. Chem. 2, 32–35.

Srivastava, K.C., 1984. Aqueous extracts of onion, garlic and ginger inhibit platelet aggregation and alter arachidonic acid metabolism. Biomed. Biochem. Acta 43, 335.

Srivastava, K.C., 1989. Effect of onion and ginger consumption on platelet thromboxane production in humans. Prostaglandins Leukot. Essent. Fatty Acids 35 (3), 183–185.

Stoilova, I., Krastanov, A., Stoyanova, A., Denev, P., Gargova, S., 2007. Antioxidant activity of a ginger extract (*Zingiber officinale*). Food Chem. 102, 764–770.

Suekawa, M., Aburada, M., Hosoya, E., 1986. Pharmacological studies on ginger. III. Effect of the spinal destruction on (6)-shogaol-induced pressor response in rats. J. Pharmacobiodyn. 9 (10), 853–860.

Tripathi, S., Maier, K.G., Bruch, D., Kittur, D.S., 2007. Effect of 6-gingerol on pro-inflammatory cytokine production and costimulatory molecule expression in murine peritoneal macrophages. J. Surg. Res. 138, 209–213.

Tsui, B., Dennehy, C.E., Tsourounis, C., 2001. A survey of dietary supplement use during pregnancy at an academic medical center. Am. J. ObstetGynecol. 185 (2), 433–437.

USDA Nutrient Database, 2013. National Nutrient Database for Standard Reference Release 25. <http://ndb.nal.usda.gov/ndb/foods/show/2954> (accessed on 27.05.15.).

Uz, E., Karatas, O.F., Mete, E., Bayrak, R., Bayrak, O., Atmaca, A.F., et al., 2009. The effect of dietary ginger (*Zingiber officinals* Rosc) on renal ischemia/reperfusion injury in rat kidneys. Ren. Fail. 31 (4), 251–260.

Verma, S.K., Singh, J., Khamesra, R., Bordia, A., 1993. Effect of ginger on platelet aggregation in man. Indian J. Med. Res. 98, 240–242.

Wang, W., Li, C.Y., Wen, X.D., Li, P., Qi, L.W., 2009a. Plasma pharmacokinetics, tissue distribution and excretion study of [6]-gingerol in rat by liquid chromatography-electrospray ionization time-of-flight mass spectrometry. J. Pharm. Biomed. Anal. 49 (4), 1070–1074.

Wang, W., Li, C.Y., Wen, X.D., Li, P., Qi, L.W., 2009b. Simultaneous determination of [6]-gingerol, [8]-gingerol, [10]-gingerol and [6]-shogaol in rat plasma by liquid chromatography-mass spectrometry: application to pharmacokinetics. J. Chromatogr. B AnalytTechnol. Biomed. Life Sci. 877 (8–9), 671–679.

We, Q.Y., Ma, J.P., Cai, Y.J., Yang, L., Liu, Z.L., 2005. Cytotoxic and apoptopic activities of diarylheptanoids and gingerol-related compounds from the rhizomes of Chinese ginger. J. Ethnopharmacol. 102, 177–184.

Weidner, M.S., Sigwart, K., 2001. Investigation of the teratogenic potential of a *Zingiber officinale* extract in the rat. Reprod. Toxicol. 15, 75–80.

White, B., 2007. Ginger: an overview. Am. Fam. Physician 75 (11), 1689–1691.

Wilasrusmee, C., Siddiqui, J., Bruch, D., Wilasrusmee, S., Kittur, S., Kittur, D.S., 2002. In vitro immunomodulatory effects of herbal products. Am. Surg. 68, 860–864.

Wilkinson, J.M., 2000. Effect of ginger tea on the fetal development of Sprague–Dawley rats. Reprod. Toxicol. 14 (6), 507–512.

Willetts, K.E., Ekangaki, A., Eden, J.A., 2003. Effect of a ginger extract on pregnancy-induced nausea: a randomised controlled trial. Aust. N. Z. J. ObstetGynaecol. 43 (2), 139–144.

World Health Organization (WHO), 2000a. WHO Traditional Medicine Strategy 2002–2005. <http://www.wpro.who.int/health_technology/book_who_traditional_medicine_strategy_2002_2005.pdf> (accessed 14.04.14.).

World Health Organization, 2000b. Traditional Medicine Strategy 2002–2005. <http://www.wpro.who.int/health_technology/book_who_traditional_medicine_strategy_2002_2005.pdf> (accessed 27.05.15.).

Wu, H., Ye, D., Bai, Y., Zhao, Y., 1990. Effect of dry ginger and roasted ginger on experimental gastric ulcers in rats. ZhongguoZhong Yao ZaZhi 15, 278–280.

Wu, K.L., Rayner, C.K., Chuah, S.K., Changchien, C.S., Lu, S.N., Chiu, Y.C., et al., 2008. Effects of ginger on gastric emptying and motility in healthy humans. Eur. J. Gastroenterol. Hepatol. 20 (5), 436–440.

Yamahara, J., Huang, Q.R., Li, Y.H., Xu, L., Fujimura, H., 1990. Gastrointestinal motility enhancing effect of ginger and its active constituents. Chem. Pharm. Bull. (Tokyo) 38 (2), 430–431.

Yamahara, J., Miki, K., Chisaka, T., Sawada, T., Fujimura, H., Tomimatsu, T., et al., 1985. Cholagogic effect of ginger and its active constituents. J. Ethnopharmacol. 13 (2), 217–225.

Yamahara, J., Mochizuki, M., Rong, H.Q., Matsuda, H., Fujimura, H., 1988. The anti-ulcer effect in rats of ginger constituents. J. Ethnopharmacol. 23, 299–304.

Yusof, Y.A.M., Ahmad, N., Das, S., Sulaiman, S., Murad, N.A., 2008. Chemopreventive efficacy of ginger (*Zingiber officinale*) in ethionine induced rat hepatocarcinogenesis. Afr. J. Tradit. Complement. Altern. Med. 6, 87–93.

Zick, S.M., Djuric, Z., Ruffin, M.T. (Eds.), 2008. Pharmacokinetics of [6]-gingerol, [8]-gingerol, [10]-gingerol, and [6]-shogaol and conjugate metabolites in healthy human subjects. Cancer Epidemiol. Biomarkers Prev. 17 (8), 1930–1936.

Chapter 26

Antimicrobials from herbs, spices, and plants

Tarik Bor[1], Sulaiman O. Aljaloud[1,2], Rabin Gyawali[1] and Salam A. Ibrahim[1]
[1]*North Carolina Agricultural and Technical State University, Greensboro, NC, United States*
[2]*King Saud University, Riyadh, Saudi Arabia*

CHAPTER OUTLINE

INTRODUCTION

Consumers increasingly demand high quality, safe food. Due to the increase in the number of foodborne outbreaks caused by pathogen microorganisms, there has been a corresponding increase in concerns over food safety. Consumers are especially concerned about the use of chemical and artificial antimicrobial compounds and preservatives that inhibit the growth of pathogens (Tajkarimi et al., 2010). Consumers' demand for maintaining nutrition and quality while continuing to provide food safety has increased the need for using alternative preservation methods to inactivate pathogen microorganisms and enzymes in food products. Foods preserved with natural additives have become popular. As a result, new methods for using natural preservatives obtained from plants, animals, or microflora have come along (Holley and Patel, 2005; Tiwari et al., 2009).

Fruits, Vegetables, and Herbs.
DOI: http://dx.doi.org/10.1016/B978-0-12-802972-5.00026-3

Natural antimicrobials are now gaining attention as a way to control microorganisms. These antimicrobials play an important role in food control by preventing microbial contamination by pathogens and by extending shelf life due to the removal of undesirable pathogens. The antibiotic resistance of pathogens can also be decreased and the immune system can be boosted through the use of natural antimicrobials (Tajkarimi et al., 2010). There are two major reasons for using antimicrobials in food models: to prevent natural spoilage (preservation) and to control the growth of microorganisms (safety). Animals, plants, and microorganisms are the major sources of natural antimicrobials. In addition to their seasoning benefits, some herbs and spices have antimicrobial effects against human and plant pathogens (Brandi et al., 2006). Food processing techniques that only employ chemical preservatives are not completely successful because the chemicals do not totally kill foodborne pathogens or stop microbial spoilage (Gutierrez et al., 2009). Recent food preservation methods such as pulsed light, high pressure pulsed electric and magnetic fields have been used for controlling pathogen and spoilage microorganisms in food (Tajkarimi et al., 2010). In this chapter, we review the antimicrobial properties of different types of herbs, spices, and their extracts. Major antimicrobial compounds of herbs and spices and their chemical composition are also discussed. The use of plant antimicrobials against pathogens in liquid and solid food models is also highlighted.

Herbs, spices, and plant extracts

Herbs and spices have been used as food additives all over the world. Not only do they improve the organoleptic properties of food, they can also increase the shelf life of food by reducing or entirely removing the number of foodborne pathogens (Lai and Roy, 2004).

Plant-derived natural antimicrobials have actually long been used for the preservation of foods. Some spices and essential oils (EOs) were used by the early Egyptians and have been used for centuries in China and India. Spices such as clove, cinnamon, mustard, garlic, ginger, and mint are still used as alternative health remedies. Spices and plant extracts have antimicrobial effects against Gram-positive pathogen microorganisms such as *Listeria monocytogenes*. These antimicrobial compounds can increase storage time and stability with active ingredients such as phenols, alcohols, aldehydes, ketones, ethers, and hydrocarbons, specifically in cinnamon, clove, garlic, mustard, and onion. The first scientific study on preservative effects of spices was conducted in the 1880s and showed the antimicrobial effect of cinnamon oil against *Bacillus anthracis* spores (Tajkarimi et al., 2010).

The majority of herbs and spices exerts antimicrobial activity against different bacteria, yeasts, and molds (Tajkarimi et al., 2010; Friedman et al., 2004, 2002; Raybaudi-Massilia et al., 2008). Phenolic compounds obtained from herbs and spices show biological activity and can be potentially used as food preservatives (Lai and Roy, 2004).

The extract of *Capsicum annuum* bell pepper prevented the growth of *Salmonella typhimurium* at 1.5 mL/100 g concentration in minced beef. For *Pseudomonas aeruginosa*, bell pepper extract showed bacteriostatic effect at 0.3 mL/100 g and bactericidal effect at 3 mL/100 g concentrations (Careaga et al., 2003). The inhibitory effects of the hydrosols of thyme, black cumin, sage, rosemary, and bay leaf against *S. typhimurium* and *Escherichia coli* O157:H7 were shown in carrots and apples. Thyme hydrosol had the highest antibacterial effect on both *S. typhimurium* and *E. coli* O157:H7 counts (Tornuk et al., 2011).

Different types of spices were grouped based on their antimicrobial activities as strong (cinnamon, clove, mustard), medium (allspice, bay leaf, caraway, coriander, cumin, oregano, rosemary, sage, thyme), and weak (black pepper, red pepper, ginger) (Zaika, 1988). Ethanol and hexane extracts of oregano, clove, sage, rosemary, and celery exerted relatively strong antimicrobial activities against *E. coli, Listeria innocua, Staphylococcus aureus,* and *Pseudomonas fluorescens*, but water extracts showed weak or no antimicrobial activity (Witkowska et al., 2013). Aqueous extracts of *Mentha* spp. have antimicrobial activities against *Bacillus fastidiosus*, *Proteus mirabilis*, *Proteus vulgaris*, *Salmonella choleraesuis*, *E. coli*, *P. aeruginosa*, *Klebsiella pneumoniae*, and *Serratia odorifera* at different concentrations (1:1, 1:5, 1:10, and 1:20) (Al-Sum and Al-Arfaj, 2013).

Green tea was particularly effective against *Bacillus cereus, S. aureus*, and *L. monocytogenes*, and rosemary had a strong inhibitory effect against *B. cereus* and *S. aureus* in tryptic soy broth (TSB). When green tea or rosemary was added to rice cakes at 1–3% concentration, the growth of *B. cereus* and *S. aureus* was significantly reduced in rice cakes after 3 days of storage at 22°C (Lee et al., 2009). Mixed extracts of *Scutellaria, Forsythia*, honeysuckle, cinnamon, and rosemary and clove oil showed strong antimicrobial effects in vacuum-packaged fresh pork from 1.81 to 2.32 log reductions in *E. coli*, *P. fluorescens*, and *Lactobacillus plantarum* counts during 28 days of storage when compared with the control (Kong et al., 2007).

Rosemary extracts and dry powders of orange and lemon were effective in controlling bacterial spoilage during 12 days of storage at 8°C (Fernandez-Lopez et al., 2005). Activin (grape seed extract) and Pycnogenol (pine bark extract) can be used as food additives to maintain the quality and safety of cooked beef (Ahn et al., 2007). Green, jasmine, and black tea aqueous extracts suppress the growth of *S. aureus* by 5.0 log CFU/mL and *L. monocytogenes* by 3.0 log CFU/mL in brain heart infusion broth (Kim et al., 2004).

The plants *Pelargonium purpureum* and *Sideritis scardica* exerted the strongest antimicrobial effects against *E. coli* O157:H7 NCTC 12900, *Salmonella enteritidis* PT4, *S. aureus* ATCC 6538, *L. monocytogenes* ScottA, *Pseudomonas putida* AMF178, and *B. cereus* FSS134 but especially on *E. coli* and *L. monocytogenes* (Proestos et al., 2013). The methanol extract of *Peganum harmala*, the EO of *Satureja bachtiarica*, the ethanol extract of *Juglans regia*, and *Trachyspermum copticum* with MIC of 105, 126, 510, and 453 μg/mL, respectively, are the most active plant extracts against *Lactococcus garvieae* from diseased *Oncorhynchus mykiss*, whereas some extracts such as *Quercus branti* Lindley and *Glycyrrhiza glabra* L had lower activity against *L. garvieae* with MIC values of 978 and 920 μg/mL, respectively (Fereidouni et al., 2013).

The addition of 5% olive or apple skin extracts reduced *E. coli* O157:H7 populations to below the detection limit and by 1.6 log CFU/g, respectively, and 1% lemongrass oil reduced *E. coli* O157:H7 to below detectable limits, whereas clove bud oil reduced pathogen bacteria by 1.6 log CFU/g. The formation of carcinogenic heterocyclic amines was reduced with the addition of olive and apple extracts by 76–85% and from 35% to 53% with clove bud oil (Rounds et al., 2012).

The aqueous extracts of *Psidium guajava*, *Citrus limonium*, *Allium sativum*, and *Zingiber officinale* were found to be active against *S. aureus*, *E. coli*, *Bacillus subtilis*, *P. aeruginosa*, and *Salmonella* species. Guava leaves had a stronger antibacterial effect against *B. subtilis* whereas *S. aureus* was inhibited more effectively with garlic cloves. Lemon leaves extract and juice inhibited the growth of *P. aeruginosa* and *E. coli*, respectively, to a high degree (Kumar et al., 2012b).

Cinnamon, clove, star anise, picklyash peel, and common fennel water extracts were mixed with chitosan at 0.2, 3.0, 0.7, 2.2, and 0.6 g/L concentrations, respectively, to design a new food preservative formula. Chilled steak samples treated with this preservative formula remained fresh after 9 days of storage (Wang et al., 2012).

Rosemary, sage, peppermint, and spearmint inhibited the growth of *B. cereus*, *Micrococcus luteus*, and *S. aureus*. Rosemary and sage showed stronger antibacterial effect than green and black teas of *Camellia sinensis* (Chan et al., 2012). *Laurus nobilis* (L.), *Rosmarinus officinalis* (L.), *Equisetum arvense* (L.), *Lavandula officinalis* (L.), and *Lavandula stoechas* (L.) leaves also showed antibacterial activity. Only aqueous extracts of *L. nobilis* showed anticandidal activity. The most sensitive bacterium was *S. aureus* and the most resistant one was *B. cereus* (Ceyhan et al., 2012).

The antimicrobial activity of cinnamon, clove, and mustard against mycotoxigenic *Aspergillus parasiticus*, *Salmonella enterica*, *L. monocytogenes*, *E. coli*, *Shigella sonnei*, *Shigella flexneri* was shown (Lai and Roy, 2004), and the application of garlic-derived organosulfur compounds in meat could enhance microbial safety (Yin and Cheng, 2003).

Clove was used to be use to prevent spoilage in meat, sirups, sauces, and sweetmeats. Cinnamon and mustard were identified as preservatives in applesauce in the 1910s. It has been reported that allspice, bay leaf, caraway, coriander, cumin, oregano, rosemary, sage, and thyme have strong bacteriostatic effects (Tajkarimi et al., 2010). EOs extracted from plants and spices have an antimicrobial effect against *E. coli* O157:H7, *S. typhimurium*, *Shigella dysenteriae*, *L. monocytogenes*, *B. cereus*, and *S. aureus* at concentrations between 0.2 and 10 μL/mL (Burt, 2004). Two percent of citric acid or up to 0.1% of cinnamon bark oil added into tomato juice and then treated with high intensity pulsed electric fields (HIPEF) caused a 5-log or greater reduction (Mosqueda-Melgar et al., 2008a,b).

In broth model systems 0.25–1.0% clove and garlic showed bacteriostatic and bactericidal activities against *E. coli* O157 and *S. enterica* serovar Enteritidis. Garlic at a 1% concentration reduced the viable cells of *S. enteritidis* in mayonnaise (Leuschner and Zamparini, 2002). The addition of fresh garlic (30 g/kg) or garlic powder (9 g/kg) into raw chicken sausage significantly reduced the aerobic plate counts and extended the shelf life of the product to 21 days (Sallam et al., 2004). Fresh garlic extract combined with ampicillin or ciprofloxacin can synergistically increase the zone of inhibition (Ankri and Mirelman, 1999; Gaekwad and Trivedi, 2013).

Allicin, an active compound, extracted from fresh garlic, in its pure form exerts antibacterial activity against a wide range of Gram-negative and Gram-positive bacteria, including drug-resistant Enterotoxigenic *E. coli* strains, antifungal (*Candida albicans*), antiparasitic (*Entamoeba histolytica* and *Giardia lamblia*), and antiviral activities (Ankri and Mirelman, 1999). Aqueous extract of garlic and garlic shoot juice in combination with nisin showed synergistic bactericidal activity against nisin resistant *L. monocytogenes* (Kim et al., 2008; Singh et al., 2001).

Turmeric (*Curcuma longa* L.) is a tropical herb which belongs to the Zingiberaceae family and is indigenous to southern Asia. Turmeric is used in foods as a condiment and in medicine as a carminative, anthelmintic, laxative and as a cure for liver ailments (Negi et al., 1999). The ethanolic extract of turmeric showed high antimicrobial activity at 3.11 and 5.65 mg gallic acid/mL extract against *E. coli*, *S. aureus*, *Saccharomyces sake*, and *Aspergillus oryzae* (Falco et al., 2011).

The total six extracts of black pepper (*Piper nigrum*) and turmeric (*C. longa*) showed antibacterial activity against *B. subtilis*, *Bacillus megaterium, Bacillus sphaericus, Bacillus polymixa, S. aureus, E. coli* and 11 molds, *Aspergillus luchuensis, A. flavus*, *Penicillium oxalicum*, *Rhizopus stolonifer*, *Scopulariopsis* sp., *Mucor* sp. (Pundir and Jain, 2010).

The ethanolic extracts of unripe banana, lemongrass, and turmeric were effective against *E. coli* ATCC25922, *E. coli*, *P. aeruginosa*, *Salmonella paratyphi*, *S. flexneri*, *K. pneumoniae*, *S. aureus*, *S. aureus* ATCC 25921, and *B. subtilis*. MIC ranged from 4 to 512 mg/mL while MBC ranged from 32 to 512 mg/mL depending on bacterial isolates and extracting solvent. *S. aureus* ATCC 25921 was killed in less than 2 h with unripe banana extract, *E. coli*, in less than 3 h with turmeric, *S. paratyphi* (Fagbemi et al., 2009), in just over 3 h with lemongrass.

Hexane extract eluted with 5% ethylacetate was most active fraction of curcumin, the yellow color pigment of turmeric, against *B. cereus*, *Bacillus coagulans*, *B. subtilis*, *S. aureus*, *E. coli*, and *P. aeruginosa* (Negi et al., 1999). Turmeric extract (1.5%, v/v) alone or combined with shallot extract (1.5%, v/v) enhanced quality characteristics and extended the shelf life of vacuum-packaged rainbow trout (*O. mykiss*) during 20 days of storage at 4±1°C (Pezeshk et al., 2011).

Cinnamon is extracted from cinnamon bark, fruit, leaf, and their EOs and many *Cinnamomum* species produce a volatile oil on distillation with different compositions and aroma characteristics (Jayaprakasha et al., 1997; Kaul et al., 2003; Negi, 2012). Bioactive fraction obtained from fruits of *Cinnamomum zeylanicum* has been used as antibacterial agent (Jayaprakasha et al., 2003). Oil of cinnamon (*C. zeylanicum*) was highly effective against *Bacillus* sp., *L. monocytogenes*, *E. coli*, *Klebsiella* sp., and the fungus *Rhizomucor* sp. (Gupta et al., 2008).

Extract of *Cinnamomum cassia* Blume (cassia bark, Chinese cinnamon) bark exerted antibacterial activity (7–29 mm/20 μL inhibition zone) against 13 bacterial species by in vitro agar diffusion method. Alcohol extracts showed a 7 mm/20 μL inhibition zone against *B.* megaterium and *Enterococcus faecalis.* Alcohol extracts of *Pimpinella anisum* (L.) (anise, aniseed) seeds were effective against *M. luteus* and *Mycobacterium smegmatus* (8 mm/20 μL inhibition zone), and *G. glabra* root extract showed various antibacterial activities (7–11 mm/20 μL inhibition zone) against tested microorganisms (Ates and Erdogrul, 2003).

The antibacterial activity of EOs extracted from nutmeg, mint, clove, oregano, cinnamon, sassafras, sage, thyme, or rosemary was determined against *B. cereus* INRA L2104 at different temperatures. Tyndallized carrot broth was used as a food model and the addition of cinnamon EO at 0.05% at refrigeration temperature (≤8°C) inhibited the growth of tested strain for at least 60 days in tyndallized carrot broth model (Valero and Salmeron, 2003). The mixture of Chinese chives (*Allium tuberosum*), cinnamon (*C. cassia*), and corni fructus (*Cornus officinalis*) extracts exhibited better inhibitory effects on the growth of *E. coli* than potassium sorbate at 2–5 mg/mL and inhibited growth of *Pichia membranaefaciens* at levels as low as 2 mg/mL concentration. The antimicrobial activity of Eos from corni fructus, cinnamon and Chinese chive was slightly enhanced with the addition of food additives such as polyphosphate and butylated hydroxyanisole (BHA). This mixed extract was effective in several food models including orange juice, guava juice, pork, milk and tea (Hsieh et al., 2001; Mau et al., 2000).

The antimicrobial activity of polyphenols, tannins, and flavonoids is well known. Pomegranate (*Punica granatum* L.) is rich in tannins which show strong antimicrobial activity. Fruits, peels, leaves, flowers, seeds, and roots of pomegranate have been widely used in herbal remedies and medicine in many countries (Negi, 2012; Al-Zoreky, 2009). The 80% methanolic extract of pomegranate peels had an inhibitory effect against *L. monocytogenes*, *S. aureus*, *E. coli*, and *Yersinia enterocolitica* and showed a more than 1 log reduction of *L. monocytogenes* in fish during refrigerated storage (Al-Zoreky, 2009). Pomegranate fruit fractions showed antimicrobial activity (inhibition zone) against *S. aureus* and *P. aeruginosa* (Opara et al., 2009). Pomegranate aril extracts had antimicrobial effects on *B. megaterium* DSM 32, *P. aeruginosa* DSM 9027, *S. aureus* Cowan 1, *Corynebacterium xerosis* UC 9165, *E. coli* DM, *E. faecalis* A10, *M. luteus* LA 2971, and three fungi, *Kluyveromyces marxianus* A230, *Rhodotorula rubra* MC12, and *C. albicans* ATCC 1023 with 30–>90 μg/mL MIC values (Duman et al., 2009). Pomegranate extract at 1% (v/v) eliminated the growth of *S. aureus* FRI 722 and inhibited enterotoxin (SE) production at 0.05% (v/v) concentration (Braga et al., 2005). The addition of pomegranate peel extract to chicken meat products extended their shelf life by 2–3 weeks during chilled storage (Kanatt et al., 2010).

Garcinia kola, commonly known as Bitter Kola, is a medium-sized tree. Different species of *Garcinia* possess antimicrobial, antioxidant, antitumorogenic, and cytotoxic activities through their secondary metabolites (Negi, 2012; Akerele et al., 2010). The crude ethanol extract of *G. kola* Heckel showed inhibitory activity against clinical bacterial isolates of *S. aureus*, *B. subtilis*, *Streptococcus viridians*, *E. coli*, *P. aeruginosa*, and *K. pneumoniae* and fungi like *Penicillium notatum*, *Aspergillus niger*, and *C. albicans*. The MIC values ranged between 2.5 and 7.5 mg/mL (Akerele et al., 2010).

Compounds extracted from *Garcinia brasiliensis* which are active against *S. aureus* and *B. cereus* were pericarp hexane extract 4.0 and 2.4 µg/mL and seed ethanol extract 10.0 and 12.6 µg/mL, respectively (Naldoni et al., 2009). Methanolic crude extract of the stem bark of *Garcinia lucida* Vesque exerted good inhibitory effect against *C. albicans* (MIC value was 64 µg/mL). Only cycloartenol obtained from dichloromethane fraction exhibited antimicrobial activity against *E. coli* and *P. aeruginosa* (Momo et al., 2011).

Pericarp extract of *Garcinia mangostana* Linn. (mangosteen) was effective against *S. aureus*, *Staphylococcus albus*, and *Micrococcus lutus* (Priya et al., 2010). The crude methanolic extracts of *Garcinia atroviridis* had an inhibitory effect against *B. subtilis* B28 mutant, *B. subtilis* B28 wild type, methicillin resistant *S. aureus, E. coli*, and *P. aeruginosa* UI 60690 at a minimum inhibitory dose of 15.6 µg/disc (Mackeen et al., 2000). The ethanol extracts of *G. kola* produced inhibition zones ranging from 8 to 18 mm against *S. aureus, P. aeruginosa, E. coli*, and *C. albicans* (Ezeifeka et al., 2004). *G. mangostana* had a strong inhibitory effect against *Propionibacterium acnes* and *Staphylococcus epidermidis* and can be used as an alternative treatment for acne (Chomnawang et al., 2005). The natural xanthones isolated from the fruit hulls of *G. mangostana* showed good inhibitory activity against phytopathogenic fungi, *Fusarium oxysporum vasinfectum*, *Alternaria tenuis*, and *Dreschlera oryzae* (Gopalakrishnan et al., 1997). The MIC exerted by the seed extracts of *G. kola* against *E. coli*, *S. aureus*, and *P. aeruginosa* ranged between 3.125 and 25 mg/mL and inhibition zones were between 4.0 and 10.5 mm. Crude ethanol extract was found to be most effective against all bacteria at different treatment regimens (Ghamba et al., 2012).

The antimicrobial activities of seven Turkish spice [cumin, *Helichrysum compactum* Boiss (HC), laurel, myrtle, oregano, sage, and thyme] methanolic extracts were investigated against *E. coli* O157:H7. Thyme and oregano showed higher inhibitory effects and their antibacterial effects varied in proportion to the concentration of extracts used (Sagdic et al., 2002). High concentrations of rosmarinic acid in methanolic extract of

Orthosiphon stamineus were closely related with the antibacterial activity of plant extract against *Vibrio parahaemolyticus*, and a similar inhibitory effect was obtained with 5% lactic acid (Ho et al., 2010).

Tea (*C. sinensis*) is a popular nonalcoholic beverage consumed by over two-thirds of the world's population due to its taste and medicinal properties. Among all tea polyphenols, epigallocatechin-3-gallate is responsible for antiinflammatory, antimicrobial, antitumor, antioxidant activities and protection from cardiovascular disease, antiobesity, and antiaging properties. Tea and its polyphenols possess antibacterial activity against *S. aureus*, *E. coli*, *Helicobacter pylori*, *Bacillus* spp., *Clostridium* spp., *Streptococcus* spp., and other bacteria, antiviral activity against influenza virus, human immunodeficiency virus (HIV), Epstein-Barr virus, Hepatitis B virus, herpes simplex virus (HSV), and other viruses, and antifungal activity against *C. albicans* and other fungi (Bansal et al., 2013). Methanolic extracts of green tea (*Camellia assamica*) at 10, 20, and 30 μL concentrations had significant antibacterial activity against *Staphylococcus* sp., *Streptococcus* sp., and *Bacillus* sp., and they were least active against *Pseudomonas* sp. and *Proteus* sp. (Kumar et al., 2012a). Ethanolic extract from green tea had potent antimicrobial activity against *Streptococcus mutans*, *Streptococcus sobrinus*, *L. monocytogenes*, *S. flexneri*, and *S. enterica* (Oh et al., 2013).

The green tea kombucha exhibited the highest antimicrobial activity against *S. epidermidis* (22 mm), *L. monocytogenes* (22 mm), and *M. luteus* (21.5 mm). The anticandidal activity of green tea kombucha was revealed by the reaction against *Candida parapsilosis* (Battikh et al., 2013). Aqueous green tea leaf extract was effective against *S. epidermidis*, *P. fluorescens*, *M. luteus*, *Brevibacterium linens*, and *B. subtilis* by disc diffusion assay (zone of inhibition ≥7 mm). MIC was determined via nitro blue tetrazolium assay (0.156–0.313 mg/mL). The extract was not toxic to Vero cell line up to a concentration of 500 μg/mL (Sharma et al., 2012).

Incorporation of green tea extract into chitosan film enhanced the antimicrobial activity of the film and therefore maintained the sensory quality and extended shelf life of pork sausages (Siripatrawan and Noipha, 2012). Aqueous and methanolic extracts of Lipton black tea in Nigeria contain tannin and reduced sugar and have antimicrobial activity against *E. coli*, *S. aureus*, *B. subtilis*, and *P. aeruginosa* at 2–10% concentrations (Funmilayo et al., 2012). Black tea and tea with milk beverages significantly reduced cariogenic oral *S. mutans* and *Lactobacillus* sp. counts (43.6–83.3%) and are thus recommended as natural anticariogenic beverages (Abd Allah et al., 2012).

Among the different teas tested, green and white tea extracts were found to be the most effective against *Campylobacter jejuni*, *E. coli* O157:H7, *S. enteritidis*, and *S. aureus*, and white tea killed all tested bacteria except *C. jejuni* 81176 within 48 h of incubation (Murali et al., 2012). Longjing tea extract reduced the *V. parahaemolyticus* count by 0.8 log MPN/g in shucked Pacific oysters and green tea treatment of oysters reduced *V. parahaemolyticus* while retarding the growth of total bacteria in oysters at 5±1°C storage (Xi et al., 2012).

Caffeine (1,3,7-trimethylexanthine) is a methylated xanthine alkaloid derivative present in plant species and has shown significant inhibitory effect against *E. coli* O157:H7 at a concentration of 0.5% (Gyawali and Ibrahim, 2012; Ibrahim et al., 2006), *Serratia marcescens*, *Enterobacter cloacae*, and *S. enterica* (Almeida et al., 2006), *S. aureus* and *Vibrio* sp. (MIC values of 192±91 and 162±165 μg/mL, respectively) (Taguri et al., 2004). Processed and fresh forms of sloe berry purees reduced *Salmonella* spp. to range of 4.24–6.70 log units within 24 h at 25°C (Gunduz, 2013).

Major antimicrobial compounds of herbs and spices

Plants have a nearly endless potential to synthesize mostly phenolic aromatic compounds or their oxygen-substituted analogs (Geissman, 1963). The majority of these compounds are secondary metabolites and approximately 12,000 have already been isolated; however, this number does not even correspond to 10% of the total number of metabolites (Schultes, 1978). In general, these materials allow plants to defend themselves against microorganisms, insects, and herbivores. Some of these materials, for example, terpenoids give the plants their characteristic scent whereas quinones and tannins are related to the plant pigment. Most of these metabolites give the plants their flavor such as the terpenoid from chili peppers and some herbs and spices used by people to marinate food produce useful medicinal compounds.

Phenolics and polyphenols

Simple phenols and phenolic acids

Simple phenols and phenolic acids are composed of a single-substituted phenolic ring (Tajkarimi et al., 2010; Gyawali and Ibrahim, 2012; Cowan, 1999). Cinnamic and caffeic acids are communal substitutes of a large group of phenylpropane-derived compounds. Tarragon and thyme both consist of caffeic acid and they are efficient against bacteria, viruses, and fungi. Catechol and pyrogallol are hydroxylated phenols proved to be toxic to microorganisms (Cowan, 1999).

Quinones

Quinones are aromatic rings with two ketone substitutions. These quinones are responsible for the browning reaction in peeled fruits and vegetables. The compound responsible for dyeing in henna is quinone. Coenzyme Q (ubiquinone) has an important role in mammalian electron transport system. Vitamin K is a naphthoquinone. Besides providing a source of free radicals, quinones bind irreversibly with nucleophilic amino acids in proteins generally causing the protein inactivation and loss of function (Cowan, 1999). Therefore quinones have potentially great antimicrobial effects. Possible targets in cells are surface-exposed adhesions, cell wall polypeptides, and membrane bound enzymes. Furthermore the quinones may also make the substrate unavailable for microorganism. Anthraquinones have antibacterial and antidepressant effects (Cowan, 1999).

Flavones, flavonoids, and flavonols

Flavones have phenolic structure containing one carbonyl group. Flavonols have extra 3-hydroxyl groups. Flavonoids are also hydroxylated phenolic compounds, but there is a C_6–C_3 unit bound to the aromatic ring. Flavonoids have antimicrobial activity through their ability to form complexes with proteins and cell walls, as explained for quinones (Cowan, 1999). Catechins inhibited *Vibrio cholerae*, *S. mutans*, *Shigella*, and other bacteria and microorganisms. Flavonoids show inhibitory effects against some viruses such as HIV, respiratory syncytial virus, herpes simplex virus type 1 (HSV-1), poliovirus type 1, and parainfluenza virus type 3. Hesperetin reduces intracellular replication of viruses. Galangin has antimicrobial activity against a lot of different Gram-positive bacteria, fungi, and viruses. Alpinumisoflavone stops schistosomal infection when administered topically (Cowan, 1999).

Tannins

They are a group of polymeric phenolic compounds which have the ability to tan leather or sedimentation of gelatin from solution, a feature known as astringency and they are present in bark, wood, leaves, fruits, and roots of the plants. Beverages containing tannins especially green teas and red wines can cure several diseases. Their mechanism of action may be related to the inactivation of microbial adhesions, enzymes, and cell envelope transport proteins. Tannins can bind to polysaccharides as well and can be toxic to filamentous fungi, yeasts, and bacteria (Cowan, 1999).

Coumarins

Coumarins are phenolic substances composed of fused benzene and α-pyrone rings. At least 1300 different coumarins have been identified.

Coumarins have antithrombotic, antiinflammatory, and vasodilatory activities. Warfarin is the most popular one and it is used as an oral coagulant and rodenticide. Coumarins may also have antiviral effects and are highly toxic in rodents. Some of the coumarins compounds have antimicrobial effects such as an inhibitory effect against *C. albicans* and thus can be used to cure vaginal candidiasis. In addition, coumarins can induce macrophages which exert a negative effect on bacterial infections. Hydroxycinnamic acids can inhibit Gram-positive bacteria and phytoalexins are assumed to have effects against fungi (Cowan, 1999).

Terpenoids and EOs

EOs have the odor of plants and are secondary metabolites that are highly enriched in substances which are called terpenes. These terpenes have predicated isoprene rings on chemical structures (Tajkarimi et al., 2010; Gyawali and Ibrahim, 2012; Cowan, 1999). Their general chemical conformation is $C_{10}H_{16}$, and their subcategories are diterpenes, triterpenes, tetraterpenes, hemiterpenes, and sesquiterpenes. When EOs are comprised of additional elements, mostly oxygen, they are called terpenoids and they are synthesized from acetate units and share their origins with fatty acids. Terpenoids are chemically in cyclic form and extensively branched. Well-known terpenoids are methanol and camphor (monoterpenes) and farnesol and artemisin (sesquiterpenes). Artemisin has been recently used as an antimalarial agent (Cowan, 1999).

Terpenoids are effective against bacteria, fungi, viruses, and protozoa. Betulinic acid can inhibit HIV. The mode of action for terpenes is not exactly understood, but it is assumed that they disrupt the membrane by the action of lipophilic compounds. Terpenoids in EOs are used to control *L. monocytogenes*. Capsaicin is an analgesic terpenoid that is present in chili peppers and is involved in a series of biological activities related to the nervous, cardiovascular, and digestive systems of human beings (Cowan, 1999).

Capsaicin can inhibit a lot of different bacteria and has bactericidal effects against *H. pylori*. Aframodial is a strong antifungal. Petalostemumol showed strong antimicrobial activity against *B. subtilis*, *S. aureus* and less activity against Gram-negative bacteria alongside *C. albicans*. Terpenoids are useful in preventing the formation of ulcers and in decreasing the severity of existing ulcers (Cowan, 1999).

Alkaloids

Alkaloids are heterocyclic nitrogen compounds. Morphine was isolated from the opium poppy *Papaver somniferum* in 1805 and used in medical applications. Codeine and heroin are both morphine derivatives. Diterpenoid alkaloids have antimicrobial effects. Solamargine is a glycoalkaloid and can be useful against HIV together with other alkaloids. Berberine is one of a considerable group of alkaloids that are effective against trypanosomes (Cowan, 1999).

Lectins and polypeptides

Peptides that could inhibit microorganisms were first discovered in 1942. These peptides generally have positive charges and are comprised of disulfide bonds. Their mode of action can be explained by the formation of ion channels in the mitochondrial membrane. Thionins are commonly present in barley and wheat and are toxic against yeasts, Gram-negative and Gram-positive bacteria whereas thionins AX1 and AX2 are only effective against fungi. Fabatin is a peptide isolated from fava beans and inhibits *E. coli*, *P. aeruginosa*, and *Enterococcus hirae*. The larger lectin molecules contain mannose-specific lectins from different plants. MAP30 from bitter melon, GAP31 from *Gelonium multiflorum*, and jacalin have inhibitory effects against viruses (Cowan, 1999).

Mixtures

In African countries, a chewing stick is used instead of a toothbrush for maintaining oral hygiene. These chewing sticks are obtained from a variety of species and they may contain different chemical compounds such as alkaloids. *Serinda werneckei* can inhibit periodontal pathogen microorganisms *Porphyromonas gingivalis* and *Bacteroides melaninogenicus* (Cowan, 1999).

Papaya secretes a milky sap called latex and included a mixture of different chemical compounds such as papain (proteolytic enzyme), carpaine alkaloid, and terpenoids. Latex is bacteriostatic to *B. subtilis*, *E. cloacae*, *E. coli*, *Salmonella typhi*, *S. aureus*, and *P. vulgaris*. Ayurveda is a type of healing practice in India that relies on single plant or mixture preparations. Preparations such as Ashwagandha, Cauvery 100, and Livo-vet have antimicrobial, antidiarrheal, immunomodulatory, anticancer, and psychotropic effects. They are potentially toxic and can cause an accumulation of high levels of lead in human blood. Propolis, or bee glue, is a crude extract with a complex chemical composition. Bee glue is collected from different trees by honeybees and contains terpenoids, flavonoids, benzoic acids and esters, and substituted phenolic acids and esters. It has antiviral activity against HSV-1, adenovirus type 2, vesicular stomatitis virus, and poliovirus (Cowan, 1999).

Other compounds

Polyamines, isothiocyanates, thiosulfinates, and glucosides have antimicrobial effects. Cranberry and blueberry juices competitively inhibit the attachment of pathogenic *E. coli* to urinary tract epithelial cells (Cowan, 1999).

Commonly used antimicrobials in the food industry include more than 1340 plants containing clearly defined antimicrobial compounds and more than 30,000 components isolated from plant oil compounds that have phenolic groups. However, characterization of features which are important in the preservation of food is only available for a few EOs (Tajkarimi et al., 2010).

In food systems, more evaluation of EOs is required. Spices and their EOs are increasingly being used for the preservation of food as natural antimicrobials in order to increase the shelf life of foods, eliminate foodborne pathogens, and improve the overall quality of food products (Tajkarimi et al., 2010).

The most common method for the production of plant-origin antimicrobials is hydro distillation, or steam distillation. Supercritical fluid extraction, as an alternative method, allows higher solubility with better mass transfer rates. Additionally, the modification of parameters like temperature and pressure allows for the extraction of different antimicrobial compounds (Burt, 2004). Medicinal and herbal plants and spices such as sage, basil, oregano, thyme, rosemary, turmeric, garlic, ginger, clove, mace, nutmeg, savory, and fennel have been used in food preservation either alone or in combination with other preservation techniques. These natural products increase the shelf life of food products or have antimicrobial effects against a wide variety of Gram-negative and Gram-positive bacteria. Factors affecting these natural additives' efficacy include pH, storage temperature, amount of oxygen, and the level of concentration and active ingredients of EOs (Burt, 2004).

In food manufacturing, spices and EOs are used as natural antimicrobials to increase the shelf life of foods, improve food quality, and remove foodborne pathogens. The aromatic oily liquids of flowers, seeds, leaves, bark, buds, twigs, herbs, wood, fruits, and roots of plants contain plant-origin antimicrobials that are extracted with different methods. EOs are composed combinations of various compounds. Some EOs such as those extracted from oregano, clove, cinnamon, citral, garlic, coriander, rosemary, parsley, lemongrass, sage, and vanillin have strong antimicrobial effects, whereas ginger, black pepper, red pepper, chili powder, cumin, and curry powder have weaker antimicrobial effects (Holley and Patel, 2005; Burt, 2004).

Chemical components of EOs

EOs can contain 20–80 different constituents at different concentrations. The main group of constituents is terpenes and terpenoids (Burt, 2004).

The monoterpenes constitute 90% of EOs and have very different structures. Oxygenated monoterpenes are more active than hydrocarbon ones (Carson and Riley, 1995). EOs also consist of terpenoids, sesquiterpenes, and diterpenes with aliphatic hydrocarbons, acids, alcohols, aldehydes, acyclic esters, or lactones (Fisher and Phillips, 2006). Plant extracts and EOs are mainly responsible for antimicrobial activities, and they can be extracted from plants and spices with different methods (Ceylan and Fung, 2004; Bajpai et al., 2008). The primary compounds of EOs can comprise 85% of the product while other compounds are generally at trace levels (Burt, 2004; Grosso et al., 2008). Plant-origin antimicrobials contain chemicals such as saponin and flavonoids, thiosulfinates, and glucosinolates. Saponin and flavonoids are found in fruits, vegetables, nuts, seeds, stems, flowers, tea, wine, propolis, and honey and usually generate soapy foam after being shaken in water. They have antimicrobial effects when they are obtained from roots, stem bark, leaves, and wood of plants such as *Avena sativa* (oat) (Tajkarimi et al., 2010). Thiosulfinates are extracted from garlic through mild procedures and have extreme antimicrobial effects against Gram-negative bacteria. Glucosinolates are found in broccoli, Brussels sprouts, cabbage and mustard powder, and account for the sharp acidic flavor of mustard and horseradish. Glucosinolates also show a broad range of activity against bacteria and fungi with direct or synergistic effects when used with other substances (Tajkarimi et al., 2010).

Commonly, the phenolic components of EOs such as citrus oil, olive oil, tea-tree oil, orange, and bergamot have a wide range of antimicrobial effects and are not classified as spices. Oils extracted from citral, garlic, clove, oregano, coriander, cinnamon, rosemary, parsley, lemongrass, sage, purple, and bronze muscadine seeds have some nonphenolic compounds as well and are effective against Gram-negative and Gram-positive bacteria (Tajkarimi et al., 2010).

Uses of plant-origin antimicrobials

Food spoilage can happen at any step from food processing to distribution. Sources of spoilage can be microbiological, physical, and chemical. Food preservation methods to control microbiological spoilage have improved remarkably recently to eliminate pathogenic microorganisms (Gould, 1996). There has been a concomitant increase in research related to the utilization of EOs and spices as natural food preservatives to improve quality and extend shelf life of food products, and reduce or remove pathogenic microorganisms (Burt, 2004; Moreira et al., 2007; Simitzis et al., 2008). Table 26.1 lists natural ingredients that have antimicrobial activity against pathogen microorganisms.

Table 26.1 Natural Ingredients Which Possess Antimicrobial Activity Against Target Pathogens

Type of Antimicrobial	MIC Value	Target Organism(s)	Reference(s)
Mint EO from *Mentha piperita*	1.2% (v/v)	*Staphylococcus aureus* and *Salmonella enteritidis*	Tassou et al. (2000)
Carvacrol, thymol, TC	1–3 mM	*Escherichia coli and Salmonella typhimurium*	Helander et al. (1998)
Carvone	10 mM		
Fingerroot extract	0.2% (v/v), 0.4% (v/v)	*Listeria monocytogenes, Bacillus cereus*, and *S. aureus*	Aktug and Karapinar (1986)
Galangal extract	8% (v/v)	*E. coli* O157:H7	Aktug and Karapinar (1986)
Fingerroot extract	10% (v/v)		
Clove, cinnamon, and mustard extracts	1% (v/v)	*E. coli* O157:H7, *S. aureus*, and *B. cereus*	Sofia et al. (2007)
Garlic	3% (v/v)		
α-Pinene, 1,8-cineole, (+)-limonene, linalool, and geranyl acetate	1 mg/mL	*E. coli, Klebsiella pneumoniae, Pseudomonas aeruginosa, Proteus vulgaris, Bacillus subtilis*, and *Staphylococcus aureus*	Sandasi et al. (2008)
Lonicera japonica Thunb. EO	62.5 μg/mL	*Listeria monocytogenes, B. subtilis*	Rahman and Kang (2009)
	125 μg/mL	*S. aureus, Salmonella enteritidis*	
	250 μg/mL	*Bacillus cereus, S. typhimurium*	
	500 μg/mL	*Enterobacter aerogenes, E. coli*	
Thyme	1000 ppm	*Vibrio parahaemolyticus*	Amiri et al. (2008)
Bay leaves	5000 ppm		
Mint	6000 ppm		
Thyme	0.05% (v/v)	*S. aureus*	Kwon et al. (2008)
Bay leaves	0.5% (v/v)		
Phenolic contents from dried fruits of cinnamon	5 mg/plate	*Salmonella typhimurium* TA100	Jayaprakasha et al. (2007)
Carvacrol	1 mM	*E. coli* O157:H7 ATCC 43895	Burt et al. (2007)
EO from *Nandina domestica* Thunb	62.5– 1000 μg/mL	*B. subtilis* ATCC6633, *L. monocytogenes* ATCC19166, *S. aureus* KCTC1916 and ATCC6538, *P. aeruginosa* KCTC2004, *S. typhimurium* KCTC2515, *S. enteritidis* KCCM12021, *E. coli* O157-Human, *E. coli* ATCC8739, *E. coli* O157:H7 ATCC43888, and *Enterobacter aerogenes* KCTC2190	Bajpai et al. (2008)
Different organic extracts of hexane, chloroform, ethylacetate, and methanol	250– 2000 μg/mL		
Carvacrol, p-cymene	7.8–800 μg/mL	*Campylobacter* spp.	Aslim and Yucel (2008)
EO and extracts from clove	0.5–5.5 mg/mL	*L. monocytogenes*	Hoque et al. (2008)
EO and extracts from cinnamon	1.0–5.0 mg/mL		

Using natural antimicrobials against pathogens in liquid food models

Clove oil and mint extract exerted strong activity at low concentrations and mild heat without pulsed electric field in tomato juice (Nguyen and Mittal, 2007). The effect of cinnamon (0% and 0.3%) in pasteurized apple juice was investigated against *S. typhimurium*, *Y. Enterocolitica*, or Enterotoxigenic *S. aureus* at 4 log CFU/mL and stored at 5°C and 20°C. Cinnamon was effective against *S. aureus* (1.2 log CFU/mL at 3 days) and *Y. enterocolitica* (0.3 log CFU/mL at 1 day). Morbidity levels were significantly greater at 20°C for all three pathogens with ~4 log CFU/mL reductions in 1 day in *Y. enterocolitica* inoculated samples with and without cinnamon, and in *S. aureus* inoculated samples with cinnamon (Yuste and Fung, 2003).

Four EOs from clary sage, juniper, lemon, and marjoram were tested against wild-type isolates of the food-related yeasts *Geotrichum candidum*, *Pichia anomala*, *Saccharomyces cerevisiae*, and *Schizosaccharomyces pombe* in malt extract medium, apple juice and milk. *S. pombe* was most sensitive yeast (MICs of 0.0625–0.125 μL/mL) and *G. candidum* was least sensitive (MICs of 0.5–2 μL/mL). Significant reduction was achieved only with the highest EO concentrations (Tserennadmid et al., 2011).

The effect of thermal treatment, applied previously, on the growth of *B. megaterium* cells was investigated in a culture medium with and without the presence of nisin, carvacrol, and thymol. When thymol and carvacrol were combined at high doses (0.6 mM), the result was a further increase in the lag phase and significant decrease in the growth rate. The combination of carvacrol and/or thymol with a previous thermal treatment killed 90% of the population, and the growth of survivors was inhibited for at least 7 days (Periago et al., 2006).

The effect of HIPEF with or without the combination of citric acid or cinnamon bark oil in apple, pear, orange, and strawberry juices against *S. enteritidis* and *E. coli* 0157:H7 was evaluated. Both of these pathogens were reduced more than $5.0 \log_{10}$ units in orange juice by only HIPEF although strawberry, apple, and pear juices were pasteurized by a combination of HIPEF with citric acid at 0.5%, 1.5%, 1.5%, respectively, or cinnamon bark oil at 0.05% and 0.1%, respectively (Mosqueda-Melgar et al., 2008a).

The effects of different concentrations (0.01–15%) of thyme (*Thymus vulgaris*), peppermint (*Mentha piperita* L.), caraway seed (*Carum carvi*), fennel (*Foeniculum vulgar*), tarragon (*Artemisia dracunculus*), and pennyroyal (*Mentha pullegium*) EOs against *S. aureus* and *E. coli* were investigated in a nutrient broth medium. Thyme EOs exerted the broadest spectrum of antibacterial effects while EOs of peppermint, caraway seed, pennyroyal, and fennel showed a moderate effect on tested microorganisms while, in contrast, tarragon EO was less efficient against both microorganisms (Mohsenzadeh, 2007).

After inoculation at a level of 4 log CFU/mL in unpasteurized apple juice *E. coli* O157:H7 could survive up to 3 days at 25°C and 19 days at 4°C. The addition of 1.25 mM carvacrol or *p*-cymene into the juice decreased the number of *E. coli* O157:H7 to undetectable levels in 1–2 days for both storage temperatures (Kisko, 2005). The effects of garlic, bay, black pepper, Origanum, orange, thyme, tea tree, mint, clove, and cumin EOs on *L. monocytogenes* AUFE39237, *E. coli* ATCC25922, *S. enteritidis* ATCC13076, *P. mirabilis* AUFE43566, *B. cereus* AUFE81154, *Saccharomyces uvarum* UUFE16732, *Kloeckera apiculata* UUFE10628, *C. albicans* ATCC10231, *Candida oleophila* UUPP94365, and *Metschnikowia fructicola* UUPP23067 and effects of thyme oil at a concentration of 0.5% on *L. monocytogenes* and *C. albicans* in apple and carrot juices during +4°C (1–5th day) were investigated. Thyme, Origanum, clove, and orange EOs had the most effective antibacterial and antiyeast activities against these microorganisms. Cumin, tea tree, and mint oils effectively inhibited the yeasts (Irkin and Korukluoglu, 2009).

EOs extracted from lemon balm, marjoram, oregano, and thyme and their MICs were investigated against *Enterobacter* spp., *Lactobacillus* spp., and *Pseudomonas* spp. through the use of agar dilution method and/or the absorbance based microplate assay in food model media based on lettuce, meat, and milk. MICs were significantly lower in beef and lettuce media than in TSB. Thyme and oregano were the most active EOs and *Listeria* strains were more sensitive to EOs than other bacteria (Gutierrez et al., 2009).

The antimicrobial effect of cinnamon was investigated against *E. coli* O157:H7 in apple juice at 8°C and 25°C. *E. coli* O157:H7 was reduced by 1.6 log CFU/mL at 8°C and 2.0 log CFU/mL at 25°C by 0.3% cinnamon (Ceylan et al., 2004). The antibacterial effect of low concentrations of *trans*-cinnamaldehyde (TC) was determined against five *E. coli* O157:H7 strains in apple juice and apple cider. The initial inoculum level for a five strain mixture was ~6.0 log CFU/mL in apple juice or cider, followed by the addition of TC at 0%, 0.025%, 0.075%, and 0.125% (v/v) levels. The inoculated apple juice samples were incubated at 23°C and 4°C for 21 days, although the cider samples were stored only at 4°C. At 23°C, 0.125%

and 0.075% (v/v) TC completely inactivated *E. coli* O157:H7 in apple juice on days 1 and 3, respectively. At 4°C, 0.125% and 0.075% (v/v) TC decreased the counts in the juice and cider to undetectable levels on days 3 and 5, respectively (Baskaran et al., 2010).

Using natural antimicrobials against pathogens in solid food models

The antimicrobial activity of EOs of oregano, thyme, basil, marjoram, lemongrass, ginger, and clove was tested *in vitro* by agar dilution method and MIC determination against Gram-positive (*S. aureus* and *L. monocytogenes*) and Gram-negative strains (*E. coli* and *S. enteritidis*). $MIC_{90\%}$ values were determined against bacterial strains in irradiated minced meat and against natural microbiota in minced meat samples. $MIC_{90\%}$ values varied from 0.05% (v/v; lemongrass oil) to 0.46% (v/v; marjoram oil) to Gram-positive bacteria and from 0.10% (v/v; clove oil) to 0.56% (v/v; ginger oil) to Gram-negative strains. Nevertheless, the $MIC_{90\%}$ values on minced meat and natural microbiota were 1.3 and 1.0, respectively, against tested microorganisms (Barbosa et al., 2009).

The physical properties and antimicrobial activities of allspice, cinnamon, and clove bud oils against *E. coli* O157:H7, *S. enterica*, and *L. monocytogenes* in apple puree film forming solutions formulated into edible films at 0.5–3% (w/w) concentrations. The antibacterial activities against these three pathogens were in the following order: cinnamon oil > clove bud oil > allspice oil. The results showed that apple-based films with allspice, cinnamon, or clove bud oils were active against these three main foodborne pathogens either with direct contact with the pathogens or by vapors emanating from films (Du et al., 2009).

Oregano and thyme incorporating soy protein edible films (SPEF) showed similar antibacterial activity against *E. coli*, *E. coli* O157:H7, *S. aureus*, *P. aeruginosa*, *and L. plantarum* in inhibition zone test. Although *E. coli*, *E. coli* O157:H7, and *S. aureus* were significantly inhibited by these films, *L. plantarum* and *P. aeruginosa* seemed to be more resistant bacteria. SPEF with oregano, thyme, and oregano plus thyme did not have significant effects on total viable counts, lactic acid bacteria, and *Staphylococcus* spp. when applied to ground beef patties, although reductions ($P < 0.05$) in coliform and *Pseudomonas* spp. counts were determined (Emiroglu et al., 2010).

The EO of cloves (10%) and cinnamon (5%) were tested against a cocktail of five strains of *L. monocytogenes* in ground chicken meat. EOs from cloves reduced all tested strains to undetectable levels within 1 day of exposure whereas EOs from cinnamon could only reduce levels by 2.0 log CFU/g within 1 day with only slight reductions or no additional decline in cell numbers during 15 days of incubation (Hoque et al., 2008).

The effect of carvacrol, cinnamaldehyde, thymol, and oregano oil on *Clostridium perfringens* growth and spore germination was investigated during the chilling of cooked ground beef. The addition of test compounds ($\geq$0.1%) into beef completely inhibited *C. perfringens* spore germination and outgrowth ($P \leq 0.05$) during cooling of the cooked beef over 12 h. Greater concentrations were required for longer chilling times. Cinnamaldehyde was significantly more effective at a lower concentration (0.5%) at the most abusive chilling rate tested (21 h) than other compounds (Juneja et al., 2006).

The addition of clove and tea tree EOs at highest concentrations (three and four times MICs) was required to inhibit the growth of *E. coli* O157:H7 in blanched spinach and minced cooked beef, respectively. The antimicrobial effect was dependent on the oil concentration, the food composition, and storage temperature (Moreira et al., 2007). The ethanolic extract of cinnamon bark (2%, w/v) inhibited the growth of *E. coli* O157:H7 and *L. innocua* by 94% and 87%, respectively. When combined with commercial antibrowning dipping solution (FreshExtend), cinnamon bark extract (1%, w/v) reduced the microbial growth significantly on apple slices stored for 12 days at 6°C in comparison to the control. The major constituent of this extract was cinnamic aldehyde (Muthuswamy et al., 2008).

The antibacterial effect of clove oil applied to the surface of ready to eat chicken frankfurters was evaluated on seven strains of *L. monocytogenes* at low (2–3 log) or high (4–6 log) inoculum levels and stored 2 weeks at 5°C or 1 week at 15°C. The growth of all seven *L. monocytogenes* strains was inhibited under either storage conditions with the addition of 1% or 2% clove oil (Mytle et al., 2006).

The effect of malic acid and EOs of cinnamon, palmarosa, and lemongrass and their main active antimicrobial substances attached to an alginate-based edible coating on shelf life and safety of fresh-cut "Piel de Sapo" melon was tested. Malic acid was effective in increasing the shelf life of fresh-cut melon from microbiological (up to 9.6 days) and physicochemical (>14 days) aspects compared with noncoated melon. The microbiological and physicochemical shelf life was up to 3.6 days and <14 days, respectively. When palmarosa oil was integrated into edible coatings at a 0.3% concentration, it seemed to serve as a good alternative for fresh-cut melon because it has been accepted by panelists, preserved fruit quality properties, inhibited the native microflora growth, and provided a significant reduction in the number of *S. enteritidis* (Raybaudi-Massilia et al., 2008).

The effect of EOs of oregano and nutmeg and storage temperature on survival and growth of *E. coli* O157:H7 has been investigated in ready to cook traditional Iranian barbecued chicken. The EOs of oregano and nutmeg had no significant inhibitory effect against *E. coli* O157:H7 in broth and ready to cook barbecued chicken (Shekarforoush et al., 2007). The effect of oregano EO supplementation on lamb meat was also tested. The results showed that incorporation of oregano EO into dietary supplements showed promising antioxidant activity by retarding lipid oxidation in lamb meat during refrigerated and frozen storage (Simitzis et al., 2008).

Thyme EOs at 0.3% concentration had a weak antibacterial activity against *E. coli* O157:H7 in TSB, negative impact on organoleptic properties of minced meat at 0.9%, and showed inhibitory activity at 0.6% against *E. coli* O157:H7 during storage at 10°C but not at 4°C. The addition of nisin into minced beef or TSB at 500 or 1000 IU/g had no effect on pathogens (Solomakos et al., 2008).

CONCLUSION

Natural antimicrobial extracts from herbs, spices, and plants can be used in food industry to prevent growth of foodborne pathogens and food spoilage microorganisms and to enhance the shelf life and stability. Due to the antioxidant and antimicrobial effects of natural ingredients, they can be a good alternative to classical food preservation methods and usage of chemical preservatives and food additives. These plant products have shown to reduce the growth of both Gram-positive and Gram-negative microorganisms including foodborne pathogens. Besides possessing antimicrobial effect on pathogenic microorganisms, herbs and spices also improve flavor, aroma, and texture of food products without affecting their sensory properties. Thus the use of plant-derived antimicrobials has a greater potential to improve the safety and quality of food products. Natural ingredients can be used in combination with other traditional food preservation methods to improve antimicrobial efficacy and ensure safety of food products.

REFERENCES

Abd Allah, A.A., et al., 2012. Antimicrobial effect of tea and tea with milk beverages on oral *Streptococcus mutans* and lactobacilli. World Appl. Sci. J. 19 (9), 1327–1334.

Ahn, J., Grun, I.U., Mustapha, A., 2007. Effects of plant extracts on microbial growth, color change, and lipid oxidation in cooked beef. Food Microbiol. 24 (1), 7–14.

Akerele, J.O., et al., 2010. Antimicrobial activity of the ethanol extract and fractions of the seeds of *Garcinia kola* Heckel (Guttiferae). Afr. J. Biotechnol. 7 (2), 169–172.

Aktug, S.E., Karapinar, M., 1986. Sensitivity of some common food-poisoning bacteria to thyme, mint and bay leaves. Int. J. Food Microbiol. 3 (6), 349–354.

Almeida, A.A.P., et al., 2006. Antibacterial activity of coffee extracts and selected coffee chemical compounds against enterobacteria. J. Agric. Food Chem. 54 (23), 8738–8743.

Al-Sum, B.A., Al-Arfaj, A.A., 2013. Antimicrobial activity of the aqueous extract of mint plant. Science 2 (3), 110–113.

Al-Zoreky, N.S., 2009. Antimicrobial activity of pomegranate (*Punica granatum* L.) fruit peels. Int. J. Food Microbiol. 134 (3), 244–248.

Amiri, A., et al., 2008. In vitro and in vitro activity of eugenol oil (*Eugenia caryophylata*) against four important postharvest apple pathogens. Int. J. Food Microbiol. 126 (1–2), 13–19.

Ankri, S., Mirelman, D., 1999. Antimicrobial properties of allicin from garlic. Microbes Infect. 1 (2), 125–129.

Aslim, B., Yucel, N., 2008. In vitro antimicrobial activity of essential oil from endemic Origanum minutiflorum on ciprofloxacin-resistant *Campylobacter* spp. Food Chem. 107 (2), 602–606.

Ates, D.A., Erdogrul, O.T., 2003. Antimicrobial activities of various medicinal and commercial plant extracts. Turkish J. Biol. 27 (3), 157–162.

Bajpai, V.K., Rahman, A., Kang, S.C., 2008. Chemical composition and inhibitory parameters of essential oil and extracts of *Nandina domestica* Thunb. to control food-borne pathogenic and spoilage bacteria. Int. J. Food Microbiol. 125 (2), 117–122.

Bansal, S., et al., 2013. Tea: a native source of antimicrobial agents. Food Res. Int. 53 (2), 568–584.

Barbosa, L.N., et al., 2009. Essential oils against foodborne pathogens and spoilage bacteria in minced meat. Foodborne Pathog. Dis., 725–728.

Baskaran, S.A., et al., 2010. Inactivation of *Escherichia coli* O157:H7 in apple juice and apple cider by trans-cinnamaldehyde. Int. J. Food Microbiol. 141 (1–2), 126–129.

Battikh, H., et al., 2013. Antibacterial and antifungal activities of black and green kombucha teas. J. Food Biochem. 37 (2), 231–236.

Braga, L.C., et al., 2005. Pomegranate extract inhibits *Staphylococcus aureus* growth and subsequent enterotoxin production. J. Ethnopharmacol. 96 (1–2), 335–339.

Brandi, G., et al., 2006. Activity of *Brassica oleracea* leaf juice on foodborne pathogenic bacteria. J. Food Prot. 69 (9), 2274–2279.

Burt, S., 2004. Essential oils: their antibacterial properties and potential applications in foods—a review. Int. J. Food Microbiol. 94 (3), 223–253.

Burt, S., et al., 2007. Carvacrol induces heat shock protein 60 and inhibits synthesis of flagellin in *Escherichia coli* O157:H7. Appl. Environ. Microbiol. 73 (14), 4484–4490.

Careaga, M., et al., 2003. Antibacterial activity of capsicum extract against *Salmonella typhimurium* and *Pseudomonas aeruginosa* inoculated in raw beef meat. Int. J. Food Microbiol. 83 (3), 331–335.

Carson, C.F., Riley, T.V., 1995. Antimicrobial activity of the major components of the essential oil of *Melaleuca alternifolia*. J. Appl. Microbiol. 78 (3), 264–269.

Ceyhan, N., Keskin, D., Ugur, A., 2012. Antimicrobial activities of different extracts of eight plant species from four different family against some pathogenic microoorganisms. J. Food Agric. Environ. 10 (1), 193–197.

Ceylan, E., Fung, D.Y.C., 2004. Antimicrobial activity of spices. J. Rapid Methods Automat. Microbiol. 12 (1), 1–55.

Ceylan, E., Fung, D.Y.C., Sabah, J.R., 2004. Antimicrobial activity and synergistic effect of cinnamon with sodium benzoate or potassium sorbate in controlling *Escherichia coli* O157:H7 in apple juice. J. Food Sci. 69 (4), M102–M106.

Chomnawang, M.T., et al., 2005. Antimicrobial effects of Thai medicinal plants against acne-inducing bacteria. J. Ethnopharmacol. 101 (1–3), 330–333.

Cowan, M.M., 1999. Plant products as antimicrobial agents. Clin. Microbiol. Rev. 12 (4), 564–582.

Du, W.X., et al., 2009. Effects of allspice, cinnamon, and clove bud essential oils in edible apple films on physical properties and antimicrobial activities. J. Food Sci. 74 (7), M372–M378.

Duman, A.D., et al., 2009. Antimicrobial activity of six pomegranate (*Punica granatum* L.) varieties and their relation to some of their pomological and phytonutrient characteristics. Molecules 14 (5), 1808–1817.

Emiroglu, Z.K., et al., 2010. Antimicrobial activity of soy edible films incorporated with thyme and oregano essential oils on fresh ground beef patties. Meat Sci. 86 (2), 283–288.

Ezeifeka, G.O., et al., 2004. Antimicrobial activities of *Cajanus cajan*, *Garcinia kola* and *Xylopia aethiopica* on pathogenic microorganisms. Biotechnology 3 (1), 41–43.

Fagbemi, J.F., et al., 2009. Evaluation of the antimicrobial properties of unripe banana (*Musa sapientum* L.), lemon grass (*Cymbopogon citratus* S.) and turmeric (*Curcuma longa* L.) on pathogens. Afr. J. Biotechnol. 8 (7), 1176–1182.

Falco, A.S., et al., 2011. Antimicrobial activity of ethanolic extracts of lemongrass (*Cymbopogon citratus*) and turmeric (*Curcuma longa*). Rev. Venez. Cien. Tecn. Ali. 2 (1), 85–93.

Fereidouni, M.S., Akhlaghi, M., Alhosseini, A.K., 2013. Antibacterial effects of medicinal plant extracts against *Lactococcus garvieae*, the etiological agent of rainbow trout lactococcosis. Int. J. Aquat. Biol. 1 (3), 119–124.

Fernandez-Lopez, J., et al., 2005. Antioxidant and antibacterial activities of natural extracts: application in beef meatballs. Meat Sci. 69 (3), 371–380.

Fisher, K., Phillips, C.A., 2006. The effect of lemon, orange and bergamot essential oils and their components on the survival of *Campylobacter jejuni*, *Escherichia coli* O157, *Listeria monocytogenes*, *Bacillus cereus* and *Staphylococcus aureus* in vitro and in food systems. J. Appl. Microbiol. 101 (6), 1232–1240.

Friedman, M., Henika, P.R., Mandrell, R.E., 2002. Bactericidal activities of plant essential oils and some of their isolated constituents against *Campylobacter jejuni*, *Escherichia coli*, *Listeria monocytogenes*, and *Salmonella enterica*. J. Food Prot. 65 (10), 1545–1560.

Friedman, M., et al., 2004. Antibacterial activities of plant essential oils and their components against *Escherichia coli* O157 : H7 and *Salmonella enterica* in apple juice. J. Agric. Food Chem. 52 (19), 6042–6048.

Funmilayo, O.O., Kamaldeen, A.-S., Buhari, A.-S.M., 2012. Phytochemical screening and antimicrobial properties of a common brand of black tea (*Camellia sinensis*) marketed in nigerian environment. Adv. Pharm. Bull. 2 (2), 259–263.

Gaekwad, V., Trivedi, N.A., 2013. In vitro evaluation of antimicrobial effect of fresh garlic extract and its interaction with conventional antimicrobials against *Escherichia coli* isolates. Int. J. Curr. Res. Rev. 5 (1), 106–114.

Geissman, T.A., 1963. Flavonoid compounds, tannins, lignins and related compounds Pyrrole Pigments, Isoprenoid Compounds and Phenolic Plant Constituents, p. 265.

Ghamba, P.E., et al., 2012. In vitro antibacterial activity of crude ethanol, acetone and aqueous *Garcinia kola* seed extracts on selected clinical isolates. Afr. J. Biotechnol. 11 (6), 1478–1483.

Gopalakrishnan, G., Banumathi, B., Suresh, G., 1997. Evaluation of the antifungal activity of natural xanthones from *Garcinia mangostana* and their synthetic derivatives. J. Nat. Prod. 60 (5), 519–524.

Gould, G.W., 1996. Methods for preservation and extension of shelf life. Int. J. Food Microbiol. 33 (1), 51–64.

Grosso, C., et al., 2008. Supercritical carbon dioxide extraction of volatile oil from Italian coriander seeds. Food Chem. 111 (1), 197–203.

Gunduz, G.T., 2013. Antimicrobial activity of sloe berry purees on *Salmonella* spp. Food Control 32 (2), 354–358.

Gupta, C., et al., 2008. Comparative analysis of the antimicrobial activity of cinnamon oil and cinnamon extract on some food-borne microbes. Afr. J. Microbiol. Res. 2 (9), 247–251.

Gutierrez, J., Barry-Rian, C., Bourke, P., 2009. Antimicrobial activity of plant essential oils using food model media: efficacy, synergistic potential and interaction with food components. Food Microbiol. 26 (2), 142–150.

Gyawali, R., Ibrahim, S.A., 2012. Impact of plant derivatives on the growth of foodborne pathogens and the functionality of probiotics. Appl. Microbiol. Biotechnol. 95 (1), 29–45.

Helander, I.M., et al., 1998. Characterization of the action of selected essential oil components on Gram-negative bacteria. J. Agric. Food Chem. 46 (9), 3590–3595.

Ho, C.-H., et al., 2010. In vitro antibacterial and antioxidant activities of *Orthosiphon stamineus* Benth. extracts against food-borne bacteria. Food Chem. 122 (4), 1168–1172.

Holley, R.A., Patel, D., 2005. Improvement in shelf-life and safety of perishable foods by plant essential oils and smoke antimicrobials. Food Microbiol. 22 (4), 273–292.

Hoque, M., et al., 2008. Antimicrobial activity of cloves and cinnamon extracts against foodborne pathogens and spoilage bacteria and inactivation of *Listeria monocytogenes* in ground chicken meat with their essential oils Report of National Food Research Institute, 729–21

Hsieh, P.-C., Mau, J.-L., Huang, S.-H., 2001. Antimicrobial effect of various combinations of plant extracts. Food Microbiol. 18 (1), 35–43.

Ibrahim, S.A., et al., 2006. Application of caffeine, 1,3,7-trimethylxanthine, to control *Escherichia coli* O157:H7. Food Chem. 99 (4), 645–650.

Irkin, R., Korukluoglu, M., 2009. Growth inhibition of pathogenic bacteria and some yeasts by selected essential oils and survival of *L. monocytogenes* and *C. albicans* in apple–carrot juice. Foodborne Pathog. Dis. 6 (3), 387–394.

Jayaprakasha, G.K., Rao, L.J.M., Sakariah, K.K., 1997. Chemical composition of the volatile oil from the fruits of *Cinnamomum zeylanicum* Blume. Flavour Fragr. J. 12 (5), 331–333.

Jayaprakasha, G.K., et al., 2003. An antibacterial bioactive fraction of cinnamon fruit, U.P. Application, Editor.

Jayaprakasha, G.K., et al., 2007. Antioxidant and antimutagenic activities of *Cinnamomum zeylanicum* fruit extracts. J. Food Compos. Anal. 20 (3), 330–336.

Juneja, V.K., Thippareddi, H., Friedman, M., 2006. Control of *Clostridium perfringens* in cooked ground beef by carvacrol, cinnamaldehyde, thymol, or oregano oil during chilling. J. Food Prot. 69 (7), 1546–1551.

Kanatt, S.R., Chander, R., Sharma, A., 2010. Antioxidant and antimicrobial activity of pomegranate peel extract improves the shelf life of chicken products. Int. J. Food Sci. Technol. 45 (2), 216–222.

Kaul, P.N., et al., 2003. Volatile constituents of essential oils isolated from different parts of cinnamon (*Cinnamomum zeylanicum* Blume). J. Sci. Food Agric. 83 (1), 53–55.

Kim, E.L., et al., 2008. Synergistic effect of nisin and garlic shoot juice against *Listeria monocytogenes* in milk. Food Chem. 110 (2), 375–382.

Kim, S., Ruengwilysup, C., Fung, D.Y.C., 2004. Antibacterial effect of water-soluble tea extracts on foodborne pathogens in laboratory medium and in a food model. J. Food Prot. 67 (11), 2608–2612.

Kisko, G., Roller, S., 2005. Carvacrol and p-cymene inactivate *Escherichia coli* O157:H7 in apple juice. BMC Microbiol. 5 (1), 36.

Kong, B., Wang, J., Xiong, Y.L., 2007. Antimicrobial activity of several herb and spice extracts in culture medium and in vacuum-packaged pork. J. Food Prot. 70 (3), 641–647.

Kumar, A., et al., 2012a. Antibacterial activity of green tea (*Camellia sinensis*) extracts against various bacteria isolated from environmental sources. Recent Res. Sci. Technol. 4 (1), 19–23.

Kumar, S., et al., 2012b. Evaluating the antibacterial activity of plant extracts against bacterial pathogens. J. Drug Deliv. Ther. 2 (4), 182–185.

Kwon, H.A., et al., 2008. Evaluation of antibacterial effects of a combination of Coptidis Rhizoma, Mume Fructus, and Schizandrae Fructus against Salmonella. Int. J. Food Microbiol. 127 (1–2), 180–183.

Lai, P.K., Roy, J., 2004. Antimicrobial and chemopreventive properties of herbs and spices. Curr. Med. Chem. 11 (11), 1451–1460.

Lee, S.-Y., et al., 2009. Inhibitory effect of commercial green tea and rosemary leaf powders on the growth of foodborne pathogens in laboratory media and oriental-style rice cakes. J. Food Prot. 72 (5), 1107–1111.

Leuschner, R.G.K., Zamparini, J., 2002. Effects of spices on growth and survival of *Escherichia coli* 0157 and *Salmonella enterica* serovar enteritidis in broth model systems and mayonnaise. Food Control 13 (6), 399–404.

Mackeen, M.M., et al., 2000. Antimicrobial, antioxidant, antitumour-promoting and cytotoxic activities of different plant part extracts of *Garcinia atroviridis* Griff. ex T. Anders. J. Ethnopharmacol. 72 (3), 395–402.

Mau, J.-L., Chen, C.-P., Hsieh, P.-C., 2000. Antimicrobial effect of extracts from chinese chive, cinnamon, and corni fructus. J. Agric. Food Chem. 49 (1), 183–188.

Mohsenzadeh, M., 2007. Evaluation of antibacterial activity of selected Iranian essential oils against *Staphylococcus aureus* and *Escherichia coli* in nutrient broth medium. Pakistan J. Biol. Sci. 10 (20), 3693–3697.

Momo, I.J., et al., 2011. Antimicrobial activity of the methanolic extract and compounds from the stem bark of *Garcinia lucida* Vesque (Clusiaceae). Int. J. Pharm. Pharm. Sci. 3 (3), 215–217.

Moreira, M.R., et al., 2007. Effects of clove and tea tree oils on *Escherichia coli* O157:H7 in blanched spinach and minced cooked beef. J. Food Process. Preserv. 31 (4), 379–391.

Mosqueda-Melgar, J., Raybaudi-Massilia, R.M., Martin-Belloso, O., 2008a. Non-thermal pasteurization of fruit juices by combining high-intensity pulsed electric fields with natural antimicrobials. Innov. Food Sci. Emerg. Technol. 9 (3), 328–340.

Mosqueda-Melgar, J., Raybaudi-Massilia, R.M., Martín-Belloso, O., 2008b. Combination of high-intensity pulsed electric fields with natural antimicrobials to inactivate pathogenic microorganisms and extend the shelf-life of melon and watermelon juices. Food Microbiol. 25 (3), 479–491.

Murali, N., et al., 2012. Antibacterial activity of plant extracts on foodborne bacterial pathogens and food spoilage bacteria. Agric. Food Anal. Bacteriol. 2 (3), 209–221.

Muthuswamy, S., Rupasinghe, H.P.V., Stratton, G.W., 2008. Antimicrobial effect of cinnamon bark extract on *Escherichia coli* O157:H7, *Listeria innocua* and fresh-cut apple slices. J. Food Saf. 28 (4), 534–549.

Mytle, N., et al., 2006. Antimicrobial activity of clove (*Syzgium aromaticum*) oil in inhibiting *Listeria monocytogenes* on chicken frankfurters. Food Control 17 (2), 102–107.

Naldoni, F.J., et al., 2009. Antimicrobial activity of benzophenones and extracts from the fruits of *Garcinia brasiliensis*. J. Med. Food 12 (2), 403–407.

Negi, P.S., 2012. Plant extracts for the control of bacterial growth: efficacy, stability and safety issues for food application. Int. J. Food Microbiol. 156 (1), 7–17.

Negi, P.S., et al., 1999. Antibacterial activity of turmeric oil: a byproduct from curcumin manufacture. J. Agric. Food Chem. 47 (10), 4297–4300.

Nguyen, P., Mittal, G.S., 2007. Inactivation of naturally occurring microorganisms in tomato juice using pulsed electric field (PEF) with and without antimicrobials. Chem. Eng. Process. Process Intens. 46 (4), 360–365.

Oh, J., et al., 2013. Antioxidant and antimicrobial activities of various leafy herbal teas. Food Control 31 (2), 403–409.

Opara, L.U., Al-Ani, M.R., Al-Shuaibi, Y.S., 2009. Physico-chemical properties, vitamin C content, and antimicrobial properties of pomegranate fruit (*Punica granatum* L.). Food Bioprocess Technol. 2 (3), 315–321.

Periago, P.M., et al., 2006. *Bacillus megaterium* spore germination and growth inhibition by a treatment combining heat with natural antimicrobials. Food Technol. Biotechnol. 44 (1), 17–23.

Pezeshk, S., Rezaei, M., Hosseini, H., 2011. Effects of turmeric, shallot extracts, and their combination on quality characteristics of vacuum-packaged rainbow trout stored at 4 ± 1°C. J. Food Sci. 76 (6), M387–M391.

Priya, V., et al., 2010. Antimicrobial activity of pericarp extract of *Garcinia mangostana* Linn. Int. J. Pharm. Sci. Res. 1, 278–281.

Proestos, C., Zoumpoulakis, P., Sinanoglou, V.J., 2013. Determination of plant bioactive compounds. Antioxidant capacity and antimicrobial screening. Focus. Modern Food Ind. 2 (1), 26–35.

Pundir, R.K., Jain, P., 2010. Comparative studies on the antimicrobial activity of black pepper (*Piper nigrum*) and turmeric (*Curcuma longa*) extracts. Int. J. Appl. Biol. Pharm. Technol. 1 (2), 491–501.

Rahman, A., Kang, S.C., 2009. In vitro control of food-borne and food spoilage bacteria by essential oil and ethanol extracts of *Lonicera japonica* Thunb. Food Chem. 116 (3), 670–675.

Raybaudi-Massilia, R.M., Mosqueda-Melgar, J., Martín-Belloso, O., 2008. Edible alginate-based coating as carrier of antimicrobials to improve shelf-life and safety of fresh-cut melon. Int. J. Food Microbiol. 121 (3), 313–327.

Rounds, L., et al., 2012. Plant extracts, spices, and essential oils inactivate *Escherichia coli* O157: H7 and reduce formation of potentially carcinogenic heterocyclic amines in cooked beef patties. J. Agric. Food Chem. 60 (14), 3792–3799.

Sagdic, O., et al., 2002. Effects of Turkish spice extracts at various concentrations on the growth of *Escherichia coli* O157:H7. Food Microbiol. 19 (5), 473–480.

Sallam, K.I., Ishioroshi, M., Samejima, K., 2004. Antioxidant and antimicrobial effects of garlic in chicken sausage. LWT-Food Sci. Technol. 37 (8), 849–855.

Sandasi, M., Leonard, C.M., Viljoen, A.M., 2008. The effect of five common essential oil components on *Listeria monocytogenes* biofilms. Food Control 19 (11), 1070–1075.

Schultes, R.E., 1978. The kingdom of plants Medicines From the Earth. McGraw-Hill Book Co., New York. p. 208.

Sharma, A., et al., 2012. Green tea extract: possible mechanism and antibacterial activity on skin pathogens. Food Chem. 135 (2), 672–675.

Shekarforoush, S.S., et al., 2007. Effects of storage temperatures and essential oils of oregano and nutmeg on the growth and survival of *Escherichia coli* O157 : H7 in barbecued chicken used in Iran. Food Control 18 (11), 1428–1433.

Simitzis, P.E., et al., 2008. Effect of dietary oregano oil supplementation on lamb meat characteristics. Meat Sci. 79 (2), 217–223.

Singh, B., Falahee, M.B., Adams, M.R., 2001. Synergistic inhibition of *Listeria monocytogenes* by nisin and garlic extract. Food Microbiol. 18 (2), 133–139.

Siripatrawan, U., Noipha, S., 2012. Active film from chitosan incorporating green tea extract for shelf life extension of pork sausages. Food Hydrocolloids 27 (1), 102–108.

Sofia, P.K., et al., 2007. Evaluation of antibacterial activity of Indian spices against common foodborne pathogens. Int. J. Food Sci. Technol. 42 (8), 910–915.

Solomakos, N., et al., 2008. The antimicrobial effect of thyme essential oil, nisin and their combination against *Escherichia coli* O157:H7 in minced beef during refrigerated storage. Meat Sci. 80 (2), 159–166.

Taguri, T., Tanaka, T., Kouno, I., 2004. Antimicrobial activity of 10 different plant polyphenols against bacteria causing food-borne disease. Biol. Pharm. Bull. 27 (12), 1965–1969.

Tajkarimi, M.M., Ibrahim, S.A., Cliver, D.O., 2010. Antimicrobial herb and spice compounds in food. Food Control 21 (9), 1199–1218.

Tassou, C., Koutsoumanis, K., Nychas, G.J.E., 2000. Inhibition of *Salmonella enteritidis* and *Staphylococcus aureus* in nutrient broth by mint essential oil. Food Res. Int. 33 (3), 273–280.

Tiwari, B.K., et al., 2009. Application of natural antimicrobials for food preservation. J. Agric. Food Chem. 57 (14), 5987–6000.

Tornuk, F., et al., 2011. Efficacy of various plant hydrosols as natural food sanitizers in reducing *Escherichia coli* O157:H7 and *Salmonella typhimurium* on fresh cut carrots and apples. Int. J. Food Microbiol. 148 (1), 30–35.

Tserennadmid, R., et al., 2011. Anti yeast activities of some essential oils in growth medium, fruit juices and milk. Int. J. Food Microbiol. 144 (3), 480–486.

Valero, M., Salmeron, M.C., 2003. Antibacterial activity of 11 essential oils against *Bacillus cereus* in tyndallized carrot broth. Int. J. Food Microbiol. 85 (1–2), 73–81.

Wang, Q.I.N., et al., 2012. Antimicrobial activities of a new formula of spice water extracts against foodborne bacteria. J. Food Process. Preserv. 36 (4), 374–381.

Witkowska, A.M., et al., 2013. Evaluation of antimicrobial activities of commercial herb and spice extracts against selected food-borne bacteria. J. Food Res. 2 (4), p37.

Xi, D., Liu, C., Su, Y.-C., 2012. Effects of green tea extract on reducing *Vibrio parahaemolyticus* and increasing shelf life of oyster meats. Food Control 25 (1), 368–373.

Yin, M.-C., Cheng, W.-S., 2003. Antioxidant and antimicrobial effects of four garlic-derived organosulfur compounds in ground beef. Meat Sci. 63 (1), 23–28.

Yuste, J., Fung, D.Y.C., 2003. Evaluation of *Salmonella typhimurium*, *Yersinia enterocolitica* and *Staphylococcus aureus* counts in apple juice with cinnamon, by conventional media and thin agar layer method. Food Microbiol. 20 (3), 365–370.

Zaika, L.L., 1988. Spices and herbs: their antimicrobial activity and its determination. J. Food Saf. 9 (2), 97–118.

Index

Note: Page numbers followed by *"f" and "t"* refer to figures and tables respectively.

B

D

E

H

I

J

K

N

T